MASSACHUSETTS GENERAL HOSPITAL

# Handbook of
# general hospital psychiatry

# MASSACHUSETTS GENERAL HOSPITAL
# Handbook of general hospital psychiatry

*Edited by*

**THOMAS P. HACKETT, M.D.**

Eben S. Draper Professor of Psychiatry,
Harvard Medical School;
Chief of Psychiatry,
Massachusetts General Hospital,
Boston, Massachusetts

**NED H. CASSEM, M.D.**

Associate Professor of Psychiatry,
Harvard Medical School;
Chief, Psychiatric Consultation-Liaison Service,
Massachusetts General Hospital,
Boston, Massachusetts

# The C. V. Mosby Company

Saint Louis    1978

Printed in the United States of America

The C. V. Mosby Company
11830 Westline Industrial Drive, St. Louis, Missouri 63141

**Library of Congress Cataloging in Publication Data**

Main entry under title:

Massachusetts General Hospital handbook of
    general hospital psychiatry.

    Includes index.
    1. Psychological manifestations of general
diseases.  2. Psychiatric consultation.
3. Psychology, Pathological.  I. Hackett,
Thomas P.  II. Cassem, Ned H., 1935-
III.  Massachusetts General Hospital, Boston.
[DNLM: 1. Hospitals, General—Handbooks.
2. Mental disorders—Handbooks.  3. Psychiatry—
Handbooks.  WM100.3 M414m]
RC49.M36        616'.001'9        78-15146
ISBN 0-8016-0931-3

TS/CB/CB  9  8  7  6  5  4  3  2

# Contributors

**Harry S. Abram, M.D.**[†]

**William H. Anderson, M.D.**
Assistant Professor of Psychiatry, Harvard Medical School;
Assistant Psychiatrist, Massachusetts General Hospital

**Jerrold G. Bernstein, M.D.**
Assistant Clinical Professor of Psychiatry, Harvard Medical School;
Assistant Psychiatrist, Massachusetts General Hospital;
Associate Medical Director, Human Resource Institute of Boston

**Carolyn B. Bilodeau, R.N., M.S.**
Psychiatric Nursing Consultant;
Former Psychiatric Nurse Clinician, Massachusetts General Hospital

**Ned H. Cassem, M.D.**
Associate Professor of Psychiatry, Harvard Medical School;
Chief, Psychiatric Consultation-Liaison Service,
Massachusetts General Hospital

**James E. Groves, M.D.**
Clinical Instructor in Psychiatry, Harvard Medical School;
Clinical Assistant in Psychiatry, Massachusetts General Hospital

**Frederick G. Guggenheim, M.D.**
Assistant Professor of Psychiatry, Harvard Medical School;
Director, Private Consultation Service,
Massachusetts General Hospital

**Thomas P. Hackett, M.D.**
Eben S. Draper Professor of Psychiatry, Harvard Medical School;
Chief of Psychiatry, Massachusetts General Hospital

**Gordon Harper, M.D.**
Co-Director, Psychosomatic Unit, Children's Hospital Medical Center
and Judge Baker Guidance Center; Assistant Professor of Psychiatry,
Harvard Medical School

[†]Deceased

**Michael Jellinek, M.D.**
Clinical Associate in Psychiatry, Massachusetts General Hospital;
Clinical Fellow in Psychiatry, Harvard Medical School

**Gerald P. Koocher, Ph.D.**
Instructor in Psychiatry, Harvard Medical School;
Staff Psychologist, Children's Hospital Medical Center;
Chief Psychologist, Sidney Farber Cancer Institute

**Anastasia Kucharski, M.D.**
Clinical Instructor in Psychiatry, Harvard Medical School;
Clinical Associate in Psychiatry,
Massachusetts General Hospital

**Aaron Lazare, M.D.**
Associate Professor of Psychiatry, Harvard Medical School;
Director, Outpatient Services, Massachusetts General Hospital

**Michel R. Mandel, M.D.**
Assistant Professor of Psychiatry, Harvard Medical School;
Director, Somatic Therapies Consultation Service,
Massachusetts General Hospital

**George B. Murray, M.D.**
Instructor in Psychiatry, Harvard Medical School;
Director, Fellowship Program in Liaison/Consultation Psychiatry,
Massachusetts General Hospital

**Suzanne O'Hara O'Connor, B.S.N., M.S.**
Psychiatric Nurse Clinician, Massachusetts General Hospital

**John E. O'Malley, M.D.**
Assistant Professor, Harvard Medical School;
Associate in Psychiatry, Sidney Farber Cancer Institute
and Children's Hospital Medical Center

**John A. Renner, Jr., M.D.**
Associate Psychiatrist, Massachusetts General Hospital;
Associate Professor of Psychiatry, Boston University School of Medicine;
Director, City of Boston Drug Treatment Program, Boston City Hospital

**Jerrold F. Rosenbaum, M.D.**
Instructor in Psychiatry and Ethel Dupont-Warren Fellow,
Harvard Medical School; Acting Director, Psychopharmacology Clinic,
Massachusetts General Hospital

**David V. Sheehan, M.B., B.Ch., B.A.O.**
Instructor in Psychiatry, Harvard Medical School;
Director, Hypnosis and Psychosomatic Clinic,
Massachusetts General Hospital

**Thomas D. Stewart, M.D.**
Clinical Instructor in Psychiatry, Harvard Medical School;
Clinical Associate in Psychiatry, Massachusetts General Hospital;
Psychiatrist, Spinal Cord Injury Service,
West Roxbury Veterans Administration Hospital

**Owen S. Surman, M.D.**
Instructor in Psychiatry, Harvard Medical School;
Assistant in Psychiatry, Massachusetts General Hospital

**James M. Vaccarino, J.D.**
Director of Legal Affairs, Massachusetts General Hospital

**Avery D. Weisman, M.D.**
Professor of Psychiatry, Harvard Medical School; Director, Project Omega,
Massachusetts General Hospital

*To Eleanor Mayher Hackett*
**T. P. H.**

# Preface

This is a handbook for professionals who work with medical and surgical patients. With few exceptions the writing is devoted to practical matters of patient care and the conduct of hospital business. Our goal was not to theorize, but rather to set down issues of importance for the psychiatrist in a general hospital.

Originally the book was intended for psychiatrists and psychiatric residents. However, as the table of contents grew and as our contributors developed their themes, the book took on a more general scope. This book contains useful information for medical students, nurses, social workers, and psychologists. It is our hope that physicians in primary care and family practice, as well as those in medical and surgical specialties, will find this a helpful guide.

It has been our privilege to work within the walls of a great teaching hospital. Since its inception, Massachusetts General Hospital has aspired to provide outstanding care for its patients and superior training for its staff and to encourage an interest in scientific inquiry. We have shared in these aspirations and have gained in the process. We are grateful to our many colleagues both in and out of our department with whom we have learned to practice medicine. We are appreciative to our patients as well as to our teachers. We are thankful for the tradition of this hospital and for its spirit, which has brought out the best in so many. Dr. Oliver Wendell Holmes says it for us:

> This Hospital has always inspired the fervid attachment of those holding any relationship to it whatsoever,—whether as citizens, proud of its benevolent services; as pupils, grateful for its teachings; or as medical officers, who have put their own work into its comprehensive fields of usefulness. It has universally fostered a feeling of affection. . . .

**Thomas P. Hackett**
**Ned H. Cassem**

# Contents

MASSACHUSETTS GENERAL HOSPITAL
# Handbook of
# general hospital psychiatry

# 1

# Beginnings: liaison psychiatry in a general hospital

## THOMAS P. HACKETT

### HISTORY

The history of general hospital psychiatry in the United States is elusive for the student who likes facts and dates neatly packaged. The seeds of liaison psychiatry were sown somewhat haphazardly whenever a medical staff member showed interest in mental disorders, whenever a disturbed patient had a medical problem, or whenever a medical patient had an emotional problem. For those interested in a more detailed account of the development of liaison psychiatry in the United States, I recommend the work of that doughty and venerable scholar, Z. J. Lipowski. He has provided an encyclopedic guide to the published information on this psychiatric subspecialty, and I commend this sensible and readable review to the student.[1-5]

If the course of consultation liaison psychiatry over the last decade is examined, one finds most activities centered around the year 1975. Before 1975 scant attention was given to the work of psychiatrists in medicine. Consultation liaison topics were rarely presented at the national meetings of the American Psychiatric Association. Even the American Psychosomatic Society, which has many strong links to consultation liaison work, rarely gave more than a nod of acknowledgment to presentations or panels discussing this aspect of psychiatry. Residency training programs on the whole were no better. In 1966 Mendel surveyed training programs in the United States to determine the extent to which residents were exposed to a training experience in consultation psychiatry.[6] He found that 75% of the 202 programs surveyed offered some training in consultation psychiatry, but most of it was informal and poorly organized. Ten years later Shubert and McKegney found only "a slight increase" in the amount of time devoted to consultation liaison training in residency programs.[7]

Despite the fact that the statistics are far from impressive in terms of growth, personal experience at Massachusetts General Hospital

1

(MGH) runs somewhat counter to the surveys. When comparing the number of lectures, teaching programs, and panels that we MGH psychiatrists are asked to give on consultation liaison topics, the demand of the last 2 years is twice that in any of the previous 18 years. Furthermore, letters requesting the names of suitable candidates to organize new consultation liaison services or to run existing ones have arrived in the last few years three times as often as before. Physicians who are well-trained in consultation liaison work are now in demand in a way they have not been throughout all my years of experience.

There are a number of reasons for this growth. One is the leadership of Dr. James Eaton, Director of the Psychiatric Education Branch of the National Institute of Mental Health (NIMH). Dr. Eaton has provided support and encouragement in establishing consultation liaison programs throughout the country. Another reason for this growth is the burgeoning interest in the primary-care specialties. Because primary-care physicians have quickly realized the relevance of psychiatry to the practice of medicine, many psychiatrists are attracted to primary-care teaching programs. The growth of liaison psychiatry has also been stimulated by the attack on psychiatry from an army of self-appointed counselors and psychotherapists, all claiming to possess the same order of skill as the psychiatrist and all demanding recognition by third-party payers. The scope and vigor of competition for patients have caused even those psychiatrists who most avidly sought a career in pure psychotherapy to start closing ranks with their fellow physicians to form a phalanx against the opposition. The medical model has become the guidon around which embattled psychiatrists are attempting to rally. Very little in the training of the psychiatrist is more germane to the medical model than consultation liaison psychiatry. For these reasons of commerce, as well as the natural growth of medicine in psychiatry, consultation liaison work has enjoyed a renaissance.

I trace the origin of organized interest in the mental life of patients at Massachusetts General Hospital to 1873 when James Jackson Putnam, a young Harvard neurologist, returned from his grand tour of German departments of medicine to practice his specialty. He was awarded a small office under the arch of one of the famous twin flying staircases of the Bulfinch Building. The office was the size of a cupboard and was designed to house electrical equipment. Putnam was given the extraordinary title of "Electrician." One of his duties was to ensure the proper functioning of various galvanic and faradic devices then used to treat nervous and muscular disorders. It is no coincidence that his office came to be called the "cloaca maxima" by the Professor of Medicine, George Shattuck. This designation stemmed from the fact that patients whose maladies defied diagnosis and treatment—in short, "the crocks"—were referred to young Putnam. With such a beginning it is not difficult for today's liaison psychiatrist to find a familiar anlage in J. J. Putnam. Dr. Putnam eventually became a Professor of Neuropathology and practiced both neurology and psychiatry. He treated medical and surgical patients who developed mental disorders. Dr. Putnam's distinguished career, interwoven with the acceptance of freudian psychology in the United States, is chronicled elsewhere.[8]

In the late 1920s, Dr. Howard Means, Chief of Medicine, appointed Boston psychiatrist Robert Herman to study patients who developed mental disturbances in conjuction with endocrine disorders. Dr. Herman's studies are hardly remembered today, although he is honored by having a conference room named after him.

In 1934 a Department of Psychiatry took shape when Stanley Cobb was given the Bullard Chair of Neuropathology and granted sufficient money by the Rockefeller Foundation to establish a ward for the study of psychosomatic conditions. Under Dr. Cobb's tutelage the department expanded and became known for its eclecticism and for its interest in the mind-brain relationship. A number of European emigrants fleeing Nazi tyranny were welcomed to the department by Dr. Cobb. Felix and Helene Deutsch, Edward and Grete Bibring, and Hans Sachs were early arrivals from the Continent. Erich Lindemann came in the mid-1930s and worked with Dr. Cobb on a series of projects, the most notable being his study of grief. This study came as a result of his work with victims of the 1942 Coconut Grove fire.

When Dr. Lindemann became Chief of the Psychiatric Service in 1954, the consultation liaison service had not yet been established. Customarily the resident assigned to night call in the emergency room saw all medical and surgical patients needing psychiatric evaluation. This was regarded as an onerous task, and such calls were often set aside until after supper in the hope that the disturbance might quiet in the intervening hours. Notes in the chart were terse and often impractical. Seldom was there a follow-up. As a result, animosity toward psychiatry grew. To remedy this Dr. Lindemann officially established the Psychiatric Consultation Service under the leadership of Avery Weisman in 1956. As Dr. Weisman's resident, I divided my time between doing consultations and learning outpatient psychotherapy. During the first year of the consultation service, 130 consultations were made. In 1958 the number of consultations increased to 370 and we organized an active research program that later became one of the cornerstones of the overall operation.

By 1960 a rotation through the consultation service had become a mandatory part of the MGH residency in psychiatry. Second-year residents were each assigned two wards. Each resident spent 20 to 30 hours a week in the consultation service for a 6-month period. Between 1956 and 1960 the service attracted the interest of fellowship students who contributed postgraduate work on psychosomatic topics. Medical students also began to choose the consultation liaison service as part of their elective in psychiatry during this period. From our work with these fellows and medical students collaborative research studies were initiated with other services. Examples of these studies are (1) the surgical treatment of intractable pain,[9,10] (2) the compliance of duodenal ulcer patients with their medical regimen,[11] (3) postamputation depression in the elderly patient,[12] (4) emotional maladaptation in the surgical patient,[13-16] and (5) the psychological aspect of acute myocardial infarction.[17]

By 1970 we had a complement of ten full-time staff members doing consultation work (nine of these supported by research grants; the tenth, by hospital salary), six residents, and a Chief Resident who was assigned full-time to the service. Growth has continued.

We now offer a fellowship program in psychosomatic medicine that has added three fellows and one full-time faculty member to our roster. A private psychiatric consultation service has been established (see Chapter 29). A somatic therapy unit has been added to evaluate and treat patients for refractory depression and chronic pain syndromes (see Chapter 4). A consultant is now assigned on a part-time basis to the renal dialysis unit. A hypnosis and psychosomatic clinic has been added (see Chapter 30). Each month several medical students rotate through the consultation liaison service. Second- and third-year psychiatric residents from other programs also come to us for training in liaison work. Our research has expanded to include major efforts on cancer, myocardial infarction, and chronic pain.

We have a liaison psychiatrist assigned to every ward in the general hospital and to the Massachusetts Eye and Ear Infirmary. In teaching we have two walk rounds a week, rounds with the Chief of the Consultation Service, Chief Resident's rounds, and a psychosomatic conference. The medical students have their own walk rounds. Each new group of residents is given a set of lecture demonstrations on hypnosis and a course in the fundamentals of liaison psychiatry. The senior staff members of the consultation liaison service give each second-year resident class a series of thirty lectures on the history of psychosomatic medicine and a view of current work in the field. A distinction must be made between a consultation service and a consultation liaison service. A consultation service is a rescue squad. It responds to requests from other services for help with the diagnosis, treatment, or disposition of perplexing patients. At worst, consultation work is nothing more than a brief foray into the territory of another service, usually ending with a note written in the chart outlining a plan of action. The actual intervention is left to the consultee. Like a volunteer firefighter, a consultant puts out the blaze and then returns home. Like a volunteer fire brigade, a consultation service seldom has the time or manpower to set up fire prevention programs or to educate the citizenry about fireproofing. A consultation service is the most common type of psychiatric-medical interface found in departments of psychiatry around the United States today.

A liaison service requires manpower, money, and motivation. Sufficient personnel are necessary to allow the psychiatric consultant time to perform services other than simply interviewing troublesome patients in the area assigned him. He must be able to attend rounds, discuss patients individually with house officers, and hold teaching sessions for nurses. Liaison work is further distinguished from consultation activity in that patients are seen at the discretion of the psychiatric consultant as well as the referring physicians. Because the consultant attends social service rounds with the house officers, he is able to spot potential psychiatric problems.

Once organized, a liaison service tends to expand. Most liaison services are appreciated and their contribution is recognized. Sometimes this brings tangible benefits such as space and salary from the departments being serviced. However, even under the best circumstances, the impact of a liaison effort seldom lingers after the effort is withdrawn. Lessons taught by the psychiatrist need constant reinforcement or they are forgotten by our medical colleagues. In a way, this is an advantage since it ensures a continuing need for our presence. Conversely, it disappoints the more pedagogical, because their students, while interested, fail to learn. I believe we must be philosophical. After all, our surgical colleagues do not insist that we learn to do laparotomies. They insist only that we be aware of the indications.

The term "psychosomatic service" has had a variable history. The term generally leaves a bad taste in the mouths of physicians. It reminds them of the 1930s, 1940s, and 1950s, when various psychosomatic schools espoused doctrines linking specific psychological conflicts or unique personality profiles with diseases designated as psychosomatic. Compounding this misunderstanding has been the term's abuse by the general public, who regard anything psychosomatic as either imaginary or nervous in origin. As a consequence, most people believe that a psychosomatic disease is not to be taken seriously. Recently the meaning of the term "psychosomatic" has undergone a metamorphosis. It has become a fashionable word in grant requests, in the titles of scholarly papers, and on the editorial pages of medical journals. To some of us psychosomatic once again means what it says—the interplay between the physical and psychological forces that are part of every disease process. It is synonymous with psychophysiological. With this in mind, some consultation liaison services have, in true Teutonic fashion, hammered together with hyphens the compound term "consultation-liaison-psychosomatic service," or more succinctly, psychosomatic-liaison service. The psychosomatic designation implies that active research is going on in the framework of liaison activities.

Whatever it is called, psychiatry in the general hospital has many facets. This book represents an effort to describe and discuss many of these facets as they have been revealed through the eye of our experience.

## PATIENT CARE, TEACHING, AND RESEARCH

The three functions provided by any consultation liaison division are patient care, teaching, and research. Each of these will be considered separately here.

### Patient care

Approaching a patient in a consultation liaison capacity is different from meeting a patient in the context of outpatient psychotherapy. The consultation patient has not necessarily asked to see a psychiatrist and may, in fact, actively resist the interview. The proper introduction of the consultant to the patient by the referring physician is crucial. If the introduction is made in a relaxed, natural way, particularly if the consultee can make it appear routine, there is seldom much resistance. If, on the other hand, the consultee is uneasy or embarrassed to have his patient seen by a psychiatrist, there is a possibility of discord in the initial contact. The liaison psychiatrist should take every opportunity to let physicians requesting consultation know how important the initial introduction is. Young house officers experience the most difficulty in requesting psychiatric consultations. Those from medical schools where psychiatry is taught well and thoroughly readily use the consultant service with minimal uncertainty or embarrassment. Others, less fortunate in their training, require time to familiarize themselves with our specialty and need our patience and goodwill along the way. By the time these young physicians finish their residency training and join the staff, they have usually assimilated enough diplomacy to make a psychiatric referral without distress to patient or consultant. They have seen firsthand that a psychiatrist offers effective care without offense to the patient. As the internist and surgeon employ the skills of the psychiatrist they recognize the limitations of our specialty as well as its many uses. Not only do they learn the problems with which the consultant can help, but also they learn the individual consultant's areas of expertise. They also learn to match a specific psychiatrist's style with the patient's temperament or problem.

There has been a growing acceptance in some hospitals of the role of psychiatry in general medicine. At Massachusetts General Hospital approximately 10% of all general hospital admissions are seen by a psychiatric consultant. This is a high percentage when compared with the national average, but it is not unique. On certain of our services, such as cardiac surgery, with its high incidence of postcardiotomy delirium, the percentage is as high as 40%. On others, such as the private consultation service (see Chapter 29), it drops to 3%. The statistics vary from month to month, depending on the energy and interest of the individual consultant and depending on the medical or surgical attending physicians who serve as visits to the wards. A Visit* who scorns psychiatric intervention is not likely to encourage house officers to call in a consultant. Despite these variations, the overall average figure remains 10%. The *MGH News* published this figure along with such reasons for consultation as pain control, depression secondary to an illness, and fear of impending surgery. This article states that the psychiatrist does not deal only with the seriously deranged or the insane. Not a small number of consultees have quoted this article to the patients they refer for consultation to assure them they are not being singled out or regarded as "mental." Unfortunately, we will have to define our role to the general public for some time to come. Our image has been variously blurred, magnified, shrunken, and

---

*Visit is a staff physician who is assigned a ward to teach residents.

distorted over the years. We must accept the task of clarifying our skills and surveying our domain with equanimity and fortitude.

Each liaison psychiatrist has a personal style. In the hope that it may be helpful to the novice consultant, I have given a brief description here of my personal approach to the consultation interview.

Generally the first visit is by way of introduction. It takes 15 minutes to peruse the chart, particularly if the patient has been hospitalized for any length of time; another 5 to 10 minutes to contact the nurse; and another few minutes to speak with a family member, if one is present. As a consequence, the initial visit may be in the nature of a sortie during which contact is established—hopefully contact that will dispel whatever alien image the patient may have of a psychiatrist.

I do my best to be friendly when I meet a patient for the first time— not effusive, not with a glad hand, nonetheless, decidedly amiable and interested. I want to learn something about this individual in a short time, and to do so I need his help. A frozen professional manner is not apt to elicit anything but hostile reserve. I seldom explain why I have come. My assumption is that this has already been discussed by the referring physician. If the patient appears confused, I try to explain my presence, but when there is uncertainty and suspicion about who requested the consultation and why, I often defer the contact until the referring physician can explain the consultation request to the patient.

I usually begin the interview by asking for a brief medical history of the illness. This assures the patient of my interest in the medical aspects of his condition, underscores my profession and allows me the chance to note how the patient's psychology has unfolded in response to the progression of symptoms. Does he include his emotional reactions to the events he describes? If so, are they appropriate? Is there evidence that his response is influenced by familial problems? What limitations or opportunities has his illness elicited? Soon the roles of people and events coincident with the illness begin to take shape. I spend the rest of my time asking questions relevant to the central issues of the apparent problem. If we unearth sensitive material about which the patient appears reluctant to talk, I seldom press the issue. Instead, I will return later in the day or the following day giving the patient time to question his physician again about my coming. To gain the patient's trust, I make a specific appointment for the second interview. By keeping the appointment, I show the patient through token behavior that I keep my promises. To further encourage trust, I am usually willing to answer most personal questions. I want the patient to know something of me.

I never take notes during the first interview and seldom in subsequent contacts unless the events of the case are complicated. Writing while talking is fine for some, but it does not fit my style. Quite consistent with my style, however, is taking a patient's pulse, listening to his chest, or examining a superficial lesion if it is called for. If I suspect that a medical diagnosis has been overlooked, I will conduct the necessary noninvasive examination.

Depending on the specific features of the case, the initial interview may last anywhere from 15 minutes to 1½ hours. I make it a point to do at least one follow-up visit while the patient is in the hospital. If this cannot be done, I often attempt to contact him by telephone to find out how he is. In any case, I discuss with the patient how often I intend to see him. If I come to believe that he will need psychotherapy as an outpatient, I will refer him to someone else if I am unable to do the task myself. I always explain the reason for this referral. It is my practice to inform patients of any shift in medication, change in plans for surgery, or indeed any alteration in care that stems from my visit. I will give them my opinions, explaining that their physician will decide how to act on my recommendations.

The consultation environment is unpredictable. The consultant may arrive on the scene only to find visitors present. A nurse or technician may come along to draw blood or record a vital function at an inopportune moment during the conversation. Finding a quiet and private spot is difficult. It requires flexibility and an understanding of hospital life. It is always best to alert the ward charge nurse that a consultant is on the way in order to advise visitors that their stay may be interrupted. A friendly nurse who knows something of the consultant's techniques is helpful in finding a corner where the patient and consultant can meet without interruption. Whenever possible I take the patient to an examining room or a vacant office. If the interview must be conducted in the presence of others, I draw the curtain about the bed and begin my questions. If I sense restraint or uneasiness, I will ask if the patient would prefer a private setting. While such requests are rare, the need for a private setting should be honored even if it means moving other patients away for an hour or two. Oddly enough, one can usually maintain the illusion of privacy behind a drawn curtain or screen.

As a matter of courtesy I sit down when interviewing or visiting patients. Long accustomed to the ritual of making rounds, many physicians remain standing as a matter of course. Standing, physicians remind me of missiles about to be launched, poised to depart. Even if this is not necessarily true, they look the part. Patients sense this and it limits conversation. In addition, when standing, the physician necessarily looks down on the patient. This disparity in height is apt to encourage the attribution of arrogance. Looking down at a patient who is prone emphasizes the dependency of the position. Sitting at the bedside equalizes station. Sitting with a patient need not take longer than standing with him.

There are two types of write-ups. One is the medical record; the second is the central or research file record (discussed in the section on research). The write-up for the patient's chart should be brief and simply written. It should contain a diagnosis and practical suggestions. Rarely is it necessary to cover more than one page of chart paper. Negative findings need not be listed. Confidential information should never be included. If the reason for the consultation request has not been put into the chart by the consultee it should be stated by the consultant if it can be done without embarrassing the patient. A brief statement of the problems should be made and the pertinent findings listed. A brief differential diagnosis and working diagnosis should be outlined followed by a list of recommendations in numerical order. Some consultants possess a fine literary style. This is commendable. Anything that emphasizes the unique merit of the consultation is apt to enhance it. A sense of humor is always valuable if it is kept in mind that the record can become part of a public document in court.

Conversation with the physician who referred the patient is more than politeness. Only a limited amount can be expressed in a note, however complete it may be. Always there are nuances of feeling and sometimes historical data as well that cannot be committed to the chart. Any exchange by telephone or in person is not only good public relations, but sound medical practice. The language used by the consultant must be compatible with the referring physician's psychiatric vocabulary.

The charge nurse on the floor is a crucial figure to consult in any evaluation of a patient on the floor. The nurse will know as much about him as anyone on the floor and perhaps more about his personality and the family interactions than his physician. The way in which the patient or his family relates to nurses may be informative. Nurses' opinions, when pertinent, should be included in evaluations, and data should be shared with them. If the patient happens to be especially troublesome, a brief visit with all of the nurses at the change of shift to ensure maximum attendance is sometimes helpful.

**Teaching**

Most liaison psychiatrists believe that teaching psychiatry to medical and surgical house officers cannot be done on a formal basis. When teaching is formalized in weekly lectures or discussion groups, attendance invariably lags. Twenty years ago Erich Lindemann, in an attempt to educate medical house officers about the emotional problems of their patients, enlisted the help of several psychiatric luminaries from the Boston area. A series of biweekly lectures was announced. Edward and Grete Bibring, Felix and Helene Deutsch, Stanley Cobb, and Carl Binger, among others, were to share their knowledge and skills. In the beginning approximately one-fifth of the medical house officers attended. Attendance steadily dwindled in subsequent sessions until finally the psychiatry residents had to be forced to attend in order to infuse the lectures with enough vitality to continue. I believe that if Sigmund Freud could have been resurrected and persuaded to hold luncheon meetings every other week for the medical staff, his reception would have been no more vigorous.

Teaching is best done at the bedside on a case-by-case basis. The exceptional house officer who wants more instruction should be given it. Primary-care physicians are more interested in psychiatry and would benefit from instruction in interview technique and other practical matters. Whenever teaching is attempted, the chief of the service involved should be approached to ensure support. Without it the most modest teaching attempt is likely to falter. The chiefs of all services should be made aware that the psychiatric consultant is willing and available to teach.

Good teaching begins with providing information in a good consultation. It can develop further in conversations between consultant and consultee. Discussion with nurses and house officers is desirable and should occur naturally. That should be the initial goal of informed consultation teaching. More formal teaching should generally be avoided, lest the reward be disappointment and unintended rebuff.

We make ourselves available to nursing students and graduate nurses, and offer continuing programs of education as requested. The same is true for social workers and, to a limited extent, for occupational therapists and physiotherapists.

Teaching medical students is a different matter. Harvard Medical School students are assigned to us only on an elective basis. Since they have chosen to study liaison psychiatry, they are usually eager for instruction. We provide them with formal teaching 2 hours a week and supervision for 1 hour a week. Small groups are also taught as needed.

The teaching of psychiatric residents rotating through the consultation service is a more complicated topic. As a general outline, each resident is supervised individually for 1 to 2 hours each week. There are weekly walk rounds with the Chief of the Psychiatric Consultation Service and with the Chief of the Psychiatric Service. There are weekly conferences with the Chief Resident and a weekly psychosomatic conference. In addition, each resident conducts a teaching group of nurses and nursing students on one floor and often supervises other groups as well.

**Research**

Research activity by the consultation liaison service is important in building bridges between medical specialties. When physicians from other services are involved in research planning and when there is dual authorship of published accounts, friendships are firmly bonded and differences fade. The general hospital population provides such a limitless legacy of research material that a consultation liaison service would be lax or unresponsive not to take advantage of it.

Small research projects are the cornerstone of larger ones. Research need not be funded through federal or state agencies. Projects can be done as "arbeits" and assigned as such to medical students during their month on the service. They can also be suggested to fellows for more extensive development over the course of the year. What begins as an "arbeit" with results and conclusions to be presented at Psychiatric Grand Rounds can, over a period of 6 months, develop into a full-fledged publication. This in turn might be the starting point for a larger investigation.

Research opportunities should include psychologists, nurses, nurse clinicians, social workers, and others who share an interest in consultation liaison work. It is important for potential researchers naive about methodology to be schooled in this before starting a project. Furthermore, it is always well to use the wisdom and advice of senior members of the team, particularly those who are skilled in methodology, before setting up a research design. In our experience psychologists are usually more adept methodologists than are psychiatrists.

A filing system should be designed to keep potential research materials readily accessible. Easy access makes follow-up both more likely and more profitable. Statistical and methodological consultation with experts in the use of computers and the statistical design of research projects is essential for those of us not gifted in this area.

Since the seed of research in liaison psychiatry is the contact between patient and consultant, the recording of this contact is central. In addition to the notes in the patient chart, the liaison psychiatrist should make what we call a context recording for each consultation encounter with patient, family, or hospital staff. This is a technique Dr. Weisman and I developed while working with dying patients. A context recording is a freely associated dictation on everything that comes to mind about the patient and the interview. It is dictated with no attempt at order in an effort to get every fact, incidental as well as obviously pertinent, into the record. No attempt is made at style, literacy, or organization. It is simply a way of putting on paper all that can be remembered. This method is especially valuable when unusual cases are prepared for journal publication.

Activity and lively thinking are the life blood of research. In order to keep the circulation flowing, research conferences must be held weekly or monthly to discuss research findings and to plan new projects. It seems congruent with liaison psychiatry to emphasize a clinical orientation toward research rather than a laboratory approach.

Once the orientation of the consultation liaison team has been pointed toward research and publication, the results usually fall easily into line. One of the distressing roadblocks en route to publication is the poor writing skill of many physicians. One or two resource people who can serve as editors and teachers can be a great help. Sometimes it is advantageous to hire a professional editor. All efforts seem worth the candle once the printed page is in the author's hand. When a service begins to develop a shelf of publications authored by various members of the team, a pride of accomplishment unfolds, compounding the excitement of the research and stimulating renewed academic effort.

## REFERENCES

1. Lipowski, Z. J.: Review of consultation psychiatry and psychosomatic medicine. I: General principles, Psychosom. Med. **29**:153-171, 1967.
2. Lipowski, Z. J.: Review of consultation psychiatry and psychosomatic medicine. II: Clinical aspects, Psychosom. Med. **29**:201-224, 1967.
3. Lipowski, Z. J.: Review of consultation psychiatry and psychosomatic medicine. III: Theoretical issues, Psychosom. Med. **30**:395-421, 1968.
4. Lipowski, Z. J.: Consultation psychiatry in a general hospital, Compr. Psychiatry **12**:461-465, 1971.

5. Lipowski, Z. J.: Consultation-liaison psychiatry: an overview, Am. J. Psychiatry **131:**623-630, 1974.
6. Mendel, W. M.: Psychiatric consultation education - 1966, Am. J. Psychiatry **123:**150-155, 1966.
7. Schubert, D. S. P., and McKegney, F. P.: Psychiatric consultation education 1976. Arch. Gen. Psychiatry **33:**1271-1273, 1976.
8. Hale, N. G.: Freud and the americans, New York, 1971, Oxford University Press.
9. White, J. C., Sweet, W. H., and Hackett, T. P.: Radiofrequency leukotomy for the relief of pain, Arch. Neurol. **2:**317-330, 1960.
10. Mark, V. H., and Hackett, T. P.: Surgical aspects of thalamotomy in the human, Trans. Am. Neurol. Assoc., pp. 92-94, 1959.
11. Hernandez, M., and Hackett, T. P.: The problem of nonadherence to therapy in the management of duodenal ulcer recurrences, Amer. J. Dig. Dis. **7:**1047-1060, 1962.
12. Caplan, L. M., and Hackett, T. P.: Prelude to death: emotional effects of lower limb amputation in the aged, N. Engl. J. Med. **269:**1166-1171, 1963.
13. Weisman, A. D., and Hackett, T. P.: Psychosis after eye surgery: establishment of a specific doctor-patient relation and the prevention and treatment of "black patch delirium," N. Engl. J. Med. **258:**1284-1289, 1958.
14. Weisman, A. D., and Hackett, T. P.: Predilection to death: death and dying as a psychiatric problem, Psychosom. Med. **23:**232-257, 1961.
15. Hackett, T. P., and Weisman, A. D.: Psychiatric management of operative syndromes. I: The therapeutic consultation and the effect of noninterpretive intervention, Psychosom. Med. **22:**267-282, 1960.
16. Hackett, T. P., and Weisman, A. D.: Psychiatric management of operative syndromes. II: Psychodynamic factors in formulation and management. Psychosom. Med. **22:**356-372, 1960.
17. Olin, H. S., and Hackett, T. P.: The denial of chest pain in thirty-two patients with acute myocardial infarction, JAMA **190:**977-981, 1964.
18. Cassem, N. H., and Hackett, T. P.: Psychiatric consultation in a coronary care unit, Ann. Intern. Med. **75:**9-14, 1971.

# 2

# Alcoholism: acute and chronic states

**THOMAS P. HACKETT**

From cases of simple intoxication, when the diagnosis can be made on the basis of breath odor and slurred speech, to the more complicated mental status of withdrawal states, alcohol is responsible for more psychiatric syndromes in general hospitals than any other substance consumed. Even when problem drinking is not in the immediate picture, a past history of alcoholism or heavy social drinking predisposes the patient to postoperative delirium and seems to lower his threshold for other types of delirium as well (see Chapter 5). Heavy drinkers have a higher than usual incidence of delirium in conjunction with fever, head trauma, and massive burns.

## DRUNKENNESS

Inebriation, by far the most prevalent toxic manifestation of drinking, is rarely discussed in the literature of liaison psychiatry. Of the conditions that come to the attention of the psychiatrist in the emergency room or overnight ward of a general hospital, few are potentially more threatening, disruptive, and dangerous. Standard medical textbooks offer little help in handling this problem even though it is the most common drug intoxication found in the United States and has been linked with all manner of violent crimes and assaults. Few sights are more frightening than that of a young and powerful man, uncontrollably drunk, mindlessly angry, yet in full possession of his motor coordination and muscular power. Loud, truculent, and unreasonable, such an individual poses a genuine menace to those about him. What are the principles of management in such a case?

### Management

For handling these individuals a regimen has been developed at MGH that has proven effective in most cases. The first principle is to

**15**

alert the hospital police or security force before starting an interview with a boisterous drunk. While police intervention is seldom required, it is reassuring to have assistance ready if one expects trouble. This is especially true if the patient may be armed or has a history of combativeness.

The second principle of our regimen is to suggest that the personal manner of the interviewer be tolerant and nonthreatening. People who possess a skill for disarming the abusive drunk seem to have little or no need to express their authority or toughness even though they may have both qualities in abundance. They can tolerate insults, threats, and oaths because they do not take them personally. Conversely, we have observed that individuals who galvanize the alcoholic person's anger and mobilize his aggression are often autocratic and rigid people whose thin sense of security is easily punctured by invective from the inebriate. The successful interviewer temporarily accepts the drunk as he is; the unsuccessful interviewer instantly attempts to make him civil. The latter effort usually backfires. In approaching the alcoholic person, a handshake of introduction should be extended. Unless the patient is known, he should be addressed by his proper name, for example, "Mr. Smith." For the time being no attempt should be made to change his behavior. Better to listen to a tirade and attempt to make sense of it than to demand that he lower his voice and talk more temperately. This is especially important if you wish to uncover a legitimate grievance or misunderstanding that, if present and cor-rectable, can quickly alleviate the patient's bellicosity.

It is advisable to avoid direct eye contact for more than a few seconds at a time. More than momentary eye contact is often taken as a challenge and becomes the prelude to combat for humans as well as for animals. The interviewer should listen to what the patient has to say seriously and appear puzzled or perplexed rather than angry or amused if the accusation or complaint is absurd. Above all, it is important to avoid any posture of belligerence. A colleague once observed that he patterned his behavior with hostile drunks after the humble-submissive posture assumed by a wolf when bested in battle. Transposed to the human habitus, this physician kept eyes downcast, fists unclenched, and shoulders stooped. Once the patient sees that the interviewer is not going to attack him, his outburst may quiet, his anger slacken.

The third principle is to offer food. Some of the more antagonistic alcoholic individuals have been soothed by the offer of coffee. If the individual is willing to leave the scene with the inducement of coffee, food, and quiet (luring him with the promise of a beer is the last resort), he should be escorted to a lobby or foyer where people are within easy calling distance. Many alcoholic persons are claustrophobic and feel trapped in small rooms. Those with underlying homosexual conflicts, sometimes found in alcoholic persons, might associate the closeness of tiny quarters with the fear of sexual advance. Furthermore, it is discomforting for most physicians to be in an enclosed area with a potentially violent person. The value of offering food, cigarettes, or drink in this case can be justified on empirical evidence only. If the patient will eat, he will lose his fight. The next step is to persuade him to take a sedative and go to bed.

As in handling other conditions of psychotic excitement, it often helps to let the patient know that his behavior is frightening.

A woman psychiatrist was called to the emergency ward to see a patient who had leaped from the examining table while a scalp laceration was being repaired. He accused the intern of deliberately trying to hurt him and the entire staff of racism. The patient was a large man with a deep, penetrating voice and a menacing manner. The psychiatrist, a tiny attractive woman, asked the others to leave— which they did reluctantly. They heard the patient thunder accusations for 3 to 4 minutes. Then quiet reigned. A shattering scream was expected, but not even a breath could be heard. Five minutes later the psychiatrist emerged and the patient was lying peaceably on the examining table, having consented to an intramuscular injection of a sedative. The psychiatric technique was simple. During a pause for breath in his ranting, she told him she was nearly speechless with fear. She reminded him that she was harmless, that she could do nothing to hurt him, and that she wanted to help him. The tremor in her voice verified her statement. He stared at her a moment. Then he muttered, "Don't want to scare nobody," and accepted the sedative.

To sedate the intoxicated individual, one must begin with a smaller dose than usual to avoid a deleterious interaction between alcohol and the agent used.[1] Once the individual's tolerance has been established, a specific dose can be safely determined. We favor the use of the benzodiazepines. If parenteral use is required, diazepam can be given intramuscularly or intravenously. Because erratic and slow absorption so often occurs in the intramuscular route, oral or intravenous use is preferred. The initial dose should be followed by a wait of from $1/2$ to 1 hour before augmenting it. The acutely intoxicated individual does not usually require hospitalization. If there is no risk of withdrawal syndrome, the patient can safely be referred to an outpatient detoxification program.

## PATHOLOGICAL INTOXICATION AND ALCOHOLIC PARANOIA
### Alcoholic coma

Alcoholic coma, although rare, is a real medical emergency. It occurs when extraordinary amounts of alcohol are consumed, often in conjunction with another drug. The main goal of treatment is to prevent pulmonary depression and respiratory arrest.

### Pathological intoxication

The disease state of pathological intoxication has been described as a condition in which the patient becomes intoxicated on very small amounts of alcohol—as little as four ounces.[2] There may be subsequent automatic behavior for which the patient is totally amnesic. This behavior may be violent and assaultive. If the alcoholic person is known to have a history of pathological alcoholism, he should be sedated heavily and confined until sobriety is assured in order to avoid possible danger to others.

The episode of pathological intoxication usually ends after prolonged sleep. It may last for only an hour or may last for days. During this time the patient is agitated, impulsive, and often aggressive. Delusions and visual hallucinations may occur. Generally the disorder is marked by hyperactivity, anxiety, or depression. Suicide attempts sometimes occur. It has been postulated that pathological intoxication is more likely to occur in borderline characters or in epileptic patients—in those individuals who tend toward emotional instability and whose pattern of defense is easily disorganized.

### Alcoholic paranoia

This condition is somewhat similar to pathological intoxication. It is a state of disorganization brought about by alcohol and made manifest by strong feelings of jealousy, antagonism, and suspicion. Sometimes the underlying disorder is homosexual in nature; when normal defenses are dissolved by alcohol, homosexual impulses emerge that, in turn, induce paranoid delusions.

The prognosis is poor for patients with pathological intoxication or alcoholic paranoia.[3] Individuals so afflicted often have a history of violence and aggression with repeated incarcerations. The liaison psychiatrist should be on the watch for the emergence of amnesia or the reversal of personality after the alcoholic session has been slept off. Although the premorbid personality of the paranoid alcoholic patient is apt to be somewhat suspicious, it is not nearly as intense or threatening as when under the influence of alcohol.

## ALCOHOLIC WITHDRAWAL SYNDROME

"Alcoholic withdrawal syndrome" is now the preferred description rather than the traditional term "delirium tremens" because the latter limits its concern to only one manifestation of the syndrome.[4] However, throughout this discussion the terms will be used interchangeably.

Until open heart surgical procedures spawned new postoperative deliria, delirium tremens was by far the most frequently encountered delirium in a general hospital. Though it was first described in medical literature over 150 years ago and has been frequently observed in general hospitals ever since, delirium tremens is misdiagnosed in an uncomfortably large number of cases.[5] It is missed because physicians tend (or choose) to forget that alcoholism is rampant among people of all possible backgrounds and appearances in the United States. Physicians also fail to suspect the patient who tends, deliberately or unwittingly, to minimize dependence on alcohol and to underestimate the amount consumed. Because 10% of the patients with uncomplicated alcoholic withdrawal syndrome and 25% of those patients who have medical or concomitant surgical complications die, it is imperative to be on the alert for this dangerous condition.

### Prediction

It is difficult to predict who will develop delirium tremens. We know that it rarely develops in patients under the age of 30 and that it seldom occurs in the absence of at least 3 years of chronic alcoholism. Although regarded as a withdrawal syndrome, there are heavy drinkers who fail to develop delirium after sudden withdrawal of ethanol. Infection, head trauma, and poor nutrition are probable contributing factors toward delirium. History of delirium tremens is an obvious predictor of a repeat episode during an enforced spell of drying out.

> One patient, a 64-year-old wharfinger, entered the hospital with recurrent gout sixteen times during a 3 year period. Each time he became tremulous and disoriented during the second night and went on to develop mild visual and vestibular hallucinations that cleared over the next 3 days. Large ships would issue through the walls or windows and the whole room would rock and sway like a wharf in a storm. The pattern was identical, including his insistence that the only alcohol he ever swallowed was a drop or two from his mouthwash.

Although delirium tremens does not always appear in alcoholic withdrawal, the withdrawal symptoms following the cessation of heavy drinking are predictable. Loss of appetite, nausea, irritability, and tremulousness are early features. The appearance of a generalized tremor, fast in frequency, becoming more pronounced when the patient is under stress, is the hallmark of the abstinence syndrome. The tremor may involve the tongue to such an extent that the patient cannot talk. The lower extremities may tremble so that the patient cannot walk. The hands and arms may shake so violently that a drinking glass cannot be held without spilling the contents. The patient will be hypervigilant, have a pronounced startle response, and complain of insomnia. Illusions and hallucinations of a mild variety may appear, producing a sense of vague uneasiness. This picture may persist for as long as 2 weeks and clear without the appearance of a delirium. Grand mal seizures ("rum fits") may occur, usually within the first 2 days. More than one out of every three patients who suffer seizures develop subsequent delirium tremens.

**Diagnosis**

If delirium tremens is to occur, it generally does so within 24 to 72 hours after withdrawal. However, there have been reports of cases where the clinical picture of delirium tremens did not appear until 7 days after the last drink. The principal features of the state are disorientation (in time or place or person in any combination); tremor; hyperactivity; marked wakefulness; fever; increased autonomic arousal; and hallucinations. Hallucinations are generally visual but may be tactile (in which case they are probably associated with a peripheral neuritis), olfactory, or auditory. Vestibular disturbances are common and often hallucinatory in nature. The patient may complain of the floor moving beneath his feet or believe he is on an elevator. The hallucinatory experience is always frightening. Animals, typically snakes, are seen in threatening poses. Mice or lice are felt and seen crawling on the skin. Once the condition manifests itself, delirium tremens usually lasts 2 to 3 days. Should it persist for a longer time, one must suspect an underlying disorder, such as infection or subdural hematoma. There are, however, a small number of individuals whose course is characterized by relapses interspersed with intervals of complete lucidity. These patients offer the consultant the most challenging diagnostic opportunities. As a rule of thumb, it is always wise to include delirium tremens in the list of differential diagnostic possibilities whenever delirium appears.

The psychiatric consultant is apt to miss the diagnosis of delirium tremens when the patient's manner, social position, or reputation belie the possibility of alcoholism. For example, the following problem arose after an emergency surgical procedure.

A 54-year-old woman was admitted to the hospital for a cholecystectomy. She was a society matron with all the attendant stereotypical characteristics. She and her surgeon were neighbors. On her third postoperative day (her fifth day without alcohol) the nurses reported that they could not keep her in bed. She got up and walked about her room in a restless, agitated fashion, constantly gazing back over her shoulder as though she feared she was being followed. Soon her peregrinations included other patients' rooms as well as the hospital corridor. She resisted violently every attempt to keep her confined to quarters. The surgeon, when called, described her as "fearful, overactive, stubborn, but polite." While she would not give any reason for her distress, she readily swallowed a 25-mg capsule of chlordiazepoxide (Librium). This produced no change in her behavior after 2 hours. She talked to herself while she paced but was able to pull herself together and to maintain a shaky semblance of poise when approached by others. Although her physician opposed psychiatric consultation, the nurses prevailed because they feared she might inadvertently hurt herself. When a house officer suggested the possibility of a "small stroke" because of the patient's long history of hypertension, the physician agreed to request psychiatric advice. After reviewing the history and noting a coarse bilateral hand tremor while observing the patient, the psychiatrist diagnosed delirium tremens. Although the patient refused to speak with him after he identified himself, the psychiatrist maintained his diagnosis because it was the most likely possibility in the absence of other signs. Her personal physician refused to accept the diagnosis, but did follow the recommended regimen of medication (100 mg of chlordiazepoxide each hour) until the patient was able to stay in bed. The medication was then reduced to a maintenance level and supplemented by 50 mg of thiamine daily. Round-the-clock special nurses were also employed. The patient awoke the following morning her normal self. It is characteristic for delirium tremens to terminate suddenly, often after a night of sound sleep.

The patient subsequently admitted drinking four to seven very dry martinis a day, each about 4 ounces. She had been doing so for the last 30 years and had gone through all of her maternity confinements without having had delirium tremens. Age may have made the difference. She refused to accept the diagnosis of delirium tremens. However, she was so frightened by her experience that she agreed to enter psychotherapy.

The consultant is also frequently misled when delirium is intermittent and the patient is examined during a lucid stage.

Exemplifying this situation is the case of a 52-year-old architect admitted for hematemesis. This patient readily admitted heavy alcohol intake, but had no difficulty in the hospital until the fourth day. He then began to gaze fixedly at a point on the ceiling and to talk in low, menacing tones to an imaginary companion. He sweated, trembled, and thrashed about so wildly that he had to be restrained in bed. He readily described auditory hallucinations of a persecutory nature. These became alarmingly vivid in the evening. The following morning a psychiatrist was called to see him and found him to be fully oriented, lucid, perfectly capable of discussing his hallucinatory experiences of the previous evening, and willing to accept the diagnosis of delirium tremens. However, he pointed out that he had never had delirium tremens before, although he had been a heavy drinker for many years. The psychiatrist noted a probable episode of delirium tremens, but observed that the patient was now lucid and ready for further diagnostic procedures. Restraints were removed. A few hours later the patient leaped out of bed, ran through the ward, upset tables, and screamed that someone was chasing him. Once again he was forcibly restrained, placed in bed, given 8 ml of paraldehyde orally and 50 mg of chlorpromazine intramuscularly. When the psychiatrist returned a few hours later, the patient's mental status was entirely normal and he could recall the violent episode. He was, in fact, so clear thinking and his mentation so intact that the psychiatrist once again suggested that restraints be removed. Within 20 minutes the patient sprang out of bed, left the ward, and almost left the hospital. After this second unexpected episode the consultant sent him to a mental hospital where he remained for the next 2 weeks with intermittent episodes of delirium.

Although this is a highly atypical course for delirium tremens, it does occur. Consultants should be wary of relinquishing restraints or discontinuing private nurses until the patient has been lucid for 24 hours.

### Differential diagnosis

The differential diagnosis must include the many types of deliria found in a general hospital (see Chapter 6). These include postoperative and post-concussive deliria as well as metabolic disorders. Two examples of the latter are: (1) impending hepatic coma and (2) acute pancreatitis. The patient with impending hepatic coma may well be disoriented and confused, but manifests decreased activity rather than agitation. Usually there are no visual hallucinations. Speech is slow and monotonous and the face masklike. Hyperphagia rather than anorexia will exist in impending hepatic coma. Physical signs such as jaundice, hepatomegaly, and fetor hepaticus from elevation of blood ammonia help determine this diagnosis.

There is a delirium that sometimes occurs in acute pancreatitis. In this condition, however, there is generally severe abdominal pain with an elevated serum amylase.

### Prognosis

The prognosis for delirium tremens is reasonably good. Death, if it occurs, usually results from acute heart failure, an infection (chiefly pneumonia), or injuries sustained during the restless period. In a small proportion of individuals the delirium may merge into a Korsakoff psychosis, in which case the patient may not regain full mentation. This is more apt to happen with closely spaced episodes of delirium tremens in the elderly.

### Treatment

As in the treatment of any delirium the prime concern must be surveillance. The patient must be watched at all times so that he cannot harm himself or others. The necessity for round-the-clock nursing care cannot be overemphasized. Although not necessarily suicidal, delirious patients take terrible unpremeditated risks. Falling from windows, slipping down stairs, and walking through glass doors are common examples of unintended lethal behavior. Restraint should never be used except for short periods. It is a point of law that when four-point restraint is used, relief must be provided to the patient every 2 hours. Usually physical restraint can be avoided by using an agent such as chlordiazepoxide 50 to 100 mg given every hour until the patient is quiet and 50 mg every 6 hours thereafter. Haloperidol (Haldol), 10 to 20 mg given orally four times daily, is often used when the patient does not respond to chlordiazepoxide. This is the case when the alcholism is secondary to a psychosis or borderline condition. Electrolyte imbalances and vitamin deficiencies must be corrected. Since the B vitamins are known to help prevent peripheral neuropathy and the Wernicke-Korsakoff syndrome, their use is vital. Thiamine, 50 mg, should be given intravenously immediately and 50 mg should be given intramuscularly each day until normal diet is resumed. A smaller amount of thiamine may be added to infusions for intravenous use. Since there is frequently a magnesium deficiency, which has been reported to produce withdrawal seizures, magnesium sulfate in a 5% sterile solution may be given in doses of four times daily for 3 days and then 1 gm daily for an additional 2 or 3 days.[6] A high-carbohydrate soft diet should be given containing from 3,000 to 4,000 calories a day with supplemented vitamins. Phenytoin (Dilantin) may be used in patients with a history of withdrawal seizures. Parenteral diazepam (Valium) has also been widely used to control seizures.

## ALCOHOLIC HALLUCINOSIS
### Diagnosis

One of the most bizarre of the alcoholic psychoses is alcoholic hallucinosis. The individual with this condition has vivid auditory illusions and hallucinations occurring in an otherwise clear sensorium. These hallucinations soon become accusatory and threatening in nature. The individual reacts with fear but is fully oriented and realizes that the voices are hallucinations. However, as the accusations persist, the patient develops ideas of persecution. Although hallucinosis is more apt to occur in the setting of alcohol withdrawl, it is by no means uncommon in individuals who continue to drink. Some authors believe that hallucinosis is programmed by a disturbance of the auditory pathways. Tinnitus is found in many patients who report hallucinosis. Curiously, when tinnitus is one-sided, the hallucinatory experience usually occurs only on that side. Olfactory hallucinations may occur with alcoholic hallucinosis, but visual hallucinations seldom occur. Alcoholic hallucinosis is much less common than delirium tremens.

The clinical picture is one in which auditory hallucinations occur in the absence of tremor, disorientation, and agitation. Usually the male patient hears voices accusing him of homosexual practices and threatening retaliation. It has been reported that in women the hallucinotic voices may vent accusations of promiscuity. Soon after the voices begin, a frightening systematized delusional system develops that may incite the patient to call the police or to arm himself. Then the individual is particularly dangerous. He is capable of making judgments based on these hallucinatory accusations and of acting with an otherwise clear mind. Suicide is a distinct danger in this condition and may occur, as in delirium, without appreciable warning.

My first patient with alcoholic hallucinosis came to the hospital on a quiet Sunday morning during my internship. The patient, a 27-year-old merchant seaman, had been listening to a local disc jockey while at a bar the previous evening. His attention was suddenly caught when he heard his name announced as a third prize winner. He had won fourteen sheep, five head of cattle, and a strawberry farm in Kansas. A taxi driver who had listened to him for 3 hours and had driven him to innumerable radio stations finally insisted on taking him to a hospital. Since this was the early 1950s, the era of the colossal giveaways, the story sounded plausible to me, especially since the patient told it in a straightforward and reasonable manner. I asked the cab driver if he had heard the announcement on the car radio. He exclaimed, "Oh no! Not you too! They all believe him instead of me. Ask him what else the voices said." I did and the seaman grudgingly admitted that the disc jockey, along with announcing his name as a winner, had accused him of homosexual acts. As he spoke he became serious and threatening. He clearly believed these voices to be real. However, he readily agreed to enter the hospital. He seemed certain that the truth of his statement would be quickly discovered if he were hospitalized. A week later he no longer heard voices and had substantially minimized the experience, just as he forgot that alcohol had caused it.

Paranoid schizophrenia is the condition that is apt to be confused with alcoholic hallucinosis. The differential diagnosis is apt to be difficult. The dominance of the auditory component of the disorder and a history of alcoholism can aid in determining the diagnosis.

**Treatment**

There is no specific treatment for alcoholic hallucinosis. Generally its course is variable ranging from weeks to months. There are reported instances in which the hallucinosis continued for years. If the individual continues to drink, recurrences are the rule.

The most important aspect of treatment is to determine whether the patient should be in a protected environment. Behavior destructive to self or to others is common enough to require commitment to a mental hospital. Sedation can be given as needed using chlordiazepoxide or chlorpromazine. Since these individuals generally feel quite normal after the disappearance of auditory hallucinations, they often insist on being discharged as soon as the voices desist. As in delirium tremens, the course can be intermittent and the patient should be kept in a hospital until a week has passed without hallucinations. He should also be vigorously warned against drinking since the hallucinotic experience is apt to return if drinking is not forsaken.

**WERNICKE-KORSAKOFF SYNDROME**

Victor, Adams, and Collins in their classic monograph *The Wernicke-Korsakoff Syndrome* state that "Wernicke's encephalopathy and Korsakoff's syndrome in the alcoholic, nutritionally deprived patient may be regarded as two facets of the same disease. These patients evidence specific central nervous system pathology with resultant profound mental changes."[7] In all of the cases reported by Victor, Adams, and Collins, alcoholism was a serious problem and was almost invariably accompanied by malnutrition. Malnutrition is thought to be the causal factor, particularly the absence of thiamine.

## Korsakoff psychosis

Korsakoff psychosis, also referred to as confabulatory psychosis, is characterized by impaired memory in an otherwise alert and responsive individual. This condition is slow to start and only gradually does the memory impairment progress. Hallucinations and delusions are rarely encountered. Curiously, confabulation, long regarded as the hallmark of Korsakoff psychosis, was exhibited in only a limited number of cases in the large series collected and studied by Victor, Adams, and Collins. Most of these patients have no insight into the nature of their illness and a limited understanding of the extent of their memory loss.

The memory deficit is bipartite. The retrograde component is the inability to recall the past and the anterograde component is the lack of capacity for the retention of new information. In the acute stage of Korsakoff psychosis the memory gap is blatant—the patient cannot recall simple items such as the examiner's first name, the day, or the time, even though he is given this information several times. As memory improves, usually within weeks to months, simple problems can be solved, limited always by the patient's span of recall.

The fact that Korsakoff psychosis patients tend to improve with time is often forgotten and too gloomy a prognosis surrounds the condition. In the Victor, Adams, and Collins series 21% recovered more or less completely, 26% showed no recovery, and the rest recovered partially. During the acute stage there is, however, no way of predicting who will improve and who will not.

The specific anatomical structures pertaining to memory that are affected in Korsakoff psychosis are the medial dorsal nucleus of the thalamus and the hippocampal formations.

### Wernicke encephalopathy

Wernicke encephalopathy appears suddenly and is characterized by ophthalmoplegia and ataxia followed by mental disturbance. The ocular disturbance, which is necessary for the diagnosis, consists of paresis or paralysis of the external recti, nystagmus, and disturbance of conjugate gaze. The patient is apt to be somnolent, confused, and slow to reply. He frequently falls asleep in midsentence. The mental impairment is described by Victor, Adams, and Collins as a global confusional state, consisting of disorientation, unresponsiveness, and derangement of perception and memory. Exhaustion, apathy, de-hydration, and profound lethargy are also part of the picture. Once treatment is started for Wernicke encephalopathy, improvement is often evident in the ocular palsies within hours. In almost all cases recovery from ocular muscle paralysis is complete within several days or weeks. In the cases reported by Victor, Adams, and Collins, about one third recovered from the global confusional state within 6 days of treatment; another third, within 1 month; and the remainder, within 2 months. The global confusional state is almost always reversible—in marked contrast to the memory impairment of Korsakoff psychosis.

**Treatment**

Recommended treatment for both conditions is identical. Victor, Adams, and Collins consider treatment to be a medical emergency. The prompt use of vitamins, particularly thiamine, prevents advancement of the disease and reverses at least a portion of lesions where permanent damage has not yet been done. Ocular palsy is notably sensitive to thiamine. Such administration is, therefore, an important diagnostic aid as well as an essential therapeutic measure. In patients who show only ocular and ataxic signs, the prompt administration of thiamine is crucial in preventing the development of an irreversible and incapacitating amnesic psychosis. In general, the treatment recommended is 50 mg of thiamine given intravenously immediately and 50 mgs intramuscularly each day until normal diet is resumed. Parenteral feedings and the administration of B-complex vitamins become necessary if the patient cannot eat. If rapid heart rate, feeble heart sounds, pulmonary edema, or other signs of myocardial weakness appear, digitalization should be started. Since these patients operate with impaired mental function, nursing personnel should be alerted to a possible tendency to wander, to be forgetful, and to become obstreperously psychotic. If the latter should occur, benzodiazepines can be given.

**Referral after hospitalization**

The disposition of individuals who are diagnosed as having either an acute or chronic alcohol syndrome is complicated. Should they be referred for psychotherapy, for disulfiram treatment, or to Alcoholics Anonymous? There is no one treatment that stands out as particularly efficacious for the alcoholic patient. The principal problem encountered by all therapeutic modalities is the problem of motivation. Most alcoholic patients in the general hospital with problems secondary to drinking have great difficulty admitting their addiction to alcohol. While they may pay lip service to the advice of their physician to seek outside help, they rarely have the tenacity to seek a therapeutic group or an individual counselor. It has been MGH practice to tell each alcoholic patient about the types of treatment programs available in the community. Alcoholics Anonymous is given equal billing with the other modalities because its success record is probably better than professionals can offer. Once the community resources have been identified and their differences described, the patient is then encouraged to contact the one with the most appeal to him. To ensure the patient's full cooperation, as well as to establish the fact that a recommendation was made, a responsible family member is informed along with the patient. It is MGH policy to insist that the patient make the first contact with the treating agency, at which time our name can be used as a referral. When we are contacted by the potential therapist, we furnish a summary of the hospital record and our recommendations. About one in five such patients actually makes contact with a treating agency. With the establishment of a hospital alcohol unit that has personnel available to interview all individuals with alcohol-related problems as noted by the consultation liaison service, the number of self-motivated referrals has increased by 20%. Whether or not this increase implies a record of more enduring sobriety remains to be seen.

**REFERENCES**

1. Hayes, S. L., and others: Ethanol and oral diazepam absorption, N. Engl. J. Med. **296:**186-187, 1977.
2. Thomson, G. N., editor: Alcoholism, Springfield, Ill., 1956, Charles C Thomas, Publisher.
3. Chafetz, M. E.: Alcoholism and alcoholic psychoses. In Freedman, A. M., Kaplan, H. I., and Sadock, B. J., editors: Comprehensive textbook of psychiatry, Baltimore, 1975, The Williams & Wilkins Co., sec. 23.3.
4. Woodruff, R. A., Goodwin, D. W., and Guze, S. B.: Psychiatric Diagnoses. New York, 1974, Oxford University Press, Inc.
5. Cutshall, B. J.: The Saunders-Sutton syndrome: an analysis of delirium tremens, Q. J. Stud. Alcohol **26:**423-448, 1965.
6. Mendelson, J. H.: Biologic concomitance of alcoholism, N. Engl. J. Med. **284:**24-32, 1970.
7. Victor, M., Adams, R. D., and Collins, G. H.: The Wernicke-Korsakoff syndrome, Philadelphia, 1971, F. A. Davis Co.

# 3

# Drug addiction

JOHN A. RENNER, Jr.

## BARBITURATES

### Abuse

In addition to the patients who attempt suicide with a barbiturate overdose, we are now seeing an entirely different group of individuals who use barbiturates as a social or recreational drug in the same manner that their elders use alcohol. The increased nonmedical use of barbiturates and such other sedative-hypnotics as methaqualone, glutethimide, and the benzodiazepines, has produced new clinical problems.

The person intoxicated by barbiturates presents many of the same diagnostic problems associated with alcohol intoxication. Slurred speech, unsteady gait, and sustained vertical or horizontal nystagmus or both occurring in the absence of the odor of alcohol on the breath suggest the diagnosis. Unfortunately, drug abusers frequently combine alcohol with other sedative-hypnotic drugs. The clinician may be misled by the odor of alcohol. The diagnosis of mixed alcohol-barbiturate intoxication will be missed unless a careful history is taken and blood and urine samples are analyzed for toxic drugs. The behavioral effects of barbiturate intoxication can vary widely, even in the same person, and may change significantly depending on the surroundings and the expectations of the user. Individuals using barbiturates primarily to control anxiety or stress may appear sleepy or mildly confused as a result of an overdose. In young adults seeking to get "high," a similar dose may produce excitement, loud boisterous behavior, and loss of inhibitions. The aggressive and even violent behavior commonly associated with alcohol intoxication may follow. The prescribed regimen for managing the angry alcoholic individual can be used equally effectively for the barbiturate abuser (see Chapter 2).

Accidental life-threatening barbiturate overdoses are becoming more common and are a special risk to individuals who are addicted to barbiturates. As tolerance to barbiturates develops, there is not a concomitant increase in the lethal dose level, as occurs in opiate addiction. As the barbiturate addict gradually increases the dosage to maintain the desired level of intoxication, the margin between the lethal dose and the intoxicating dose becomes smaller. Although the opiate addict may be able to double the regular dose and still avoid fatal respiratory depression, as little as a 10% to 25% increase over the usual daily dosage may be fatal to the barbiturate addict. Thus, a barbiturate overdose should always be considered as potentially life-threatening, especially for drug abusers. Different signs and symptoms may be observed, depending on the drug or combination of drugs used, the amount of time since ingestion, and the presence of such complicating medical conditions as pneumonia, hepatitis, diabetes, heart disease, renal failure, or head injury. At first the patient appears lethargic or semicomatose. The pulse rate is slow but other vital functions are normal. As the level of intoxication increases, the patient becomes unresponsive to even painful stimuli, reflexes disappear, and there is a gradual depression of circulation and rate of respiration. Pupil size is not changed by barbiturate intoxication, but secondary anoxia may cause fixed, dilated pupils. In persons who have adequate respiratory function, pinpoint pupils usually indicate an opiate overdose or the combined ingestion of barbiturates and opiates. Such patients should be observed carefully for increased lethargy and progressive respiratory depression. Appropriate measures for treating overdoses should be instituted as necessary. Patients may walk into an emergency room and later lapse into a coma; they should never be left unattended until all signs of intoxication have cleared.

Because there is no cross-tolerance between narcotics and barbiturates, special problems are presented by methadone maintenance patients who continue to abuse barbiturates or other sedative-hypnotics. If a barbiturate overdose is suspected, the methadone patient should be given a narcotic antagonist to counteract any respiratory depression caused by methadone. We recommend naloxone (Narcan), 0.4 mg given intramuscularly or intravenously, because it is a pure narcotic antagonist and has no respiratory depressant effect even in large doses. If the respiratory depression does not improve after treatment with naloxone, the patient should be treated for a pure barbiturate overdose.

**Withdrawal**

The barbiturate withdrawal syndrome can present a wide variety of symptoms including anxiety, insomnia, hyperreflexia, diaphoresis, nausea, vomiting, and sometimes delirium and convulsions. As a general rule, individuals who ingest 600 to 800 mg per day of secobarbital for more than 45 days will develop physiologic addiction and show symptoms after withdrawal. Minor withdrawal symptoms usually begin within 24 to 36 hours after the last dose. Pulse and respiration rates are usually elevated, pupil size is normal, and there may be postural hypotension. Fever may develop and dangerous hyperpyrexia can occur in severe cases. Major withdrawal symptoms such as convulsions and delirium indicate addiction to large doses (900 mg or more of secobarbital).

Grand mal convulsions, if they occur, are usually seen between the third and seventh day, though there have been cases reported of convulsions occurring as late as 14 days after the completion of a medically controlled detoxification. Because of the danger of convulsions, barbiturate withdrawal should be carried out only on an inpatient basis. Withdrawal convulsions are thought to be related to a rapid drop in the blood barbiturate level. Treatment should therefore be carefully controlled so that barbiturates are withdrawn gradually with minimal fluctuation in the blood barbiturate level. Theoretically, this should decrease the danger of convulsions. Treatment with phenytoin will not prevent convulsions due to barbiturate withdrawal though it will control convulsions due to epilepsy.

Delirium occurs less frequently than convulsions but rarely appears unless preceded by convulsions. It usually begins between the fourth and sixth days and is characterized by both visual and auditory hallucinations, delusions, and fluctuating levels of consciousness. The presence of confusion, hyperreflexia, and fever help distinguish this syndrome from schizophrenia and other nontoxic psychoses.

**Treatment for withdrawal**

Several techniques are available for managing barbiturate withdrawal. The basic idea is to withdraw the addicting agent slowly to avoid the danger of convulsions. First, the daily dosage that produces mild toxicity must be established. Since barbiturate addicts tend to underestimate their drug use it is dangerous to accept the patient's history as completely accurate. Treatment should begin with an oral test dose of 200 mg pentobarbital, a short-acting barbiturate. If no physical changes occur after 1 hour, the patient's habit probably exceeds 1200 mg of pentobarbital per day. If the patient shows only nystagmus and no other signs of intoxication, the habit is probably about 800 mg per day. Evidence of slurred speech and intoxication, but not sleep, suggests a habit of 400 to 600 mg per day. The patient can then be started on the estimated daily requirement divided into four equal doses administered orally every 6 hours. Should signs of withdrawal appear, the estimated daily dosage can be increased by 25% following an additional dose of 200 mg pentobarbital given intramuscularly.

After a daily dose that produces only mild toxicity has been established, the pentobarbital dosage can be decreased each day by 10% of the established daily dosage. An alternative method is to switch the patient from pentobarbital to an equivalent dose of the longer-acting phenobarbital (30 mg phenobarbital equals 100 mg pentobarbital or secobarbital) once the daily dose is established and then withdraw the phenobarbital 30 mg per day. At MGH we recommend this latter method since the use of a long-acting barbiturate produces fewer variations in the blood barbiturate level and should produce a smoother withdrawal.

**Inpatient management and referral**

Barbiturate addicts can present a variety of psychological management problems. Effective treatment requires a thorough evaluation of the patients' psychiatric problems and the development of long-term treatment plans prior to discharge. Treatment for withdrawal or overdose presents an opportunity for effective intervention in the addicts' frequently self-destructive life-style. This opportunity should not be neglected. Drug abuse patients have a reputation for deceit, manipulation, and hostility. They frequently sign out against medical advice. It is rarely acknowledged that these problems are usually caused by inadequate attention to the patient's psychological needs. Most of these problems can be eliminated by effective medical and psychiatric management. The patient's lack of cooperation and frequent demands for additional drugs are often due to anxiety and to the all-too-real fear of withdrawal seizures. This anxiety will be greatly relieved if the physician thoroughly explains the withdrawal procedure and assures the patient that the staff knows how to handle withdrawal and that convulsions will be avoided if the patient cooperates with a schedule of medically-supervised withdrawal.

We sometimes fail to realize that the patient's tough, demanding behavior is a defense against a strong sense of personal inadequacy and a fear of rejection. Addicts have been conditioned to expect rejection and hostility from medical personnel. The trust and cooperation necessary for successful treatment cannot be established unless physicians show by their behavior that they are both genuinely concerned about the patient and medically competent to treat withdrawal. Physicians can expect an initial period of defensive hostility and "testing" behavior and should not take this behavior personally. Patients need to be reassured that their physician is concerned about them.

If the patient manifests signs of a serious character disorder and has a history of severe drug abuse, the setting of firm limits is necessary to ensure successful detoxification. Visitors must be limited to those individuals of known reliability. This may mean excluding spouses and other relatives. Family counseling should be started during hospitalization and should focus on the family's role in helping the patient develop a successful long-term treatment program.

Hospital passes should not be granted until detoxification is completed; however, passes with staff members as escorts should be used as much as possible. An active program of recreational and physical therapy is necessary to keep young easily bored patients occupied.

The story of a man, aged 21 years, who was hospitalized after having a grand mal seizure illustrates several of the problems that may occur.

> The son of an eminent attorney, the patient described several years of episodic barbiturate and alcohol use and admitted to 3 months of daily barbiturate use after dismissal from college for failing grades. Three days before the patient's seizure, his father discovered that the young man had been ingesting secobarbital tablets taken from the medicine cabinet. The patient agreed to stop using barbiturates but did not realize that he was addicted. After admission to the hospital the young man became a serious management problem. He demanded additional medication and refused to obey hospital regulations. Twice he left the floor without permission and on one occasion he returned obviously "high." A discussion with his physician became an angry shouting match. The patient denied any extra drug use and insisted that he be permitted to leave the ward. He threatened to file a lawsuit for violation of his civil rights. In consultation the patient was hostile and provoked. He denied having any psychiatric problems and suggested that his physician was trying to have him committed to a mental hospital. The patient's hostility disappeared after the psychiatrist indicated that he had no interest in committing him but was concerned that his arguments with his physician and the nurses were interfering with his medical treatment. Once reassured that the psychiatrist did not think he was crazy, he admitted his fear of having more seizures. He did not know what to expect during detoxification and was too frightened to admit his fears to his physician. He finally admitted that he was meeting friends in the hospital cafeteria and

they were giving him extra drugs. A meeting was then arranged between the patient and his physician. The physician explained the detoxification procedure in detail including possible causes of seizures and the need for diagnostic tests. The patient was relieved to hear this information and readily agreed to appropriate limitations on visitors and hospital passes. The remainder of his hospitalization passed without incident and he agreed to continue seeing the psychiatrist after his discharge.

In some situations patient management is easier if the patient does not know the exact dosage schedule for withdrawal. A placebo may be given for 3 or 4 days following the final dose. This procedure should be used *only if the patient agrees to it in advance.* It works best with anxious, insecure patients who are able nonetheless to trust their physician, but is clearly contraindicated if the patient is paranoid or incapable of trusting the physician.

Since treatment for detoxification or for an overdose rarely cures an addict, referrals for long-term outpatient or residential care should be made early in the treatment process. Ideally the patient should meet the future therapist prior to discharge. If transferring to a halfway house or residential program the patient should move there directly from the hospital. Addicts are not likely to execute plans for follow-up care without strong encouragement and support.

## NARCOTICS

With the growing number of narcotic addicts in our major cities, the secondary treatment of addiction is becoming commonplace on medical and surgical units. Proper management of such patients necessitates knowledge of Food and Drug Administration (FDA) regulations, appropriate techniques for using methadone, and community treatment resources.

The classic signs of opiate withdrawal are easily recognized and usually begin 8 to 12 hours after the last dose. The patient generally admits the need for drugs and will show sweating, yawning, lacrimation, tremor, rhinorrhea, marked irritability, dilated pupils, and increased respiratory rate. More severe withdrawal signs occur 48 to 72 hours after the last dose and include tachycardia, hypertension, nausea and vomiting, insomnia, and abdominal cramps. Untreated, the syndrome subsides in 5 to 10 days. Withdrawal symptoms are similar in patients addicted to methadone, but they may not appear until 30 to 48 hours after the last dose, and will abate over 2 to 4 weeks.

FDA regulations define methadone maintenance as any treatment with methadone that extends beyond 21 days. Addicts cannot be maintained unless they show physiologic evidence of current addiction (withdrawal signs) and can document a 2-year history of addiction. They must be withdrawn from the narcotic within 21 days if their addiction history is less than 2 years. The only exception to this rule is for the addict who is hospitalized for the treatment of a medical, surgical, or obstetrical condition. Under these circumstances, the physician has the option of maintaining the addiction of any addict for the duration of the primary illness. We at MGH strongly recommend that the addiction be maintained until the addict has fully recovered from the presenting illness and that the addict be given the option of drug withdrawal treatment prior to discharge.

Establishing the appropriate dose of methadone for a street addict is a trial and error process. Since the quality of street heroin is never certain, the addict's description of the size of the current habit is of minimal value. The safest guide to dosage is to monitor the patient's pulse, respiration, and pupil size. After the presence of withdrawal is documented, a hard-core addict should receive 20 mg methadone orally. Only if the patient is well known as a heavy user should the starting dose be as high as 30 mg. A relatively young patient or a patient who describes a small habit can begin treatment with 10 mg given orally. If vital signs have not stabilized or if withdrawal signs reappear after 2 hours, an additional 5 or 10 mg can be given orally. It is rare to give more than 40 mg during the first 24 hours.

> One woman aged 17 years, admitted for evaluation of fever of undetermined origin and associated epigastric distress requested large doses of methadone and claimed to have a heroin habit costing $200 a day. Further history revealed that she and her husband had been addicted for less than 3 months and were both relatively naive heroin users. After she began to show signs of opiate withdrawal, she was given 10 mg methadone orally; an additional 5 mg was given 10 hours later when her respirations were noted to again be more than 18 per minute. The following day she remained comfortable after a single dose of 15 mg. Later it was discovered that she had regional enteritis.

The addict should be maintained on a single daily oral dose that keeps him or her comfortable and that keeps respiration and pulse rates within normal ranges. The dose should be reduced 5 or 10 mg if the patient appears lethargic. If the street addict is to be withdrawn from drugs immediately, his methadone can be reduced 10% to 15% a day. If the drug habit has been maintained in the hospital for 2 or more weeks, or if the patient had been using methadone before admission, detoxification should proceed more slowly. The dose can be reduced 5 mg per day until 20 mg per day is reached. Further dose reduction should occur at the rate of 5 mg every 3 or 4 days. Chances for successful withdrawal treatment will be enhanced if the patient is aware of the dose and is able to choose the withdrawal schedule within limits established by the physician. By involving the patient in the treatment process and by using a flexible withdrawal schedule, the physician can keep withdrawal symptoms at a tolerable level. Rigid adherence to a fixed schedule of doses is less likely to achieve success and may lead to premature termination of treatment.

If a patient is already in a methadone maintenance clinic prior to admission to the hospital, the methadone dose should be confirmed by the clinic staff and should not be changed without consultation with the clinic physician responsible for the patient's treatment. Under no circumstances should such a patient be withdrawn from drugs unless there is full agreement among the patient, the hospital physician, and the methadone clinic staff on this course of action. Such detoxification is not likely to be successful, particularly if the patient is under stress from some concurrent medical or surgical condition. Withdrawal from drugs may complicate the management of the primary illness. The option of detoxification should not be considered until the patient has fully recovered from the condition that necessitated hospitalization.

Maintenance patients should be continued on daily oral methadone. If parenteral medication is necessary, methadone can be given in doses of 5 or 10 mg intramuscularly every 8 hours. This regimen should keep the patient comfortable regardless of the previous oral dose. An alternative method is to give one-third of the daily oral dose intramuscularly every 12 hours. As soon as oral fluids can be tolerated, the original oral dose should be reinstated.

A common problem is determining the appropriate dosage of an analgesic for patients on methadone maintenance.

> A 28-year-old woman was hospitalized for the treatment of acute renal colic. Four years previous to this she had been hospitalized for similar symptoms that subsided after she passed a kidney stone. During the year prior to her second hospitalization the patient was in a methadone maintenance program and was receiving 60 mg methadone daily. She was doing well in treatment and for the last 6 months was working regularly as a secretary. A psychiatrist was asked to see the patient because she was threatening to sign out of the hospital.

She claimed that she was receiving no effective relief for her pain and that she wished to obtain heroin to treat herself. The nurses described her as constantly complaining, demanding, and attempting to manipulate additional doses of narcotics. A review of her chart revealed that she was receiving doses of 5 mg morphine, approximately half the usual analgesic dose in such situations, with strict orders not to repeat the dose sooner than every 4 hours because of her history of drug abuse. Her physician had assumed that she would require lower doses of morphine because she was taking methadone. After consultation, the physician accepted the psychiatrist's recommendation that the usual dose of 10 mg morphine be given every 2 hours as circumstances required because the patient would probably metabolize any narcotic more rapidly than normal. This regimen effectively controlled the patient's pain and she suddenly became more cooperative. There was no recurrence of her "manipulative" behavior or other management problems. Two days later she passed several renal stones; she was discharged several days later. Her physician had not realized that her "demands and manipulations" were legitimate requests for effective doses of analgesics.

The analgesic effect of methadone is minimal in maintenance patients and, at best, lasts only 6 to 8 hours. If control of pain is required addicts should be given normal doses of other narcotics in addition to their methadone. Because of cross-tolerance, a maintenance patient will metabolize other narcotics more rapidly and may therefore require more frequent administration of analgesics than nonaddicted patients. Pentazocine (Talwin) is contraindicated for such patients; because of its narcotic antagonist effects, this analgesic will produce withdrawal symptoms in opiate addicts.

Discharge planning should be initiated as quickly after admission as possible. For patients not already in treatment, a week or more may be required to arrange admission to a drug-free residential program or to a methadone maintenance clinic. Since a serious illness usually causes an addict to reexamine his behavior and possibly choose rehabilitation, the physician should emphasize the need for long-term treatment. No addict should be discharged while still on methadone unless he is returning to a maintenance program or specifically refuses detoxification. Even when a physician discharges a patient for disciplinary reasons, medical ethics necessitate that the patient be withdrawn from methadone before discharge. Hospital physicians cannot legally give addicts methadone for administration at home.

## MIXED DRUG ADDICTION

Increasing numbers of patients are addicted to a combination of drugs including barbiturates, alcohol, and opiates. Accurate diagnosis is difficult because of confusing, inconsistent physical findings and unreliable histories. Blood and urine tests for drugs are required to confirm the diagnosis. The patient who is addicted to both opiates and barbiturates should be maintained on methadone while the barbiturates or other sedative-hypnotics are withdrawn. Then methadone can be withdrawn in the usual manner.

Behavioral problems should be dealt with as previously described. The firm setting of limits is essential to the success of any effective psychological treatment program. Some patients who overdose or present medical problems secondary to drug abuse such as subacute bacterial endocarditis and hepatitis are not physiologically addicted to any drug despite a history of multiple drug abuse. Their drug abuse behavior is usually associated with severe psychopathology. These patients should receive a thorough psychiatric evaluation and may require long-term residential treatment.

## AMPHETAMINES
### Abuse

Stricter federal controls on the production and distribution of amphetamines have reduced the number of amphetamine abusers to a few. Routine medical evaluation may uncover the most common type of amphetamine abuse treated in the general hospital. This is the patient who began using amphetamines to control obesity and later became a chronic amphetamine abuser. The patient quickly develops tolerance and may use 100 mg or more a day in an unsuccessful effort to control weight. This amphetamine abuse can be treated by abruptly discontinuing the drug or by gradually tapering the dose, whichever is more acceptable to the patient. In either case, the patient should be shown a more appropriate program for weight control.

A more serious problem is the patient who develops a severe psychological dependence on amphetamines and may present the same symptoms seen in younger "street drug" abusers. Typical complaints associated with amphetamine intoxication include anorexia, insomnia, anxiety, hyperactivity, and rapid speech and thought processes (speeding). Adrenergic hyperactivity, such as hyperreflexia, tachycardia, diaphoresis, and dilated pupils responsive to light may be seen. Fortunately, more severe symptoms such as hyperpyrexia and hypertension are relatively rare. Patients may also manifest stereotyped movements of the mouth, face, or extremities.

The other classic syndrome seen in either acute or chronic amphetamine intoxication is a paranoid psychosis without delirium.

While typically seen in young people using methamphetamine intravenously, it can also occur in individuals using dextroamphetamine or other amphetamines orally on a chronic basis. The paranoid psychosis may occur with or without other manifestations of amphetamine intoxication. The absence of disorientation distinguishes this condition from most other toxic psychoses. This syndrome is clinically indistinguishable from an acute schizophrenic reaction of the paranoid type and the correct diagnosis is often made only in retrospect, based on a history of amphetamine use and a urine test positive for amphetamines.

**Treatment**

Amphetamines can be withdrawn abruptly. If the intoxication is mild, the patient's agitation should be handled by *reassurance alone.* The patient should be "talked down" much as one would handle an LSD reaction. If sedation is necessary, benzodiazepines are the drugs of choice. Phenothiazines should be avoided. They increase the patient's agitation because they heighten the patient's sense of dysphoria. However, major tranquilizers must be used in cases of severe hypertension or hyperpyrexia. Chlorpromazine, 25 to 50 mg given intramuscularly, or haloperidol, 2.5 to 5.0 mg given intramuscularly, will reverse these life-threatening conditions. If adrenergic hyperactivity is severe, the patient should be given propranolol, 20 to 40 mg orally or 1 to 2 mg intravenously; but this medication should not be used if the patient has diabetes, asthma, or organic heart disease.

Most signs of intoxication will clear in 2 to 4 days. The major problem then is appropriate psychiatric management of postamphetamine depression. In mild cases this will be manifested by feelings of lethargy with the subsequent temptation to use amphetamines again for "energy." In more serious cases, the patient may become suicidal and will require inpatient psychiatric treatment. The efficacy of antidepressants in such cases has not been adequately documented. Even with support and psychotherapy, most patients will experience symptoms of depression for 3 to 6 months following the cessation of chronic amphetamine abuse.

**SUGGESTED READINGS**

Ellinwood, E. H., editor: Current concepts on amphetamine abuse, U.S. Department of Health, Education, and Welfare publication no. (HSM) 72-9085, National Institute of Mental Health, Washington, D.C., 1972.

Fultz, J. M., and Senay, E. C.: Guidelines for the management of hospitalized narcotic addicts, Ann. Intern. Med. **82:**815-818, 1975.

Green, A. I., Meyer, R. E., and Shader, R. I.: Heroin and methadone abuse— acute and chronic management. In Shader, R. I., editor: Manual of psychiatric therapeutics, Boston, 1975, Little, Brown and Co.

Shader, R. I., Caine, E. D., and Meyer, R. E.: Treatment of dependence on barbiturates and sedative-hypnotics. In Shader, R. I., editor: Manual of psychiatric therapeutics, Boston, 1975, Little, Brown and Co.

Smith, D. E., and Wesson, D. R.: Phenobarbital technique for treatment of barbiturate dependence, Arch. Gen. Psychiatry **24:**56-60, 1971.

Smith D. E., and Wesson, D. R.: Diagnosis and treatment of adverse reactions to sedative-hypnotics, U.S. Department of Health, Education, and Welfare Publication No. (ADM) 75-144, National Institute on Drug Abuse, Washington, D.C., 1974.

# 4

# The pain patient: evaluation and treatment

**THOMAS P. HACKETT**

## THE NATURE OF PAIN

Trying to separate functional from organic factors in long-standing pain is both vexing and unprofitable. Nevertheless, it is a task all too frequently requested of liaison psychiatrists. The physician's preoccupation with ferreting psychological issues out of the pain he cannot cure and his desire to implicate them as causal is well known. Like the ritual "washing of hands" by the Roman tribune eager to absolve himself of responsibility, the request to separate psyche from soma is often a symbolic write-off. The psychiatric consultant must be prepared for this when asked to evaluate a patient with unexplained pain.

Emotional conditions can unquestionably produce pain—a pain that hurts just as much as the pain from a tumor or a gunshot wound. It is equally certain that the severity of pain resulting from either gunshot or tumor can increase or decrease as a function of the patient's apprehensiveness. The most important lesson to remember about pain is that it hurts, whatever its cause. With the exception of six specific conditions that will be described later, pain is rarely generated and maintained by psychological forces alone. It is nevertheless important to weigh the psychological forces bearing on pain. This chapter is designed to give the consultant a basis for evaluating the psychological components of pain. In particular it will attempt to describe the limits of the psychiatric assessment of pain and to offer a framework for consultation when the request is to "rule out the functional."

Long-standing pain is difficult to assess largely because of the limits of our model for pain. Most of what we learn about pain in medical school is based on the concept of acute pain. The patient in acute pain moans, writhes, sweats, begs for help, and gives every appearance of being in great distress. Those in the vicinity of someone in acute pain feel an urgency to help. When pain persists over days and weeks the individual adapts to it often without realizing that he does so. This adaptation means that the pain becomes bearable without seeming to change in intensity. How this happens is not fully known. The sensation may become intermittent or the sufferer more capable of using distraction. Whatever the reason, the patient learns to accommodate the pain so that he can appear in society without making those around him uncomfortable. The patient becomes able to sit in the physician's examining room complaining of agonizing pain while giving little or no evidence of being in agony. It is ironic that the capacity to adapt to severe pain is often the patient's undoing. It causes the examiner to doubt the patient's veracity as a reporter. The sufferer now finds himself in the position of having to prove that he is in pain. He feels on trial. The physician who begins to doubt that the patient is in pain should remember Wilder Penfield's maxim—believe that pain exists when the patient says so unless the patient is a known malingerer. Generally physicians who have had pain syndromes themselves are in a much better position to assess and to treat long-standing pain in others.

It is helpful in the evaluation of pain to remember some simple definitions. Mersky states that pain should be defined operationally. "Commonly this implies a disagreeable sensation and tissue damage; and if not, it implies a response by the patient with terms corresponding to those used where there is tissue damage."[1] Ryle, with wry succinctness, says that "pain is a sensation of a special sort which we ordinarily dislike having."[2] The definition I favor comes from a British writer, Peter Fleming: "If you come to think about it, physical pain has many singularities. Of all human experience, it is, as long as it lasts, the most absorbing; and it is the only human experience which, when it comes to an end, automatically confers a real if not perhaps a very high kind of happiness. It is also the only experience this side of death which is by its nature solitary. But the oddest thing about it is that despite its intensity, and despite its unequalled power over mind and body, when it is over, you cannot remember it at all."[3]

Pain can be divided into two components—the original and the reactive. The original component has also been called the primary or organic or "tissue" component. It is the felt sensation. The reactive component, known also as the processing or secondary component, is the psychological response to the felt sensation. This subdivision is far too simple because it implies that both components must be present and yet distinct in the experience of pain. We know this is not true. Pain can be experienced centrally. However, for the sake of this chapter's thesis, the two-part model is appropriate. One could speculate, using this model, that if Van Cliburn or Michael DeBakey had a door slammed on his hand, the pain might be more severe than if the same accident happened to a psychiatrist. The fingers of the pianist or surgeon are the source of livelihood, self-esteem, and pride; as such the reactive component would be considerable. By biting his tongue severely, a psychiatrist might similarly muster a large reactive component in the ensuing pain.

Our main focus will be on the reactive or psychological component of pain, not only because it falls to us naturally, but because it can be altered by distraction, reduced by suggestion, or augmented by fear. Although there is some relationship between the primary sensation and the secondary component, it is by no means direct and linear. We cannot say that the larger the amount of tissue damaged, the greater the psychological effect. Other factors intervene.

**Pathological versus experimental pain**

There are two general types of pain—pathological and experimental. Familiarity with the difference between experimental and pathological pain is important to the understanding of the reactive component of pain. Pathological pain is pain associated with injury, as with laceration, myocardial infarction, or renal calculus. Experimental pain is produced in the laboratory by a variety of means ranging from electrical shock to compression of the Achilles tendon. One would think that both sensations might be equally uncomfortable given a strong enough stimulus. However, the curious nature of pain is such that these experiences are quite different. The difference depends entirely on the reactive or psychological component of pain. An experimental subject experiencing laboratory pain knows that he can bring his discomfort to a halt by crying out. He knows the dimensions of his pain—that it signals no imminent catastrophe, no distant incapacity. Pathological pain in dramatic contrast, is by nature, an alerting mechanism heralding the presence of danger. The difference between experimental and pathological pain is nowhere better demonstrated than in their dramatically different responses to morphine. Massive wounds sustained in accidents or in battle can be made painless by small doses of morphine. In contrast, individuals in severe experimental pain would be no more apt to respond to 15 mg of morphine sulfate than to parenteral sterile saline. Morphine appears to exert its effect not on the primary component of pain, but on the reactive. We are indebted to Henry Beecher[4] for illuminating research on this subject.

Another example of the importance of the psychological nature of the painful experience also comes from Beecher.[4] In his study of soldiers shot down at Anzio, all of them seriously wounded yet mentally clear, two-thirds did not want morphine. In fact most of them denied having any pain. The wound meant relief from combat, an honorable reprieve from mortal peril. In a civilian population suffering far less tissue trauma as the result of abdominal surgery (cholecystectomy), Beecher found that four out of five wanted medication to relieve their pain. The soldier, thankful to have escaped alive from the battlefield, regarded his wound with a feeling akin to pleasure. The civilian following major surgery regarded the incident as both disruptive and depressing. Beecher assumed from this that "there is no simple, direct relationship between the wound per se and the pain experience. The pain is in very large part determined by other factors and of great importance here is the significance of the wound." This background will give the reader some idea of the practical importance of psychological factors in the experience of pain. It can also be seen that the presence of massive tissue damage need not be accompanied by a commensurate amount of pain. The lesson is that neither the presence nor absence of organic pathology offers much in the way of a guide to the measurement of pain suffered.

Face to face with an individual in chronic pain, the physician with customary skepticism generally takes steps to convince himself of the presence of authentic pain. He first searches for an objective assessment of pain. For the most part this is a futile search, rendered all the more absurd by the very subjective nature of pain. There is a myth that an instrument exists by which the presence of pain can be verified. Although investigators are working on methods to objectify and standardize the experience of pain (usually by comparing known amounts of induced laboratory pain with the patient's pain), the techniques are still experimental. For the purpose of this chapter, it can be said that no such instrument is in clinical use.

The second step the physician usually takes is to find an independent observer. This crude assay consists of asking the nurses on duty or the patient's spouse whether or not the sufferer has periods when there seems to be no pain. This step is self-defeating. Even in spells of acute pain, moments can go by when the individual, through distraction, may appear not to suffer. In chronic pain long stretches of time pass with no display of discomfort. Furthermore, most family observers are far from objective. Nurses, unless especially trained, are equally inaccurate observers.

**Pain and the placebo**

The physician then moves to the use of placebos. In the entire field of medicine few phenomena are as misunderstood as is the placebo trial. Despite an abundance of excellent research on the topic, most of which has been published in widely read journals and textbooks, people still regard the placebo test as a means of separating functional from organic pain. To compound this error, many of those who conduct placebo trials do so in such an unscientific fashion that they lose whatever useful information might have been gained.

To begin with, it is known that approximately 33% of a population in pain will obtain relief from an inert substance just as if they were given an analgesic.[4] Evans and Hoyle in 1933 used sodium bicarbonate to treat individuals suffering from angina pectoris. In 38% of their subjects they found this agent to be just as effective as nitroglycerin.[5] Similar studies have been conducted in various parts of the world and the placebo response is found in about 33% of whatever population is tested. The placebo response is a normal aspect of personality and cannot be linked with any type of psychopathology. Hysterics, depressed patients, and neurotics are no more apt to be placebo reactors than are so-called normal people. Following surgery about one patient out of three obtains pain relief from saline or some other inert substance and is therefore considered placebo positive. Some investigators believe that a much higher proportion of the population could respond to placebos if suggestion were supplied as well. There is reason to believe that this is correct. Whether the pain is from a metastatic malignancy or is part of involutional melancholia, relief will come to the placebo reactor. Consequently, the only thing learned from a placebo trial is whether or not the patient is placebo positive. The trial is of no assistance in separating psychogenic from organic pain.

The timeworn custom of slipping in a few saline shots for morphine and calling this deception a placebo trial demonstrates only the ignorance of the perpetrator. If a shot of sterile saline is substituted for one out of six injections of meperidine and the patient responds to this fake shot by obtaining relief, the nature of his pain will be questioned. In fact, his relief is based on the conditioned response. Having been taught to associate the needle stick with surcease of pain, the patient learns to react to the needle and the inert substance just as Pavlov's dog learned to react to the ringing bell. Any of us, placebo reactor or not, would be apt to respond in the same way. In a valid placebo trial, the inert substance must be given to the patient in a randomized manner along with the usual narcotic under double-blind conditions for at least 5 days. Without this control the placebo trial is useless. Furthermore, one of the chief hazards of placebo use is that the patient feels tricked. If he discovers that placebos have been used (as he generally does), it is natural for him to feel on trial and wrongly accused. To prevent this it is advisable to tell the patient beforehand that over the next few days the pain medication will be changed a number of times in an effort to find the most effective drug. He should be told that two or more agents will be used. To exclude any hint of trickery, I prefer to avoid inert substances and use diazepam or oxazepam instead. An explanation of the double-blind system should be given. Depending on the patient's intelligence and interest, a more complete explanation of placebo response can be offered. The point is to avoid trickery and the best way to do so is to include the patient in the plot. One palatable way to present the information is to describe the placebo as a power of the mind. Like hypnosis, it can reduce discomfort without the risk of developing drug dependency or addiction. It is desirable to be placebo positive; this should be explained to the patient. In our experience the only value in identifying the placebo responder is a therapeutic one. Such patients can, with safety and efficiency, use nonaddicting agents over a long period with considerable success.

## PAIN AND THE PSYCHIATRIC CONSULTANT

All too frequently it is only after everything else has been tried, including the use of placebos, that the physician finally calls in the psychiatrist to assist in the evaluation of the patient with chronic pain. The psychiatrist enters the room in the dust left by the other physicians departing the scene for more interesting and salvageable cases. Calling in the psychiatrist is the final tactic used to assess the patient's pain.

The psychiatric consultant should be brought into the case early and ought to be introduced as a regular member of the medical team. The referring physician should take care to ensure that the patient does not interpret the need for a psychiatrist as a sign that his veracity is in doubt. It should be explained that a psychiatrist is routinely asked to evaluate all patients with long-standing pain (which indeed should be the case). As a general rule when the referring physician is comfortable in using the services of a psychiatrist, the patient accepts the examination without protest. It is only when the psychiatrist is called in at the end of a long, frustrating, and unprofitable hospitalization that the patient balks and protests.

Once the psychiatrist has entered the evaluative arena, what can be expected? To the inexperienced psychiatrist this is often a baffling and frustrating task that grows in complexity with each new attempt to find a resolution. There are a few simple things that can be done without getting bogged down in functional versus organic speculation. The diagnosis or elimination of the most common psychiatric conditions associated with pain is often sufficient.

**The psychiatric examination**

While interviewing the patient with a chronic pain syndrome requires no special psychiatric skill, it does demand that the examiner pay close attention to detail and to the patient's style of discourse. Some psychiatrists insist that the individual avoid discussion of pain or any aspects of the painful experience. Instead, they focus exclusively on life history and various events that may have psychodynamic significance. In my experience this approach puts the patient on the defensive and brings out all of his stubbornness. I prefer to have the patient focus on his pain. I take a detailed history of when and how it began and inquire about the various treatments received and the personalities of the physicians involved. Throughout all interviews, I look for fluctuations in the course of pain. Under what circumstances did it improve? Under what circumstances did it exacerbate? Was it the medication that helped or did the physician's manner make the difference? How long were remissions and what life events coincided with exacerbations? It is often valuable to go over the same material more than once, particularly when life circumstances intersect the course of pain and alter it for better or worse. I do this not so much to make a dynamic formulation as to gather facts that will make it possible to predict fluctuations in pain that might otherwise seem inexplicable. As one comes to understand how a patient's pain is shaped by his life, it is sometimes possible to modify the pattern in a small way and thereby reduce suffering.

Since many patients have extensive histories of pain, and delight in regaling the examiner with their odyssey through clinics, spas, and hospitals, I often ask them to write a detailed account of their pain from its onset to the present time. Included in this, I request information on all medication—those that helped and those that did not—complete with side effects and the reasons for discontinuing those that were stopped. In subsequent sessions I make forays and then excursions into the patient's mental life from earliest memory to the present.

I am interested in the individual's family experience with pain. If it is possible, I have the patient draw a family tree specifying on each limb the diseases, particularly the pain syndromes, which may have been present. Chronic pain seems to run in families—not just potentially painful diseases such as cancer, but also chronic pain conditions such as low-back syndrome, headache, "bowel colic," arthralgia, and the like. My overall scheme is to learn how the individual's family has coped with disease and with pain, as these undoubtedly influence the patient's experience. Similarly, I acquaint myself with the ethnic background of the person in pain. Several authors have made valuable contributions toward understanding the cultural determinants of the painful experience.[6]

### Six psychiatric conditions that commonly present with pain

I am particularly interested in identifying six psychiatric conditions that are known to present with pain as the chief complaint. Recognizing these disorders in the pain patient or ruling them out is a major accomplishment; often it is the only contribution the psychiatrist can make for the pain patient. The six conditions are: depression, hysteria, compensation neurosis, schizophrenia, malingering, and the pain prone person as described by Engel.[7]

**Depression.** Depression is by far the most common of the six psychological conditions that present with pain as the initial symptom. The depression is, more often than not, an involutional state and the individual has a background of obsessive, rigid, inflexible traits common to people who develop mid-life depressions. Sometimes family history will disclose menopausal or climacteric depressions in relatives and pain is frequently a part of the clinical picture.

The head is the most common site, but chest pain, low-back pain, rheumatic pain, and abdominal pain are all found. In fact, there is no specific type of pain to signal the presence of an underlying depression. Clues to the diagnosis of depression are the absence of objective physical or laboratory findings and the presence of a precipitating incident (such as a loss) that the patient refuses to acknowledge as such. Supporting diagnostic features are those of any depression: loss of libido—or in the case of the male, diminished potency—sleep disturbance, appetite change, lassitude, apathy, and loss of interest in work. A preoccupation with death, their own or the death of others, is pathognomonic of depression. Much of this information may have to come from a spouse because the typical patient in this category will focus all attention on pain and either deny or minimize the importance of a loss or even the presence of symptoms other than pain. It is not unusual to make the diagnosis by the fact that the pain improves with antidepressant medication.

The treatment of these depressions is similar to that offered for any depressive disorder (see Chapter 10). There is only one difference. A program of treatment may be carried out and successfully completed without the patient's ever admitting or realizing that he was depressed. The therapist must always acknowledge that the patient has genuine pain and must not force psychological insights no matter how trenchant they may be. As will be mentioned subsequently, insight-oriented psychotherapy has limited value in the treatment of patients in pain. The more somatic the physician's orientation, the more success he is apt to achieve. The antidepressants, both tricyclic and monoamine oxidase inhibitor compounds, are valuable. Support and encouragement must be given along with attention to symptomatic relief with nonnarcotic analgesics and other appropriate aids such as hydrotherapy or physiotherapy. If relief or a cure cannot be obtained through the methods described here within 6 months, electroconvulsive therapy should be considered. This is especially helpful when the depression is involutional in nature.

In the treatment of a pain syndrome caused by depression, the danger of suicide should always be kept in mind. Even when the patient does not hint that his thoughts turn in this direction, the therapist should regularly inquire about thoughts of suicide. Individuals with tic douloureux and cluster headaches are said to have a higher incidence of suicide than patients with other painful conditions.

While depression may be a primary cause of pain, it is far more apt to be the result of long-standing pain. Indeed, it is unusual to find an individual with a chronic pain syndrome who is not depressed. Usually such a person readily admits feeling "down" and "sad" about the limitations imposed on life by the pain. This type of reactive depression does not carry the toll of vegetative symptoms that is typical of the primary depression, nor is it usually as severe. When chronic pain strikes an individual who is characterologically depressed, the pain may then become the nucleus of what was previously a formless despondency, but that is not always the case. In any event, in such a case one gets a history of depression antecedent to pain.

There are two main ways in which reactive depression can be

differentiated from primary or causal depression in long-standing pain:

1. The patient with reactive depression is willing to acknowledge being depressed. Those with a primary depression seldom admit being depressed and never admit that such depression might cause or contribute to the pain itself.
2. Vegetative signs and symptoms are well represented in primary depression and less so in reactive depression.

These are imperfect differential diagnostic points, but they can serve as crude guidelines.

**Hysteria.** Conversion hysteria was thought by Freud to be a common cause of pain. He was quick to highlight the symbolic meaning of the pain and to point out that the choice of symptom was determined by underlying conflicts as well as by the precipitating event. The physician may suspect that conversion mechanisms are responsible for the symptoms of pain if the patient can be diagnosed as a hysteric according to principles elucidated in Chapter 7. The difficulty with the diagnosis of conversion hysteria is that it is used far too carelessly by psychiatrists and nonpsychiatrists and through this loose application has lost relevance as a disease entity. Even when the pain patient is a known hysteric, there are three criteria that should be present before the pain can be explained on this basis:

1. The symptom must have either a symbolic or specific meaning for the patient.
2. There must be a figure of identification on whom the symptom is modeled.
3. The pain should follow no known anatomical pathway.

The treatment of pain in the patient with hysteria is in no way different from the treatment of hysteria in general. One must only remember that the pain itself must never be dismissed as "unimportant to the central problem—which is emotional." To dismiss the pain is tantamount to losing the patient or the patient's cooperation. Frequently the most successful treatment of the patient with hysteria combines psychotherapy with other therapy. Thus, infrared heat therapy, hydrotherapy, and physiotherapy can be used as well.

**Psychosis.** Schizophrenia, organic psychoses, dementias, and hypochondriasis can all present with the symptom of pain. The pain will be delusional in nature, often bizarre in both distribution and quality, and usually one part of a mosaic of symptoms which together form the picture of psychosis. Rarely will pain be the only symptom. It is also rare to have pain as the presenting symptom of schizophrenia. I have been referred four such cases in the last 10 years. In each case the pain was linked to a delusion of persecution. Pathological pain does, of course, occur in patients with psychosis, dementia, or hypochondria. When this occurs, how does one detect it? The denial of pain, or its significance, is common in schizophrenic patients. This accounts for the unusually large number of silent myocardial infarctions, perforated duodenal ulcers, and ruptured appendices found in mental hospitals. In my experience, when pain is part of a delusional system or represents a fixed idea of the hypochondriac or the demented patient, the sufferer is not eager to have the discomfort removed. In fact, the patient may balk at the suggestion of cure. The physician dealing with psychotic patients must be always vigilant for limps, grimaces, splinting of extremities, and other external indicators of pain.

**Compensation neurosis.** Compensation neurosis applies to an individual with chronic pain when the amount of distress seems unduly amplified in terms of the discernible pathology or when it persists long past the time most psysicians, insurance adjustors, and union stewards think it should. In almost every case the patient has filed a claim for financial compensation. Some psychiatrists consider the term a fiction derived for the convenience of management to pejoratively label unwanted claimants. When the pain is feigned, the individual is called a malingerer. The pain of an individual with compensation neurosis is not feigned. It may seem out of proportion to the injury. It may tax professional mettle not to suspect that the patient is pretending, but it is important to keep in mind that the hurt is real.

Typically, the patient with compensation neurosis is a blue-collar worker who has overworked to compensate for an underlying need to be taken care of. He is a hyperattainer who holds down more than one job and provides abundantly for his family. He considers himself to be a loyal employee and union member, a patriot, a churchgoer, and a family man. He then sustains an industrial accident. The injury may be trivial or major. Whatever the extent, he develops an incapacitating pain that prevents him from resuming the role of provider. He joins the ranks of the dependent. Because he has a history of hard work and accomplishment, because he genuinely enjoyed his active life and takes no conscious relish in being on the dole, he assumes his new role with a sense of entitlement. When he fails to be rehabilitated in the generous allotment of time provided by management, he incurs their enmity. Next he exhausts the patience of his union and, soon thereafter, in a domino effect, of his wife, his children, and his friends. He is left with an attorney to bolster him. His pain symbolizes the sum of frustration he has endured and becomes a badge of the long hours he has toiled, of the vacations he has postponed, and of the sacrifices he has vainly made for others. Receiving compensation has become the only reward for his suffering. The issue of pain has been transformed into an issue of pride. It has become not only a question of hurt, but of hurt feelings.

In this age of litagation, a lawyer often appears on the scene not far behind the surgeon. As a consequence, nearly every case involves the possibility of some form of compensation. As costs escalate, so lawyers proliferate. Compensation neurosis can be suspected in any case where the pain patient is represented by more than one attorney.

Therapy is often impossible until the legal issues are settled. A transient euphoria usually develops when the case closes favorably. Invariably this is followed by a depression. An exploration of the depression often reveals a long history of dissatisfaction with some aspect of life—marriage, work, or something of major importance. Counseling sometimes helps.

**Malingering.** The malingerer is a pretender. In order to obtain an end—money, privilege, or the avoidance of an unpleasant duty—the malingerer fakes a complaint. He will seldom undergo painful laboratory procedures for diagnostic reasons. This separates the malingerer from the person with Münchausen's syndrome. More often than not the correlation between the symptom and the goal will be uncomplicated and linear. Malingered pain is more apt to be found in federal hospitals, Veteran's Administration installations, and service hospitals than in general hospitals. Of all the conditions described so far it is the only pain that is not felt.

The malingerer is not so much treated as discovered. Every specialty has its array of covert techniques to reveal the faker. The most practical means of diagnosing the malingerer is to rule out organic pathology through the usual examinations and tests and also to find, through a careful scrutiny of background (particularly old service records), evidence of similar behavior in the past. Like lying, malingering tends to be a character trait used in times of stress from early adolescence through senium. Once revealed, psychotherapy can be offered, but I imagine that the results would be negligible.

**The pain prone person.** The pain prone person was described by Engel in a brilliant study of psychogenic pain.[7] Such a patient is characterized by a conscious or unconscious sense of guilt for which pain serves as atonement. A background of suffering and defeat with an intolerance of success is found in these patients, along with a tendency to solicit pain as with accident proneness or multiple surgery. Such patients tend to develop pain as a replacement for loss. Pain, rather than more predictable or appropriate emotions, occurs in response to stressful conflicts. The location of pain is said to be determined by unconscious identification with a love object. The psychiatric conditions sometimes found in the background of these individuals include conversion hysteria, depression, hypochondriasis, and paranoid schizophrenia.

There is no specific type of treatment available for the pain prone person. As reported by Engel, they are difficult to treat. Since a variety of psychiatric diagnoses are included under the heading of pain prone person, therapy should be structured to suit the individual.

### Chronic pain syndromes

When each of the six foregoing conditions has been ruled out, the physician often still has a patient suffering from a variety of emotional problems that may contribute to or even cause pain. However, there is not sufficient evidence to call this pain entirely functional. It is the unusual chronic pain syndrome that does not contain a combination of both psychological and physical components and it is important to be able to give the referring physician some idea of the relative significance of each to the patient's pain. While there are few rules of thumb that apply in all cases, I have developed a scale called the Madison Scale. Madison is an acronym composed of the first initial of seven characteristics that, in my opinion, correlate with psychogenicity of pain. For those interested in quantification, each characteristic can be rated on a 0 to 4 scale. The higher the total score, the greater the importance of psychological factors.

**M** *Multiplicity.* This means the pain is either in more than one place or is of more than one variety. It also means that when one pain disappears through a therapuetuc effort, another will replace it.

**A** *Authenticity.* Patients with pain having a high psychological titer often seem more interested in your acceptance of their pain as genuine than they are in receiving a cure for it. They want to be believed. I have found this to be especially true for the pain that masks a depression.

**D** *Denial.* Chronic pain patients often deny the presence of emotional problems. This denial can be highlighted when they give an exaggerated account of marital or family harmony. They paint a rosy picture of domestic bliss even in the face of impending divorce. Should they admit the occasional presence of anxiety or depression, it is with the proviso that these affects never influence the intensity of their pain. Pathological pain is a fluctuating state. It is highly sensitive to the influence of fear, anger, sadness, and tranquility. When a pain is reported to be unresponsive to these emotions, I question its nature.

**I** *Interpersonal relationships.* During the course of an interview the individual may grimace or spontaneously complain of pain when someone's name is mentioned—someone who has something to do directly, indirectly, or symbolically with the patient. Similarly, if that person should walk into the room during the interview, the patient will give evidence of being in immediate distress such as pressing the nurse call button. Yet, when the patient's attention is drawn to this relationship, the connection will be discounted.

**S** *Singularity.* Singularity means that there has never been a pain like this. The following statements demonstrate singularity: "I am sure you've never encountered a pain like this in your large practice, Doctor." "I have never heard of a pain like this nor has any other physician who has treated me." It is a singular and unusual pain, one that puts the patient into a special category.

**O** *"Only you."* This is perhaps the most pernicious factor in the Madison Scale in terms of the future of the physician-patient relationship. It reads, "Only you can help me, Doctor." When the patient, soon after meeting you, presents you with a white charger complete with lance and banner bearing the cross of St. George, you should immediately imagine the scores of other physicians who stand behind you in serried ranks with horses crippled, lances bent, and pennons torn.

**N** *Nothing helps-or-no change.* This means that the pain does not change from hour to hour, day to day, or year to year. If anything, it only gets worse. Nothing helps, including drugs. It defies all that is known about the nature of pathological pain. Distraction, suggestion, chemical interference, barometric pressure, circadian influences, and political upheaval fail to alter the patient's perception of the discomfort. Like the national debt, it remains forever present, and if a change should occur, it invariably is toward the red. When asked "Why do you take so many medications?" the answer will be something like, "What else is there to do? If I don't take them I will be worse off." When reminded of the statement that, "nothing helps," the answer is, "Something is better than nothing," or some equally meaningless cliché. All pathological pain changes for better or worse during a 24-hour period. Distraction plays a role as does mood. Appropriate pain medication invariably helps. In the absence of relief, either spontaneous or drug induced, the nature of the patient's pain is questionable. If medication, properly given, does not help, the consultant should consider another type of distress—more psychological than physical. For example, some patients following surgery require an inordinately large amount of narcotic to control their postoperative pain. When this becomes excessive, for example, 100 mg meperidine every hour, I have found that such patient often have a fear that something like a malignancy was discovered and that they were not told. If the fear is known, reassurance can be given and the pain will decline. Individuals who are unprepared for the severity of postoperative pain are most susceptible to such situations. So much pain, they reason, must have a special cause.

These are no more than clues to guide the practitioner in the search for factors that may help in the recognition of underlying psychological issues. When the Madison Score is above 15, some form of psychiatric intervention should be considered.

## TREATMENT OF PAIN
### General principles

After all of the psychiatric conditions have been ruled out, most of the chronic pain syndromes can be treated by general practitioners. However, if psychiatrists desire to treat them, they also can do so. The principles are the same. To begin with, the patient should never be branded as suffering from "imaginary pain." The physician must take every means to assure the patient that there is no question about the degree of suffering involved. Although psychological factors may play a role—more important in some, less in others—this by no means diminishes either the quality or quantity of pain the patient endures. To this end the physician should always be willing to discuss the pain and to take active measures in suggesting remedies that might be helpful.

With a pain patient I invariably spend at least half of each inpatient visit discussing the complaint itself. Its relation to the weather, to the intervening events between visits, and to the patient's health in general are subjected to scrutiny. If warranted, I suggest simple remedies in addition to medication. The application of poultices, unguents, rubifacients, astringent lotions, splints, and hot packs can provide variety to the treatment plan. Massages, rubdowns, and chiropractic manipulation can also be helpful as long as the practitioner is known and trusted. Certainly hydrotherapy and physiotherapy have their place in our therapeutic armamentarium. While these manipulations may seem like humbug or chicanery, some may have intrinsic value in soothing pain and all share equally in the task of providing tangible evidence of the physician's active interest.

The second principle of management is to assure the patient that treatment will continue even if there is no immediate improvement. One of the fears expressed by many patients in chronic pain is of abandonment—that if they do not improve, the physician will see them no more or will refer them to someone else.

While not requiring a cure, it is important for the physician to be ever hopeful that the condition will remit or that some method will be discovered to reduce discomfort. The physician should guard against being affected by the patient's sense of discouragement. Great patience is required of the physician who treats the pain patient. Don Lipsitt has described the so-called crock clinics that are usually dumping grounds for chronic pain patients.[8] These are clinics where individuals are free to return for unlimited periods with no expectation of improvement. The symptom, whether pain or something else, is a "ticket" to establish contact with a physician. As long as the relationship is maintained, the patient seldom decompensates and rarely goes on to find more complex and dangerous treatments. The crock clinic model is a good example to follow in treating the chronic pain patient.

The third principle of treating chronic pain is to avoid surgery. Very few procedures on the central nervous system are definitive in the cure or control of pain and most carry with them a tax that is sometimes worse than the pain. Not only is pain surgery to be approached skeptically, but any type of surgery for the chronic pain patient should be regarded with great care before advising the patient to proceed.

**Medication**

Many of the patients evaluated will be receiving narcotic medication regularly on an outpatient basis. The medication should be changed to a nonnarcotic analgesic if at all possible. At best, this is a difficult job requiring a good therapeutic alliance. The process should be a joint endeavor, something that the physician and the patient accomplish together. In my experience, success is most likely if substitution rather than withdrawal is the goal. For example, instead of tapering down and eventually omitting meperidine, one might substitute aspirin or acetaminophen (Tylenol) along with diazepam, and add a cocktail at supper and a night cap at bedtime as an additional incentive for each substitution or dose reduction. The most important ingredient in the regimen will be the enthusiasm and support of the physician and his pleasure at progress. Behavioral compensations can be used adjunctively. Each period spent without the narcotic can be rewarded in a way that pleasures the patient such as by seeing a movie, eating an ice cream cone, or flying a kite.

When one fails to switch off the narcotic, the next step is to attempt to use the least addictive preparation possible. Codeine and methadone are the best choices. Usually, the change from parenteral medication to oral can be made by increasing the dose by half initially and then reducing it to a standard oral dose. Social sanctions are so strongly opposed to injected medication and the morbidity is so much greater that patients sometimes make the transition without demurring. Issuing an effective oral preparation in sufficient quantity is the most crucial factor. Lectures to the pain patient on the dangers of addiction are largely unnecessary. Most of the risk-centered lectures are for the benefit of the practitioner rather than for the patient. As the smoker knows the risk of smoking, so the pain patient knows the danger of addiction.

Rules of usage should be established early in the course of treatment. If, for example, a patient requires meperidine for low-back pain and has been unable to substitute a nonnarcotic or codeine, then a daily limit should be placed on the amount consumed. Since some days are apt to be less painful than others, a weekly maximum should be established, and finally a monthly maximum. Usually 400 mg per day is the average with meperidine or 120 mg of codeine. It should be explained that these maximums must never be exceeded and that the patient is expected to bear the pain rather than to go beyond the amount jointly agreed on. To run over the monthly allotment would mean a period of reassessment in the hospital. Of course, the patient could resort to nonnarcotic analgesics such as aspirin and acetaminophen during times of drug drought, but nothing stronger. Any individual on a chronic pain medication should be offered a drug rotation when one narcotic is switched to another, as from meperidine to codeine. The idea of enforcing a drug holiday on pain patients has always seemed totally onesided to me. An invention by physicians for physicians, it imposes a needless hardship on the patient without accomplishing anything.

One of the keys to the successful use of narcotics for chronic pain is to supply an adequate potentiator. Potentiators are drugs that are given in conjunction with the narcotic to prolong and intensify the reaction. Promethazine has long been a popular potentiator. It is usually given in doses of 12.5 mg, but I have found that 25 mg given three or four times daily is apt to be more beneficial. Other phenothiazines have been used as potentiators as have benzodiazepines, antihistamines, butyrophenones, and amphetamines.[9] Many individuals dislike the sense of grogginess that comes with the use of a narcotic. Adding 5 mg of dextroamphetamine once or twice a day with the narcotic can add to its effectiveness as well as reduce its sedative effect. Like narcotics, the amphetamines have been taken by many individuals over years without causing addictive behavior. Individuals who are prone to addiction are usually recognized early in the course of treatment.

The tricyclic antidepressants[10] and the monamine oxidase inhibitors[11] have been used successfully in the treatment of cluster headaches and other pain syndromes. The exact nature of this action is not known. One surprising finding is that a considerable improvement in pain can be obtained with a dose of tricyclic antidepressant that falls far beneath its therapeutic range for the treatment of depressions. It has been thought that these drugs relieve pain only in cases where pain is a symptom of an underlying depression. While this is a logical inference, I have treated people successfully with the tricyclics and the monamine oxidase inhibitors who showed no evidence of depression, either clinically or with projective tests.

### Education

The education I refer to here has to do with the ward personnel, not directly with the patient. For reasons that are unclear, medical people, be they physicians or nurses, view the patient who is in constant need of pain medication with suspicion. Even if the patient is a terminal cancer victim soon to die, medical caretakers still worry about the danger of addiction. Why they do so taxes the imagination, but the fact that they do is easily confirmed by asking the hospitalized patient. Marks and Sachar did this and found that 32% of the respondents said they were in severe discomfort; 41% were in moderate discomfort.[12] The authors surveyed the house officers responsible for their care and found that they believed that patients should be pain free. Why this blatant discrepancy between their belief and the fact of their care? Marks and Sachar attributed it to an underestimation of the effective dose, an overestimation of the medication's duration of action, plus an exaggerated notion of the danger of addiction. I would add to this the failure in the system of education to be acutely aware of the patients' suffering. Physicians are taught that 50 to 100 mg of meperidine every 2 to 4 hours is the proper amount of narcotic to prescribe for severe pain. Rarely are they told to vary the amount depending on the patient's body weight and previous tolerance for the drug. In the list of priorities for the care of patients, patients' state of comfort occupies a place near the bottom.

It has been my experience to have dealt with three physicians who held a very hard line in dispensing narcotics to postoperative patients and others in pain. I would frequently quarrel with them on what seemed to be their indifference to suffering. All claimed that the danger of addiction far outweighed the transient discomfort their narcotic skinflinting caused. Over the years each of these physicians entered the hospital with pain as the chief symptom, one with a cervical disc, another with a lumbar disc, and a third with postherpetic neuritis. All were chastened by their experience and emerged with a far more liberal policy of dispensing opiates and opiate derivatives.

My experience with these physicians prompts me to suggest a new requirement for receiving a Doctor of Medicine degree—a period spent as an inpatient with a painful condition to learn firsthand the experience of having someone else tell you how much pain you are having and determining how much pain medication you need. The same should be required for the matriculation of nurses.

When the amount of medication a patient requires for the management of pain becomes a cause célèbre on the ward, the liaison psychiatrist would be well advised to call a meeting of the house staff, attendents, and nurses, so that all biases and suspicions can be brought into the open. Medical personnel are far more apt to underestimate the amount of narcotic required for a given pain than to overestimate it. In either case, their opinions are usually based more on misinformation or folklore than on fact. Once these are aired and the true issues exposed to daylight, the patient usually benefits. Somehow all medical personnel believe that it is an indulgence to give any more than the usual amount of pain medication, whether the individual weighs 140 lbs or 340 lbs. Medical personnel often make no allowance for differences in body weight, disposition, or tissue tolerance. The liaison phychiatrist can uncover these factors and also some of the hidden agendas, programmed unwittingly by prejudice, which usually work against good patient care.

**Psychotherapy**

With the exception of depression, hysteria, and compensation neurosis, psychodynamic psychotherapy when offered as the sole treatment has, in my experience, rarely been successful in alleviating chronic pain. While I have known practitioners who claim success with individuals suffering from low-back syndrome, from migraine, and from other nonspecific painful conditions, their record is far from illustrous. Psychotherapy, however, when used in conjunction with the treatment methods mentioned earlier, might well produce significant benefit, particularly if insight can be given on some of the underlying interpersonal relationships that contribute to pain. An axiom used by those who conduct psychotherapy with chronic pain patients is that providing insight as to why the hurt is there is a great boon to the physician's morale that may, in turn, make the patient feel better for a time. I agree. Rarely does insight alone, no matter how illuminating, relieve pain. Supportive, eclectic, common-sense general-practitioner-type management is what is called for.

### Hypnosis

The use of hypnosis in chronic pain syndromes has been discussed at length in the literature. The best summary has been published recently under the able coauthorship of Ernest and Josephine Hilgard.[13] Hypnosis depends almost entirely on the patient. Only about one in four subjects is able to achieve a state of concentration of sufficient magnitude for lasting pain control. I have used a system of teaching individuals autohypnosis for the control of pain similar to the technique developed by Erickson.[14] It is a method worth looking into as long as the physician knows its limitations and is patient enough and experienced enough in the techniques to give it full therapeutic trial.

### Pain units (inpatient)

A large number of pain clinics and inpatient milieu units have been started around the United States largely following the example of Fordyce's group in Seattle.[15,16] They use a variety of techniques, centering around behavior modification, milieu therapy, group therapy, relaxation techniques, relearning techniques, and other types of social feedback systems. Their success rate is promisingly high, but more time and thorough follow-up studies are needed to evaluate the long-term effectiveness of their approach.

### Acupuncture

Acupuncture received a wide vogue in the United States, but its flame is currently sputtering. Some studies have demonstrated its effectiveness on pain[17,18]; others have shown it to be of little or no value.[19] Acupuncturists have specialized skills. They are quick to spot those individuals who have refractory pain syndromes and to refer them elsewhere. Acupuncture is certainly no panacea.

### Electroconvulsive shock therapy

Electroconvulsive shock therapy has been used by some practitioners, particularly in long-standing pain that is accompanied by depression and is refractory to other forms of treatment. When properly done with judicious case selection, electroconvulsive shock therapy has favorable and long-lasting results. It is the belief of those most skilled in this technique that the mechanisms they are treating in pain patients are those of depression[20] (see Chapter 11).

## Surgery

There are two types of surgery to be considered. The first type consists of exploratory procedures designed to investigate through direct visualization whether an anatomical structure might be producing the pain in question. The decision to perform this type of procedure will be determined by the medical and psychological circumstances.

The second type of surgery is pain surgery or surgery directed against the central or peripheral nervous system solely for the purpose of removing or easing pain. It need have no connection with the pain's cause and is palliative at best. Rhizotomy, chordotomy, tractotomy, and cingulumotomy are some of the procedures used. Dorsal column stimulators have recently come into use as well.

Contrary to general belief, in the proper hands, some of the central procedures performed stereotactically using radiofrequency lesions, such as dorsalmedial thalamotomy, cingulumotomy, and limited frontal leukotomy, do not carry a high psychiatric morbidity. Personality changes, mental dulling, and memory impairment are rare. The benefit provided in the relief of pain is, however, dissapointingly short-lived. If pain is reduced, it usually returns within 6 months. As a consequence, the use of such procedures should be limited to pain caused by terminal malignant diseases.

Pain surgery is seldom a desirable alternative. Pain is an elusive sensation which appears to use many pathways other than the traditional conduits of painful sensation. Melzack believes that chronic pain, in contrast to acute pain, has multiple determinants and that there are no specific pain pathways for this phenomenon.[17] To exemplify this, let me close with the account of an extraordinary case.

> R. C. was a 28-year-old mechanic who was thrown from his motorcycle on the way to his wedding. An injury resulted to his brachial plexus, as well as to his left arm, which required an amputation at the shoulder. He developed severe phantom limb pain within 2 weeks of the surgery. Six months later the stump was revised and a neurectomy performed. The pain remained unaltered. The nerve

was then severed further into the stump with similar result. A rhizotomy was then performed that was unsuccessful, followed by a chordotomy with the same outcome. The patient was then put in individual psychotherapy for a year. There was no improvement. He was then hospitalized and given hypnotherapy, group therapy, and massive doses of phenothiazines and then antidepressants. None of these measures produced improvement. After six sessions of ECT the pain was only intensified. A higher cervical chordotomy was performed without success, and then a mesocephalic tractotomy, again with no relief. He next had both dorsomedial thalamic nuclei ablated using stereotactic electrocautery. During the course of this procedure an electrode slipped and entered his mesencephalon resulting in a 2 week coma. He emerged from this with personality intact but still with his original pain. Then electrolytic lesions were made bilaterally in the inferior mesial quadrant of the frontal lobes in stages. The pain remained. He then had a left radio frequency amygdalotomy, followed by a left cingulumotomy. The pain continued as before. There was no change in his personality as noted by his therapist or his wife. The pain remained 4 years after the accident, just as pristine as it was 2 weeks after the injury. The house in which pain lived had been destroyed, but the sensation, like a stubborn revenant, remained to haunt the patient and his physicians.

Pain continues to be one of man's most important and complicated sensations. In this chapter I have deliberately avoided speculation and have used theory only when it was essential for understanding. My intention was to stay close to what is clinically applicable.

**REFERENCES**

1. Mersky, H., and Spear, F. G.: Pain: psychological and psychiatric aspects, Baltimore, 1967, The Williams & Wilkins Co.
2. Ryle, G.: Concept of mind, London, 1949, The Hutchinson Publishing Group, Ltd.
3. Fleming, P.: My aunt's rhinoceros and other reflections, New York, 1958, Simon and Schuster, Inc.
4. Beecher, H. K.: Measurement of subjective responses, New York, 1959, Oxford University Press.
5. Evans, W., and Hoyle, C.: The comparative value of drugs used in the continuous treatment of angina pectoris, J. Med. 2:311-338, 1933.
6. Zobrowski, M.: People in pain, San Francisco, 1969, Jossey, Bass, Inc., Publishers.
7. Engel, G. L.: Psychogenic pain and the pain prone patient, Am. J. Med. 26:899-918, 1959.
8. Lipsitt, D. R.: Medical and psychological characteristics of "crocks," J. Psychiatry Med. 1:15-25, 1970.
9. Forrest, W. H., and others: Dextroamphetamine with morphine for the treatment of postoperative pain, N. Eng. J. Med. 296:712-715, 1977.

10. Lance, J. W.: Mechanism and management of headache, London, 1973, Butterworth & Co. (Publishers), Ltd.
11. Anthony, M., and Lance, J. W.: Monoamine oxidase inhibition in the treatment of migraines, Arch. Neurol. **21:**263, 1969.
12. Marks, R. M., and Sachar, E. J.: Undertreatment of medical inpatients with narcotic analgesics, Ann. Intern. Med. **78:**173-181, 1973.
13. Hilgard, E. R., and Hilgard, V. R.: Hypnosis in the relief of pain, Los Altos, California, 1975, William Kaufmann, Inc.
14. Erickson, M.: In Haley, J. (editor): Advance techniques of hypnosis and therapy, New York, 1967, Grune & Stratton, Inc.
15. Fordyce, N. E., and others: Operant conditioning in the treatment of chronic pain, Arch. Phys. Med. Rehabil. **54:**399-408, 1973.
16. Fordyce, N. E., and others: Case histories and shorter communications: an application of librium modification technique to a problem of chronic pain. In Weisenberg, M., editor: Pain: clinical & experimental perspectives, St. Louis, 1975, The C. V. Mosby Co.
17. Melzack, R.: How acupuncture can block pain. In Weisenberg, M., editor: Clinical and experimental perspectives, St. Louis, 1975, The C. V. Mosby Co.
18. Katz, R., Kao, C. Y., Spiegel, H., and Katz, G. J.: Pain, acupuncture, hypnosis. In Bonica, J. J., editor: Advances in neurology, Vol. 4, International symposium on pain, New York, 1974, Raven Press.
19. Smith, G., and others: Unpublished data.
20. Mandel, M. R.: Electroconvulsive therapy for chronic pain associated with depression, Am. J. Psychiatry, **132:**632-636, 1975.
21. White, J. C., and Sweet, W. H.: Pain and the neurosurgeon, Springfield, Ill., 1969, Charles C. Thomas, Publisher.

**SUGGESTED READINGS**

Melzack, R.: The puzzle of pain, New York, 1973, Basic Books, Inc., Publishers.
Sternback, R.: Pain patients (traits and treatments), New York, 1974, Academic Press, Inc.
Weisenberg, M.: Pain, clinical and experimental perspectives, St. Louis, 1975, The C. V. Mosby Co.

# 5
# The surgical patient

OWEN S. SURMAN

## THE SURGICAL EXPERIENCE
### Surgery as a life stress

Surgery is a common life stress often met with emotional difficulty. The exact incidence of psychiatric complications is unclear. Titchener and Levine reported that more than a third of 142 general surgical patients had problems of psychological adjustment after convalescence.[1] As surgery becomes more complex, emotional sequelae mount. Kimball, for example, reported that all open heart surgery patients experienced some degree of impaired cognitive function in the early postoperative period.[2]

Virtually all patients approach surgery with a degree of fear. Furthermore, as Titchener warns, looks can be deceiving. The "sweetly cooperative patient" who represses anxiety may have greater postoperative distress than the patient who openly expresses fear.[3] Emphasis in this section is placed on the short-term postoperative outcome. It is during this period that the psychological impact of surgical intervention is most clearly in evidence.

The stress of surgery arises from several sources. Deutsch emphasizes the threat of death and bodily injury.[4] Other factors include metabolic stress, separation from family, financial hardship, and the forced dependency of the surgical setting. Attitudes, both conscious and unconscious, toward the involved organ system and the nature of the patient-surgeon relationship play an added role.[5]

The degree of difficulty with which patients face surgery varies widely. Of central importance are the types and effectiveness of coping skills that the individual has developed. Ability to adapt to discomfort, to form trusting relationships, and past responses to stress all provide clues to the manner in which the patient might react to surgery.

Janis emphasizes that "the stress experience tends to arouse apparently outgrown modes of response to childhood danger."[6] The threat of bodily harm brings back childhood fears of parental punishment and abandonment. This results in an emergence of aggression and in increased dependency with the surgeon placed in the dual role of villain and benefactor. The patient often experiences childlike fantasies of mutilation as well as compensatory images of increased affection from family, physician, and medical staff.

### Factors in postoperative adjustment

**Identification with others.** One important factor affecting the psychological outcome of surgery is the patient's identification with others. Abram and Gill described two patients with carcinoma who respectively underwent a mastectomy and a resection of carcinoma of the antrum.[7] In the postoperative period the mastectomy patient fared well, as had her sister who had undergone the same surgery. The patient with antral carcinoma developed a postoperative psychosis. She feared that she would die, as had a cousin who had been afflicted with the same disease.

**Social setting.** Social forces also play a prominent role in the response to surgery. Stable family relationships and a network of social supports are important aids to good postoperative adjustment.

**Age.** Titchener and Levine reported a 50% incidence of disabling postoperative depression in those who were age 65 and over.[1] At the other end of the age scale Levy reported that among 124 children undergoing surgical procedures those in the 1 to 3 year age group had the greatest difficulty with pain and separation anxiety.[8] Among the elderly, fear of infirmity and loss of independent function are a predominate concern in the United States; in early childhood, lack of understanding, threat of parental separation, and insufficient coping skills add to the impact of the surgical stress.

**Type of surgery.** The nature of the surgical procedure is still another predictor of the types of difficulty that patients will encounter. The frequent occurrence of postcardiotomy delirium has been the subject of numerous studies,[9-18] the results of which point to cerebral anoxemia as the major etiological factor.

Loss of sexual potency is a frequent complication of prostatectomy in middle-aged and elderly men. Finkle and Prian found that 16% of these patients who were potent prior to surgery lost erectile competence as a result of surgical and psychological factors.[19]

Mastectomy and pelvic procedures in women are commonly followed by depression associated with the impact of these procedures on sexual identity and self-esteem.[20,21]

The occurrence of phantom limb sensation and phantom limb pain following amputation has been studied and reported by Ewalt, Melzack, and others.[22,23] Simmel, in her study of patients with leprosy (Hansen's disease), found that phantoms do not result from absorption of digits unless surgical amputation is performed. Thus a "stable cognitive schema" seems essential to the phantom experience.[24]

Hackett and Weisman refer to the frustration of imperfect communication among those undergoing laryngectomy.[25] The same authors studied the frequent incidence of "black patch delirium" among elderly patients who experienced sensory deprivation from bilateral eye masking after cataract surgery.[26]

Sutherland and others describe the fastidious and compulsive behavior of cancer patients following colostomy.[27]

The psychological outcome of renal transplantation varies with the degree of surgical success.[28] Special problems at times result from change in self-image and from the uncertainties of graft survival.[29,30] Posttransplant encephalopathy is an infrequent but important complication. Immunosuppression with high dose steroids is a major contributing factor (see Chapter 19).[31,32]

## PREDICTORS OF POSTOPERATIVE MORBIDITY AND MORTALITY

Several variables in the postoperative period may predispose to adverse postoperative sequelae such as depression, psychosis, delirium, increased surgical morbidity, and death.

### Preoperative anxiety

The relationship of preoperative levels of anxiety to postsurgical outcome has been a major focus of attention. Janis, in a study of thirty general surgical patients, rated preoperative levels of anxiety as extremely high, extremely low, or moderate. Those with moderate anxiety had the best postoperative emotional adjustment. This group felt generally confident about surgery and made efforts to learn about its effects. Patients with extremely low anxiety used denial and optimism to such an extent that they were poorly prepared to deal with the normal exigencies of the recovery process. Those with extremely high anxiety could not gain comfort from reassurance.[6] Titchener and Levine reported similar findings in their larger series of 200 patients.[1]

Abram and Gill attempted to predict which of twenty-eight general surgical patients would have postoperative psychological difficulty. A favorable outcome was most likely among those with realistic expectations and low anxiety. Notable is their finding of a 50% incidence of medical complications among those with postoperative emotional problems. Those who did well psychologically had no complications.[7] Lipowski commented on the ambiguity of the term "anxiety" and reviewed the controversy between those who propose a curvilinear relationship between preoperative anxiety and postoperative difficulty and those who describe a linear relationship.[33] Patients with low anxiety states are viewed by some as overly optimistic deniers whose failure to recognize the real stresses of surgery leads to later complications.[1,6] Other observers have viewed low preoperative anxiety as a favorable finding which may be associated with the patient's realistic appraisal of surgical outcome.[7,34]

Methodological considerations in preoperative and postoperative psychological assessment were reviewed by Wolfer and Davis. There are variations among reported studies in the nature of preoperative assessment, in the selection of outcome criteria, in the size and type of surgical sample, in the definition of variables, and in the quality of medical and nursing care. Wolfer and Davis used a wide variety of measures to assess the impact of anxiety on the postoperative course of 146 surgical patients and found almost no significant correlations.[35]

## Dependency

For many patients, illness, especially chronic illness, means an increased reliance on others. For some, this "sick role" carries the benefit of being cared for; it allows the gratification of underlying dependency needs, should these be present. In a two-part prospective and retrospective study Knox found that women with a good response to mitral valvotomy had a history of good marital and sexual adjustment. A poorer medical outcome was found among those with evidence of marked dependency and sexual maladjustment.[36]

Kennedy and Bakst established six psychological profiles among 148 patients undergoing cardiac surgery. Serious medical complications were most frequent among those who were disease dependent and among those who sought good health, but were panicky about surgery. Patients in the best prognosis group desired good health and recognized without fear the risk of surgery.[34]

## Depression and denial

Kimball investigated fifty-four patients undergoing open heart procedures and divided them into four groups based on preoperative psychological assessment. The highest incidence of mortality and morbidity was among those with high levels of preoperative depression and among those who denied anxiety but nonetheless demonstrated evidence of emotional distress. Patients who expressed moderate uneasiness and confidence and who demonstrated a capacity to cope with the stresses of life had the best outcome.[37] The prognostic value of Kimball's preoperative grouping was reconfirmed in a subsequent study of 180 cardiac surgery patients. Kimball and his coworkers found that the groups in which patients denied anxiety and were depressed had an increase in short-term postoperative complications and postoperative mortality.[38]

Important questions remain. Is denial a negative attribute in the preoperative patient as suggested by Janis and by Kimball,[6,37,38] or is it a positive attribute as in Kennedy's and Bakst's good prognosis group who blocked out fear?[34]

### Evidence of preoperative central nervous system impairment

Another potentially valuable predictor is evidence of central nervous system impairment in the preoperative patient. Kilpatrick and others found that patients who had a fatal outcome to cardiac surgery had had significant measurable preoperative impairment of concentration and abstract thinking. The specific psychological measurements were suggestive of mild organic brain disturbance. Using the results of psychological tests the authors were able to predict survivors and nonsurvivors with more than 90% accuracy.[39]

### Summary

These studies present a tentative picture of the patient who presents a good surgical risk. The good-risk patient (1) is intellectually intact, (2) copes well with stress, (3) has a low to moderate level of preoperative anxiety, (4) acknowledges the risks of surgery, (5) is confident of a favorable outcome, (6) has adjusted well to his illness, (7) has a strong motivation for good health, (8) has realistic expectations, and (9) is free of depression.

### PREDICTORS OF POSTOPERATIVE DELIRIUM
#### Definition

Postoperative delirium is a serious surgical complication. The hallmark of delirium is a clouding of consciousness varying in degree from mild cognitive impairment to severe disorientation, agitation, and perceptual distortion. Delusions may be present along with hallucinations in all sensory modalities. The mental state usually clears within 24 to 72 hours. A valid incidence of postoperative delirium is impossible to state since criteria for recognition vary widely. What is clear is that certain situations herald a substantially increased risk that delirium will occur. Alcoholism, trauma, and age were the three factors most often associated with delirium in Titchener's and Levine's series. Those over age 65 had a 25% incidence of delirium. Titchener and Levine noted that aging patients were especially intolerant of isolation and immobilization. The incidence of delirium among older patients was related inversely to the number of their hospital visitors.[1]

**Predisposing factors**

Lipowski reported the primary predisposing factors in delirium to be age (over 50), alcohol or drug addiction, and cerebral damage, regardless of cause or age at which it was sustained.[40] History of postoperative delirium is another factor cited by Tucker.[41] Morse and Litin selected a group of sixty patients identified by the surgical staff as delirious and compared them to a control group of fifty-seven patients. The groups were matched for sex and type of operation, but not age, since the delirium patients were older. Psychological factors discriminating between the two groups included the following:

Alcoholism
Depression
Family history of psychosis
Organic brain syndrome (at any time)
Preoperative insomnia
History of postoperative psychosis
Retirement adjustment problems
Functional gastrointestinal disturbance

All of the above factors were more prevalent among those who were delirious. Denial of fear and higher socioeconomic group were more frequent among control patients. The incidence of delirium was unrelated to marital status or to preoperative evidence of functional psychosis.[42]

The high incidence of delirium following cardiac surgery has led to a vigorous search for predictive factors. The relationship between age and delirium has almost invariably been confirmed.[10-14,18] The relationship between preoperative brain damage and postsurgical delirium has also been confirmed.[11,14,17] However, there has been some disagreement about other predictive factors.

Egerton and Kay found a relationship between family history of psychosis and delirium, but, unlike Morse and Litin, found that marital instability is an additional predisposing factor.[11] Layne and Yudofsky, also in contrast to Morse and Litin, found that less anxiety is evident among those who become delirious and postulated that denial is a predisposing factor.[43] Rubenstein and Thomas found that a history of psychiatric disorder increases the likelihood of delirium, but has no effect on the mortality of patients undergoing cardiac surgery.[44] Blachly arrived at opposite conclusions.[10]

### Effects of preoperative intervention

In three controlled studies attempts were made to influence the incidence of delirium through preoperative psychiatric intervention. Lazarus and Hagens compared patients undergoing similar open heart procedures by the same operative team at two Milwaukee hospitals. The authors played an active supportive role with patients at the public facility but not with control patients at the private facility. The incidence of postoperative delirium was 33% for control patients and 14% for experimental patients.[45] Layne and Yudofsky later reported a reduction of almost 50% in the incidence of postoperative delirium among cardiotomy patients who had had one preoperative psychiatric visit.[43] In a later study undertaken at MGH, twenty patients scheduled for mitral valve surgery were seen preoperatively by a psychiatrist and instructed in the use of autohypnosis. Twenty control patients received routine preoperative preparation. While the results were not statistically significant, there was a tendency for those seen more than once prior to surgery to have a lower incidence of delirium.[18]

The major problem thus far in research on postoperative delirium is the lack of uniform criteria for diagnosis. Also, some researchers have relied on medical records rather than on direct psychiatric examination for case detection.[42,45] The timing of postoperative assessment and the nature of surgical and nursing care are also important. Statistical analysis of multiple variables leads to the possibility of chance positive findings.[42] Finally, important variables such as age may have influenced outcome studies of psychiatric intervention.[43,45] The type of surgery is still another variable. Rabiner and others, for example, have shown that delirium is more prevalent among those patients undergoing cardiac valve surgery than among those having coronary artery bypass surgery.[46] Despite these shortcomings the work to date has yielded some consistent findings pertinent to clinical practice.

**Summary**

Delirium is most likely to occur after surgery in the presence of CNS insult, advancing age, and alcohol or drug addiction. In at least two studies routine preoperative psychiatric interviews were said to reduce the incidence of delirium following surgery.[43,45]

## MANAGEMENT OF PREOPERATIVE PSYCHOLOGICAL STATES
### Psychosis

A notable finding in the study by Morse and Litin was the lack of correlation between preoperative functional psychosis and postoperative delirium.[42] By itself psychosis is no contraindication to surgery. A problem may arise if the impending surgery is part of a delusional scheme. Thus, it is important to investigate the psychosis. Bizarre appearance and style of communication should alert the surgeon to a need for psychiatric evaluation. The patient should be asked what he believes to have caused his illness, what result he expects from surgery, and if he has an explanation for the principal symptoms.

One young man was referred for psychiatric examination following repeated requests for orthopedic treatment. Aside from his rather vague presentation of symptoms and his notably withdrawn and quiet manner there had been no obvious evidence of psychosis. The psychiatric interview focused on his complaint of chronic knee pain. When asked if he thought his body was changing in any way, he replied that his pelvis was becoming larger. When questioned further he said that he was becoming a woman.

It is important to determine if there is a history of psychiatric treatment with hospitalization or treatment with psychoactive drugs, and if so, what the past difficulties were. When a diagnosis of functional psychosis is established, the family should be contacted to assist in providing supportive care, should this be needed.

After consultation with the anesthesiologist the physician should prescribe antipsychotic medication and administer it throughout the course of hospitalization. Daily visits by the psychiatrist are necessary for both patient and staff. The staff should be advised on the best approach to the patient's care.

For the most part, psychotic patients will respond well to the structured regimen of the surgical unit and can be treated in a direct candid manner. At times there may even be an improvement in psychological status following surgery. However, psychotic patients do present special problems:

1. Informed consent must be managed with help from relatives and the hospital attorney.
2. It may at times be difficult to separate somatic delusions from physical symptoms. Proper assessment requires close collaboration between the psychiatrist and surgical staff.
3. The risk of suicide is always present in a psychotic depression; thus, precautions in the form of round-the-clock special nurses are usually warranted.
4. Antipsychotic drugs may cause familiar complications. Choice of medication should focus on the patient's drug history (what agents have been most successful) and the relative side effects of the antipsychotic drugs. Aliphatic-substituted phenothiazines, such as chlorpromazine, cause the greatest hypotensive effects. Piperazine-substituted phenothiazines such as trifluoperazine (Stelazine) and butyrophenones such as haloperidol (Haldol) cause the highest incidence of extrapyramidal neurological complications. Haloperidol, because of its antipsychotic potency and its relative freedom from respiratory and cardiovascular side-effects, is gaining many adherents.

**Depression**

The presence of depression should warn of an increased surgical risk. Most often a depressive disorder will be recognized in a single interview. The patient may be silently withdrawn or restless and agitated. Severe depression tends to present a mask-like facies and a dour, unchanging mood. Vegetative changes such as anorexia, weight loss, and sleep disturbance, especially with early morning awakening, are of diagnostic importance. Inquiry into the patient's surgical expectation may reveal disinterest or frank despondency about surgical outcome. This despondency is an important clue to the existence of depression in the absence of other signs and symptoms. A history of depression is of diagnostic value and signals a risk of postoperative depression even in the absence of mood disturbance in the period immediately prior to surgery. In manic-depressive disease, surgery has been known to precipitate a depression.

If the depression is severe, surgery should be postponed when possible. Tufo and Ostfeld report an alarmingly high postoperative mortality among open heart surgery patients who were clinically diagnosed as depressed before surgery.[47] Psychiatric referral is definitely indicated when moderate to severe depression is detected before surgery. The patient may require antidepressant drugs throughout hospitalization. Again the anesthesiologist should be informed. If the patient is in an involutional state or presents a severe suicidal risk, electroconvulsive therapy should be considered.

A preoperative depression can be related to the prospects of surgery. Such prospects may be based on misconceptions that will give way to proper explanation. Careful inquiry may reveal a secret fear that surgery will unearth some dreaded underlying condition such as cancer. There need be no logic to this other than the identification with a relative or friend who suffered this fate. The patient may believe that surgery will cause maiming or dismemberment in some unpredictable way. These preoperative fantasies can contribute to depression and can often be relieved by discussion, explanation, and reassurance.

Elderly patients are particularly likely to become depressed when facing surgery. Titchener and Levine point out the following factors:

1. Most aged persons fear that illness will be followed by a decline in personal status.
2. Elderly patients are exposed to a different, uncertain environment in which the caregiving personnel may be viewed as lacking patience and understanding.
3. There is the fear that surgery will impair the patient's independence and level of adaptation.

Titchener and Levine advise that these adverse, albeit realistic, fears may be alleviated by a combination of frequent encouragement, familiarization with hospital surroundings, avoidance of immobilization, and frequent visits by relatives and acquaintances.[1]

### Alcoholism and drug addiction

Alcoholism and drug addiction may have grave impact on surgical outcome. The effects of acute withdrawal are a major consideration. Delirium tremens, for example, is currently associated with a mortality of 15%.[48] Addiction to barbiturates and related depressants is also associated with the risk of withdrawal. The withdrawal syndrome may be complicated by convulsions and delirium, either or both of which add to operative morbidity. A second consideration is that persons suffering from alcohol or drug addiction often have poor nutrition. Consequently, they have a reduced ability to handle stress and are therefore more prone to infection and delay of wound healing and repair. Third, delay in obtaining treatment is common; thus, their overall condition may be more grave at the time of surgery. Finally, this group of patients arouses considerable anger in the surgical staff. Indeed this factor in itself does not help the prognosis.

Several years ago while interning in a city hospital I observed a man in his forties admitted with bleeding esophageal varices. The patient was depressed, belligerent, and uncooperative. When efforts were made to pass a Sengstaken-Blakemore tube to stop the bleeding the patient fought off both the admitting intern and surgical resident. Finally the patient issued an ultimatum. He insisted that he be operated on under anesthesia or he would sign out. The staff was equally insistent on conservative management. Psychiatric consultation was not considered. Instead the patient was angrily informed that a sign-out would mean certain death. He responded to this with indifference. Subsequent attempts to talk him out of leaving proved fruitless. He was offered transfer to another institution but declined. His wife pleaded with him to stay but he refused. Two days later he returned to the emergency room—dead on arrival.

An alternative to the sign-out might have been impossible under the circumstances, but the house officer had a wellknown aversion to alcoholic patients.

The most important point in managing the alcoholic patient or drug addicted patient is that treatment be delivered in a nonjudgmental fashion. Psychiatric and social service consultations will prove helpful in dealing with the difficulties common to this group, providing a thorough social history, and arranging for follow-up care.

If surgery is elective and the addicted patient is motivated for psychiatric treatment, arrangements may be made for detoxification in an appropriate facility and surgery can be delayed. Otherwise, the patient's drug dependent state should be maintained at least until after surgery. Levels of barbiturate requirements for those addicted to depressant drugs can be established by giving a test dose of pentobarbital and finding the amount sufficient to produce a mild intoxication.[49] Alcohol patients may be treated with a benzodiazepine or with intravenous alcohol, 50 ml of 95% ethyl alcohol in 1 liter of dextrose and water at the rate of 10 drops per minute. Thiamine and B-vitamin supplements should be added. For narcotic addiction daily requirements are best established by oral administration of 10 to 20 mg of methadone after withdrawal signs appear.[49] Higher levels of drugs will be necessary for postoperative analgesia. All of these methods should be under the close supervision and control of a psychiatrist (see Chapter 3).

### Anxiety

Detection of anxiety is based on objective manifestations of worry, autonomic arousal, self-report by the patient, empathy on the part of the surgeon, or the report of a third party such as a relative or nurse.[50] As in the case of depression, anxiety may be acute in onset and related to fear of surgery. It may also represent a chronic emotional disorder or personality trait. The patient is the first source of information, but social mores and personality may not allow the patient to acknowledge distress. Informing patients that anxiety about surgery is normal opens the way to further inquiry. It is wisest to ask not if they are worried, but what worries they have. For some, anxiety may focus on a specific aspect of surgery or anesthesia. One patient, who awaited mitral valve replacement had a morbid fear of endotracheal intubation. The patient was desensitized of the phobia by hypnosis after two brief sessions. The rest of the hospital stay was psychologically uneventful.

For others, anxiety may be caused by misconception. The average patient knows little anatomy. One woman scheduled to have an exploration of a pelvic mass asked if her menses would cease after a hysterectomy. A technique for discovering misconceptions is to have patients draw pictures of what they think the problem is and of the surgery planned.

It is important to determine prior surgical experience, particularly any difficulties with surgery that are now avoidable. For example, childhood surgical experiences may form a basis for an induction-mask phobia. By explaining the use of preoperative medication, having the anesthetist meet the patient, and offering the use of pentothal given intravenously, this fear may be averted.

So-called anniversary reactions may occur on or near specific dates with which the patient associates an earlier loss or trauma. Assisting the patient to reconstruct such associations may have a pronounced effect on reducing anxiety.

It can help to know how the patient has dealt with past stresses. Unusual anxiety in response to ordinary life stress may reflect long-standing emotional difficulty. This is especially likely when the patient is unable to form a trusting relationship with the surgeon or does not respond to reassurance. If this is the case, an underlying paranoia may exist. Scrutiny may reveal a covert thought disorder, a marked depression, or cerebral impairment.

Surgeons themselves can inadvertently become a source of anxiety. This is especially likely when surgeons attempt to reduce their own anxiety with an unnecessarily detailed account of risks in the name of informed consent. Alternatively, they may err in the direction of adopting an overly paternal "leave it to me" approach that leaves the patient with insufficient knowledge of what to expect. Liaison psychiatrists soon learn the styles of the surgeons they deal with and develop the necessary skill to explain these idiosyncrasies to patients. Some patients may also be predisposed toward viewing surgery as a form of passive assault. This may even take on a sexual connotation with the surgeon viewed as the aggressor. One patient who became delirious after cardiac surgery had a delusion that she had been raped.

To reduce preoperative anxiety the surgeon should give the patient enough information to form a judgment about the procedure and an idea of the postoperative course. Fears should be identified and openly discussed. Minor tranquilizers such as benzodiazepines (for example, diazepam, chlordiazepoxide) can be used but should never replace reassurance and psychological support. Since diazepam has a half-life of 30 hours, the surgeon prescribing it should be alert to the danger of oversedation and confusion. The amount of drug can be titrated according to the patient's need. Some patients may require 40 mg of diazepam daily while others may become semicomatose with this amount of drug. The nursing staff should be taught to observe whether levels of sedation are sufficient.

Sleep is extremely important in the preoperative period and may necessitate far more hypnotic than one would expect, especially if the patient has been using sleeping pills for a long period. It is important to find out what the patient has been accustomed to taking for sleep and to be guided by this rather than by standard doses. If the patient prefers a small amount of alcohol given as a "nightcap" instead of a hypnotic, this should be considered.

Finally, psychiatric referral is advisable for those whose anxiety is not reduced and for those who deny anxiety in the face of clinical evidence to the contrary. These are the patients who present a higher surgical risk.

### Hex or predilection to death

These are the patients that Kimball refers to as "sanctioned suicides."[37] These patients display no fear or concern, but report a certainty that surgery will be followed by their death.

> Hackett and Weisman described the case of an immigrant Greek farmer who displayed none of the signs of depression, but stated simply that he would die after subtotal gastrectomy. The patient accepted his self avowed fate with equanimity and interpreted his illness as an act of God. Three days after an uncomplicated procedure the patient developed an atrial flutter and died. A large mural thrombus occluding the pulmonary valve was found at autopsy.[51]

As described by Hackett and Weisman the patients who have a genuine predilection to death are neither anxious nor depressed. They are fully convinced that death will come using surgery as its vehicle. They have a reason to die about which there is no apparent conflict. Their commitment to death is so convincing that the examiners come to share it. In cases of this sort, the mortality is nearly 100%. Whether such accounts represent coincidence or a causal relationship is difficult to assess. A related phenomenon is the taboo death or voodoo death seen in primitive cultures. An exceptionally high incidence of fatal illness has also been noted among the elderly after admission to state mental institutions and among prisoners of war. Frank has reviewed these findings and refers to theories of adrenal overexcitation and excess vagal activity as possible physiologic mediators.[52]

Surgery should be avoided if possible when patients quietly accept what they regard as a fated postoperative death.

## Denial

The controversy concerning the relationship of denial to surgical outcome is discussed earlier in this chapter. One problem centers around the use of the term "denial." A distinction can often be made between those who report an absence of fear but have a realistic outlook and those whose apparent calm is a false facade. When denial is concomitant with clinical evidence of anxiety or false expectation the physician should be alert to potential problems. Such a patient might deny having concern to the physician but constantly seek reassurance from spouse or nurses. If this is the case, a psychiatric consultant should be requested.

## Paranoid states

There are some individuals who encounter life stress with a primitive style of projection. Anxiety becomes externalized and blame is centered on some aspect of the environment. These patients are not psychotic and can at times be engaging and likable when all is going well. There are a few clues.

1. The surgeon should be alerted by patients who are overly ingratiating but quick to blame their former physicians.
2. Prior litigation is another clue.
3. Unusual apprehension about certain aspects of physical examination is yet another. For example, those who seriously question the necessity of a routine rectal examination or simple venipuncture may harbor paranoid tendencies.
4. Paranoid tendencies should be suspected of those who are

preoccupied with trivial details such as the exact time of surgery or the anesthetist's middle initial.

The paranoid patient is best managed by helping the staff realize that in fact this patient's suspicions are not directed toward them alone but represent a way of coping with stress in general. Great care should be taken to explain everything in detail to this patient. Any questions should be answered thoroughly and nothing be withheld that might later be used against the physician. Familiarity with the surgical setting and contact with others who have had similar treatment can reduce anxiety and suspicions. When a patient's paranoid behavior leads to staff tension and disruption of ward procedure, psychiatric consultation should be requested.

### The polysurgical patient

At times surgery may be sought as a means of resolving unconscious conflicts. Abram warns that the surgeon may unwittingly become a partner in a destructive relationship whereby the patient undergoes a series of unnecessary procedures in a futile attempt to resolve unconscious conflicts.[53] Menninger refers to the penchant of some patients for repeated operations as "polysurgical addiction." He cites as an example a patient who underwent twenty-eight surgical procedures. Among the unconscious motives explored by Menninger were (1) avoidance of some event more feared than surgery, (2) search for love through submission and punishment (masochism), (3) an ungratified wish for childbearing, and (4) wish for injury (castration) as a means of becoming worthy and accepted.[54]

### Disturbance of consciousness

The important relationship between preoperative central nervous system dysfunction and postoperative complications is discussed earlier in this chapter. The observation by Morse and Litin of an association between preoperative insomnia and postoperative delirium is notable.[42] At times the patient who appears anxious, depressed, and restless will on close inspection reveal evidence of cognitive impairment. A brief mental status examination should test immediate memory, attention span, and general orientation. An innocuous way for the examiner to inquire about hallucinations is to ask the patients if they have dreams and if these sometimes occur in the daytime when the eyes are open. Function of memory and attention can be tested by digit span, serial sevens, and recall of current events concerning treatment or hospitalization. Folstein and others have described a "mini-mental state" examination. The test requires 5 to 10 minutes to administer and includes a series of eleven questions.[55] (see Chapter 6).

If there is cerebral insufficiency a thorough search should be made for an underlying reversible etiology. Psychological management is similar to that described earlier for the aged. The staff should be instructed to visit the patient frequently to provide friendly interchange in which orientation and support are offered. The patient should be escorted around the room and the ward repeatedly until familiar. Unfamiliar people should always be introduced and different situations always anticipated so the patient is prepared for them.

## GENERAL PRINCIPLES OF PREOPERATIVE PSYCHOLOGICAL MANAGEMENT
### Studies of preoperative psychological intervention

Two studies by Egbert and others demonstrate the effectiveness of preoperative teaching by the anesthetist. In one study of 218 patients, the relative value of a preoperative visit or administration of pentobarbital alone or both was judged. Each patient in the group visited by the anesthetist was told the time of surgery, the anesthesia, and the individual medical condition. Those who received a visit and no pentobarbital were more adequately prepared than those who received pentobarbital alone. Those who received both pentobarbital and a preoperative visit were the most adequately prepared.[56]

In a study of patients undergoing intra-abdominal procedures, a control group of fifty-one patients was told nothing of the postoperative pain control, while a study group of forty-six patients was told that postoperative pain was normal to experience. The study group was also shown how to relieve tension by taking a deep breath and allowing the abdominal wall to relax. The patients were instructed to request medication if a reasonable level of comfort was not achieved. Patients in the study group requested far less narcotic analgesic postoperatively and appeared more comfortable and in better physical and emotional condition than did patients in the control group.[57]

Earlier reference was made to studies by Lazarus and Hagens[45] and Layne and Yudofsky[43] who demonstrated a 50% reduction in the incidence of postoperative delirium among cardiac surgery patients who had a preoperative visit by a psychiatrist. As also noted, we at MGH were unable to demonstrate a statistically significant benefit from brief preoperative psychiatric intervention combined with instruction in autohypnosis.[18] In our study of postcardiotomy delirium we were impressed by the changing role of the nursing staff. Lazarus and Hagens describe a tendency for nurses to avoid communication with patients following surgery for fear of disturbing them.[45] Notable in our experience was the extensive preoperative teaching and postoperative support that patients routinely received from the nursing staff. It is likely that this factor along with improvement in surgical techniques has reduced the severity of postoperative delirium. These changes in the surgical environment may have obviated the need for routine preoperative intervention by a psychiatrist and might explain discrepancies in the studies.

Other investigators have also noted the benefits of preoperative psychological support for surgical patients. Kennedy and Bakst told their patients "I'll see you in the recovery room this afternoon," thus emphasizing their belief in a successful outcome by making an appointment.[34] Fox, Rizzo, and Gifford describe a suprisingly intense relationship which surgical patients developed with a psychiatrist and use this as a means of mitigating fears about surgery with apparent emotional benefits postoperatively.[58] Operative and preoperative uses of hypnosis have been studied for their effect on pain reduction and improvement in postoperative convalescence.[59-61] The actual value of hypnosis in reducing pain and discomfort after surgery remains to be proved.[18]

The essential point to be made is that regardless of the agent (nurse, anesthetist, surgeon, or psychiatrist) or the techniques employed (teaching, hypnosis, or psychotherapy), preoperative psychological support seems to have an important effect on postoperative outcome.

### Management and intervention

**Education.** The patient must be told what discomforts to expect, including drains, catheters, nasogastric tubes, intravenous tubing and other surgical articles . The patient should be told to expect pain; it is normal. The patient should be taught how to ask for pain medication by signal in case an endotracheal tube prevents speech. The physician must be certain that the patient has no fantasies or misconceptions and is aware of the risk of complications.

**Anticipation.** The patient must be assured that apprehension after surgery is normal and that moving about in bed, coughing, or deep breathing will not reopen the incision. The patient must also be taught that it is normal to be confused when awakening from anesthesia, to misinterpret events, and to be suspicious. This transient state of mind is commonly called the intensive care syndrome and will desist within hours or days. The patient should be reminded that the physician will make visits in the intensive care unit. It can even be suggested that the presence of the physician will recall the conversation about delirium and suspicions and will reduce anxiety. If possible, it is advisable to take the patient to the intensive care unit before surgery, to introduce the nurses there, and to explain the equipment so that the patient is familiar with the landscape.

**Reassurance.** The patient should be assured that the physician will be in the recovery room after surgery, that he will receive adequate medication for pain, that he need have no fear of addiction to postoperative analgesics. A visit with someone who has undergone a similar procedure and who can describe it in a reasonable way is likely to be most helpful.

Psychological support and reassurance is based on information gained from the patient, relatives, and nursing staff. It is important to reassure only what the patient needs reassurance about, not what the physician thinks is required. The same is true of support. So often caregivers tend to reassure themselves in the name of serving the patient. The hospital staff is there to help with any problems that may be encountered. They are allies, not adversaries.

**Sedation.** Hypnotic and sedative agents should be used judiciously as an adjunct to direct psychological support. It is important to stress the adjunctive nature of tranquilizers and to deemphasize their use as the primary means of easing the patient's mind.

## POSTOPERATIVE PSYCHIATRIC COMPLICATIONS
### Complications of anesthesia

Psychiatric complications of anesthesia include prolonged drowsiness, sleep disturbance, bad dreams, hallucinations, and awareness during surgery. Mostert has presented a review of this subject. He notes that dreams can occur with all anesthetics, especially ketamine, which is a potent hallucinogen, and that hallucinations can be avoided by simultaneous administration of benzodiazepines.[62] The problem of awareness is unresolved. While it is generally agreed that patients may partially awaken in light planes of anesthesia, it remains unclear as to whether adequate levels of anesthesia suppress all memory. Evidence of awareness during deep EEG-monitored ether anesthesia was presented by Levinson. Ten patients were purposely presented with an alarming comment during surgery. One month later, Levinson hypnotized and regressed these subjects to the time of their operative experience. Nine gave evidence of conscious recall.[63] One obvious reason for possible false positive findings is fantasy. Lewis and others induced light plane anesthesia in ten subjects with thiopentone and nitrous oxide (76.4%) maintenance. Subjects were presented with a tape recording that included a poem, a list of low-frequency words, and a fire bell accompanied with the exclamation, "That's a fire bell!" When able to respond to questions, patients were studied for recall. They were studied again at 1 hour, and again at 48 hours. There was no indication of awareness.[64]

This subject is of considerable importance and worthy of continuing investigation. For the time being one can only advise caution about discussion in the operating room. Mostert advises special care when the patient presents a history of recall from prior surgery or when shock demands minimal anesthesia.[62]

### Postoperative delirium

Some predictive psychological factors relative to the occurrence of delirium have been discussed. Delirium is a form of encephalopathy (see Chapter 6). Delirium tremens secondary to alcohol withdrawl is a commonly encountered form. The clinical picture in other types of postoperative delirium is variable. Clouding of consciousness may at times be subtle. The patient may appear quietly withdrawn but otherwise unremarkable except to close scrutiny. As physicians come to know more about delirium and confusional states they realize that the prototypes are only the most obvious cases. Many patients are quietly confused and disoriented during their entire stay in the surgical intensive care unit and no one is the wiser.

In these obvious cases of postoperative delirium the onset and manifestations are dramatic. Mental status examination will reveal a varying degree of disorientation, perceptual distortion, and lability of mood. Delusions, often paranoid, may occur coupled with hallucinations that are classically visual. The patient will be agitated and may interfere with vital support systems. Difficulties are encountered in respiratory care. Failure to mobilize the patient sets the stage for embolism.

A distinction from postoperative functional psychosis is at times difficult. The essential distinguishing feature is that delirium represents an alteration in the level of awareness. Memory, attention, responsiveness, and orientation are impaired and the clinical picture tends to fluctuate. Engel and Romano point out that "a generalized slowing in the EEG is a *sine qua non* of delirium" and the final arbiter between delirium and functional psychosis.[65] Others disagree (see Chapter 6).

The approach to the delirious postsurgical patient involves a search for all identifiable causes of organic brain dysfunction. The cause may be metabolic, infectious, endocrinic, hematologic, cardiovascular, toxic, or traumatic. At times a simple cause may be overlooked.

> A man in his middle fifties was referred for psychiatric consultation soon after surgical treatment for a fractured femur. He was severely disoriented, agitated, and confused. There was no evidence of past psychiatric disorder. After it was suggested that a careful study of systems might reveal the source of the problem, a young medical student noted that the patient's hematocrit had fallen and questioned the possibility of a fat embolus. That was the final diagnosis.

Other frequent postoperative complications that should be considered in the presence of delirium are infection, pulmonary embolus, pneumonia, and sedative overload.

> An elderly asthmatic woman was disoriented in time and place during a 24-hour period without discernible cause. Her list of medications included an order for diazepam, 5 mg at bedtime. When the diazepam was discontinued she returned to full orientation and had no further difficulty. The problem was an atypical response to a generally useful sedative.

Frequently delirium occurs in the apparent absence of specific metabolic disturbance. The incidence following cardiac surgery has been reported at 13% to 100%.* Sensory deprivation in the surgical intensive care unit has been thought to be a contributing factor.[10-12,14-16] Close inspection reveals a high incidence of neurologic findings.† These are frequently missed by the primary attending physician.[66-68] Neuropathological findings at autopsy disclose evidence of ischemic brain damage.[9,13,47] As noted previously, age is an important factor. Gilman and others concluded that the disorder results from diminished cerebral blood flow and that preexistent cerebrovascular disease is the most significant contributing factor.[13,47,67] The primary point to be made then is that delirium is prima facie evidence of insult to the central nervous system.

The following is a case of delirium concomitant with postoperative depression.

> T. A., a retired military man in his late fifties, was admitted for a coronary artery bypass graft following two myocardial infarctions in the preceding year and the development of intractable angina. A few days after cardiac surgery, T. A. developed an embolism to his right

---

*See references 2, 10 to 12, 14, 17, 18, 43, 45, and 66.
†See references 10, 13, 45, 47, 67, and 68.

leg and returned to the operating room for a thrombectomy. Consultation was requested when he became withdrawn and depressed and evidenced the same frequently intermittent angina encountered prior to surgery. The nursing staff reported that he was exceedingly dependent, used nitroglycerin in large amounts, failed to cooperate with instructions, and once made a sexual advance to a nurse.

Psychiatric evaluation showed the patient to be tearful and depressed with labile affect. He expressed fears of death and of becoming helplessly dependent on his family. He was proud of his career as an enlisted man and longed to return home, especially since his son would soon leave for a military academy. Further questioning revealed a general amnesia for the events following cardiac surgery. With great embarrassment he reported that he had been experiencing "bad dreams" consisting of vivid visual hallucinations. Since surgery his confusion had abated; however, he continued to sleep poorly and suffered radiating angina in periods of increased anxiety.

T. A. expressed considerable relief when reassured that he was not losing his sanity as he feared and that confusion of some degree was expected after this procedure. His sleep disturbance was explained to him as related to fears of dying, which others frequently experience. Diazepam was started in a dosage of 2 mg given four times per day. T. A. was instructed in a relaxation technique that would reduce angina and improve sleep.

A few days after the initial consultation, T. A.'s status improved considerably. Episodes of angina became less frequent and his level of anxiety diminished. Although still mildly depressed, he slept well and had no recurrence of "bad dreams."

The treatment of postoperative delirium includes observation and special nursing to ensure against suicide.[69,70] Sedation rather than restraint should be used. Benzodiazepines are safe and useful in the management of anxiety and agitation. When behavior becomes obstreperous and uncontrollable haloperidol is the drug we prefer. The staff should be taught how to reassure the patient and how to augment reality testing. The psychiatrist should visit the patient one or more times daily. These brief visits can be very helpful to the patient, family, and staff. One patient who became severely disoriented and paranoid following onset of an anoxic encephalopathy later commented that he recalled almost nothing of this experience but the visits of the psychiatrist whom he referred to as his "best friend." Round-the-clock orientation should be instituted along with low lights, soft music if desired by the patient, clock, and calendar. The patient's close relatives should be reassured that the delirium is common and transient. They should be encouraged to remain at the bedside, especially if the patient is paranoid and suspicious of the attending staff. The patient's misperceptions must be countered by patient clarification and by the reassurance that his confusion will clear in a short time. The importance of effective reorienting techniques was well demonstrated in a controlled study by Budd and Brown.[69] They found that there is a significant reduction in the incidence of postcardiotomy delirium for patients who receive a specific nurse-administered postoperative reorientation procedure.

Depression frequently accompanies delirium and tends to improve as the sensorium clears. Surgeons and students should avoid bedside discussions on daily rounds. These are often the seedbeds of confusion.

**Postoperative psychosis**

The distinction between delirium and postoperative functional psychosis has been discussed. Functional psychosis may be seen as a continuation of a prior psychopathological state or may occur de novo. Titchener and others noted psychotic depression to be the most common form following surgery, especially among patients who were isolated, lonely, and lacking in close relationships.[70]

Management of acute postoperative psychotic disturbance is essentially the same as the treatment previously described for preoperative psychosis and delirium. The use of major tranquilizers and psychological support will often lead to a rapid resolution. At times the disorder becomes chronic.

**Depression**

Postoperative depression is generally an easy diagnosis to make. The patient appears depressed, admits to being depressed, and has the usual vegetative signs. Masked depression should be considered as a diagnostic possibility when the patient is anxious and withdrawn after surgery, reports inexplicable, persisting pain or other obscure somatic complaints, and has sleep and appetite disturbance as well. In the differential diagnosis, anxiety, psychosis, delirium, and undiagnosed organic disease should be considered.[38,71] Delirium is ruled out if the sensorium is intact. Psychosis can usually be eliminated if there is no thought disorder. Anxiety states may mimic depression. At times there are patients who are simply too frightened to move. The patient's mental status will improve rapidly once the fears subside.

Depression is a common reaction to loss. As earlier noted, it is frequently seen following pelvic surgery in women, mastectomy, enterostomy, amputation, and also with rejection and steroid complications in transplant surgery. The loss entailed in surgery may include (1) a body part, (2) self-esteem, (3) sexual function, (4) independent social function, or (5) ability to pursue gainful employment. Other possible causes of depression are (1) reactivation of a preexistent depressive disorder, (2) failure of surgery to meet expectations, (3) identification with others who had poor surgical outcome, and (4) absence of adequate social support. As noted previously the aged are especially predisposed to postoperative depression. Medical complications of depression arise in many cases. Some of these complications are failure at early ambulation, impairment of respiratory function, and malnutrition. These conditions predispose to atelectasis, infection, and pulmonary embolism. Later in the postoperative course depression may interfere with rehabilitation and with the return to effective social function. Prolonged convalescence in elderly patients who became depressed following lower limb amputation is described in a study by Caplan and Hackett.[72]

The treatment of depression necessitates the use of psychotherapy, psychopharmacology, and social intervention. In their study of noninterpretive intervention Hackett and Weisman describe psychotherapy promoting increased hope by stressing those areas in which the patient feels a sense of competence and control.[25,73]

Use of central nervous system stimulants such as amphetamines and methylphenidate should be considered to assist the patient who is lethargic, withdrawn, and inactive. Antidepressant drugs such as the tricyclics and monoamine oxidase inhibitors are also useful. It is important to remember that there is often a long delay in the response to antidepressants and that side effects may occur, particularly in the elderly and in those with cardiovascular impairment. Also, antidepressant and stimulant drugs should not be combined, particularly monoamine oxidase inhibitors with the risk of hypertensive crisis.

The goodwill of family and close friends can be used to provide encouragement and boost morale. If there is no social support the therapist can assist the patient by establishing contact with patient visiting groups and societies linked with particular illnesses. The social worker can be particularly helpful in assisting with social and economic pressures that impede recovery. If the patient has strong religious ties, the appropriate clergy can be of assistance.

Depressed patients often regress and depend on the nursing staff. This demanding dependency is apt to be frustrating on a busy ward. The staff will become understandably resentful when the patient's call light is on continuously. Consultation is most effective when this issue is addressed. The psychiatric consultant can assist the nursing staff in the development of behavior-modification approaches that encourage the patient toward a gradual increase in activity. When attention is consistently on what the patient fails to accomplish, regression and dependency are increased. The psychiatric nurse clinician can often assist the nurses with the patient who "just won't cooperate."

It is important to let the patients know that they are depressed, that this is a common occurrence after surgery, that they may not feel quite themselves for a while, and that depressions subside. The physician should recognize that depressed patients tend to blame themselves for failing to live up to the surgeon's expectations and that this is also frequently accompanied by fear that the physician will become disinterested.

Most importantly, depression should be recognized and treated early to avoid prolonged convalescence.

**Continued pain**

There are wide individual differences in the degree of pain experienced following surgery. Egbert and others noted that morphine intake following major abdominal surgery may range from none to 95 mg on the first postoperative day.[74] Factors which influence the pain experience include (1) type of surgery, (2) mood, (3) social interactional factors, and (4) adequacy of prescribed analgesia.

Attention should first be given to the order sheet. Many physicians are reluctant to provide adequate analgesics from fear of narcotic addiction and lack of knowledge of analgesics. Marks and Sachar dramatically emphasize the tendency of physicians to inadvertently undermedicate their patients. They conducted interviews with thirty-seven patients admitted to the medical services with pain as a significant symptom. They found 32% of these patients were in "severe distress" from pain; 41%, in "moderate distress;" and 27%, in "minimal distress"—despite the fact that the house officers involved believed in full pain control and had ordered analgesics. The physicians had underestimated the necessary dose or had chosen an ineffective preparation. Marks and Sachar estimate a less than 1% incidence of addiction following the administering of 100 mg of meperidine every 4 hours for 10 days.[75] Hackett discusses medical prejudice in the treatment of pain and reports addiction in only eight of more than 230 patients given narcotics for chronic pain.[76]

More satisfactory pain control can often be achieved by allowing the patient to determine the interval between doses. The patient then has more self-control and a better state of analgesia will result. With this approach, the patient usually requires less medication than if the narcotic were ordered in the conventional way.

There is no need to terminate narcotic orders early in the postoperative course. Mild withdrawl symptoms may occur when narcotics are stopped after several doses have been given daily for 1 to 2 weeks. This does not signify addiction.[49,75] When prolonged analgesia is required methadone is the favored choice because of its potency in oral administration, low addiction potential, and its long action.

When an increase in either amount or frequency of analgesic does not control postoperative pain, it is a good idea to look for a possible psychological cause. The most common cause is depression (see Chapter 4). This possibility should be discussed with the patient's relatives, the nursing staff, and the patient. There may be an obvious but unrecognized reason for the depression. Psychotherapy, clarification, or an antidepressant may make a substantial difference.

The patient may fear that coughing will reopen the operative incision. Fear of death may lead to insomnia and lowered pain tolerance. Evidence of withdrawl or displeasure on the part of the medical staff may compound the problem. The patient should be told that some pain is a normal part of the healing process and that coughing and turning will cause no danger but will hurt for a while. Potentiating an analgesic with an anxiolytic drug is sometimes helpful. Other potentiators are phenothiazines (especially promethazine), butyrophenones (haloperidol), and the amphetamines. Hypnosis can also relieve postoperative pain through both relaxation and the direct suggestion of analgesia. Most importantly, the physician should give time in appropriate doses. For both inpatients and outpatients frequent brief visits by the attending staff often lead to fewer complaints of pain.

## SUMMARY

Surgery is a form of life stress. Many emotional factors are common to the surgical experience. Specific surgical procedures have been studied for their postoperative psychological effects. Psychological variables such as depression, anxiety, dependency, denial, and cognitive impairment appear to be of predictive value in assessing operative outcome. The management of preoperative states (psychosis, depression, addiction, anxiety, denial, paranoid states, cognitive impairment) involves first their recognition and then the appropriate therapy and psychopharmacological intervention. Patients who manifest severe depression, predilection to death, or polysurgical predisposition are especially poor surgical candidates.

General principles of preoperative psychological intervention include education, anticipation of postoperative difficulties, reassurance, sedation, and psychiatric consultation where indicated. Postoperative complications include delirium, functional psychosis, depression, and continued pain. The question of awareness under anesthesia is unresolved.

The point of view from which surgery is discussed emphasizes the recognition and treatment of psychopathological states. This has been a one-sided presentation and does not reflect our enthusiasm about modern surgery and its capacity to better our lives. We have invariably found our association with the surgical staff to be meaningful and productive.

One point of particular importance is the very special relationship between the surgeon and patient. This relationship represents a vital and powerful tool. Its value in assisting the healing process cannot be overstated.

## REFERENCES

1. Titchener, J. L., and Levine, M. L.: Surgery as a human experience, New York, 1960, Oxford University Press, Inc.
2. Kimball, C. P.: Psychological responses to the experience of open heart surgery, I. Am. J. Psychiatry **126:**348, 1969.
3. Titchener, J. L.: Psychiatry and surgery. In Freedman, A. M., and Kaplan, H. I., editors: Comprehensive textbook of psychiatry, vol. I, Baltimore, 1967, The Williams and Wilkins Co.
4. Deutsch, H.: Some psychoanalytic observations in surgery, Psychosom Med **4:**105, 1942.
5. Abram, H. S.: Psychiatry and surgery. In Freedman, A. M., Kaplan, H. I., and Sadock, B. J. editors: Comprehensive textbook of psychiatry, vol. II, Baltimore, 1975, The Williams & Wilkins Co., pp. 1759-1765.
6. Janis, I. L.: Psychological stress, New York, 1958, John Wiley & Sons, Inc.
7. Abram, H. S., and Gill, B. F.: Predications of post-operative psychiatric complications, N. Engl. J. Med. **265:**1123, 1961.
8. Levy, D.: Psychiatric trauma of operations in children and a note on combat neurosis, Am. J. Dis. Child. **69:**7, 1945.
9. Brierly, J. B.: Neuropathological findings in patients dying after open-heart surgery, Thorax **18:**291, 1963.
10. Blachly, P. H., and Starr, A.: Post-cardiotomy delirium, Am. J. Psychiatry **121:**371, 1964.
11. Egerton, N., and Kay, J. H.: Psychological disturbances associated with open-heart surgery, Br. J. Psychiatry **110:**433, 1964.

12. Kornfeld, D. S., Zimberg, S., and Malm, J. R.: Psychiatric complications of open-heart surgery, N. Engl. J. Med. **273**:287, 1965.
13. Gilman, S.: Cerebral disorders after open-heart operations, N. Engl. J. Med. **272**:489, 1965.
14. Heller, S. S., and others: Psychiatric complications of open-heart surgery. A re-examination, N. Engl. J. Med. **283**:1015, 1970.
15. Abram, H. S.: Psychological reaction to cardiac operation. A historical perspective, Psychiatry Med. **1**:277, 1970.
16. Blacker, R. S.: The psychosis of open-heart surgery. With a note on the sense of awe, J. A. M. A. **222**:305, 1972.
17. Kimball, C. P.: The experience of open-heart surgery, III. Toward a definition and understanding of post cardiotomy delirium, Arch. Gen. Psychiatry **27**:57, 1972.
18. Surman, O. S., Hackett, T. P., Silverberg, E. L., and Behrendt, D. M.: Efficacy of psychotherapy for patients undergoing cardiac surgery, Arch. Gen. Psychiatry, **30**:830, 1974.
19. Finkle, A. L., and Prian, D. V.: Sexual potency in elderly men before and after prostatectomy, J. A. M. A. **196**:125, 1966.
20. Lindemann, E.: Observations on psychiatric sequelae to surgical operations in women, Am. J. Psychiatry **124**:132, 1941.
21. Daly, M. J.: Psychological impact of surgical procedures on women. In Freedman, A. M., Kaplan, H. I., and Sadock, B. J., editors: Comprehensive textbook of psychiatry, vol. II, Baltimore, 1975, The Williams & Wilkins Co. pp. 1477-1480.
22. Ewalt, J. R., Randall, G. L., and Morris, H.: The phantom limb, Psychosom. Med. **9**:118, 1947.
23. Melzack, R.: The puzzle of pain, New York, 1973, Basic Book, Inc., Publishers.
24. Simmel, M. L.: Phantoms in patients with leprosy and in elderly digital amputees Am. J. Psychiatry **69**:529, 1956.
25. Hackett, T. P., and Weisman, A. D.: Psychiatric management of operative syndromes, II. Psychodynamic factors in formulation and management, Psychosom. Med. **22**:5, 1960.
26. Weisman, A. D., and Hackett, T. P.: Psychosis after eye surgery: establishment of specific doctor-patient relationship in prevention and treatment of black patch delirium, N. Engl. J. Med. **258**:1284, 1958.
27. Sutherland, A. M., Orbach, C. E., Dyk, R. B., and Bard, M.: Psychiatric impact of CA and cancer surgery, I. Adaptation to dry colostomy, Cancer, **5**:857, 1952.
28. Abram, H. S.: The psychiatrist, the treatment of chronic renal failure and the prolongation of life: III. Am. J. Psychiatry. **128**:84-89, 1972.
29. Castelnuovo-Tedesco, P.: Organ transplant, body image, psychosis, Psychoanal. Q. **42**:349-363, 1973.
30. Christopherson, L. K., Gonda, T. A.: Patterns of grief: end stage renal failure and kidney transplantation, Transplant. Proc. **5**:105l-1056,1973.
31. Blazer, D. G., II, Petrie, W. M., and Wilson, W. P.: Affective psychosis following renal transplant, Dis. Nerv. Syst. **37**:663-667, 1976.
32. Abram, H. S., and Buchanan, D. C.: Organ transplantation: psychological effects on donors and recipients, Surg. Rounds **1**:22-25, 1978.

33. Lipowski, Z. J.: Physical illness and psychopathology, Int. J. Psychiatry Med. **5**:483, 1974.
34. Kennedy, T. A., and Bakst, H.: The influence of emotion on the outcome of cardiac surgery. A predictive study, Bull. N. Y. Acad. Med. **42**:811, 1966.
35. Wolfer, J. A., and Davis, C. E.: Assessment of surgical patients. Preoperative emotional conditions and postoperative welfare, Nurs. Res. **19**:403, 1970.
36. Knox, S. J.: Psychiatric aspects of mitral valvectomy, Br. J. Psychiatry **109**:656, 1963.
37. Kimball, C. P.: A predictive study of adjustment to cardiac surgery, J. Thorac. Cardiovasc. Surg. **58**:891, 1969.
38. Kimball, C. P., Quinlan, D., Orbone, F., Woodward, B.: The experience of cardiac surgery, V. Psychological patterns and predictions of outcome, presented at the 9th European Conference on Psychosomatic Research, April 30, 1972, Vienna, Austria.
39. Kilpatrick, D. G., Miller, W. C., Allain, A. N., Huggins, M. B., and William, L. H.: The use of psychological test data to predict open heart surgery outcome: a prospective study, Psychosom. Med. **37**:62, 1975.
40. Lipowski, Z. J.: Delirium, clouding of consciousness and confusion, J. Nerv. Ment. Dis. **145**:227, 1967.
41. Tucker, W. I.: The prevention and management of toxic psychosis (postoperative psychosis), Lahey Clin. Bull. **13**:268, 1964.
42. Morse, R. M., and Litin, E. M.: Postoperative delirium. A study of etiologic factors, Am. J. Psychiatry **126**:388, 1969.
43. Layne, O. J., Jr., and Yudofsky, S. C.: Postoperative psychosis in cardiotomy patients. The role of organic and psychiatric factors, N. Engl. J. Med. **284**:518, 1971.
44. Rubenstein, D., and Thomas, J. K.: Psychiatric findings in cardiotomy patients, Am. J. Psychiatry **126**:360, 1969.
45. Lazarus, H. R., and Hagens, T. H.: Prevention of psychosis following open-heart surgery, Am. J. Psychiatry **124**:1190, 1968.
46. Rabiner, C. J., Willmer, A. E., and Fishman, J.: Psychiatric complication following coronary bypass surgery, J. Nerv. Ment. Dis. **160**:342-348, 1975.
47. Tufo, H. M., Ostfeld, A. M., Shetielle, R.: Central nervous system dysfunction following open-heart surgery, J. A. M. A. **212**:1333, 1970.
48. Victor, M., and Adams, R. D.: Alcohol. In Harrison, editor: Principles of internal medicine, New York, 1974, McGraw-Hill Book Co., p. 676.
49. Jaffe, J. H.: Drug addiction and drug abuse. In Goodman, L. S., and Gilman, A.: The pharmacologic basis of therapeutics, New York, 1970, Macmillan Publishing Co., Inc. pp. 276-310.
50. Hackett, T. P., Cassem, N. H., and Wishnie, H.: Detection and treatment of anxiety in the coronary care unit, Am. Heart J. **78**:727, 1969.
51. Weisman, A. D., and Hackett, T. P.: Predilection to death. Death and dying as a psychiatric problem, Psychosom. Med. **23**:232-256, 1961.
52. Frank, J.: Persuasion and healing, New York, 1969, Schocken Books Inc.
53. Abram, H. S.: Psychological aspects of surgery, International Psychiatry Clinics, **4**:2, 1967.
54. Meninger, K. A.: Polysurgery and polysurgical addiction, Psychoanal. Q. **3**:173, 1934.
55. Folstein, M. F., Folstein, S. E., and McHugh, P. R.: "Mini-mental state", a

practical method of grading the cognitive state of patients for the clinician. J. Psychiatr. Res. **12**:189, 1975.

56. Egbert, L. D., Bartlet, G. E., Tarndorf, H.,and Beecher, H. K.: The value of preoperative visits by the anaesthetist, J. A. M. A. **185**:553, 1963.

57. Egbert, L. D., Battit, G. E., Welch, C. D., and Bartlett, M. K.: Reduction of postoperative pain by encouragement and instruction of patient, N. Engl. J. Med. **270**:825, 1964.

58. Fox, H. M., Rizzo, N. D., and Gifford, S.: Psychological observations of patients undergoing mitral surgery, Psychosom. Med. **16**:186, 1954.

59. Kolouch, F. T.: Hypnosis and surgical convalescence: a study of subjective factors in postoperative recovery, Am. J. Clin. Hyp. **7**:120, 1964.

60. Werbel, E. W.: Use of posthypnotic suggestion to reduce pain following hemorrhoidectomies, Am. J. Clin. Hypn. **6**:133, 1963.

61. Marmer, M. J.: Hypnoanalgesic and hypnoanaesthetics for cardiac surgery, J.A.M.A. **171**:512, 1959.

62. Mostert, J. W.: States of awareness during general anaesthesia, Perspect. Biol. Med. **19**:68, 1975.

63. Levinson, B. W.: Br. J. Anaesth. **37**:544, 1965.

64. Lewis, S. A., Jenkinson, J., and Wilson, J.: An EEG investigation of awareness during anaesthesia, Br. J. Psychiatry **64**:413, 1973.

65. Engel, G. L., and Romano, J.: Delirium, a syndrome of cerebral insufficiency, J. Chronic Dis. **9**:260, 1959.

66. Gilberstadt, H., and Sako, Y.: Intellectual and personality changes following open-heart surgery, Arch. Gen. Psychiatry **16**:210, 1967.

67. Javid, H., and others: Neurological abnormalities following open-heart surgery, J. Thorac. Cardiovasc. Surg. **58**:502, 1969.

68. Silverstein, A., and Krieger, H. P.: Neurologic complication of cardiac surgery, Arch. Neurol. **3**:601, 1960.

69. Budd, S. and Brown, W.: Effect of a reorientation technique on post cardiotomy delirium, Nurs. Res. **23**:341, 1974.

70. Titchener, J. L., Zwerling, I., Gottschalk, L., and Levine, M.: Psychosis in surgical patients, Surg. Gynecol. Obstet. **102**:54, 1956.

71. Murray, H. W., Moore, J. O., and Luff, R. D.: Disseminated aspergillosis in a renal transplant patient: diagnostic difficulties re-emphasized, Johns Hopkins Med. J. **137**:235, 1975.

72. Caplan, L. M., and Hackett, T. P.: Prelude to death. Emotional effect of lower limb amputation in the aged, N. Engl. J. Med. **269**:1166, 1963.

73. Hackett, T. P., and Weisman, A. D.: Psychiatric management of operative syndromes, I. The therapeutic consultation and the effect of non-interpretive intervention, Psychosom. Med. **22**:267, 1960.

74. Egbert, L. D., Lamden, S., and Hackett, T. P.: Psychological problems of surgical patients. In Eckenhoff, J. B., editor: Science and practice in anaesthesia, Philadelphia, 1965, J. B. Lippincott Co., pp. 15-20.

75. Marks, R. M., and Sachar, E. J.: Undertreatment of medical inpatients with narcotic analgesics, Ann. Int. Med. **78**:173, 1973.

76. Hackett, T. P.: Pain and prejudice: why do we doubt that the patient is in pain? Med. Times **99**:130, 1971.

# 6

# Confusion, delirium, and dementia

**GEORGE B. MURRAY**

A consultation/liaison psychiatrist spends much time in a general hospital with the problem of diagnosing and suggesting treatment for confusion, delirium, and dementia. This chapter is not intended to be a literature review or an exhaustive study of either delirium or dementia. It is intended primarily as a guide for the liaison psychiatrist in a "what to look for" and a "what to suggest" approach. It presupposes some familiarity with confusion, delirium, and dementia.

The consulting psychiatrist is often asked by medical and surgical specialists to determine the mental clarity of a particular problem patient. It is sometimes difficult to assess whether a patient is mildly confused, delirious, demented, or psychotic secondary to a functional disorder. With the increase of longevity and a proportional increase in the elderly hospital population, confusion, delirium, and dementia are more frequently observed. The incidence of Alzheimer's disease (now considered to include what used to be called senile dementia) with organic dementia was estimated at 40% to 58% of persons over age 65 in 1970. This means about 350,000 to 510,000 persons afflicted.[1]

Not infrequently the psychiatrist is called when there is a management or behavioral problem with a patient. However, it is also true that many patients are quietly demented, delusional, or delirious. Since these patients, perduring quietly in their disorder, present no problem to the managing staff, the psychiatrist is never called. The liaison psychiatrist who spends time on specific wards occasionally sees patients who are cryptic psychotics. Intervention usually results in better management for those patients. A major function of the liaison psychiatrist is to differentiate confusion, delirium, and dementia, insofar as possible, and to distinguish them from other entities such as depression. To help in this differentiation some middle level explanatory theory and terminological clarification are in order.

## SOME MIDDLE LEVEL THEORY

The term "middle level theory" is used to indicate that what follows is neither at the stark, nonarguable, fact level; nor is it at the cartesian, clear and distinct, burnished level of universals. What follows lies between these two poles and is an attempt at some heuristic generalities.

In the *Diagnostic and Statistical Manual of Mental Disorders,* second edition, of the American Psychiatric Association, the diagnostic nomenclature includes a classification called "organic brain syndromes." (In the proposed third edition this classification will probably be altered.) Organic brain syndromes are described with the following symptoms:

1. Impairment of orientation
2. Impairment of memory
3. Impairment of all intellectual functions such as comprehension, calculation, knowledge, learning, and others
4. Impairment of judgment
5. Lability and shallowness of affect

Under this diagnostic label, confusion, delirium, and dementia fit as more specific elements of the organic brain syndrome. Physicians often use the designations of acute organic brain syndrome and chronic organic brain syndrome (COBS) to make a rough distinction between what could more particularly be called delirium and dementia. The transient or acute organic brain syndrome would be roughly equivalent to an acute confusional state or delirium, whereas the chronic brain syndrome would be roughly equivalent to dementia. To use the jargon of engineering, this is not all "clean and neat" but rather "quick and dirty." This "organic brain-syndrome" terminology has, however, served the medical profession at least passably well in the past. I will not use the phrase "organic brain syndrome" in this chapter. Confusion, delirium, or dementia will be the terms used here in the hope that they are more helpful clinically and even possibly more specific.

Dementia can be described as the spectrum of mental states resulting from disease of the human cerebral hemispheres. This emphasizes that dementia is not a singular condition but a broad spectrum of dysfunction. Dementia can range from a barely discernible deviation from normal to virtual cerebral death.[2] This is a working definition of dementia and not everyone would agree with it. Engel and Romano[3] maintain that the distinction between delirium and dementia is an arbitrary one, established by convention, with the main criterion of reversibility versus irreversibility. This leads to the philosophically "higher level theory" question of whether or not a dementia such as that found in normal pressure hydrocephalus can truly be such if it is reversible. It is not my intent to attempt resolution of such problems here. The definition of delirium presents obvious problems. Because there is controversy over the essence of delirium, confusion exists in the literature with the terminology of the concept of delirium, for example, acute brain syndrome, acute confusional state, toxic psychosis, and infectious-exhaustive syndrome, to name a few. Psychiatrists Romano and Engel,[4] supported by Lipowski,[5] believe that delirium could be described as a reversible global impairment of cognitive processes. The operative words here are "reversible" and "global." Neurologists Adams and Victor[6] try to describe delirium more specifically. They propose delirium as a special type of confusional state characterized by gross disorientation in the presence of alertness and vigilance. This would include disorders of perception and such symptoms as excessive alertness, intense agitation, and frenzied excitement. Their concept uses delirium tremens as its paradigm.

Adams and Victor also distinguish an acute confusional state with three divisions.[6] They would prefer to call most deliria acute confusional states and use the following three divisions:

1. A delirium, in a narrow sense, that is either hyperkinetic or hypokinetic (so-called quiet delirium), keeping delirium tremens as the prime analogue
2. A primary mental confusion that may or may not be distinguishable from
3. A beclouded dementia that may be the result of some other disease

The opinion of Romano and Engel, however, is that delirium embraces the whole spectrum of acute confusional states.[4]

In summary, I would suggest that as one approaches the patient clinically, a graded framework be kept in mind, that is, acute confusional states versus delirium versus dementia (possibly reversible versus irreversible). "Acute confusional state" is a term used to describe the afflicted patient's mental status, especially if history or laboratory data are not available on the patient. Chédru and Geschwind[7] have characterized the principal feature of the acute confusional state as a reduction of attention. An easy tendency to shift attention may also be found. Other symptoms, such as disorientation, changes in mood, and hallucination, are not essential for the diagnosis. Delirium is the term used to describe more dramatic reversible global impairment of cognitive processes than the more descriptive acute confusional state. The clinician does not know if the impairment is reversible a priori, of course, but two hints that may be helpful in labeling it delirium or acute confusional state rather than dementia are (1) a correctable metabolic imbalance as shown by the patient's laboratory data, such as a blood urea nitrogen (BUN) of 97 mg/100 ml, or a hypercalcemia of 19.4 mg/100 ml, and (2) use of a rule of thumb clinical judgment which posits that deliria are more often due to impairment of general attentional mechanisms while dementias are usually caused by a deterioration of intellectual capacity (secondary to "neuron burn-out") occurring in relatively clear consciousness.[8] For the liaison psychiatrist the final judgment remains clinical, depending on theoretical bias, available information, and experience.

## CHARACTERISTICS OF DELIRIUM

In every delirium or acute confusional state there is reduction in the level of cognition or a clouding of consciousness. This is accompanied by relatively generalized slowing of the electroencephalogram (EEG).[3] As a reversible psychiatric syndrome three elements are usually found:

1. The individual is awake and usually capable of responding verbally.
2. Evidence of impairment of thinking, memory, perception, and attention exists. This tends to fluctuate over time.
3. There is an impaired ability to comprehend both the environment and internal perceptions in accordance with the individual's past experience and knowledge, that is, defective reality testing.[5]

Writing impairment (dysgraphia) is the most sensitive indicator of consciousness impairment according to Chédru and Geschwind.[7] In thirty-four acutely confused patients, they found thirty-three to have writing impairments. Writing was impaired in its motor, spatial, and linguistic aspects. Motor impairments included letters clumsily drawn, and reduplication of strokes in letters as M and W; spatial impairments included inability to align letters properly and orient the lines upward or downward; linguistic errors appeared primarily in spelling. All dysgraphia disappeared when the confusion cleared.

There are three possible outcomes for a delirium: complete recovery, progression to irreversible amnesic syndrome (primary memory loss) or dementia, or progression to irreversible coma and death. A delirium may last anywhere from minutes to months, but the average does not exceed 1 week.

Consciousness is roughly that state that allows cognitive processes to occur. This is neither a philosophical nor a neurophysiological description, both of which are problems for "higher level theory." Cognitive processes include perceiving, thinking, and remembering. The content of cognitive processes is thought to be the result of higher cerebral function and therefore requires the integrity of the hemispheres. Another aspect of consciousness is arousal. Arousal is more general in nature than awareness, and has been likened to the gain control on audio systems. It is thought that the ascending reticular activating system, especially from pons to midbrain and thalamus, is important in this state.[9] Interruption of the reticular activating system can result in unconsciousness. It is my bias that an important key in determining whether delirium or dementia is present is the feature of arousal. The delirious person tends to show high or low levels of arousal over time and unstable variation in the gain or volume of arousal.

What is the substrate or mechanism of delirium? This is not clearly known. Neurology demonstrates that brain cuts do not show any pathological changes of significance in delirium as such. There are at least three different physical mechanisms suggested. One is a withdrawal phenomenon such as that seen in withdrawal from ethyl alcohol or barbiturates. Withdrawal is thought to trigger a release of inhibitory functions. A second type is that of ingestion of toxins, for example scopolamine, or a toxin present in an infectious disease. A third type of physical mechanism could be destructive lesions such as those found in acute inclusion body encephalitis.

Are there any specific types of delirium? This depends to a great extent on one's point of view. One may contend that all delirium is the same or that there are different types of deliria, depending on whether one tends to be a "lumper" or "splitter" in using diagnostic categories. Probably the basic agreement would be that most deliria are phenomena due to multiple organic or psychogenic causes. Stressors, internal and external, act on the mind-brain complex to produce delirium. To call a delirium toxic is clinically helpful but not scientifically satisfying. Various deliria have been described in association with internal and external stressors: for example, lesions in limbic structures as hippocampus and cingulate gyrus have an associated agitated delirium[10]; cerebrovascular disease has elicited deliria[11]; personality dissociation may manifest hallucinations, release of primary process material, and agitation. For a helpful, thorough "grocery list" of the causes of delirium see Aita.[12]

Several clinical features of delirium follow[5,13]:

1. The onset of delirium can be rapid or slow. There may be mild transient symptoms, disturbed sleep, or nightmares.

2. Patients can be aware of the dysfunction and may use the defenses of denial, projection, conversion, or withdrawal to master the feelings this dysfunction may incur. Patients may therefore make it more difficult for the psychiatric examiner by denying to themselves and to the examiner what they are really experiencing.

3. Nocturnal exacerbations may occur possibly due to a decrease in sensory stimuli. The phenomenon of "sundowning" is common in general hospitals. A soft night-light, a calendar, and a clock in the room can provide a modicum of orienting input. Some older people report that soft background radio music during the night is reassuring to them. Although the causes of "sundowning" are not known, it is thought to be due to decreased sensory input and possibly to be connected with circadian rhythms.

4. Disorientation is not an absolute for diagnosis. Patients may be oriented, especially in the early states, and still be delirious. They may mistake unfamiliar persons or places for the familiar. They may believe they are in their local hospital and act perfectly reasonable otherwise. They may confuse what should be familiar names. It is important for the physician to do a formal mental status examination of patients, that is, to press the patients for specific answers to questions and not accept general answers.

5. The patients' grasp of the environment may be faulty. This grasp is the product of complex cognitive processes usually impaired by delirium. For example, patients may know they are in the hospital, but may believe it is primarily for a follow-up gastrointestinal series for their duodenal ulcer whereas, in fact, they have been admitted for bleeding esophageal varices and knew it at the time of admission.

6. Attention and arousal are key areas. There may be a selective central influence related to the reticular activating system important in serving up sufficient arousal to guarantee attention. It is not fully clear whether selective or global attention impairment can be of diagnostic significance. Geschwind's group has argued[14] that the main deficit in the acute confusional state is in the function of selective attention. Usually there is an inverse correlation between attention and distractibility—as one increases, the other decreases. Attention needs a certain amount of arousal; too little or too much impairs attention.

7. Thinking is an effort for delirious patients. Bizarre thoughts may intrude into the patients' conversation or general thought stream.

Delirious patients tend to be more concrete than abstract. Psychotic patients with formal thought disorders can be quite abstract rather than concrete. Delusions may appear but are usually transient. They may change in response to environmental stimuli. They are usually unsystematized and persecutory, in contradistinction to the neatly formed paranoid delusions of the patient who has paranoid schizophrenia or paraphrenia. Because of the jumbled and poorly linked thought processes, the examiner may wonder if a formal thought disorder exists.

8. The patient with delirium commonly has perceptual impairment or illusions. It helps me to consider illusions as a sort of premature and improper labelling of percepts. Visual illusions tend to predominate.

9. Hallucinations have been estimated to vary from 39% to 100% in delirious patients.[5] They are probably less common in the older person than the younger person. Visual hallucinations predominate over auditory or sensory hallucinations. Auditory hallucinations are particularly predominate in paranoid schizophrenia and are often cited as the major mode of hallucination in so-called alcoholic hallucinosis.

10. In delirium, short-term memory is impaired. As demonstrated by Hebb,[15] a certain amount of arousal is required in order to remember. The graph of the memory arousal correlation is a bell-shaped curve; too little arousal gives no memory, a certain amount gives peak memory, and intense arousal decreases memory. In most deliria there is either not enough or too much arousal. Katz, Agle, De Palma, and DeCosse differentiate global and selective cognitive impairment; global is associated with hypokinetic delirium and selective is associated with hyperkinetic delirium. In their experience, global impairment was due more often to an organic lesion, whereas a selective impairment was due more often to environmental stress.

11. The affects most commonly found in deliria are anxiety, fear, and depression, alone or in combination.

12. Psychomotor behavior may be slowed or agitated. Agitation may take the form of picking at the sheets or some bizarre type of behavior such as trying to find the toilet in the clothes closet.

Differentially, acute confusional states or fully developed deliria may result from meningitis, postictal states, drug intoxications, metabolic problems, pulmonary embolism, carcinoma, withdrawal states, fever, pneumonia, congestive heart failure, myocardial infarction, urinary tract infections, postoperative states, hypothermia, dehydration, lack of sleep, other underlying medical problems, and external, environmental stress.

## CHARACTERISTICS OF DEMENTIA

Dementia is more easily diagnosed if it is seen longitudinally. When seen once or over a relatively brief time it can be difficult to diagnose. This difficulty is compounded when there is no opportunity to discuss the patient with family members or others who can give some historical background and commentary on how the patient has behaved. Early behavioral characteristics seen in demented persons include:

1. A lack of initiative
2. An increase in irritability over and above former normal behavior
3. Some loss of interest in various areas of their lives
4. Impaired performance

This last characteristic comes to the attention of the family often in the form of the inability of patients to "hold their liquor" as they used to. It is not uncommon for a family member to say that grandfather becomes silly or irascible after only one drink. Evolution of dementia may be a slow process taking from 3 to 8 years. Some of the late characteristics are:

1. Distractibility
2. Inability to think clearly and intellectual fatigue
3. Lack of perseverance in tasks he is performing
4. Defective memory (although this may be an early sign also)
5. Alteration in mood, especially depression, and lack of insight

It is difficult to correlate EEG slowing with the characteristics found in dementia. In their presenile dementia series, Nott and Fleminger[17] found 67% of their patients had abnormal EEGs. Recently Albert, Feldman, and Willis[18] have described subcortical dementia especially as seen in progressive supranuclear palsy. It is distinguished from cortical dementia by impaired timing and activation. Subcortically demented persons have been described as forgetful, but with a good memory; they are slow to present the searched-for memory item.

Clinically there are two basic types of dementia, the treatable and nontreatable. The most important treatable type of dementia is normal pressure hydrocephalus in which there is the triad of (1) ataxia, (2) dementia, and (3) urinary incontinence.[19] Dementia due to normal pressure hydrocephalus can present with symptoms of depression such as apathy, inattentiveness, agitation, and poverty of thought.

Another treatable form is pseudodementia,[20] in which the patient, usually middle-aged or elderly, is in fact substantially depressed and not demented. Without going into the pharmacology of why it works, it is often helpful to try a suspected pseudodemented patient on a clinical trial of amphetamine or methylphenidate. If the patient responds to the amphetamine or methylphenidate, a strong suspicion arises that he is not demented and therefore is treatable. A course of tricyclic antidepressants, if not contraindicated, can be instituted with some hope of success. Clearly, correct diagnosis is important here since normal pressure hydrocephalus and depression are treatable entities.

Although with deliria structural changes are rarely seen, senile dementia, Alzheimer's disease, and Pick's disease do show structural neuroanatomical correlates. The neuropathology of these diseases has been shown to consist primarily in neurofibrillary tangles, senile plaques, and granulovacuolar changes in the cortex. There is growing evidence that limbic structures also show severe alteration with distinctive patterns in Alzheimer's presenile dementia and senile dementia.[21] If the bulk of the brain is taken into consideration, there appears to be some loss of neurons. The tendency today is to consider senile dementia and Alzheimer's disease as two results of the same process. There is a direct relationship between the severity of the senile dementia and the number of plaques. Neurofibrillary tangles are thought to be a reliable index of previous mental malfunction; they occur only exceptionally in the cerebral cortex of nondemented persons. There are cases reported with apparent dementia but no distinctive pathological correlates.[22]

Two recent tools may well be critical in our clinical ability to determine dementia. Computerized axial tomography (CAT) of the head is now in use in the larger medical centers. CAT scanning can be valuable in determining ventricular enlargement and cerebral atrophy,[23] thereby minimizing the use of the invasive technique of pneumoencephalography. Regional cerebral blood flow is also promising as a technique to demonstrate underlying dysfunction in dementia.[24]

Differentially, dementia may result from degenerative causes such as Alzheimer's disease and Huntington's chorea, metabolic causes such as myxedema and Wilson's disease, vitamin deficiencies such as lack of vitamin $B_{12}$, neoplastic causes such as glioma and metastasis, mechanical causes such as trauma ("punchdrunk syndrome"), vascular causes such as collagen diseases and arteriosclerosis, toxic causes such as alcohol and absinthe, and infectious causes such as general paresis and Creutzfeldt-Jakob disease.[25]

## APPROACH TO THE PATIENT

An important point to determine in approaching the patient is whether the consult is of an urgent type or allows some leisure on the part of the consultant. This means the consultant has to know why he is being called—a point not always clear in large teaching hospitals. Is he being called because the patient is such a management problem that he is tying up two or three nurses during each shift, or is it that the principal physician would like to have some help selecting a sedative for the patient's management? If the consult does not need urgent attention, it is important to check the chart of the patient. This means more than just riffling through the chart. The consultant must look in the chart for various key items:

**Previous psychiatric intervention.** Check for previous psychiatric hospitalization. If found, what were the diagnoses, hospital course, prognosis, discharge medications, and follow-up? Was there ever any psychiatric evaluation? A history or previous physical may mention this. (In teaching hospitals more than one history and physical examination report are usually in the chart—the medical student's usually being the most thorough.)

Some hospitals have social service units and a case history written by the social worker may be present. Usually this is an invaluable aid, especially concerning the patient's relationships with family. The consultant has to judge whether a full reading or quick scan is sufficient. The use of clinical judgment in which the psychiatrist has been schooled during his first postgraduate year (internship) will expedite this decision.

**Vital signs.** Check for hypotension and possible anoxic changes. Hypertension over long periods can produce small lesions which affect behavior slowly, yielding such symptoms as mood lability, drive reduction, insomnia, and impaired judgment. Was this a febrile course? What was the highest recorded temperature?

**Operative procedures and use of anesthesia.** Surgery is traumatic and postoperative confusion is not a rarity. The consultant should check the anesthesiologist's chart not only to notice blood loss and replacement, but, more importantly, to evaluate the blood pressure readings taken during surgery. A mild hypoxia may be well tolerated by the young without detectable behavioral consequence. In the elderly, however, a mild hypoxia may produce subtle mental changes and discrete motor changes such as intermittent darting of the tongue to one side. Such subtle changes may go unrecognized in the hospital during the postoperative period.

Surgery itself, or time on the respirator, may induce inappropriate antidiuretic hormone secretion and thereby cause a relative hyponatremia that can effect mental changes. This hyponatremia need not necessarily be drastically reduced. It is now known that sodium concentration of 125 mEq/L effects mental changes.[26] It is entirely possible that the idiosyncratically sensitive brain may show mental changes at sodium concentration of 130 mEq/L.

**Unusual specific conditions.** Is the patient undergoing hyperalimentation? If so, what is the nature of the diet, for example, FreAmine? Is the patient undergoing chronic renal dialysis? How often? Has the patient ever had seizures during dialysis (generally indicating an electrolyte imbalance)?

**Nurses' notes.** Speaking to the nurses in charge of the patient gives a more longitudinal window on patient behavior. Since the consultant is usually not present during all three nursing shifts, it is useful to peruse the nurses' notes for possible significant behavioral observations.

**Laboratory values.** Unhappily, consulting psychiatrists often do not even skim "the numbers" on the patients they are asked to see. One of the functions of a consultant is to come in fresh—not close to or heavily invested in a specific diagnosis. Coming in fresh, the consultant may notice high or low normal laboratory test values and his suggestions may lead to the repetition of a study with positive results.

Scanning "the numbers" over the hospitalized period gives an idea whether, for example, the patient's BUN is normal or whether there is a trend up or down. The brain is a sensitive organ and can vary in its individual sensitivity to calcium, sodium, or other electrolytes. Therefore borderline high or low normal values may be a key to mildly confusional states or incipient deliria. A nonexhaustive list of laboratory values with a sampling of pathological states associated with each is given here. The consultant may do well to keep these in mind:

Hemoglobin (Hb)—anemia, dehydration?
White blood cells (WBC)—infection?
Red blood cells (RBC)—anemia?
Mean corpuscular volume (MCV)—vitamin $B_{12}$ deficiency?
Blood urea nitrogen (BUN)—starvation, dehydration, uremia?
Magnesium (Mg)—weakness, depression?
Calcium (Ca)—endocrine disorder?
Sodium (Na)—hyponatremia?
Potassium (K)—weakness, depression?

Ammonia ($NH_3$)—hepatic encephalopathy, precoma?
Arterial blood gases (ABG) ($Pa_{O_2}$, $Pa_{CO_2}$, pH) if taken—carbon dioxide narcosis?
Osmolality if taken—both serum and urinary, hyponatremia?
Input and output—if not critical can be checked in rough way with the nursing staff

Familiarity with the basic elements of brain function in the critically ill can prepare the consultant better for intensive care unit consultation.[27]

**Medications.** This topic is vast and could be the subject of a paper in itself (see Chapters 26 and 27). Consultants should know what medications and what dosages the patients are presently using. Medications may be responsible for a decompensated mental state. It is necessary also to understand such pharmacology in order to make intelligent recommendations for further medication management of the patient. For example, although obstetricians and gynecologists have for years been using a combination of meperidine (Demerol) and promethazine (Phenergan) for pain management, other physicians, especially general surgeons, have not been clinically aware of the potentiating effect of phenothiazines with the use of narcotic analgesics. This potentiation allows decreased doses of narcotics for the alleviation of pain. Although most general psychiatrists are aware of this, they may not be aware of the newer information (yet to be clearly established) that the more antihistaminic phenothiazines such as promethazine (Phenergan) and the diphenylmethanes such as hydroxyzine (Vistaril, Atarax) appear to have a greater potentiating effect than the aliphatic phenothiazines such as chlorpromazine.[28]

Psychiatric side effects of drugs is another subject in itself (see Chapter 27). Although the general psychiatric consultant is not necessarily a pharmacologist with "grocery lists" of side effects at the ready, some clear side effects mentally tucked away will help him to be a more intelligent consultant. Placebos can have side effects that are primarily the usual vague symptoms that psychiatrists, internists, and family practitioners are familiar with, such as drowsiness, weakness, lightheadedness, tension, palpitations, headaches, and restlessness.

A sampling of some medications with possible side effects relevant to confusion, delirium, and dementia are:

**Anticholinergics.** Atropine-like compounds have many uses in medicine, and side effects, especially deliria, are not as rare as once thought.[29] Thioridazine has the most anticholinergic action of the phenothiazines. Tricyclics have atropine-like effects.

**Carbidopa.** At least two cases of delirium have been reported using a carbidopa-levedopa treatment regime.[30] I have also observed depression clinically after introduction of carbidopa.

**Levodopa (L-dopa).** Chronic L-dopa use has been associated with dementia (although the dementia may well be due to the underlying Parkinson's disease) and it has also been associated with agitated confusion in 60% of the patients in one series.[31]

**Digitalis glycosides.** Occasionally the first symptom of cardiac glycoside intoxication is confusion or delirium.

**Pentazocine.** Neuropsychiatric reactions are the most common side effects of this medication, with bizarre feelings, hallucinations (more often visual than auditory), disorientation, and agitation in from 7% to 10% of users.[32,33]

**Steroids.** Initiation of, and withdrawal from, high-dose steroids can provoke mental changes. Of those patients receiving 40 mg or less of prednisone 1% may have mental changes; of those receiving 80 mg or more, 18% may have mental changes.[34] Some mental changes due to steroids may not show up for 10 to 15 days.

## MENTAL STATUS EXAMINATION

Some formal mental status examination should be performed. The time or the cooperation may not be available to perform a complete psychiatric mental status examination of the type given in an inpatient psychiatric unit. A formal examination that can be easily repeated allows for better follow-up and assessment of progress or decline. Some psychiatrists use a technique called JOMAC, an acronym meaning to take a cursory view of *j*udgement, *o*rientation, *m*emory, *a*ffect, and *c*onsciousness or the intellect. I recommend the mini-mental status examination by Folstein, Folstein, and McHugh.[35] This is a mini-mental examination by which several parameters are tested and the patient's status is numerically graded (see p. 106). There are only eleven questions that concentrate on the cognitive functions and these can be given in 5 to 10 minutes. The examination can be repeated often and can serve as a numerical key recordable in the chart to show progress or decline. Jacobs, Bernhard, Delgado, and Strain[36] have also made available a brief questionnaire adapted specifically for diagnosis of various organic mental syndromes in the medically ill. The mental status examination is one of the psychiatrist's powerful tools used to assess the affective state. Nonpsychiatrists are not as precise in differentiating delusion from hallucination, dissociation from psychosis, or hypomania from joviality.

Patient _____
Examiner _____
Date _____

### "MINI-MENTAL STATE"*

| Maxi-<br>mum<br>score | Score | |
|---|---|---|

**Orientation**

5    ( )    What is the (year) (season) (date) (day) (month)?

5    ( )    Where are we: (state) (county) (town) (hospital) (floor).

**Registration**

3    ( )    Name 3 objects: 1 second to say each. Then ask the patient all 3 after you have said them. Give 1 point for each correct answer. Then repeat them until he learns all 3. Count trials and record.

Trials _____

**Attention and Calculation**

5    ( )    Serial 7's. 1 point for each correct. Stop after 5 answers. Alternatively spell "world" backwards.

**Recall**

3    ( )    Ask for the 3 objects repeated above. Give 1 point for each correct.

**Language**

9    ( )    Name a pencil, and watch (2 points)
Repeat the following "No ifs, ands or buts." (1 point)
Follow a 3-stage command:
"Take a paper in your right hand, fold it in half, and put it on the floor" (3 points)
Read and obey the following:

#### Close your eyes (1 point)

Write a sentence (1 point)
Copy design (1 point)
Total score
ASSESS level of consciousness
along a continuum _____

Alert     Drowsy     Stupor     Coma

---

*From Folstein, M. F., Folstein, S. E., and McHugh, P. R.: "Mini-mental state," a practical method for grading the cognitive state of patients for the clinician, J. Psychiatr. Res. **12**:189-198, 1975. Copyright 1975, Pergamon Press, Ltd.

# INSTRUCTIONS FOR ADMINISTRATION OF
## MINI-MENTAL STATE EXAMINATION
### Orientation

(1) Ask for the date. Then ask specifically for parts omitted, e.g., "Can you also tell me what season it is?" One point for each correct.

(2) Ask in turn "Can you tell me the name of this hospital?" (town, county, etc.). One point for each correct.

### Registration

Ask the patient if you may test his memory. Then say the names of 3 unrelated objects, clearly and slowly, about one second for each. After you have said all 3, ask him to repeat them. This first repetition determines his score (0-3) but keep saying them until he can repeat all 3, up to 6 trials. If he does not eventually learn all 3, recall cannot be meaningfully tested.

### Attention and calculation

Ask the patient to begin with 100 and count backwards by 7. Stop after 5 subtractions (93, 86, 79, 72, 65). Score the total number of correct answers.

If the patient cannot or will not perform this task, ask him to spell the word "world" backwards. The score is the number of letters in correct order. E.g. dlrow = 5, dlorw = 3.

### Recall

Ask the patient if he can recall the 3 words you previously asked him to remember. Score 0-3.

### Language

*Naming:* Show the patient a wrist watch and ask him what it is. Repeat for pencil. Score 0-2.

*Repetition:* Ask the patient to repeat the sentence after you. Allow only one trial. Score 0 or 1.

*3-Stage command:* Give the patient a piece of plain blank paper and repeat the command. Score 1 point for each part correctly executed.

*Reading:* On a blank piece of paper print the sentence "Close your eyes", in letters large enough for the patient to see clearly. Ask him to read it and do what it says. Score 1 point only if he actually closes his eyes.

*Writing:* Give the patient a blank piece of paper and ask him to write a sentence for you. Do not dictate a sentence, it is to be written spontaneously. It must contain a subject and verb and be sensible. Correct grammar and punctuation are not necessary.

*Copying:* On a clean piece of paper, draw intersecting pentagons, each side about 1 in., and ask him to copy it exactly as it is. All 10 angles must be present and 2 must intersect to score 1 point. Tremor and rotation are ignored.

Estimate the patient's level of sensorium along a continuum, from alert on the left to coma on the right.

## DIFFERENTIATING DELIRIUM FROM DEMENTIA

In differentiating delirium a key clinical observation is the patient's arousal. The demented person generally, not always, tends to have about the same degree of arousal for 1, 2, or several days. The patient with delirium does not continue to have the same level of arousal. He may wax or wane—sometimes more aroused, sometimes less aroused. This is a major distinction between delirium and dementia. Attention, obviously, is linked to arousal, but there are different types of attention. A demented person may be sufficiently aroused, but may be distracted by some persistent thought or sensory input and not attend to the matter at hand. The delirious patient is also often distracted, but it may have a different quality in that the "gain" of his arousal, tends to vary, either turned down or up. The delirious patient gives the impression of being oblivious to or, conversely, jumpy in response to all environmental stimuli. The delirious person's arousal and correlative attention tends to vary more than that of the demented person, who generally maintains a constant amount of arousal with a constant amount of inattention.

If the patient is thought to be demented, a simple Set Test by Isaacs and Kennie[37] can be performed to aid in diagnosis. This test asks the patient to name as many items as possible in four general categories such as animals, colors, fruits, and towns. One point is given for each different item named. Naming less than fifteen out of the possible forty or more items indicates dementia. A score of 15 to 24 indicates possible dementia.

It is my opinion that the psychiatrist may "lay on of the hands." Much information about delirium and dementia may be gathered by examining the patient and by asking him to perform various tasks as elements of a neurological examination. Some tests show cortical release phenomena. The most prominent of the various physical signs associated with dementia are the grasp, glabellar, blink, palmomental, Babinski, and sucking reflexes.[38] Recently the nuchocephalic reflex[39] has been shown in individuals more than 16 years of age to be directly correlated with diffuse cerebral dysfunction. This reflex becomes inhibited at age 4 and in dementia it may be disinhibited or released. Testing for this reflex is a relatively simple maneuver. The patient is asked to stand up and close his eyes. The examiner stands behind him. The examiner briskly turns the patient's shoulders to the left while the patient keeps his eyes closed. If the head turns to the side of the turned shoulder, the response is a normally inhibited reflex; if the head maintains the original straight-ahead position during the shoulder turn, the response is a disinhibited reflex correlated with loss of higher cortical function.

Asking the patient to perform simple commands (such as left hand on right elbow, right hand on left elbow, left hand on left elbow) and observing how the commands are executed may be revealing. If there is undue hesitation or confusion in carrying out such commands, a suspicion of organic disease must be entertained. Testing for reproduction of "kinetic melodies"[40] may well give information substantiating a frontal lobe dysfunction. "Kinetic melodies" is a term Luria uses to describe the performance of complex movements generalized in time. All good drummers have excellent control of kinetic melody. As a test for frontal lobe function, the examiner has only to "play" left and right fingers on a desk in a pattern such as RRL, LLR and ask the patient to repeat it. One can progress the difficulty to a paradiddle, such as RLRR, LRLL. The degree of difficulty experienced in performing these kinetic melodies gives a rough estimate of frontal lobe dysfunction.

Any suspicion of hepatic precoma should prompt the examining psychiatrist to test extended arms for asterixis. Asterixis is not specific for hepatic disease and is seen in a variety of metabolic diseases such as chronic pulmonary disease. The important point is that the patient's arms may be outstretched for as long as 30 seconds before there is a lapse.

If it is not clearly evident in the psychiatrist's mind whether the patient is delirious or demented, some laboratory tests can be suggested. Although EEGs are rarely ordered for this type of differential diagnosis, on occasion they may be helpful. A CAT scan, if available, can demonstrate cortical atrophy. If not already ordered, so-called crazy chemistries are very helpful. These include BUN, blood ammonia, sugar, magnesium, calcium, and electrolytes. Calcium concentrations above 15 mg/100 ml are not infrequently coupled with mental disturbance with paranoid trends.[41] It may also be helpful, if suspicion is aroused, especially in emergency room consultation, to obtain blood and urine specimens for toxic screens of substances that the patient may have ingested and denies.

In diagnosing dementia the psychiatrist must be sure to have distinguished it from pseudodementia.[20] There are dementias without signs of depression and depressions without signs of dementia; most difficult, especially in the elderly, are patients who have symptoms and signs of both entities. Shader and co-workers[42] have developed an assessment scale of eighteen symptoms. This can be helpful in diagnosing early senile dementia, deterioration, and depression. Hypothyroidism may cause depression; unless the diagnosis is clear without it, clinically warranted thyroid studies are in order. On occasion the usual thyroid studies will be normal or low normal; it may then be of advantage to get a thyroid-stimulating hormone (TSH) level in order to determine whether the thyroid gland is involved.

When discussing delirium and dementia, the mental changes seen in a Wernicke-Korsakoff syndrome should be mentioned. Initial symptoms of this syndrome may take the form of a mild delirium, but more frequently there is global confusion, dullness, and apathy. According to Victor, Adams, and Collins,[43] a few patients will present with an amnesic confabulatory (Korsakoff) psychosis and may not have any ocular or ataxic signs of Wernicke's syndrome. If such a patient is referred to the psychiatrist owing to mental symptoms, it is important to treat the patient as quickly as possible with 50 mg of thiamine intravenously followed by 50 mg intramuscularly daily just as if the patient presents with ocular and ataxic signs. Initial global confusion and apathy also respond to thiamine. Two points come to mind with regard to delirium tremens and withdrawal. The first is that delirium tremens can be seen in the patient who continues to drink, but who has suffered some type of trauma.[44] The second is that anesthesia for surgery (such as perforated gastric ulcer or portacaval shunt) can delay the expected onset time of withdrawal delirium tremens. Ten days after surgery a febrile, tachycardic alcoholic patient with incipient confusion may be having an onset of withdrawal rather than an occult pulmonary infectious process. A thorough history and mental status examination may be quite helpful in this differential diagnosis.

Delirium and dementia usually have organic causes. However, clinical experience leads to the conclusion that there are deliria resulting from so-called functional or nonorganic causes. Such deliria can result from dissociation or another form of hysterical psychogenic process. A formal thought disorder can generally be clinically distinguished from the cognitive disorder of delirium by two points:

1. Formal thought disorder often gives the examiner an impression of a "secret-logic-code" linking the loosely associated thought content.
2. There is consistency of the arousal and attention level in formal thought disorder.

Some theorists maintain that all deliria are organic and that those without a presently known biological cause will have one eventually. Postoperative deliria have been described often; it is not clear at present that all are due to biological causes; therefore, environment[45] and inner psychological dynamics are said to play a role (see Chapter 5). Future research may show such biological causes for deliria such as brain edema secondary to hyponatremia.[46,47]

Various names have been given to environmental deliria such as "recovery room" delirium.[48] Hackett, Cassem, and Wishnie[49] urge caution in attributing psychiatric difficulties in an intensive care unit to the "intensive care syndrome." The studies of Holland, Sgroi, Marwit and Solkoff[50] do not support the theory that the intensive care unit environment causes psychological disturbances as such.

Clinical experience seems to indicate that external stressors are involved in the development of various deliria. Three relationships that should be examined when assessing confusion, delirium, and dementia are the intrapersonal (or inner experience of self), the interpersonal (such as the interplay between staff or significant others and patient), and the impersonal (such as the possible effect of hardware on the patient).[51]

**MANAGEMENT**

Once the diagnosis is made, the next step is the management. In some urgent cases time is not available for comfortable diagnosis and the physician may have to manage the patient on the basis of a quick provisional impression. An example of this is the patient in a postictal confusion from temporal lobe epilepsy who attempts to "bull" his way out of the hospital. Intervention is obviously necessary with this patient before a more studied diagnosis can be made. In general, however, the diagnosis is known and there are four areas of concern in management.

1. Treatment of the underlying cause when possible (as in delirium)
2. Orientation of the patient
3. Human contact with the patient, such as staff interactions, visits by relatives, visits by psychiatrist
4. Medication whether used for chemical restraint, anxiety reduction, or delirium treatment as with physostigmine for delirium caused by some anticholinergic agent

As stated in the previous section, the underlying cause of a delirium may be organic or possibly external stressors. Postoperative delirium is not unusual and, if watched and diagnosed as such, with correction of any metabolic abnormalities, will generally pass with time. If possible, sedative or hypnotic drugs should not be used in order to avoid masking mental abnormalities. If the delirious patient does become a behavioral problem as with increased agitation, it may be necessary to use medication in behavior management. Psychopharmacological measures may be indicated to keep the patient from such activity as pulling out intravenous tubing.

At this point it is also important to discuss the patient's behavior with the staff. Nurses may know what does and does not scare or reassure the patient. Staff personnel inexperienced in the handling of delirious, behaviorally irritating patients will benefit from instructive intervention by the psychiatrist. Staff toleration of unusual or disruptive behavior is relative. Degree of toleration is proportional to acquired skill in dealing with such aggravations as boisterous, agitated, or threatening and bellicose behavior. Toleration is also proportional to the amount of leisure or the degree of overwork under which the staff operates. The consultation/ liaison psychiatrist can aid the staff with specific skills in understanding interpersonal dynamics.

The liaison psychiatrist's assessment of the staff influences, consciously or unconsciously, the recommendations or prescriptions of medication for agitation. It may influence the type as well as the dosage of medication. Before any drug is given, adequate provision for nursing observation and medical resuscitation must be assured. Adequate oxygenation and assessment of cardiovascular function and general metabolic state are more than just desirable before giving quieting medications.

If the patient is mildly obstreperous and agitated, I would suggest a rial of a benzodiazepine, for example, 5 mg of diazepam given intramuscularly, preferably in the deltoid muscle for better absorption. Depending on the awareness and arousal level of the patient, the dose can be titrated up or down with observation. If the patient is unmanageable, a phenothiazine or butyrophenone may be preferred. For elderly patients I prefer to use haloperidol. For the unmanageable patient 5 to 10 mg given intramuscularly if oral is not possible, will usually be sufficient. Haloperidol has been used intravenously although this is not indicated on the package insert. Doses of 40 to 60 mg have been injected intravenously over time with good results. It is especially helpful in agitated postcardiotomy patients who endanger their lives by their agitation and for whom restraints are not feasible.

In the management of demented and delirious patients with some awareness, the following aspects are helpful:

1. Familiarity appears to be a key feature in orientation. Things become familiar sooner when a warm affect is associated with a piece of the environment. Familiar items from home may help to warm up the strange hospital surroundings.

2. Every room should have a night light (situated so as not to cast moving shadows), calendar, clock, and, if possible, a quiet radio for background reality cueing. Orientation devices and low level sensory input seem to help stave off external stressor type deliria. Many demented persons report that they appreciate the radio.

3. Attention should be paid to the nonverbal communications of the patient. Visits to the patient should be cheering and not exciting. Intensive care units have found frequent short visits are preferable to fewer long visits.

4. There should be encouragement of active inquiry on the staff's part—that is, "Mr. Jones, do you know what day this is?" "Do you know where you are?" and so on, especially for geriatric patients who tend to commit "sins of omission."

5. The patient should be given only one stimulus at a time. This is obviously more time consuming, but ordinarily recognizing the need for more time makes the psychiatrist and staff more patient. One stimulus at a time means not asking a patient to do anything else until the previously requested task is completed. To do otherwise tends to confuse the demented patient and can scare a delirious patient, especially if the delirium is due to a toxic substance such as an anticholinergic, where visual focusing is a problem.

6. Instructions should always be given in a slow-paced manner so that the patient is able to process the information. One may have to repeat the instructions, so they should not be too complicated.

7. Procedures should be explained to the patient in the simplest possible way unless he does not wish to hear the facts. Too often procedures are not explained at all, especially to mildly confused or demented patients. The psychiatrist may have to make the explanation and should be prepared for such explanations as how and why an intravenous pyelogram is taken or what a "commando" procedure for cancer is.

8. Addressing an elderly demented patient by first name under the guise of great care-giving is infantalizing. It both emphasizes the patient's incapacity to perform and further reduces what little dignity remains.

9. Some believe that using the first name with the delirious patient may be necessary or helpful in gaining the patient's attention.

## SUMMARY

An attempt has been made in this chapter to aid the consultation/ liaison psychiatrist in the practical diagnosis and management of confusion, delirium, and dementia. Making the correct diagnosis is dependent on knowing signs and symptoms. Therefore some of this chapter is devoted to the various conceptions of confusion, delirium, and dementia. There is active discussion and argument today about the definitive features of these three states. In an attempt to be of pragmatic assistance to the clinician I suggest approaches and management of the patient suffering from observable impairment of orientation, memory, intellectual functions, judgment, affect, or any combination of these impairments.

## REFERENCES

1. Katzman, R.: The prevalence and malignancy of Alzheimer disease, Arch. Neurol. **33:**217-218, 1976.
2. Wells, C. E.: The symptoms and behavioral manifestations of dementia. In Wells, C. E., editor: Dementia, Philadelphia, 1971, F. A. David Co. pp. 1-12.
3. Engel, G. L., and Romano, J.: Delirium, a syndrome of cerebral insufficiency, J. Chronic Dis. **9**(3):260-277, 1959.
4. Romano, J., and Engel, G. L.: Physiologic and psychologic considerations of delirium, Med. Clin. North Am. **28:**629, 1944.
5. Lipowski, Z. J.: Delirium, clouding of consciousness and confusion, J. Nerv. Ment. Dis. **145**(3):227-255, 1967.
6. Adams, R. D., and Victor, M.: Delirium and other acute confusional states. In Thorn, G. W., and others, editors: Harrison's principles of internal medicine, ed. 8, New York, 1977, McGraw-Hill Book Co., pp. 145-150.
7. Chédru, F., and Geschwind, N.: Writing disturbances in acute confusional states, Neuropsychologia **10:**343-353, 1972.
8. Folstein, M. F., and McHugh, P. R.: Phenomenological approach to the treatment of "organic" psychiatric syndromes. In Wolman, B. J., editor: The therapist's handbook, New York, 1976, D. Van Nostrand Co. pp. 279-286.
9. Plum, F., and Posner, J. B.: Diagnosis of stupor and coma, ed. 2, Philadelphia, 1972, F. A. Davis Co., pp. 2-25.
10. Medina, J. L., Rubino, F. A., and Ross, E.: Agitated delirium caused by infarctions of the hippocampal formation and fusiform and lingual gyri, Neurology **24:**1181-1183, 1974.
11. Horenstein, S.: Effects of cerebrovascular disease on personality and emotionality. In Benton, A. L., editor: Behavioral change in cerebrovascular disease, New York, 1970, Harper & Row, Publishers, 1970, pp. 171-194.
12. Aita, J. A.: Everyman's psychosis—the delirium, Neb. Med. J. **53:**424-427, 1968.
13. Pincus, J. H., and Tucker, G. J.: Behavioral neurology, New York, 1974, Oxford Book Co., Inc., pp. 118-120.

14. Mesulam, M.-M., Waxman, S. G., Geschwind, N., and Sabin, T. D.: Acute confusional state with right middle cerebral artery infarctions, J. Neurol. Neurosurg. Psychiatry **39**:84-89, 1976.
15. Hebb, D. O.: Drives and the C.N.S. (conceptual nervous systems), Psychol. Rev. **62**:243-254, 1955.
16. Katz, N. M., Agle, D. P., DePalma, R. G., and DeCosse, J. J.: Delirium in surgical patients under intensive care, Arch. Surg. **104**:310-313, 1972.
17. Nott, P. N., and Fleminger, J. J.: Presenile dementia: the difficulties of early diagnosis, Acta Psychiatr. Scand. **51**:210-217, 1975.
18. Albert, M. L., Feldman, R. G., and Willis, A. L.: The "subcortical dementia" of progressive supranuclear palsy, J. Neurol. Neurosurg. Psychiatry **37**:121-130, 1974.
19. Rosen, H., and Swigar, M. E.: Depression and normal pressure hydrocephalus, J. Nerv. Ment. Dis. **163**:35-40, 1976.
20. Post, F.: Dementia, depression, and pseudodementia. In Benson, D. F., and Blumer, D., editors: Psychiatric aspects of neurologic disease, New York, 1975, Grune & Stratton, Inc., pp. 99-120.
21. Hooper, W. W., and Vogel, F. S.: The limbic system in Alzheimer disease, Am. J. Pathol. **85**:1-20, 1976.
22. Todorov, A. B., Go, R. C. P., Constantinidis, J., and Elston, R. C.: Specificity of the clinical diagnosis of dementia, J. Neurol. Sci. **26**:81-98, 1975.
23. Fox, J. H., Ramsey, R. G., Huckman, M. S., and Proske, A. E.: Cerebral ventricular enlargement: chronic alcoholics examined by computerized tomography, J.A.M.A. **236**(4):365-368, 1976.
24. Gustafson, L., and Risberg, J.: Regional cerebral blood flow related to psychiatric symptoms in dementia with onset in the presenile period, Acta Psychiatr. Scand. **50**:516-538, 1974.
25. Katzman, R., and Karasu, T. B.: Differential diagnosis of dementia. In Fields, W. S., editor: Neurological and sensory disorders in the elderly, New York, 1975, Stratton Intercontinental Medical Book Corp., pp. 103-134.
26. Arieff, A. I., Llach, F., and Massry, S. G.: Neurological manifestations and morbidity of hyponatremia: correlation with brain water and electrolytes, Medicine, **55**(2):121-129, 1976.
27. Siesjö, B. K., Carlsson, C., Hägerdal, M., and Nordström, C.-H.: Brain metabolism in the critically ill, Crit. Care Med. **4**(6):283-294, 1976.
28. Momose, T.: Potentiation of postoperative analgesic agents by hydroxyzine. In Bonica, J. J., editor: Considerations in management of acute pain, Hosp. Pract. pp. 22-27, 1977.
29. Granacher, R. P., and Baldessarini, R. J.: Physostigmine: its use in acute anticholinergic syndrome with antidepressant and antiparkinson drugs, Arch. Gen. Psychiatry **32**:375-380, 1975.
30. Lin, J. T-Y., and Ziegler, D. K.: Psychiatric symptoms with initiation of carbidopa-levodopa treatment, Neurology, **26**:699-700, 1976.
31. Sweet, R. D., and others: Mental symptoms in Parkinson's disease during chronic treatment with levodopa, Neurology **26**:305-310, 1976.
32. Miller, R. R.: Clinical effects of pentazocine in hospitalized medical patients, J. Clin. Pharmacol. **15**:198-205, 1975.
33. Wood, A. J. J., and others: Medicines evaluation and monitoring group: central nervous system effects of pentazocine, Br. Med. J. **1**:305-307, 1974.

34. Boston Collaborative Drug Surveillance Program: Acute adverse reactions to prednisone in relation to dosage, Clin. Pharmacol. Ther. **13:**694, 1972.
35. Folstein, M. F., Folstein, S. E., and McHugh, P. R.: "Mini-mental state," a practical method for grading the cognitive state of patients for the clinician, J. Psychiatr. Res. **12:**189-198, 1975.
36. Jacobs, I. W., Bernhard, M. R., Delgado, A., and Strain, J. J.: Screening for organic mental syndromes in the medically ill, Ann. Intern. Med. **86:**40-46, 1977.
37. Isaacs, B., and Kennie, A. T.: The set test as an aid to the detection of dementia in old people, Br. J. Psychiatry **123:**467-470, 1973.
38. Paulson, G. W.: The neurological examination in dementia. In Wells, C. E., editor: Dementia, Philadelphia, 1971, F. A. Davis Co., pp. 13-33.
39. Jenkyn, L. R., and others: The nuchocephalic reflex, J. Neurol. Neurosurg. Psychiatry **38:**561-566, 1975.
40. Luria, A. R.: Frontal lobe syndromes. In Vincken, P. J., and Bruyn, G. W., editors: Handbook of clinical neurology, vol. 2, New York, 1969, John Wiley & Sons, Inc., pp. 725-757.
41. Sachar, E. J.: Endocrine factors in depressive illness. In Flach, F. F., and Draghi, S. C., editors: The nature and treatment of depression, New York, 1975, John Wiley & Sons, Inc., pp. 397-411.
42. Shader, R. I., Harmatz, J. S., and Salzman, C.: A new scale for clinical assessment in geriatric populations: Sandoz clinical assessment—geriatric (SCAG), J. Am. Geriatr. Soc. **22:**107-113, 1974.
43. Victor, M., Adams, R. D., and Collins, G. H.: The Wernicke-Korsakoff syndrome, Philadelphia, 1971, F. A. Davis Co.
44. Cryer, P. E., and Kissane, J.: Delirium and fever, Am. J. Med. **58:**265-271, 1975.
45. Nadelson, T.: The psychiatrist in the surgical intensive care unit. I. Postoperative delirium, Arch. Surg. **111:**113-119, 1976.
46. Deutsch, S., Goldberg, M., and Dripps, R. D.: Postoperative hyponatremia with the inappropriate release of antidiuretic hormone, Anesthesiology, **27:**250-256, 1966.
47. White, W. A., and Bergland, R. M.: Experimental inappropriate ADH secretion by positive pressure respirators, J. Neurosurg. **36:**608-613, 1972.
48. Frank, K. A., Heller, S. S., and Kornfeld, D. S.: A survey of adjustment to cardiac surgery, Arch. Intern. Med. **130:**735-738, 1972.
49. Hackett, T. P., Cassem, N. H., and Wishnie, H. A.: The coronary care unit: an appraisal of its psychological hazards, N. Engl. J. Med. **279:**365, 1968.
50. Holland, J., Sgroi, S. M., Marwit, S. J., and Solkoff, N.: The ICU syndrome: fact or fancy, Psychiatry Med. **4:**241-249, 1973.
51. Hackett, T. P., and Weisman, A. D.: Psychiatric management of operative syndromes. II. Psychodynamic factors in formulation and management, Psychosom. Med. **22:**356-372, 1960.

# 7

# Hysteria

**AARON LAZARE**

---

This chapter reviews what is known about conversion reaction (hysterical neurosis, conversion type, or conversion disorder) in general hospital practice. Since I will be critically assessing the diagnostic criteria, conversion reaction is broadly defined at this point as *a symptom that represents a loss or alteration of sensory or voluntary motor functioning and that resembles medical illness although no known medical disorder explains the symptom.* This clinical condition is important because of its incidence (5% to 16% of hospitalized patients seen in formal psychiatric consultation[1-5]), because of the difficulty in establishing the diagnosis, and because of the attendant problems of patient management.

The importance of the conversion reaction is matched by the semantic and conceptual confusion surrounding it and its relationship to other hysterical phenomena. This confusion is attested to by the titles of several recent articles: "Hysteria—Multiple Manifestations of Semantic Confusion,"[6] "The Hysterical Character in Psychoanalytic Theory: Evolution and Confusion,"[7] and "Hysteria: The Consultant's Dilemma—Twentieth Century Demonology, Pejorative Epithet, or Useful Diagnosis?"[8] Perhaps as a result of this semantic and conceptual confusion, psychiatrists interested in the subject write about conceptual issues, leaving little time and energy for empirical studies. Without the data from these studies, physicians are left with authoritative but unscientific recommendations about the diagnosis and treatment of hysteria.

In this chapter, I will attempt (1) to clarify some of the conceptual confusion by distinguishing conversion reaction from five other clinical phenomena that have been referred to as "hysterical," (2) to present a critical analysis of the empirical data on the differential diagnosis of conversion reaction, and (3) to review what has been written on the hospital management of patients with conversion reaction.

## HYSTERICAL PHENOMENA

This section will review the historical development and contemporary meaning of "conversion reaction." This condition will then be
contrasted with five other clinical conditions that may be referred to as
hysterical: psychophysiological reactions, dissociative states, hysteria
or Briquet syndrome, the hysterical personality, and hysterical psychosis.

### Conversion reaction

Freud's work on what is now called conversion reaction (also
referred to as conversion hysteria or hysterical neurosis, conversion
type) was the beginning of psychoanalysis itself. In his early papers he
considered the classic hysterical symptoms of blindness, convulsions,
contractures, and disturbances in sensation. Freud believed these
symptoms to be psychogenic.

For Freud, the symptoms could be explained by traumatic events,
repression, and disturbed sexuality. More specifically, following a
traumatic event, the painful and unacceptable memory was said to be
repressed or dissociated from the mainstream of consciousness while
the affect was converted to a somatic symptom rather than verbalized
at the time of the trauma. The symptom itself was said to be a
meaningful symbolic expression of the sexual wish as well as a
protection against the conscious awareness of the wish. To the degree
that the symptom was effective protection against anxiety, the patient
would have "la belle indifférence," an attitude of indifference despite
extensive disturbances in function.

In contrast, Charcot and Janet explained the disorder as a hereditary degenerative process of the nervous system. Both Charcot and
Janet, nevertheless, appreciated the importance of psychological factors in the understanding of hysteria.

The predisposition to conversion was originally thought to be actual
sexual seduction occurring in childhood, and the trauma leading to the
conversion was believed to be of a sexual nature. The personality of
such patients was described as "hysterical." With further developments in psychoanalytical theory, the idea of a predisposition to
hysteria based on childhood sexual traumas was relinquished and
replaced by "a fixation in early psychosexual development at the level
of the Oedipus complex, with a failure to relinquish the incestuous tie
to the loved parent."[9] Since such developmental fixations are characteristic of relatively healthy patients suffering from oedipal-genital
conflicts, the mistaken conclusion was drawn that hysteria did not

occur in patients suffering from pregenital conflicts. This is no longer accepted. It is now generally believed that patients dealing with preoedipal drives also use conversion. Some psychoanalysts deal with this semantic-conceptual problem by limiting the word "hysterical" to those conversion reactions associated with oedipal-genital conflicts.[10] For general psychiatrists, conversion reactions and hysterical symptoms are synonymous.

During the past 2 decades there has been renewed interest in hysterical symptoms.[11-14] One important approach has been to attempt to understand the conversion reaction as "a kind of nonverbal communication couched in a protolanguage that arises in and is conditioned by the specific setting of the doctor-patient relationship."[11] The so-called secondary gain, or what the patient is able to get from the outside world, is seen as more important than the primary gain, or what the symptom accomplishes within the patient's mind. Recent concepts of the conversion reaction also deemphasize the conflicts over sexual issues and emphasize the importance of dependency needs and aggressive drives.

From the historical development of the concept of conversion reaction have come these criteria for diagnosis: emotional stress prior to the onset of symptoms, hysterical personality, la belle indifférence, the symptom as symbolism, the symptom as communication or secondary gain, and disturbed sexuality.

### Psychophysiological symptoms

The psychophysiological disorders, like the conversion reactions, are bodily disorders thought to be related to psychological disturbances. They include peptic ulcer, essential hypertension, bronchial asthma, migraine, rheumatoid arthritis, hyperthyroidism, regional enteritis, and ulcerative colitis. These conditions were often lumped together with conversion reactions until the 1930s when Alexander formulated separate descriptions. The psychophysiological disorders are said to differ from conversion reactions because:

1. They involve mainly the autonomic neuroendocrine outflow systems.
2. They have no symbolic meaning and serve no psychological function; they result from the failure of psychological defense and coping mechanisms.[15]
3. There is gross pathology in the involved organ system.

Recently the distinction between the conversion reactions and the psychophysiological disorders has again become blurred. Several investigators believe that the psychophysiological symptom can have symbolic meaning and Engel has called attention to several conversions involving structures not innervated by the sensory or voluntary nervous system.[16] Barnett conducted a chart study of 109 patients in order to compare many variables among sixty-three patients with psychophysiological disorders (limited to nine diseases including the eight listed above plus angina or arrhythmia when there was firm consensus on the psychosomatic contribution) and forty-six patients with conversion reactions.[17] There were many significant differences. Patients with psychophysiological reactions were (1) more intelligent, (2) less apt to be referred for psychiatric consultation because of the symptom itself, (3) less apt to have multiple complaints, (4) more apt to cite occupational or financial stress, (5) more apt to be an oldest child, (6) less apt to be an only child, (7) apt to have more siblings of the same sex, (8) apt to show greater insight, (9) apt to have more overt depression, (10) apt to show more repression of affect, (11) less apt to display histrionic traits, (12) less apt to show indifferent affect, (13) less apt to show signs of thought disorder, and (14) less apt to be characterized in terms of primary and secondary gain and symptom symbolism. This study gives strong support for distinction between these two clinical entities.

**Dissociative states**

The dissociative states, also referred to as hysterical neurosis, dissociative type, include the clinical phenomena of somnambulism, amnesia, fugue, trance, and multiple personality. These conditions are said to be similar to the conversion reactions; both have grossly defective repressive functions that lead to "exaggerated and pathological process of exclusion. Some segment of reality, internal or external, gets separated off from the rest of the personality organization."[18] The differences between the two hysterical conditions are striking. In the conversion reaction, there is a circumscribed loss of function while the rest of the personality is little affected. The symptom also has value for its symbolic expression. In dissociative states, large segments of internal and external reality are involved, and the symptoms, which serve to deny reality, often lead to an increase rather than a decrease in anxiety.[13]

**Hysteria—Briquet syndrome**

A group of psychiatrists at Washington University in St. Louis first described a syndrome referred to as hysteria or Briquet syndrome.

This starts early in life, occurs primarily in women, and is characterized by recurrent symptoms in many organ systems. The symptoms that are dramatically described by the patient include varied pains, menstrual disorders, sexual maladjustment, headaches, anxiety symptoms, frequent conversion reactions, excessive hospitalizations, and excessive operations. The conversion reaction may constitute an important part of the syndrome but is not synonymous with the syndrome. Those who support the usefulness of the concept of Briquet syndrome argue that it follows a predictable course, clusters in certain families, and is associated with sociopathy, "suggesting that the two conditions may arise from similar etiologies and pathogenetic factors."[19,20] Those who criticize the concept regard it as a "fictitious syndrome"[6] or believe that the absence of psychodynamic considerations in the conceptualization of Briquet syndrome makes the concept limited.[11]

**Hysterical personality**

Textbooks of psychiatry at the turn of the century described personality traits that were found in association with conversion reaction symptoms. These traits, which eventually included excitability, emotional instability, overreactivity, self-dramatization, attention-seeking, immaturity, vanity, and unusual dependence,[21] came to be called the "hysterical personality" or "hysterical character." Factor analytic studies demonstrate that most of these traits cluster together mathematically.[22,23] Although these personality traits first came to the attention of clinicians because of their association with hysterical symptoms, it is currently believed that patients with conversion reactions may have any personality traits.

Considerable confusion now exists among psychoanalysts and between psychoanalysts and general psychiatrists over the meaning of "hysterical character." Since "hysterical" has referred to problems relating to the oedipal-genital level of development, patients with the hysterical traits already described who are suffering from preoedipal pathology should not, according to many analysts, be referred to as "hysterical personalities." Terms such as "histrionic," "infantile," "hysteroid," "primitive," and "borderline" have been proposed as alternatives. This leads to the confusing situation of a clinician referring to a patient with striking hysterical traits as not really hysterical. The physician must be aware of this semantic confusion in order to make sense out of clinical discussions involving the term "hysterical personality."[7]

## Hysterical psychosis

"Hysterical psychosis" is a term that currently has no official status, but is still used by many clinicians. Hollender and Hirsch characterize the syndrome as manifested by hallucinations, delusions, depersonalization, and bizarre behavior.[24,25] The thought disorder is sharply circumscribed and transient, lasting no longer than 1 to 3 weeks and finally sealing off, so that there is "practically no residue."[24] If affect is altered, it is volatile, not flat. The disorder is apt to be encountered in patients with hysterical personalities. Hollender and Hirsch discuss three processes responsible for the hysterical psychosis. One process consists of culturally sanctioned behavior that is tolerated or supported and may represent good reality testing in the sociocultural context. Another consists of "appropriation of psychotic behavior." In this process the patient assumes a psychotic role as a communication to others. The assumption of the role may represent an unconscious identification with a psychotic person and an attempt to establish rather than lose contact with reality. The third process is a true psychosis. It is said to occur primarily in patients with hysterical personalities who, under particular circumstances, are vulnerable to ego disruption.

Critics of the concept of hysterical psychosis argue that the first two processes are not true psychoses. The third is a psychosis, but the prefix "hysterical" adds nothing to the diagnosis.

## THE DIFFERENTIAL DIAGNOSIS OF CONVERSION REACTIONS

The primary request of a referring physician is usually for confirmation that the patient is suffering from a conversion reaction (or is "hysterical") rather than suffering from organic disease. The secondary request may be for management and disposition.

The diagnosis of conversion reaction is made by demonstrating (1) the absence of organic pathology and (2) the presence of several criteria that, combined, support the diagnosis of conversion reaction. These diagnostic criteria are derived from theories about hysterical phenomena and from clinical experience. They are commonly accepted and extensively published. Studies of the validity of these criteria, however, are few and must be interpreted according to the methods of investigation—including the clinical setting, the selection of patients, the sample size, the experience of the consulting physician, and the prospective or retrospective design of the study. A summary of the methods used in each of the studies is presented to help the reader assess the findings.

**Ziegler and Paul, 1954.**[26] This is a 20 to 25 year follow-up of sixty-six female patients who were given a final diagnosis of "psychoneurosis hysteria" when discharged from the Boston Psychopathic Hospital between 1927 and 1932. Each patient was seen by one or more staff psychiatrists. The follow-up consisted of interviews of patients and families and record reviews conducted by the investigators.

**Chodoff and Lyons, 1958.**[27] This is a retrospective study of records of seventeen consecutive inpatients initially evaluated by Lyons and discharged from a Veterans Administration hospital in Washington, D.C., between October, 1954, and 1956 with the diagnosis of conversion reaction.

**Gatfield and Guze, 1962.**[28] This is a 3 to 10 year follow-up of thirty-seven patients who were discharged from a neurology and neurosurgery service between 1950 and 1957 with a diagnosis of conversion reaction. Patients with pain were excluded from the study. The results are based on twenty-four patients who were interviewed by the investigators.

**Stephens and Kamp, 1962.**[29] This is a retrospective study based on clinical records of 100 inpatients who were treated at the Henry Phipps Psychiatric Clinic sometime during the periods of 1913 to 1920 or 1945 to 1960.

**Ziegler, Imboden, and Meyer, 1960 to 1963.**[1,12,30] This is a retrospective study based on the clinical records of 134 consecutive inpatients and outpatients who had conversion reaction as diagnosed in consultation by two of the authors at Johns Hopkins Hospital during a 4 year period in the 1950s.

**Slater and Glithero, 1965.**[31] This is a 7 to 11 year follow-up study of ninety-nine inpatients who received the diagnosis of hysteria at the National Hospital in England in 1951, 1953, or 1955. One-third to one-fourth of the diagnoses were made by psychiatrists; the remainder, by neurologists. Histories could be traced for eighty-five of the original ninety-nine patients. Of the eighty-five, twelve had died by the time of the study. Follow-up was performed by Slater and Glithero.

**Lewis and Berman, 1965.**[32] This is a retrospective study based on clinical records of all patients whose discharge diagnosis included conversion hysteria when they were released from Wisconsin General Hospital in 1963. There were fifty-seven such patients out of 16,000 discharges. Forty-five of the fifty-seven had had psychiatric consultation. Twelve were diagnosed by internists and neurologists.

**Raskin, Talbott, and Meyerson, 1966.**[33] This is a prospective study of fifty patients referred from the inpatient and outpatient neurological services of Mount Sinai Hospital and Columbia-Presbyterian Medical Center between August, 1964, and January, 1965, whenever a conversion reaction was considered in the differential diagnosis. "If the presenting problem was primarily pain or seizures the patient was excluded because of the difficulty in making a definitive diagnosis in such cases." The study is a comparison between thirty-two patients who were diagnosed as having conversion reactions and seven who had organic illness. Eight patients whose conditions were still undiagnosed and three patients who had hysterical elaborations of organic pathology were not included in the study. Each patient was interviewed for 1 to 4 hours by one of the investigators.

**McKegney, 1967.**[2] This is a retrospective study based on clinical records of all patients who received a diagnosis of conversion reaction when they were seen in formal psychiatric consultation between June 30, 1964, and June 30, 1966, at the Yale-New Haven Medical Center. Of 1,052 patients seen in psychiatric consultation, 144 received the diagnosis of conversion reaction. These were all inpatients, almost all of whom were referred by the medical or surgical services. All consultations were initially performed by nine advanced psychiatric residents and one staff psychiatrist.

**Barnett, 1971.**[17] This is a retrospective study based on clinical records of forty-six patients with conversion reactions and sixty-three patients with psychophysiological symptoms who were seen in consultation by second- and third-year psychiatric residents in 1967 or 1968.

**Stefansson, Messina, and Meyerowitz, 1976.**[4] The data presented in this paper were derived from records of sixty-four patients hospitalized between 1960 and 1969 on medical, surgical, and gynecological services of a university hospital and diagnosed by third-year psychiatric residents as having conversion or probable conversion symptoms.

Of these eleven studies, four provide follow-up data,[26,28,31,33] seven provide data on hysterical phenomena based on retrospective chart review,[*] and one is a prospective study of hysterical symptoms based on direct patient examination.[33] In the eleven studies care is variously

---

*See references 1, 2, 4, 12, 17, 27, 29, 30, and 32.

provided in medical or psychiatric settings and diagnosis of conversion reaction is made variously by a neurologist, internist, psychiatrist, or psychiatric resident.

**Absence of an organic cause for the symptom**

The first criterion for the diagnosis of conversion hysteria is the absence of organic pathology to explain the symptom. Since the hysterical process can mimic any organic process and can affect any part of the nervous system, such a criterion may be difficult to document. The diagnostician can be more confident when there is "inconsistency with the somatic process"[15]; that is, when the motor or sensory pathways affected do not follow the neurological pathways, but rather follow the patient's perconceived notions about how the human body functions. For neurological symptoms, DeJong[34] has reviewed the various behavioral observations and clinical tests that may be used in the examination of suspected cases of hysteria.

The responsibility for a careful medical work-up rests with the referring physician. The psychiatrist's interest and knowledge about diagnostic procedures, however, provide insurance that the patient has received appropriate medical scrutiny, particularly when the referral is made in part as a result of the referring physician's frustration with unsuccessful treatment or because of the patient's unpleasant personality.

All clinicians who make the diagnosis of conversion hysteria should be humbled by several follow-up studies that indicate that an original diagnosis of hysteria is frequently in error. Of Slater and Glithero's seventy-three patients, twenty-two (30%) were later found to have organic disease that was missed at the time of admission. These include duodenal and gallbladder disease, Takayashu syndrome, meningitis serosa circumscripta, cortical atrophy, presenile dementia, generalized vascular disease, old brain injury, epilepsy, renal carcinoma, and brainstem angioma. Of Gatfield and Guze's twenty-four patients five (21%) were later found to have organic illness that included tabes, degenerative neurological disease, basal ganglia disease, brain tumor, and dementia. Of Ziegler and Paul's sixty-six patients, five (8%) were later found to have epilepsy. In addition, nine of twenty-two (41%) patients who subsequently became psychotic had a childhood history of rheumatic fever, chorea, or influenza, whereas one of twenty-two (5%) patients interviewed by the authors and found not to be psychotic had a similar history. These findings suggest the possibility that organic brain disease was a factor in the etiology of the more seriously ill group. In the study of Stefansson, Messina, and Meyerowitz, eight of sixty-four (13%) patients diagnosed as having conversion reactions were subsequently found to have organic disease including brain tumor, ureter stone, and cancer of the pancreas. In the study of Raskin, Talbott, and Meyerson, of fifty patients initially referred with the possibility of conversion reaction, seven (14%) were suffering from organic pathology that included cerebrovascular accident, brain tumor, dystonia musculorum deformans, multiple sclerosis, phenothiazine reaction, and transverse myelopathy. From these studies, it may be concluded that of all hospitalized patients who receive a diagnosis of conversion reaction, from 13% to 30% will be patients with misdiagnosed organic illness.

Three factors may account for these missed diagnoses:

1. The initial examination may have been incomplete.

2. In its early stages, the organic lesion may have produced symptoms either atypical of the organic process or not associated with other symptoms necessary to establish the diagnosis. Some of the transitory symptoms of early multiple sclerosis are an example.

3. An organic disease may have released hysterical reactions or general disturbances in personality that may be called "hysterical."[31,35]

To complicate matters further, there is a high incidence of concomitant organic disease in hospitalized patients who receive a diagnosis of conversion reaction; that is, the organic disease and the conversion reaction exist side by side. A common example is the patient with epilepsy who also has conversion seizures. In Slater and Glithero's sample, nineteen of eighty-five (22%) patients had both conversion reactions and organic disease. Whitlock[36] found that 62.5% of the patients with hysterical symptoms suffered from significant coexisting or preceding brain disorder as compared to 5.5% of the patients in the control group. The presence of organic illness, therefore, provides no assurance that there is no conversion reaction. Conversely, the presence of a conversion reaction provides no assurance that there is not an organic condition.

Relative assurance that the symptom cannot be explained on an organic basis is insufficient to establish the diagnosis of conversion reaction. This is not a diagnosis of exclusion. The psychiatric consultant needs to establish a combination of several positive findings in the categories that follow to increase the certainty of correct diagnosis.

**Previous conversion reactions, undiagnosable physical symptoms, Briquet syndrome**

An important criterion for the diagnosis of conversion reaction is a previous history of conversion reactions or incapacitating physical symptoms without organic cause. When such patients have multiple symptoms in a frequency and combination that meet the criteria for Briquet syndrome, the chances of the symptoms in question being a conversion reaction become much greater. In Raskin's study,[33] twenty-six of thirty-two (81%) patients with conversion reactions had a previous history of multiple somatic symptoms involving various organ systems, in contrast to two of seven (29%) patients whose symptoms were organic in origin. Nineteen of the thirty-two patients with conversion reactions had enough concomitant symptoms to warrant a diagnosis of "hysteria" (Briquet syndrome) or a partial form of this syndrome. Only one of the seven patients with organic disease had "hysteria." In Gatfield and Guze's[28] sample of twenty-four patients, five of the ten patients who initially appeared to have conversion reactions but did not fall into the "hysteria–possible hysteria group" turned out to have a neurological disorder or dementia. None of the fourteen patients with "hysteria–possible hysteria" developed organic disease. Perley and Guze suggest on the basis of previous work that if a diagnosis of "hysteria" is established, "no other explanation for the presenting symptoms is likely to develop in about 90% of the cases."[37]

The empirical data described suggest that the presence of a Briquet syndrome (or partial Briquet syndrome) or a previous history of conversion reactions is an important diagnostic criterion of conversion reaction.

**Associated psychopathology**

The incidence of concomitant psychiatric pathology in patients with conversion hysteria is so great that its presence is supportive of the diagnosis. In Lewis and Berman's fifty-seven patients, four were addicts, twelve suffered from depression, ten had anxiety reactions, four were sociopathic, and eight were schizophrenic or schizoid. These diagnoses accounted for thirty-eight patients (67%).[32] In Ziegler and Paul's follow-up of sixty-six patients, twenty-two (33%) had a subsequent diagnosis of psychosis upon readmission to a psychiatric hospital. Of the twenty-two, there were twelve diagnosed cases of schizophrenia, nine of manic-depression, and one "psychosis with psychopathic personality."[26] In Stephen and Kamp's study of 100 patients, eight were thought to have an underlying psychotic condition, three not thought to be schizophrenic were later admitted to a state hospital with a diagnosis of schizophrenia, and thirty-nine were believed to be depressed even though depression was not considered the primary difficulty. Of the thirty-nine depressed patients, two were subsequently admitted to a state hospital for depressive psychosis and one received private treatment for depression but committed suicide.[29] Of the original 100 patients, then, fifty had some concomitant psychopathology (total 50%).[29] Of Ziegler and Imboden's 134 patients, fifty-nine (44%) suffered from concomitant psychiatric conditions—forty from depression and nineteen from incipient schizophrenia. In the depressed group, the depressive features were usually overshadowed by the conversion reaction.[30] Of McKegney's 144 patients, thirty-two (22%) suffered from overt depression and fifty-one (35%) from covert depression.[2] Of Slater's group of eighty-five patients with conversion hysteria, four committed suicide. Of his thirty-two patients still alive and showing no evidence of organic disease, two developed schizophrenia, eight "have shown themselves liable to cyclothymic depression," and one had a severe depressive illness.[31]

Barnett found psychosis in 11% and neurosis in 28% of his cases.[17] Finally, in the Stefansson study, thirty-two (50%) were described as depressed.[4]

Based on these studies, the conclusion can be drawn that hospitalized patients with a diagnosis of conversion hysteria will be diagnosed as having schizophrenia or depressive illness in 33% to 50% of the cases. Follow-up will show incidence of psychiatric hospitalization and suicide well above normal. The presence of other psychiatric illness is, therefore, strongly supportive of the diagnosis of conversion reaction.

### Symptom model

It is generally believed that patients unconsciously model conversion symptoms on their own previous illnesses or on the illnesses of significant figures in their lives, usually from childhood.

In support of this, Barnett found that 61% of the conversion patients reflected either a similar organic illness ar a similar illness in the immediate childhood family.[17] In Raskin's prospective study, which included thirty-two patients with conversion reactions, five of the patients with conversion reactions had exact models in significant figures, six patients had previous histories of physical disease mimicked by the conversion reaction, and two patients had important life experiences involving the affected body part.[33] Lewis and Berman noted only two of fifty-three cases where identification with a significant person was mentioned.

A model for the conversion reaction, therefore, is probably a useful diagnostic criterion.

### Emotional stress prior to the onset of symptoms

Emotional stress prior to the onset of the symptom is believed by most investigators to be a necessary, but not sufficient, criterion for the diagnosis of conversion hysteria. Engel[15] points out that the patient with conversion reactions is usually oblivious to any relationship between the symptom and life events. Conversely, a patient's insistence on a psychic origin for the symptom strongly favors an organic cause.

Despite the common agreement as to the importance of past events, there is only one study attempting to document this. In Raskin's prospective study, twenty-six of the twenty-eight (93%) patients with conversion reactions had precipitating stresses, whereas two of the seven (29%) patients with organic illness had precipitating stresses.[33] The judgment of stress was based on a detailed psychiatric history that examined the interplay between the nature of the stress and its complications, past responses to stress, and changes in the patient's life situation that undermined the usual defenses. Emotional stresses included immediate or impending object losses, increased burdens such as caring for invalid relatives, impending marriages or increasing sexual intimacy, intense family battles, childbirth, and threat of lawsuit.

On the basis of available data, emotional stress prior to the onset of symptoms may be a useful diagnostic criterion. Further studies are required.

### Hysterical personality

In the study of Raskin, Talbott, and Meyerson[33], the investigators used the American Psychiatric Association diagnostic manual[21] and the criteria of Chodoff and Lyons[27] to assess the presence of hysterical personality. In their sample of thirty-two patients with conversion reactions, ten had hysterical personalities and an additional six had a mixed hysterical-obsessive personality (total 50%). Three of seven (43%) of the patients with organic diseases had hysterical personalities. Stephens and Kamp[29] found nine of 100 (9%) patients with conversion reactions to be hysterical and an additional fourteen to be emotionally unstable. In Lewis and Berman's[32] series of fifty-seven cases more than 50% were diagnosed as having hysterical personality disorders. Chodoff and Lyons[27] found three (18%) hysterical personality disorders in seventeen patients with conversion reactions, while Barnett[17] found that 7% of the patients with conversion reactions had a hysterical personality.

On the basis of the studies described, the presence of the hysterical personality is of no value in the diagnosis of conversion reactions.

## La belle indifférence

The importance of la belle indifférence as a diagnostic criterion of conversion reactions is agreed in most clinical papers on the subject. Raskin, Talbott, and Meyerson,[33] in the only controlled prospective study, found la belle indifférence in thirteen of thirty-two (41%) patients with conversion reactions as compared to three of seven (43%) patients with organic illness. In Lewis and Berman's[32] retrospective study they found indifference to symptoms mentioned in the records of only four of fifty-seven (7%) cases. In many more cases, they point out, just the opposite was present. The patients were deeply interested in their ailments.

It may be concluded on the basis of the available data that la belle indifférence is of no value in the diagnosis of conversion reactions.

## Symptom as symbolism (primary gain)

"The primary gain refers to the effectiveness of the conversion symptom in providing a satisfactory symbolic expression for the repressed wishes."[15] The symbolic nature of the symptom, then, is supposedly at the heart of the syndrome, and in this regard the conversion reaction differs fundamentally from the psychophysiological condition.

Limited empirical data do not unequivocally support the value of the symptom as symbolism in establishing a diagnosis of conversion reaction. Raskin and investigators say they "did not feel that they had sufficient data to draw conclusions about the symbolic content."[33] Lewis and Berman "found not a single instance in which the physician described a symptom and expressed directly what he thought it symbolized. . . .Thus, for ordinary diagnostic purposes, the criterion of symbolism seems of little utility."[32] In Barnett's study, on the other hand, 22% of the conversion patients showed clear primary gain and 15% showed clear symbolism, whereas of the psychophysiological patients 3% showed clear primary gain and 0% clear symbolism.[17]

The empirical data on the value of the symptom as symbolism or primary gain is mixed and further study is required.

## Symptom as communication (secondary gain)

Raskin, Talbott, and Meyerson found that both conversion and organic symptoms had secondary gain. Thirty-one of thirty-two patients with conversion symptoms and all seven of the patients with organic conditions demonstrated secondary gain.[33] Lewis and Berman's survey indicates that "clearcut manipulation of the environment via the symptom is by no means an omnipresent feature of cases diagnosed as conversion hysteria, even in those cases diagnosed as having hysterical personalities."[32] Barnett, on the other hand, found that 74% of the patients with conversion reactions showed clear secondary gain in contrast to 27% of the patients with psychophysiological illness.[17]

The empirical data on the value of secondary gain in establishing the diagnosis of conversion reactions are mixed and require further study.

## Disturbed sexuality

Disturbed sexuality is not generally used to diagnose conversion hysteria, partly because there are few empirical data on the relationship between hysteria and disturbed sexuality and partly because contemporary interest in hysteria is in the nonsexual areas. However, the findings of Lewis and Berman[32] that "6 of the 46 women had overt, unmistakable incestual experiences or conflicts, and five more had such problems so near the surface that little inference was necessary to find them. . ." and that "the males in our series appeared no less preoccupied with sexual and oedipal problems than the females" cannot be ignored. Barnett found three patients (7%) with conversion reactions who reported sexual seduction in childhood. My own clinical experience is consistent with Lewis and Berman's findings. The importance of disturbed sexuality for the diagnosis of conversion reactions deserves further empirical study.

## Sibling position

Sibling position, like disturbed sexuality, is not commonly used to support the diagnosis of conversion hysteria. Two studies, however, suggest that it might be useful diagnostically. Ziegler, Imboden, and Meyer[1] found that patients with conversion reactions are the youngest child in the family or the youngest child of the same sex 35% more often than would have been predicted by chance. Patients in these family positions are said to be more apt to be immature and dependent, two traits ascribed to patients with conversion hysteria. Stephens and Kamp report similar findings.[29] Barnett, however, found patients with conversion reactions to be the youngest in the family equally as often as patients with psychophysiological reactions.

The value of sibling position for the diagnosis of conversion reaction deserves further study.

## MANAGEMENT

There are only a few authors who suggest guidelines or provide clinical anecdotes on the treatment process. Most authors choose not to discuss treatment or to relegate such a discussion to a brief afterthought. When treatment is discussed, recommendations range from psychoanalysis to the acknowledgment that no treatment is effective. Three reasons for this state of affairs are:

1. The preoccupation with the conceptual confusion over hysterical phenomena has distracted clinicians from studying the treatment process.
2. There may be a particular lack of success in engaging and treating many patients with conversion reactions.
3. Patients suffering from conversion reactions form a very heterogeneous group including "normal" individuals with transient conversion reactions, patients with Briquet syndrome, patients who are severely depressed or who are schizophrenic, and patients involved in cases of financial compensation.

Acknowledging the limited information about management and treatment, I will review the recommendations of others and share some of my own experiences.*

### Establishing or suggesting the diagnosis

In suggesting the probability or even the possibility of a diagnosis of conversion hysteria, the psychiatrist can make a considerable contribution to patient care. Dangerous or expensive diagnostic procedures that may be clinically unnecessary can be postponed, perhaps indefinitely. Further psychiatric evaluation, treatment, contact with hospital staff, or even time itself may be the appropriate intervention. The attending physician is thus relieved of pressure from the patient's family and ward staff to "do something." The psychiatrist also

---

*See references 1, 8, 9, 13, 32, and 38.

supports the attending physician by sharing the responsibility for managing these very difficult patients.

**Working with the hospital staff**

Once it is established or suspected that the patient is suffering from hysterical phenomenon and not from organic disease, the hospital staff is apt to respond in nontherapeutic ways. Often, even prior to the psychiatric consultation, the patient's behavior is provocative, demanding, shallow, manipulative, phony, unreasonable, bitchy, or childish. The psychiatrist can be helpful (1) by calling attention to the patient's premorbid strengths and by explaining the regressive nature of the behavior, (2) by explaining the cultural determinants of the behavior—if there are any, (3) by explaining the dynamics of the symptom, showing how, given the patient's background, social situation, and psychological resources, this is the only possible response—maladaptive as it is, (4) by providing a behavioral analysis for the staff, defining the pathological events, the antecedent and reinforcing conditions, and possible therapeutic interventions, (5) by involving the staff in treatment strategies, and (6) by providing support for the staff in dealing with their day-to-day frustrations while providing therapy for the patient regardless of their feelings.[8]

**Specific interventions**

The type and effectiveness of the intervention vary considerably from patient to patient. Patients for whom psychiatric help is apt to be most effective are those with a good premorbid adjustment, few if any conversion reactions in the past, good object relations, an obvious and traumatic stress, distress over symptoms, and accessibility to feelings. Patients who reject psychiatric care and for whom it is of little value are those with long histories of hysterical symptoms (some of whom meet the criteria for Briquet syndrome) that have effectively controlled those around them and that perhaps entitle them to some kind of compensation or pension.

Cadoret and King,[38] in discussing treatment for the group least amenable to treatment, encourage support of the patient and family by the family physician in an attempt to prevent the complications of frequent surgical operations, drug dependence, marital separation or divorce, and suicide attempts. They note that few patients with conversion reactions who are referred to a psychiatrist persist with treatment. Patients and their families can be supported by knowing what to expect and which symptoms are not medically serious.

Ziegler, Imboden, and Meyer[1] noted a great deal of refractoriness to psychotherapy in their patients who continued to insist that their problems were neither emotional nor psychological. Attempts to convince the patients otherwise resulted in their seeking help elsewhere. The investigators believe there is greater success with those who accept psychiatric hospital treatment.

McKegney referred 31% of those patients with diagnosed conversion reactions for outpatient psychotherapy. It was his impression that most patients did not follow through with this plan.

Behavioral techniques may constitute a useful approach for certain populations.[39-41] Research in this area is promising.

My own experience with patients who have conversion reactions less deeply entrenched is similar to that of Rabkin.[13] The psychiatric consultant works somewhat obliquely, talking about the patient's life situation without hinting at a confrontation over the symptom. An adversarial relationship must be avoided. The patient cannot be expected to say, "You are right. It is all in my mind." I tell the patients I do not know what is causing their symptom, but that I would like to get to know them and understand their situation. During the course of the subsequent psychodynamic interview, I listen for the possible meaning of the symptom as symbolism, as social communication, as a way of dealing with unbearable affect. It may be useful to help the patients verbalize directly what they have been unable to express except through their bodies and bear whatever affects have been intolerable. If the patient is asking symbolically for particular social responses such as caring, it might be useful to meet with the family or ward staff so that these needs can be provided. It is the unusual patient who will understand the symptom as part of a recurrent neurotic conflict and will then want to pursue intensive psychotherapy.

The following case report illustrates some of these therapeutic issues.

**History.** The patient was a 32-year-old married mother of two who suffered from multiple sclerosis. She was referred by her neurologist for psychiatric evaluation. The specific problem was her inability to move her legs, for which there was no clear neurological reason. At the time of referral, the patient had been hospitalized on a neurology ward for 3 weeks.

The patient had been ill for 6 years, beginning soon after her husband returned from Vietnam. She noticed falling, impaired vision, a speech impediment, and "looking like a lush and a dope addict." The patient stated, nevertheless, that she had nothing to complain about, was lucky to be able to rely on herself, and considered herself a wealthy individual. She never discussed her illness with her husband and avoided accepting help from husband, children, relatives, or friends. She felt she had done a good job with her illness and that she deserved a "gold star." Her most difficult moments were related to her loss of function over simple activities such as writing a check. She dealt with her tensions by crying alone or by banging her head against the wall. There was no clear psychological precipitating event prior to the paralysis except a case of flu that lasted 1 month and that sapped some of her energy.

The patient had been married 13 years. Her husband, a pipe fitter and plumber, was described in glowing terms. Her children, ages 12 and 13, were bright and, like the husband, were said to be wonderful people.

The patient was reared by her paternal grandparents for the first 4 years of her life while her mother was hospitalized with catatonic schizophrenia. From 4 to 13 years of age the patient stayed in a convent where she learned to rely on only herself. At 13 years of age she began to live with her parents only to find that her father had cancer. He died 2 years later. Her father, whom she "adored," also taught her to be independent. Her mother was considered a "leech," a weak, demanding person. The mother did not speak to the patient for 2 years until the patient's current hospitalization.

**Intervention.** After initially expressing concern that she would give me a headache, grief, or aggravation by talking about herself, the patient relaxed and rather enjoyed my inquiry into the story of her illness and her life. She was particularly relieved when I reassured her that she wasn't schizophrenic, but rather neurotic like the rest of us. I gently probed into her superindependent posture, and she made it clear that this area was not to be tampered with. I also sensed that she would be outraged if I were to suggest that there was a psychological cause for her paralysis. After this visit, I urged the nursing staff to be particularly supportive to her. We met for a second visit the next day, at which time the patient freely talked with appropriate affect about her difficult life. Near the end of the hour she said she believed the paralysis was lifting and that she would be able to walk again within 2 to 3 days. Her prognosis was correct.

This was a woman of considerable psychological strength who had overcome many obstacles to be able to marry, rear children, and achieve happiness. She had learned to be independent through the lessons of her father and her nine years in the convent, where normal dependence was not rewarded. Being given to or being cared for reminded her of her mother, who behaved in a child-like, demanding, unacceptable way. Her independence and need to be strong, together with her relative social isolation (no siblings, no grandparents, unavailable mother), made her neurological illness difficult to bear. I speculated that she was particularly overwhelmed just prior to the paralysis and that her symptom was, unconsciously, her only way of calling for help and accepting some caring. Her warm acceptance of my two interviews and her acceptance of my name and telephone number should she wish more interviews after discharge was indirect evidence of her need to have someone be interested in her without demanding anything in return or forcing her to acknowledge her need. Once her dependent needs were satisfied, she could relinquish the symptom.

## CONCLUSION
### Hysterical phenomena

Most clinicians would have no difficulty in distinguishing conversion reactions from any of the other phenomena that are sometimes referred to as hysterical if the concepts were clearly defined. The distinction between hysterical phenomena is, in fact, so clear and their relationship to one another is so tenuous that one wonders why they are or have been referred to as hysterical. The reasons, I believe, are primarily historical. I agree with Chodoff that "the diagnosis has become a balloon filled with air rather than substance. . .It is a fossil encrusted with and obscured by successive layers of meaning."[11] The clinician, however, must know history so as not to be bewildered and confused by it. For clinical purposes each of the hysterical phenomena should be considered as a distinct clinical phenomenon.

In the April 15, 1977, draft of DSM-III,[42] the five conditions described in this chapter as "hysterical" are no longer referred to as hysterical. Hysterical psychosis is now "brief reactive psychosis"; hysterical personality is now "histrionic personality disorder"; hysteria (Briquet syndrome) is now "somatization disorder (Briquet syndrome)"; hysterical neurosis, dissociative type, is now "dissociative disorder"; and hysterical neurosis, conversion type, is now "conversion disorder."

### Differential diagnosis of conversion reaction

Based on current knowledge, the diagnosis of conversion reaction for an unexplained physical symptom is most probable when (1) a careful medical examination reveals or suggests no organic process to explain the symptom, (2) there is a previous history of conversion reactions, undiagnosable physical symptoms, or Briquet syndrome, and (3) there is associated psychopathology, especially depression, schizophrenia, or incipient psychosis. Symptom model and emotional stress prior to the onset of symptom may be useful criteria. Hysterical personality, la belle indifférence, symptom as symbolism (primary gain), symptom as communication (secondary gain), disturbed sexuality, and sibling position do not appear to be useful diagnostic criteria. The psychiatric consultant must take into account that even when careful medical examination suggests no organic disease, in a significant number of cases an organic process will become evident in the future. The presence of coexisting organic process does not rule out the possibility of a conversion reaction.

Of the presumed criteria for the diagnosis of conversion reactions, the most useful (previous conversion reactions or Briquet syndrome and associated psychopathology) are unrelated to the psychodynamic literature on hysteria. Of the criteria for the diagnosis of conversion reactions derived from theories about hysteria, only two (symptom model and prior emotional stress) may be valid according to available empirical data.

There are two possible explanations for these findings. The first is that current theory about conversion reactions and the derivative diagnostic criteria are invalid. The second is that the current theory, for the most part, is sound and the derivative diagnostic criteria are valid, but the research design has been inadequate to assess validation.

In support of the second explanation, there are considerable limitations to the empirical studies described in this chapter.

1. The studies are few.
2. Most studies are retrospective and based on chart review. The frequency of la belle indifférence, hysterical personality, primary gain, or secondary gain cannot be assessed by reviewing a chart written by someone who may not have been interested in these aspects of the patient's pathology or personality.
3. The assessments of the patients are performed by clinicians of varying degrees of experience and with varying prejudices as to what phenomena ought to be associated with conversion reactions.
4. For the most part, assessments of variables such as hysterical personality, depression, and la belle indifférence are not operationally defined.
5. Most of the studies do not use a control group. Even if the percentage of patients with conversion reactions who have hysterical personalities is known, the psychiatric consultant needs to know the percentage of hysterical personalities in a

control group of persons with organic disease, psychophysiological reactions, or no illness (depending on the hypothesis to be tested).

It is my own judgment, based on clinical experience with patients with conversion reactions and on research experience successfully validating psychoanalytical concepts by nonpsychoanalytical techniques,[22,23] that the theory about conversion reactions and the derivative diagnostic criteria is, for the most part, valid. Its clinical usefulness, however, is considerably limited without reliable operational definitions of the variables in question and without unequivocal research support for their validity in distinguishing conversion reactions from other clinical conditions. There are over ten articles on the clinical and conceptual aspects of conversion reactions for every empirical study. The time has come for a shift in emphasis.

## REFERENCES

1. Ziegler, F. J., Imboden, J. B., and Meyer, E.: Contemporary conversion reactions: a clinical study, Am. J. Psychiatry **116:**901-910, 1960.
2. McKegney, F. P.: The incidence and characteristics of patients with conversion reactions. I: A general hospital consultation service sample, Am. J. Psychiatry **124:**542-545, 1967.
3. Brownsberger, C. N.: Hysteria—a common phenomenon, Am. J. Psychiatry **123:**110, 1966.
4. Stefansson, J. G., Messina, J. A., and Meyerowitz, S.: Hysterical neurosis, conversion type: clinical and epidemiological considerations, Acta Psychiatr. Scand. **53:**119-138, 1976.
5. Lipowski, Z. J., and Kiriakos, R. Z.: Borderlands between neurology and psychiatry: observations in a neurological hospital, Psychiatry Med. **3:** 131-147, 1972.
6. Cleghorn, R. A.: Hysteria—multiple manifestations of semantic confusion, Can. Psychiatr. Assoc. J. **14:**539-551, 1969.
7. Lazare, A.: The hysterical character in psychoanalytical theory: evolution and confusion, Arch. Gen. Psychiatry **25:**131-137, 1971.
8. Lewis, W. C.: Hysteria: the consultant's dilemma—twentieth century demonology, pejorative epithet, or useful diagnosis?, Arch. Gen. Psychiatry **30:**145-151, 1974.
9. Nemiah, J. C.: Hysterical neurosis, conversion type. In Freedman, A. M., Kaplan, H. I., and Sadock, B. J., editors: Comprehensive textbook of psychiatry, vol. I, ed. 2, Baltimore, 1975, The Williams & Wilkins Co., pp. 1208-1220.
10. Rangell, L.: The nature of conversion, J. Am. Psychoanal. Assoc. **7:**632-662, 1959.
11. Chodoff, P.: The diagnosis of hysteria: an overview, Am. J. Psychiatry **131:**1073-1078, 1974.
12. Ziegler, F. J., and Imboden, J. B.: Contemporary conversion reactions, Arch. Gen. Psychiatry **6:**37-45, 1962.

13. Rabkin, R.: Conversion hysteria as social maladaptation, Psychiatry **27**:349-363, 1964.
14. Szasz, T.: The myth of mental illness, New York, 1961, Harper & Row, Publishers.
15. Engel, G.: Conversion symptoms. In McBride, C. M., editor: Philadelphia, 1970, J. B. Lippincott Co., pp. 650-668.
16. Engel, G.: A reconsideration of the role of conversion in somatic disease, Compr. Psychiatry **9**:316, 1968.
17. Barnett, C.: Conversion reactions and psychophysiologic disorders: a comparative study, Psychiatry Med. **2**:205-220, 1971.
18. Cameron, N.: Personality development and psychopathology: a dynamic approach, Boston, 1962, Houghton Mifflin Co., chap. 10.
19. Guze, S. B., and Perley, M. J.: Observations on the natural history of hysteria, Am. J. Psychiatry **119**:960-965, 1963.
20. Guze, S. B.: The validity and significance of the clinical diagnosis of hysteria (Briquet's syndrome), Am. J. Psychiatry **132**:138-141, 1975.
21. Diagnostic and statistical manual of mental disorders, vol. II, New York, 1968, American Psychiatric Association.
22. Lazare, A., Klerman, G. L., and Armor, D. J.: Oral, obsessive, and hysterical personality patterns: an investigation of psychoanalytic concepts by means of factor analysis, Arch. Gen. Psychiatry **14**:624-630, 1966.
23. Lazare, A., Klerman, G. L., and Armor, D. J.: Oral, obsessive, and hysterical personality patterns: replication of factor analysis in an independent sample, J. Psychiatr. Res. **7**:275-290, 1970.
24. Hollender, M. H., and Hirsch, S. J.: Hysterical psychosis, Am. J. Psychiatry **120**:1066-1074, 1964.
25. Hirsch, S. J., and Hollender, M. H.: Hysterical psychosis: clarification of the concept, Am. J. Psychiatry **125**:909-915, 1969.
26. Ziegler, G. K., and Paul, N.: On the natural hysteria in women: follow-up study of twenty years after hospitalization, Dis. Nerv. Syst. **15**:301-306, 1954.
27. Chodoff, P., and Lyons, H.: Hysteria, the hysterical personality and "hysterical conversion", Am. J. Psychiatry **114**:734-740, 1958.
28. Gatfield, P. D., and Guze, S. B.: Prognosis and differential diagnosis of conversion reactions: a follow-up study, Dis. Nerv. Syst. **23**:623-631, 1962.
29. Stephens, J. H., and Kamp, M.: On some aspects of hysteria: a clinical study, J. Nerv. Ment. Dis. **134**:305-315, 1962.
30. Ziegler, F., Imboden, J., and Rodgers, D.: Contemporary conversion reactions. III: diagnostic considerations, J.A.M.A. **186**:307-311, 1963.
31. Slater, E., and Glithero, E.: Follow-up of patients diagnosed as suffering from "Hysteria," J. Psychosom. Res. **9**:9-13, 1965.
32. Lewis, W. D., and Berman, M.: Studies of conversion hysteria. I: operational study of diagnosis, Arch. Gen. Psychiatry **13**:275-282, 1965.
33. Raskin, M., Talbott, J. A., and Meyerson, A. T.: Diagnosed conversion reactions, J.A.M.A. **197**:530-534, 1966.
34. DeJong, R. N.: The neurological examination, ed. 3, New York, 1967, Harper & Row, Publishers.
35. Merskey, H., and Buhrick, N. A.: Hysteria and organic brain disease, Br. J. Med. Psychol. **48**:359-366, 1975.

36. Whitlock, F. A.: The aetiology of hysteria, Acta Psychiatr. Scand. **43:**144-162, 1967.
37. Perley, M. J., and Guze, S. B.: Hysteria: the stability and usefulness of clinical criteria, N. Engl. J. Med. **266:**421-426, 1962.
38. Cadoret, R. J., and King, L. T.: Psychiatry in primary care, St. Louis, 1974, The C. V. Mosby Co.
39. Dickes, R.: Brief therapy of conversion reactions: an in-hospital technique, Am. J. Psychiatry **131:**584-586, 1974.
40. Kass, D., Silvers, F., and Abrams, G.: Behavioral group treatment of hysteria, Arch. Gen. Psychiatry **26:**42-50, 1972.
41. Hersen, M., Gullick, E. L., Matherne, P. M., and Harbert, T. L.: Instructions and reinforcement in the modification of a conversion reaction, Psychol. Rep. **31:**719-722, 1972.
42. The Task Force on Nomenclature and Statistics: Diagnostic and statistical manual of mental disorders, vol. III, New York, April 15, 1977, The American Psychiatric Association.

# 8

# Extreme manifestations of anxiety in the general hospital: phobic states, obsessive-compulsive neurosis, and anxiety neurosis

DAVID V. SHEEHAN

Anxiety and fear spare no human faced with danger. While examining anxious patients, physicians recall their own experience with anxiety and use it as a model to provide help and comfort. "Remove the threat and the adaptive anxiety response will pass" is the well-worn strategy for coping with normal response-to-danger anxiety. However, there exists a group of distinct anxiety syndromes that are not mere exaggerations of normal response-to-danger anxiety, but are quite beyond the experience of normal people. They are devastatingly intense and crippling. They have a bewildering array of presentations. As ubiquitous mimics of medical illness, they invite the physician to frequent and costly examinations. The final reward is usually puzzlement and helplessness for the physician and, for the patient, a reassurance-tranquilizer package and guilty embarrassment at being misunderstood. Approximately 10% to 15% of all patients seen in general medical practice are recurrently anxious, hypochondriacal, hysterical, obsessive, or fearful. They are rarely calmed and are always and at all hours in need of attention. The physician's frustration is compounded by the patient's insistence that the anxiety is often without apparent source—occurring spontaneously for no good reason—and is therefore all the more frightening. In the past decade psychiatry has made significant strides toward delineating these common syndromes more precisely and toward treating the symptoms effectively without resorting to traditional animistic theories that explain all but help none.

## PHOBIC STATES

The best known manifestations of extreme anxiety are the phobic states. A phobia is defined as a fear that is out of proportion to the situation, is beyond voluntary control, cannot be rationalized, and leads to avoidance of the feared stimulus.

### Significance

The total incidence of phobias in the general population is 76.9 per 1,000 people. Of these, 2.2 per 1,000 are severely disabled.[1] The incidence of phobia as a main complaint in psychiatric practice is 2% to 4%.[2] Approximately 10% of the patients seen in general practice have phobic anxiety even when this is not the main presenting symptom.

### Classification and definition

The purpose of any classification system is to organize phenomena into groups with common attributes. In psychiatry the disorders that make up a group might have symptoms, signs, pathophysiology, and a similar response to treatment in common. Several methods for classifying phobias exist ranging from the literary trend of assigning long names derived from classical Greek to every type of phobic situation to the more modern scientific classification of Marks.[2] Marks classifies phobias by differences in clinical picture, demography, psychophysiological response, and psychological testing.

Following Marks' method and guided by the principle of finding an effective treatment regimen for each patient, psychiatrists may classify phobic states as (1) phobic anxiety state (agoraphobia, illness phobia, and polyphobia), (2) social phobia (fear restricted to social activities, that is, eating, vomiting, writing in public), and (3) specific mono-symptomatic phobias. These three groups require different treatment approaches.

#### Phobic anxiety state (agoraphobia, illness phobia, polyphobia)

*Definition.* The term "agoraphobia" was first used by Westphal[3] in 1871 to describe fears of being in public places—for example, streets or shops. The term derives from the Greek root "agora" meaning a place of assembly. Many other fears are usually present, but this is the most constant and disabling in the constellation of clinical features. Knowing a patient is frightened of crowded places or leaving home helps predict that other symptoms will be present like fear of fainting or losing control, panic attacks, depersonalization, exhaustion, obsessions, and a multiple of anxiety symptoms. This syndrome has received many labels, notably anxiety hysteria,[4] phobic-anxiety-depersonalization syndrome,[5] phobic anxiety state,[6] and panphobic syndrome. Illness phobias are included in this category since they are usually associated with a variety of other anxiety symptoms and with panic attacks that maintain the fear.

Transient concerns that a particular lump or mole is malignant or that a new symptom is a foreboding of a serious illness are common and normal. However, when such fears of illness are persistent and adequate reassurance and explanation does not calm the patient's hypochondriacal concerns, special therapeutic techniques are required to help the patient. Illness phobias may be found as part of many psychiatric disorders, notably depression and schizophrenia. Frequently these illness phobias are part of an anxiety syndrome or agoraphobia. The concerns are usually triggered by anxiety symptoms or panic attacks and become a conditioned response to anxiety.

Although there is no specificity in the precipitating stresses, it is not uncommon to find these patients involved in a mourning process. The type of illness may be dictated by the illness suffered by the lost, loved person. When anxiety symptoms are prevalent, they can be successfully treated like agoraphobia. When illness phobia is circumscribed and without any other associated symptoms, systematic desensitization is the treatment of choice, as in specific phobias.

*Epidemiology.* This most common and distressing phobic disorder makes up approximately two-thirds of all phobic patients seen in hospital practice.[2,7] Of the general population it is estimated that sixty-three people per 1,000[1] have agoraphobia. Women make up two-thirds of these patients.[2]

Agoraphobia usually begins in early adult life. The mean onset age is 24 years.[2,7] Sixty-five percent of these cases begin when the patient is between the ages of 15 and 29. In this respect it differs from specific phobias that begin when the patient is 30 to 40 years of age. Curiously, there is a long delay (often several years) before these patients seek psychiatric treatment. Most first consult their physician for treatment of physical symptoms.

Most studies find that agoraphobic individuals have a stable family background,[2,7] in contrast to sociopathic individuals, for example. Their marriages tend to be stable. On the other hand, the incidence of neurosis among relatives of agoraphobic individuals is significantly higher than in control groups. Agoraphobic patients have high incidence of enuresis, fears, and night terrors as children.[2,7] Agoraphobic individuals are found among all socioeconomic groups, all educational backgrounds, and all premorbid personality types. The role of genetic inheritance in the etiology of agoraphobia is still unresolved. For anxiety states the concordance rate among monozygotic twins is significantly higher than for dizygotic twins.[8,9] However, there is no report in the literature of monozygotic twins concordant for agoraphobia. Nineteen percent of agoraphobic patients have a close relative with agoraphobia.[2,7]

Sexual disorder, especially orgasmic dysfunction, is more common among women who have agoraphobia than among normal controls, but similar in frequency to that found in other neuroses like anxiety neurosis, hysteria, and obsessive-compulsive neurosis.[2] The sexual disorder often antedates the onset of the phobia but may also be secondary to it. Such patients may report that sexual excitement precipitates a panic attack. Subsequent avoidance behavior and fear would hardly be surprising.

*Clinical features.* Most patients identify a major life change, for example, illness, a death, childbirth, or acute stress, as the source of their condition. Some identify a time, such as the anniversary of a loss, when it first started. There is no specificity in events that precipitate phobic disorders, and the events probably act as nonspecific stressors. However, some of these generalized phobias start suddenly for no apparent reason. This observation cannot be lightly dismissed. The presence or absence of a precipitant has little apparent effect on the subsequent course of the disorder.

Agoraphobia has a chronic fluctuating course with periodic exacerbations and incomplete remissions. The onset of phobic behavior may be sudden or slow, but is almost always preceded by panic attacks and anxiety. Usually these patients are suddenly overcome by terrifying anxiety or panic. The patients become faint, with weak, rubbery legs and a nauseous, sinking sensation in the abdomen, as if on the deck of a ship in high seas. The heart may begin to race and thump loudly, the mouth becomes dry, and a lump in the throat gives the sensation of choking. These individuals are unable to catch a breath and have trouble breathing normally; they attempt to compensate by taking rapid, shallow breaths with the result that hyperventilation may follow. Frequently the surroundings seem to fade away or become more distinct. Sometimes everything appears louder and closer than usual. Individuals may tremble all over, and even suffer transient mutism, blindness, paralysis, or paresthesia. These patients usually believe that they are losing control, going insane, or going to die. This unspeakable and unknowable terror may immobilize patients temporarily, but it is usually accompanied by a flight response to a safe place—"I had to drop everything and get away. I wanted to run and run and run until I got away from that feeling." These feelings of acute anxiety last for seconds or minutes. Only rarely do they last hours, and then they are usually repeated short attacks. I have seen cases where several hundred such episodes occurred in a single day. At times the episodes occur without much outward demonstration of distress and patients, often very ashamed of their condition, able to hide such experiences from family and friends for years.

Such episodes often lead patients to medical consultation in the course of which they may collect an impressive array of diagnoses ranging from hypoglycemia to Menière's disease. Physical examinations reveal nothing abnormal and patients are repeatedly dispatched with little reassurance and prescriptions for minor tranquilizers. Repeated panic attacks intensify the hypochondriacal concerns and increase the frequency of physician visits in spite of reassurance.

> One individual visited the hospital emergency room each week for electrocardiography. After months of these repeat performances, he found he had stretched the patience of the interns and was no longer welcome. Then he came each evening and sat on the bench outside the emergency ward so that if the anticipated myocardial infarction occurred, he would have immediate care. Although he had good insight into this behavior and joked about his "seat of safety," it was only after considerable therapeutic effort that he gave it up permanently.

Retreat to a safe place or person often brings relief from the attack. This causes dependency on close friends and relatives. Before avoidance behavior develops, it is not possible to differentiate agoraphobia from anxiety neurosis.

Phobic avoidance begins after a particularly severe panic attack that leaves the patient helpless. The scene of the attack is most often the first situation avoided. Gradually the anxiety attacks and flight responses occur in other situations and quickly new phobias are developed. Sometimes the phobia generalizes until the individual is restricted to one piece of furniture in one room of the house and becomes alarmed outside this narrowly defined limit.

> One patient first developed terrifying panic during a tornado. The fear generalized to tornado watches, then thunderstorms, then dark clouds, and later, any clouds or a bad weather forecast. Eventually, even storms or low pressure systems developing in the Caribbean caused such alarm that the individual had to carry a weather radio

and pressure gauge everywhere. Later this person could not leave the house "just in case," and had to have all windows open, even in icy weather, as a precaution to minimize the damage when the tornado came.

Agoraphobic patients may have years of medical and even psychiatric consultation focusing on one or another aspect of their anxiety state without ever questioning their phobic behavior. Many are frightened of being left alone and need constant company even when they are housebound. Travel is accompanied by elaborate planning and preparation. Subways, trains, tunnels, and crowded traffic particularly must be circumvented. If a route has hospitals, physicians and a friend's home at intervals along the way, or if it allows for rapid escape, it is deemed safer. The aisle seat in a theater or church is always more comfortable for the same reason. Confinement of any kind, for example, in a dentist's or hairdresser's chair, an elevator, or a swimming pool, is intolerable. The corner store is still more popular with agoraphobic individuals than the large supermarket where they fear getting lost or having to wait in line. They find bright lights distressing and are often more comfortable in the dark. Places that are very open, wide, or high, such as highways, parks, squares, and bridges, are especially avoided.

Paradoxically, there are occasionally transient and dramatic switches in phobic behavior. One woman, housebound for 6 years, drove her son to the hospital emergency ward when he suffered a deep laceration and was bleeding heavily. She was surprisingly composed through the episode, but within 24 hours was again housebound.

Most patients carry their "security blankets" with them to provide relief in the event of sudden panic. Smelling salts, small bottles of vodka, and minor tranquilizers are particularly popular. Suddenly finding themselves without this article of security precipitates great alarm. A few patients become transiently alcoholic or addicted to drugs in an attempt to control their anxiety.

Almost any stress can aggravate agoraphobia. Physical illness, confinement to bed, psychological stress, or even loss of practice in going may be followed by increased restriction of activities. Between attacks, chronic tension, low-grade, free-floating anxiety, and anticipatory anxiety are the rule. After the panic attacks, some patients feel exhausted or depleted for hours or days. When willpower and positive motivation do not yield results, depression may set in. Crying spells, hopelessness, early insomnia, helplessness, worthlessness, irritability, and even mild suicidal ideas may emerge. These are associated with deterioration of the agoraphobic condition. However, many of these patients do not report depression, confirming Burton's[10] observation that "some indeed are sad and not fearful; some fearful and not sad; some neither fearful nor sad; but both. . . ."

The incidence of depersonalization and derealization varies in different studies perhaps because of lack of agreement on a precise definition. Forty percent of agoraphobic individuals experience periods of feeling all or some of their bodies or minds do not belong to them. They feel detached, unreal, or outside their surroundings (depersonalization). They may sense things around them as unreal, artificial, or strange (derealization).[2,7] This experience usually lasts seconds or minutes.

Obsessive thoughts such as harming others by stabbing or injuring their children and compulsive rituals such as counting, checking, or washing, are frequent for these phobic patients. Many obsessions are more precisely described as phobias. When obsessions and compusions are severe, the prognosis is poor.

Agoraphobia usually has a chronic fluctuating course with repeated relapses and incomplete remissions. Only 20% of the patients have periods of complete remission from their agoraphobia.[2]

**Social phobias**

*Definition.* The fears of those with social phobias are restricted to social activities such as eating, speaking, writing, drinking, or vomiting in the presence of other people. Unlike agoraphobic individuals, they usually have few associated psychiatric symptoms and little generalized anxiety without any apparent source. Some, however, tend to resemble those with a mild agoraphobia. As a group they are placed between those who have agoraphobia and specific phobia since they possess some of the characteristics of each.

*Epidemiology.* Social phobias make up approximately 8% of all phobias. Approximately two-thirds of the sufferers are women. Social phobias are among the most common phobias in men. They have an age of onset similar to agoraphobia, that is, when the patient is 15 to 30 years old, rarely beginning before puberty or after 40. About 50% have or have had other major psychiatric symptoms like depression or severe anxiety, and almost 20% have an alcoholic or drug addiction problem resulting from their attempts to control their fears. Curiously, in the Maudsley sample of patients with social phobias, many more came from "broken homes" (34%) than did patients with agoraphobias and specific phobias.[2]

*Clinical features.* The onset may be slow and insidious without any one clearcut precipitant, or sudden and swift after a traumatic experience (for example, vomiting at a meal may sensitize the patient to develop a social phobia in this setting). Invitations to eat with friends become a cause for anticipatory anxiety and even elaborate preparations like fasting. Even the arrival of such an invitation in the mail may precipitate terrifying panic. In the feared situation the patient perspires profusely, trembles until unable to hold eating utensils steadily, and feels nausea and constriction in the throat. Food fads develop since certain foods are more likely to precipitate a vomiting attack. Before the meal these persons may carefully explore escape routes and the closest bathroom to the dining area. They engage in extensive catastrophizing thought that serves to aggravate and maintain the symptom. As a result, their social activities become increasingly restricted. Those who are polysymptomatic with more generalized anxiety, panic attacks, or depression, spontaneous fluctuations in galvanic skin response (GSR), and slow habituation may be given the same therapy as agoraphobic patients. Those with circumscribed fears, few associated anxiety symptoms, rapid habituation, and few spontaneous fluctuations in GSR are best given desensitization therapy alone, as are specific phobia patients.

**Specific phobias**

*Definition.* These patients have monosymptomatic phobias with little generalization. They fear a different cluster of items and situations than those with agoraphobia and social phobia. Their fears are restricted to one specific focus. For example, fears of an animal, driving, heights, needles, darkness, physicians, therapy, thunderstorms, or flying are particularly common. These patients have few associated psychiatric symptoms and no generalized anxiety or spontaneous panic attacks.

*Epidemiology.* Although such fears are common in the general population, these individuals request treatment less frequently than those with agoraphobia or social phobia. In general, these phobias, in contrast to agoraphobia, begin before puberty—especially the animal phobias. In children the incidence of these phobias is equal for boys and girls, but by puberty women have the highest incidence.[12] Specific phobia patients tend to come from stable, happy families without many phobias. They are otherwise unremarkable in socioeconomic status, intelligence, education, childhood, or marital adjustment.[2,7]

*Clinical features.* Usually this group has few associated psychiatric symptoms, and no generalized anxiety or spontaneous panic attacks. Traumatic experiences can frequently be identified, although these are at times long lost to memory. Once established, such fears generalize;

for example, a cat phobia may generalize to all furry animals, to furry hats, to anyone who has contact with a cat or cat accessories, or to phonetically related words like bat or rat. Such patients frequently have other minor fears, but, otherwise, their fears are specific and circumscribed.

If the phobic object or situation is common in the person's environment, the disability may be crippling.

> A woman living in California had a terror of earthquakes. After minor tremors she would sleep outside for days and suffer severe insomnia and nightmares. She would very reluctantly agree to live inside again only after consultation with local seismologists. Because she was unable to drive across any geological faults, her movement was restricted. After moving east she suffered no further disability.

The physician is often surprised at the excessive vigilance of these patients. They go to extraordinary lengths to screen for any evidence of the phobic object.

> A 45-year-old man with a severe phobia of needles came to me only after several calls to ensure that no needles were present in the office and that no blood test or physical examination would be required as part of the evaluation procedure. His alarm returned after he noticed a paper on my desk on the use of intramuscular, long-acting, psychotropic drugs.
>
> He had avoided all physician contact for 15 years in the fear that they would recommend hospitalization, ask for blood tests, or brandish a needle during the course of examination. He identified an "assault" by a physician with a needle when he was 10 years old as the original precipitant. Years later, seeing his terminally ill son receive intravenous feeding and frequent injections with pain resulted in a significant intensification of his fears. It was only very reluctantly that he allowed his family to see physicians lest they suffer an injection.
>
> As a result of his avoidance of physicians he had renal stones, intermittent hematuria, dental caries, and gingivitis that resulted in frequent abscesses and loosening of most of his teeth. However, he preferred to suffer chronic pain rather than go to a dentist or be admitted for medical care. He was short of breath, especially at night, and had been told years before that he might get subacute bacterial endocarditis and cardiac valvular damage from his chronic infections. Several prior attempts at treatment with psychotherapy, tranquilizers, and even hypnotherapy, had failed, leaving him discouraged.
>
> Six sessions of systemic desensitization in imagination followed by three sessions of densensitization in vivo with needles brought complete relief and also the possibility for the much-needed medical and dental care. There was no relapse or symptom substitution. Indeed, the patient reported losing peripherally related anxiety, depression, and other psychosomatic symptoms as a consequence of treatment.

## Psychophysiology of phobic states

The psychophysiological differences among those who have agoraphobia, social phobia, or specific phobia have implications for treatment. Agoraphobic individuals who are very anxious and have spontaneous panic attacks show spontaneous fluctuations in GSR.[13] For normal individuals at rest attached to a galvanometer, the tracing is flat and smooth with infrequent small spikes. For agoraphobic individuals at rest, the tracing shows multiple large and small fluctuations—as if the autonomic nervous system were firing spontaneously or in status epilepticus. Individuals with specific phobias do not have spontaneous fluctuations in GSR.[13] Those with social phobias who have panic attacks and generalized anxiety as a group resemble agoraphobic patients, although some with more circumscribed fears do not have spontaneous fluctuations in GSR.[13]

They differ also in habituation response. This measure of GSR determines the rate at which a person's autonomic nervous system becomes accustomed to a novel sound or stimulus. Agoraphobic patients and most social phobic patients with overt anxiety and spontaneous fluctuations in GSR habituate slowly, while individuals with specific phobias, and some with social phobias who have little overt anxiety and no spontaneous fluctuations in GSR habituate rapidly.[13] Systematic desensitization depends on a normal habituation response to be effective. Consequently this treatment is most effective for those who have specific phobias or social phobias with few spontaneous fluctuations and who habituate normally on GSR.[13] Conversely, it works poorly (as does psychotherapy) for those with agoraphobias.[13]

## Treatment

**Insight-oriented psychotherapy and psychoanalysis.** Until 1958, insight-oriented psychotherapy and psychoanalysis were the principal treatments prescribed for phobic disorders. The results were unpredictable and phobias were considered chronic conditions with a poor prognosis. Phobias were believed to be symbolic displacements of underlying fears or unresolved conflicts.[14] It was feared that treating or removing the symptoms directly would result in the underlying conflict manifesting itself in another form. For this reason therapy was directed at identifying and resolving the underlying conflicts.[14] Frequently, however, when insight into the origins, causes, and consequences of the phobia was achieved and the conflicts were resolved, the embarrassed therapist and disappointed patient found the phobic behavior had not altered in the slightest degree. These techniques and imaginative speculations are still practiced by some trained during the psychoanalytical era and are now only of historical interest. Many carefully controlled studies find insight psychotherapy not significantly superior to placebo therapy in the treatment of any phobias, and even inferior to placebo therapy on some measures.[15-17]

**Hypnotherapy, learning theory, systematic desensitization, and behavior modification.** Hypnotherapy was practiced by pragmatic therapists with more rapid results. Watson and Rayner[18] demonstrated that a phobia was acquired and generalized according to the principles of learning theory. They conditioned Little Albert to fear a white rat and later, by generalization, other furry objects, and proposed methods by which the conditioning could be overcome or unlearned. In a series of experiments Wolpe[19-22] demonstrated that phobias could be learned or conditioned directly and that although conflict could lead to a phobia it was not necessary for its induction. Learning theory holds that a previously neutral object gains the ability to trigger anxiety by being associated first with an unconditioned, anxiety-provoking stimulus. The subsequent avoidance behavior is maintained by negative reinforcement.

Wolpe described a behavior modification technique—a systematic desensitization for the treatment of phobic states—that produced excellent results in uncontrolled studies.[20] Gelder and Marks[23-26] compared different treatment modalities in a controlled study of phobic patients and found desensitization superior to individual and group psychotherapy. No symptom substitution occurred.[1] Others confirmed this.[27-29] A variety of behavior modification techniques subsequently proliferated in the literature, including flooding and response prevention,[30] shaping,[31] prolonged exposure,[32] implosive therapy,[33] aversion relief,[34] paradoxical intention,[35] and modeling.[36] In controlled comparison studies desensitization is generally found to be the most effective technique, although the question remains open. In a series of studies between 1965 and 1968 Gelder and Marks[17, 24-28] found that those responding well to the behavior therapies had specific circumscribed phobias and few associated symptoms. Agoraphobic patients responded poorly.

For treatment purposes we at MGH divide phobic patients into two categories:

1. Those with agoraphobias, social phobias, and illness phobias who are usually polysymptomatic, polyphobic, and very anxious, with spontaneous panic attacks, spontaneous GSR fluctuations, and a slow habituation rate on GSR
2. Those with specific circumscribed phobias, some social phobias

with few associated symptoms, no spontaneous panic attacks, no spontaneous fluctuations on GSR, and a normal rapid habituation response

Patients in the first group require drug treatment and subsequent behavior therapy. The drug controls their anxiety syndrome and panic attacks and restores their habituation response to a more normal range. Then they become better candidates for behavior therapy. Patients in the second group are resistant to drug treatment. They respond well to the behavior therapies, particularly systematic desensitization, which depends on a normal habituation response. Desensitization is essentially a therapy of habituation. Hypnotherapy is probably effective to the extent that it resembles one of the other behavior therapies in technique.

**Drugs in the treatment of phobic anxiety states.** The minor tranquilizers are comforting without being curative or predictably effective. Their value in the treatment of these patients is greatly overrated. Major tranquilizers may aggravate the symptoms and there is no good evidence to warrant their continued use in phobic patients. Propranolol (Inderal) has some value in blocking the peripheral symptoms in these patients, particularly tachycardia. Because of their addiction potential, barbiturates both oral and intravenous, are best avoided as a primary treatment for these patients. There is no good evidence that they are more effective than placebos in the treatment of agoraphobia. Neither is there good reason at this time to recommend injections of acetylcholine.[2]

Two drugs are primarily effective in the treatment of these patients[37]: the monoamine oxidase inhibitors, of which phenelzine dihydrogen sulfate is the most widely used and studied, and the tricyclic antidepressants, of which imipramine and chlorimipramine are the most studied. Both of these drugs are significantly more effective than a placebo ($P < .01$) in a double-blind, controlled trial on chronic agoraphobic patients.[37] Both drugs have disadvantages. While receiving phenelzine dihydrogen sulfate patients are restricted to a low tyramine diet (no cheese, wine, beer, etc.) to avoid a transient hypertensive reaction. As a result physicians are reluctant to prescribe these drugs. However, these patients are so hypochondriacal and obsessive that they usually take extreme precautions with these drugs. One of my patients insisted on being on the low tyramine diet for 8 months before starting phenelzine dihydrogen sulfate, in case "any molecules remain in my body." She returned to work full-time after 6 weeks on phenelzine dihydrogen sulfate and after a 5 year absence from work. Most patients who have used both imipramine and phenelzine dihydrogen sulfate prefer phenelzine dihydrogen sulfate because it is subjectively more pleasant to take, particularly after the fourth week. The anticholinergic and other side effects of imipramine, including orthostatic hypotension and sedation, make management more difficult for the physician during the initial phase of treatment. Without a larger sample it is difficult to say if there is a significant difference in the effectiveness of these drugs for agoraphobic individuals. In our sample, those being given phenelzine dihydrogen sulfate consistently achieved lower scores overall on phobic scales, a finding that parallels our clinical impression.[37]

Phenelzine dihydrogen sulfate is given as 15 mg orally three times per day for the first 2 to 3 weeks. All patients are given a list of proscribed foods and drugs. Hypotension, insomnia, and a detached sedated feeling are the most frequent side effects in the first 2 weeks. After the second week these are replaced by a euphoric, energized, optimistic outlook. The dose is increased to 15 mg given orally four times per day if more symptom reduction is necessary. Hypotension and insomnia are useful guides in the search for the optimal dose. Control of anxiety symptoms may appear as early as 2 weeks or as late as 6 weeks and the effect appears to improve with time. Patients are given therapeutic doses of the drug for 6 months or more—until they are confident about functioning normally without the drug—and then the drug is withdrawn gradually in 4 weeks. Relapses are common after the drug is discontinued, although our findings are not as pessimistic about this as are those of others.[38] Several patients in our series continue to function well after being drug free for up to 1 year. Imipramine is prescribed at doses of at least 150 mg per day with a 1 week buildup to this dosage. Troublesome side effects are common, but with adequate preparation of the patient and encouragement it is rarely necessary to deviate from the dosage schedule in the first weeks of treatment. If adequate symptom reduction—especially of panic attacks—is not achieved after 3 weeks, the dose is increased to 200 mg per day and later even to 250 mg per day. Many (about 40%) of our patients have required these higher doses for optimal results. Hypotension, dry mouth, excessive perspiration, muscle twitching, constipation, and sedation are the most frequent side effects reported. Cardiac toxicity (PR, QRS, and QT prolongation, heart block, tachyrhythmias) makes some physicians understandably concerned about prescribing this drug in therapeutic doses.[39-41] If patients fail to respond to either drug, they usually respond to other monoamine oxidase inhibitors or tricyclic compounds. Depression or vegetative signs of depression do not appear to predict a good response to these drugs in agoraphobic patients.[37] After 4 to 6 weeks of treatment with these drugs the number of phobias diminish and the few remaining central fears and avoidance behavior can be reduced with behavior therapy, such as systematic desensitization.

**Behavior therapy.** The essence of most behavioral techniques in the treatment of phobic states is graduated exposure to the phobic object. This graduated exposure may be accomplished using any of several techniques described here. Most of these initially involve the exposure sequence in imagination followed by real-life exposure. These methods are the most commonly used:

1. Graduated exposure in imagination during relaxation as in
   a. Wolpe's systematic desensitization using a muscle relaxation technique[21,22]
   b. Methohexital-assisted systematic desensitization, 1 to 3 ml of a 2.5% solution given slowly over a 40 minute session[42]
   c. Augmented respiratory relief (or respiratory relief alone)
   d. Systematic desensitization using carbon dioxide and oxygen 30% to 70% carbon dioxide at 10 liters per minute (one inhalation) before each series of scene exposures[22]
2. Graduated exposure with intensification in imagination to an anxiety-provoking level, allowing the anxiety to peak out and drop, as in flooding[30]
3. Graduated exposure in imagination alone without increasing anxiety or decreasing it[22]
4. Graduated exposure in imagination during the "reflex" relief-relaxation period on termination of an aversive stimulus (for example, electric shock) as an aversion relief therapy[34,45]

When conducting the in vivo graduated exposure there is some evidence that prolonged exposure yields better results than exposure for shorter periods.

In practice, Wolpe's systematic desensitization is the simplest technique to master and at this time the safest, most predictably effective, and most widely used. The technique involves the graduated exposure to phobic stimuli along a hierarchy while the patient is experiencing deep muscle relaxation. The phobic stimuli are first imagined and later actually experienced. The patient is first trained to tense the muscles of the legs, abdomen, shoulders, neck, head, and arms as vigorously as possible and then to let the tension go as completely as possible. By practicing this regularly the patient achieves more effective and rapid relaxation. Hierarchies are then constructed for each of the patient's phobias. Scenes involving gradual confrontation with the phobic stimulus are constructed in detail. For example:

|                                                              | SUDS |
| ------------------------------------------------------------ | ---- |
| Scene 1: You are 100 yards from the cat.                     | 20   |
| Scene 2: You are 50 yards from the cat.                      | 40   |
| Scene 3: You are 10 yards from the cat.                      | 70   |
| Scene 4: You are 1 yard from the cat.                        | 90   |
| Scene 5: The cat is crawling over you as you lie still.      | 100  |

Then a subjective distress score (SUD score) on a scale of 0 to 100 is assigned to each scene by the patient. In the example the anxiety or distress score increases as the phobic stimulus is approached. In desensitization itself, the relaxed patient is asked to visualize the scene with the lowest SUD score as vividly as possible for 10 seconds. This sequence is repeated with time-out periods for relaxation between visualizations. With each presentation the SUD score associated with the scene drops (because of habituation) and is recorded. When the SUD score on any scene is zero or very low, the procedure is repeated for the scene with the highest SUD score—until little or no anxiety is attached to any scene. Then the patient is gradually exposed to the actual phobic stimulus in real life, and avoidance and escape behavior is prevented. This consolidates the gains made with systematic desensitization in imagination. If a patient is desensitized twice successfully in therapy sessions and returns with a relapse, a search for a life situation or other factors maintaining the phobia is usually rewarded. When this is manipulated, progress is then maintained. The graduated exposure in life to the phobic stimulus should be supervised and conducted by the therapist when possible to ensure satisfactory results.

Other techniques, for example, flooding[30] may be particularly useful in certain cases. The procedural details are reviewed in several textbooks on behavior therapy and in original papers. The slow, intravenous use of a 2.5% solution of methohexital shortens treatment time and ensures better relaxation and toleration of the phobic stimulus by the patient.[42] One milliliter (25 mg) is given very slowly intravenously at the outset. A profound muscle relaxation and mental calm results and desensitization is conducted in the usual manner. Since the drug has a very short duration, 5 to 10 mg are given slowly intravenously every few minutes to maintain relaxation at optimal levels without interfering with mental alertness. The patient should remain alert and be able to cooperate easily with the procedure. Five to ten minutes after the needle is withdrawn the patient feels normally alert and recovered from the effects of the drug. Patients should be questioned about allergies to barbiturates, about respiratory and cardiac disease, and about porphyria before the drug is administered, and the physician should have a laryngoscope and airway tube present during the procedure.

Here is an example of the successful combining of drug therapy and behavior therapy.

> While crossing a walkway overpass near the hospital on his way home from work, a 40-year-old retarded hospital employee was suddenly overwhelmed by an impulse to throw himself into the traffic below. The accompanying panic was so strong that he became phobic to that overpass—with the result that he could not take the train home. He walked to his home several miles from the hospital. In spite of interpretations, insight, and encouragement from his therapist, his phobia continued to generalize. First he could use no streets within view of the overpass; then he could use no exits that opened on those streets; later he was obsessed all day anticipating leaving the hospital; and, finally, he began to avoid work. He was referred for behavior therapy. During his first session a hierarchy of phobic scenes was constructed. Using intravenous methohexital he successfully reduced his SUD score on half of the hierarchy scenes to zero. During session two his progress was maintained with no relapse of SUD score and he was desensitized, again with methohexital, to the remaining scenes. At this point I brought the patient to the overpass (during rush hour traffic) and accompanied him across. Physical reassurance was offered at the start and gradually with praise and encouragement he became more independent until he would cross alone with comfort. This took 40 minutes. He was encouraged to stop, watch the traffic pass below him, and enjoy the breeze and view. He used the overpass alone that evening to return home and has used it twice daily without incident or relapse for a year since. His only comment now is "It seems silly now that I should have been so frightened about a thing like that."

## OBSESSIVE-COMPULSIVE NEUROSIS
### Definition

This disorder is characterized by the persistent intrusion of unwanted thoughts or impulses into the patients' conscious awareness or by persistent irresistible compulsions to carry out actions against their will. The obsessive thoughts may be single words, or a complex sequence of ideas or thoughts. The obsessive thoughts or compulsive acts are frequently accompanied by panic or strong anxiety. Individuals feel strongly compelled to counteract or resist the idea or impulse. They experience the obsession or compulsion as foreign or ego alien and retain their insight in perceiving them as irrational.

## Epidemiology

Transient obsessive-compulsive symptoms are common in the general population. The estimated maximum prevalence in the general white population is less than .05%.[46] Men and women appear to be affected equally and as many as 50% of all obsessive-compulsive patients are said to remain unmarried.[46] Although it may start at any age, it is primarily a condition of adolescence and early adult life. Most cases start before the mid-twenties. In contradistinction to anxiety neurosis patients and phobic patients, obsessive-compulsive patients seek treatment at a much earlier age for their symptoms.[47] In 85% of the cases, the duration of the acute obsessive-compulsive flareup was less than 1 year. Approximately one-third of these patients have had two or more such episodes. It is considered a chronic disorder with a remitting course. The concordance among monozygotic twins is higher than among dizygotic twins, even when reared apart—a finding suggesting genetic influences.[44]

## Clinical features

Thoughts, images, or words may persistently intrude into patients' minds against their will. Although this may occur spontaneously, triggering stimuli for the obsession can often be identified. Sixty percent of these patients have multiple rather than single obsessions. For example, after his father's death a man of 28 was deeply distressed by the recurrent, obsessive, mental image of his father standing naked before him and by the compulsion to embrace him. He was unable to banish this recurrent thought. A patient obsessed with thoughts that his medication was contaminated with dirt or diseases from the staff and other patients presented major management problems while he was a medical inpatient requiring drug treatment. It is striking to note the frequency with which dirt, contamination, aggression, and sex are the focus of obsessive preoccupation. Religion, order, safety, and numbers also frequently recur as the substance of an obsession.

Obsessions may also be irrational impulses to some sort of action. Although the feelings are very compelling and patients fear that they will lose control and act on the impulse, they usually do not. Common examples include the impulse to scream or shout obscenities during a quiet church service or the impulse to jump off a bridge. It is hardly surprising that such obsessions frequently lead to phobic avoidance of the situation or of the object triggering the impulse.

Compulsions, on the other hand, are obsessional motor acts. They are repetitive acts that must be performed, however useless or irrational. Resisting them causes alarming anxiety. Seventy-five percent of obsessive-compulsive patients have compulsions.[48] Of those with compulsions, fewer than 10% have multiple compulsions.[48] When the compulsion is socially acceptable, or at least not entirely unacceptable, the patient may yield to or carry out the compulsive act directly (a yielding compulsion). A 32-year-old business executive felt compelled to repeatedly check the medication he was taking. He would carry the bottle at all times and frequently take it out, read the letters carefully, take out a pill, and check the color, markings, and odor of the pill before replacing it.

When the primary obsession or compulsive impulse is socially unacceptable, the compulsive act usually involves an attempt to counteract, neutralize, control, contain, or undo the consequence of the feared and unacceptable urge. Such compulsive acts may serve as atonement for some real or imagined thought or action the patient feels guilty about. A 28-year-old woman was obsessed with the thought that she would take her clothes off in a public place. She developed a ritual of constantly checking the buttons and zippers on her clothes to ensure that they were properly closed. A 40-year-old man was obsessed by an impulse to strike people he met. To contain the impulse he developed a hand clasping ritual behind his back which intensified when he met people. Seventy-five percent of these patients are frequently plagued by doubt. This doubt reinforces their need to repeat the compulsive act endlessly.[48] After turning off the gas or closing the door, they return repeatedly only seconds later to check again just in case. When the compulsion is an already lengthy or highly complex sequence, this doubt can lead to crippling repetition and disability. The presence of compulsions in an obsessive-compulsive neurosis makes the prognosis poorer.

The role of obsessional personality traits like orderliness, cleanliness, need for control, punctuality, inflexibility, lack of imagination, painful accuracy, and attention to detail have been overemphasized in obsessive-compulsive neurosis. The presence of the neurosis may accentuate these obsessive traits during the acute phase of the disorder. Obsessions and compulsions are found in other psychiatric disorders—including schizophrenia, anxiety states, phobic states, depression—and sometimes also in organic disease states such as postencephalitic states, temporal lobe lesions, oculogyria, and possibly basal ganglia disease.

## Treatment

Few systematic studies have been made to clarify the natural course of obsessive-compulsive disorders and the percentage of cases that spontaneously recover. As a result it is difficult to evaluate the anecdotal reports of treatment successes.

**Psychotherapy.** There are no controlled studies to suggest that psychotherapy is any more effective than placebo therapy in the treatment of obsessive-compulsive neurosis. Although there are some case reports of recovery or improvement during the course of psychotherapy, it is not easy to ascribe the recovery directly to the therapist's intervention. Psychoanalytic theory posits that these patients suffer from a conflict between an id impulse and a superego retaliation for the impulse. In the process of this struggle the ego is weakened. In more simplistic terms, there is a conflict between rage and obedience, in which the self has little voice. The focus of psychotherapeutic treatment is to weaken the superego pressure or the retaliation against the aggressive impulses while strengthening the patient's ego to come to terms with the aggressive impulses. However, it is now generally conceded that obsessive-compulsive patients respond poorly to psychotherapy and it is no longer the treatment of choice.

**Behavior therapy.** Learning theory holds that previously neutral obsessional thought gains the ability to trigger anxiety by occurring first in association with an unconditioned, anxiety-provoking stimulus. In this way the obsession becomes a conditioned stimulus for anxiety. Later, at a second evolutionary stage, the patient finds that a certain compulsive ritual reduces the anxiety associated with the obsessional thought. Repeated performance of this ritual and its success in reducing the anxiety results in reinforcement of the compulsive act. The compulsion then becomes established and fixed.

The behavior therapies attempt to undo and reverse these two stages. When the compulsion is absent (25% of cases[48]), only one stage needs unlearning. Consequently, the procedure is simpler and easier, and the prognosis is better. When obsessions and compulsions are present together, a two-pronged approach is necessary. Otherwise the obsessions and anxiety may remit, but the compulsions will continue.

Although controlled studies using the behavior therapies for this disorder are still few, the results are superior to, and more rapid, predictable, and stable than, psychotherapy. In spite of this, many cases resist or only partially respond to behavior therapies. In the past few years new techniques and variations have proliferated and provide the therapist with a large, versatile armamentarium with which to treat obsessive-compulsive neurosis. The behavioral technique may be overt (at the level of overt behavior), as in in vivo exposure and response prevention, or covert (in imagination), as in thought stopping, covert assertion, covert extinction, or covert negative reinforcement.

*Overt techniques.* The choice here is exposure and response prevention. The patient is exposed to the anxiety-provoking obsession in a graduated manner along a hierarchy. This graduated exposure may be accomplished using any of these techniques:

1. Exposure in imagination during relaxation as in
   a. Wolpe's systematic desensitization using a muscle relaxation technique[21,22]
   b. Methohexital-assisted systematic desensitization, 1 to 3 ml of a 2.5% solution given intravenously very slowly[42]
   c. Respiratory relief[43]
   d. Augmented respiratory relief using carbon dioxide and oxygen mixtures[43]
   e. Systematic desensitization using carbon dioxide and oxygen (30% to 70% carbon dioxide) at 10 liters per minute (one inhalation) before each series of scene exposures[22]
2. Exposure with intensification in imagination to an anxiety-provoking level, allowing the anxiety to peak out and drop (as in flooding)[30]
3. Exposure in imagination alone without increasing anxiety or decreasing it[22]
4. Exposure in imagination during the "reflex" relief-relaxation period on termination of an aversive stimulus (for example, electric shock) as an aversion relief therapy[45]

When the exposure procedure is successful in imagination (that is, the SUD score is 0 on all items), it is necessary to repeat the sequence with actual exposure to ensure success.

The concomitant use of modeling is unnecessary and provides no advantage. These procedures treat the obsession. Response prevention is used to treat the compulsion. It is used concomitant with overt behavioral techniques when compulsions are present. The patient is prevented from completing the ritual. This may be done in a graduated manner, for example, gradual reduction of the length of the ritual or number of times it is repeated. Sometimes total response prevention is used. With improvement and confidence the patient is taught to incorporate the response prevention and to use it as a self-control technique.

An 18-year-old boy was obsessed with the idea that he and others would be contaminated by semen and therefore constantly engaged in ritual washings. He was gradually exposed to the semen in imagination and later in vivo. At the same time he was actively prevented from engaging in washing rituals. The water supply to his wash basin was cut off and his necessary washing to remain presentably clean was supervised and restricted. He made an impressive improvement and returned to work after fifteen sessions.

Response prevention may be very anxiety-provoking at first, and the patient may violently resist it, but persistence by the therapist is rewarded.

I favor relaxation-assisted systematic desensitization and response prevention because it is as effective as other techniques and more pleasant for the patient. However, aversion relief may be very useful in cases where all else fails. This technique was first used by Thorpe and others[49] in the treatment of single phobias and subsequently modified by Solyom[50] in the treatment of an obsession.

A chronic obsessive-compulsive patient with fears of contamination was undergoing treatment in our clinic. She had an obsessive crisis when she was unexpectedly exposed to a particularly "dirty" situation and as a result felt that she, her clothes, her place of work, and, indeed, everything had become hopelessly contaminated. This lasted 2 days and resulted in complete isolation and 6 hours of a washing ritual without relief. She stopped eating, became acidotic, and could not return to work. Increased tranquilization failed to provide the necessary relief. When examined she was very frightened. Wolpe's muscle relaxation technique and hypnosis failed to bring any relaxation. She had difficulty concentrating because of repeated obsessions. For this reason, thought stopping and covert negative reinforcement were ineffective. Aversion relief was used. A short hierarchy was constructed for the immediately threatening items. She was instructed to picture herself as dirty and contaminated and engaging in her washing ritual. During this imagery and for 3 seconds after it ceased she received a continuous aversive electrical stimulus to her right forearm as a contingent punishment for her thought and ensuing behavior. After 10 seconds, when I signaled "now," she switched the imagery to a scene where she was exposed to dirt and contamination, yet did not feel dirty or contaminated or feel a need to engage in ritual washing. On successfully accomplishing this cognitive set, she said aloud, "I am clean," whereupon the aversive stimulus ended immediately. She continued to visualize this positive exposure for 20 seconds of relief without the maladaptive compulsive thought (and later for longer periods). If she felt dirty and contaminated, anxiously fearful, and compelled to ritual washing in less than 20 seconds, she indicated so and the aversive stimulus returned. The procedure was repeated. In this way, the anxiety thought, "I am dirty and contaminated and must engage in ritual compulsive washing to relieve the anxiety it causes me," was punished. The opposite thought, "I am exposed to this dirt and contamination, but not anxious about it and feel no need to engage in compulsive washing to rid myself of it," was associated with relief from punishment (shock). The obsessive-compulsive thought was punished, while escape from this thought was rewarded by relief from the shock. This procedure is designed to eliminate or decrease the strength of the maladaptive thought while rewarding the more normal, adaptive thought and consequently increasing its strength.

After several repetitions, her anxiety level (SUD score) began dropping and was impressive after 30 minutes when she reported feeling calmer and back in more control again. It was surprising even to me that so much aversive stimulation could have resulted in anxiety reduction. In spite of my reluctance to persist beyond a certain point, the patient was insistent that I continue, since it was resulting in continual improvement. Following $1\frac{1}{2}$ hours of this procedure the patient had a meal in the hospital cafeteria without prompting, returned home, did not engage in rituals that evening, and returned to work the next day with a satisfactory degree of comfort.

Additional behavioral treatment was necessary as follow-up, of course, to reduce the symptoms further. However, the aversion therapy had been successful where other measures had failed. It had prevented further physical illness, isolation, and psychiatric hospitalization.

*Covert techniques.* These techniques parallel the overt techniques in that there is exposure and response prevention at a covert, imagination level. The particular obsessive-compulsive ritual often dictates which technique is most appropriate. Of the covert techniques, thought-stopping is now the most widely used.[22,27,51,52] As with all forms of behavior therapy, a detailed behavioral analysis and description must first be elicited from the patient. The immediate antecedents and consequences of the symptom in question are especially important. Here is an example of the thought-stopping technique:

> A 35-year-old woman with Hodgkin disease became obsessed with the thought that during chemotherapy injections she was inadvertently contaminated with a virulent illness. Although she was reassured repeatedly, and although she realized it was absurd, the thought persisted.
>
> *Step 1.* The therapist stopped the patient's overt obsession/compulsion. The patient closed her eyes and imagined the target obsession coming insistently to mind, verbalizing the thoughts leading up to and into the obsession. At the start of the obsession the therapist shouted, "Stop!" forcefully. The patient was startled. Asked what happened, she reported the obsession stopped. This was repeated until the obsession was stopped effectively by this method.

*Step 2.* The therapist stopped the patient's covert obsesssion/compulsion. The sequence of step 1 was repeated, but instead of verbalizing the thoughts, the patient thought them. She signaled by raising a finger when she began to think one of the obsessive thoughts. The therapist shouted "Stop!" This was repeated until the thoughts were blocked.

*Step 3.* The patient overtly stopped her covert obsession/compulsion. The patient verbalized the thoughts to herself and shouted, "Stop" when the obsession began. At first, the patient said "stop" in a feeble, polite tone of voice. She was encouraged by modeling to shout it forcefully, assertively, and aggressively. This mastered, she repeated it until the obsession was blocked.

*Step 4.* The patient covertly stopped her covert obsession/compulsion. She said "stop" to herself by tightening the vocal chords and moving the tongue forward. This was repeated forcefully under supervision until the obsession was blocked. The patient was then encouraged to practice this regularly at home and to keep records of the response. Practice in target situations is encouraged.

A similar procedure using an aversive stimulus instead of "stop" is effective, although less pleasant. At this time it is difficult to determine whether the implicit punishment in shouting "stop," the patient's assertion while shouting, or a combination of the two is the prime stimulant toward recovery. Similar results may be obtained if patients wear a rubber band around their wrist, stretch it, and let it go against the anterior surface of the wrist when they wish to stop thought.

**Drugs.** Major and minor tranquilizers are widely prescribed for obsessive-compulsive neurosis to minimize associated anxiety. The minor tranquilizers are comforting to these patients without either curing or alleviating the central symptoms. Nor is there good evidence for the efficacy of major tranquilizers, which may even aggravate the symptoms. They are best reserved for obsessive patients with a concomitant psychotic disorder. Two groups of drugs are more predictably effective—the tricyclic antidepressants (in therapeutic doses) and the monoamine oxidase inhibitors. There are probably two types of obsessive patients, just as there are two types of phobic patients. One type has severe associated anxiety symptoms, spontaneous fluctuations in GSR, and slow habituation responses. These patients respond indifferently to behavior therapy. They require drug therapy to bring their spontaneous panic under better control so that they can habituate more normally to behavior therapy. The other type has more circumscribed symptoms, no spontaneous GSR fluctuations, and normal habituation patterns. This distinction is useful in clinical management, but remains to be documented accurately. A sizable literature exists attesting to the efficacy of chlorimipramine (unavailable in the United States). It is similar in efficacy to the other tricyclic drugs except that it has a more potent effect on serotonin metabolism than to the others. No double-blind, placebo-controlled studies have yet been published showing clorimipramine more effective than the other tricyclic drugs for this or for phobic anxiety states. I have found imipramine (150 mg per day) effective in a series of severe obsessive-compulsive patients. It appears to reduce significantly the anxiety and panic associated with the original obsessive thoughts and usually leads to a reduction in frequency and intensity of obsessions.

> A woman had spent several hours each day for 55 years without a remission doing elaborate calculating rituals. These obsessive thoughts were accompanied by overwhelming panic and fear that she would not find the correct solution. She carried a book of mathematical tables to facilitate her calculations. She had had countless treatments and medications through the years to no avail and had given up all hope of recovery. She came for help because her failing memory made the ritual more difficult, prolonged, and anxiety-provoking. After 4 weeks of therapy with 150 mg of imipramine per day the panic attacks ceased and the obsessions diminished to less than 5 minutes per day. They continued to diminish weekly. Behavior therapy (covert assertion and thought stopping) and hypnotherapy led to further improvement so that the symptoms occurred only rarely, and then were not compelling. After 4 months she had overcome her disability and traveled out of state to visit family and friends, staying overnight away from home and socializing easily for the first time. After 8 months of using imipramine she felt optimistic enough to gradually withdraw from the medication. The symptoms began to reappear after 3 weeks. After 10 weeks she began to take 150 mg imipramine per day again. At 6 month follow-up she had achieved and maintained her former level of improvement.

One novel behavioral technique used here to withdraw the patient from her mental calculation ritual and to bypass her mild memory lapse was the use of an electronic pocket calculator. This reduced the number of calculations and the time required to get the correct solution and helped break up the original mental sequence by substituting a new one until thought-stopping enabled more effective resistance to the impulse.

The use of intravenous infusions is warranted only in resistant cases and then only in young, physically healthy patients. These drugs may cause considerable damage to the heart and should be used only under careful medical supervision. This procedure is also reported to be effective for agoraphobia.[53] The patient is given infusions 5 days per week (Monday to Friday) for 3 weeks. Fifty milligrams of chlorimipramine is diluted in 150 ml of normal saline (5% dextrose is reported to be more irritating locally) and is given with a no. 23 butterfly needle during a 2 hour period. The dosage is increased by 50 mg daily to 300 to 350 mg while the time of the infusion is increased to 7 hours. Lunch may be served during the infusion. Patients are usually sleepy by afternoon. Constant medical supervision is essential and electrocardiographic monitoring advisable. Resuscitation and cardiac arrest equipment and drugs should be on hand. On weekends the patient takes the Friday dose orally. After maximal improvement the large dose is discontinued in favor of an oral maintenance dose of 50 mg three times per day. Appropriate behavior therapy may be conducted during these intravenous infusion sessions.

Both imipramine and, to a lesser extent, phenelzine dihydrogen sulfate are effective in reducing obsessive-compulsive symptoms in anxious patients with phobic symptoms.[37] They were both significantly more effective than placebo in a double-blind study I conducted.[37] However, the reduction in obsessive-compulsive scores is incomplete and not as impressive as the reduction in anxiety, phobic anxiety, depression, or somatization scores for these patients. The usual dietary and drug restrictions are necessary as with all monoamine oxidase inhibitors. The personality of such patients—their care and attention to detail—makes them particularly suitable candidates for these drugs with dietary and drug restrictions. Dally[54] reported that the monoamine oxidase inhibitors were not generally useful in pure obsessional states while Annesley[55] and Jain, Swinson, and Thomas[56] reported cases of obsessive-compulsive neurosis that responded well to phenelzine dihydrogen sulfate.

Bauer and Novak[57] found doxepin and amitriptyline were effective in a double-blind controlled study. Ananth and others[58] found doxepin useful in doses of 300 mg daily.

Although these drugs have some merit in the treatment of true obsessive-compulsive neurosis, a satisfactory antiobsessive drug is not yet available. The treatment most likely to be effective is using a combination of a tricyclic antidepressant and flooding and response prevention.

**Leukotomy and electroconvulsive therapy.** In cases of severe chronic debilitating obsessive-compulsive neurosis unresponsive to other treatments, leukotomy—usually selective—may be considered. There is evidence that it lessens the intensity of both obsessions and compulsions, often providing complete relief.[59] Since it causes an irreversible lesion it cannot be undertaken lightly and is considered a treatment of last resort.[60]

There is no satisfactory evidence that electroconvulsive therapy is a predictably effective treatment for patients with obsessive-compulsive neurosis. Indeed, it may sometimes aggravate the condition and is best avoided. It is most likely to be effective in those patients with concomitant vegetative signs of depression.

## ANXIETY NEUROSIS
### Definition

Anxiety neurosis is a condition that has a central feature of anxiety even to the point of panic and that is usually associated with such somatic symptoms as palpitation, tachycardia, hyperventilation, faintness, and exhaustion. This syndrome has appeared over the past 2 centuries under several diagnostic labels, including Da Costa syndrome, cardiac neurosis, neurasthenia, irritable heart, and effort syndrome. The clinical features described under these headings suggest that all are manifestations of the same disorder.

### Epidemiology

Surveys suggest that at any time 2% to 5% of the population and as many as 10% of the patients in hospital practice are suffering from this disorder.[61-65] The incidence is equal for men and women. Although it may occur at any age it is characteristically a disorder of young adults and has a mean age of onset of 25 years.

Slater and Shields[66,67] found a concordance of 50% in monozygotic twins for anxiety neurosis, even when the twins were reared apart. In dizygotic twins the concordance for anxiety neurosis was only 4%, with strong anxiety traits occurring in 13%.

### Clinical features

Myers[8] first described the condition in detail in 1870 while in the British Campaign in India. Da Costa,[9,68] a Philadelphia physician, described the case of a Union Army private who suffered from the condition during the Civil War. He noted the connection between the exacerbations in the cardiac symptoms and the timing of various battles. Since then, anxiety neurosis has been associated with soldiers, stress, and heart disease through many wars.[69]

Anxiety neurosis is a polysymptomatic disorder with few objective signs. A careful history usually uncovers many symptoms, although the patient may exhibit few. The site of the presenting symptom usually dictates which specialist the patient seeks. Those with tachycardia and chest pain are usually seen by the cardiologist, while those complaining of dizzy spells, headaches, unsteadiness, or paresthesia are likely to consult a neurologist. Sighing respiration, episodes of tachypnea, or hyperventilation are common. Such patients complain of breathing difficulties and of being unable to get a full breath. This is sometimes associated with left mammary chest pain that occurs when the patient is resting and may last acutely for minutes or as a dull pressure for weeks. There may be hyperawareness of heartbeat and even premature beats and tachycardia. A faint feeling, dizziness, and an unsteadiness or giddy sensation or rubbery feeling in the legs give a feeling of impending collapse. Trembling, excessive perspiration, a choking sensation, and hyperventilation are all common symptoms reported by these patients. The anxiety or panic attacks may be followed by excessive sleeping and fatigue for hours or days.

There are no reliable clinical signs to guide the examiner, although brisk reflexes, moist palms, and tachycardia are frequently seen. Hypoglycemia, thyrotoxicosis, pheochromocytoma, carcinoid syndrome, Meniere disease, and even tuberculosis and brucellosis have similar presenting symptoms.

A careful search for significant life changes or events in the period immediately preceding the onset of the symptoms is often rewarded. Typical precipitants are losses of all kinds—death or loss of a friend or relative, loss of a job, financial loss, and life-threatening stress and illness. Although it is often easy to identify stresses and emotional factors that aggravate the condition, it is not always possible.

The condition has a chronic course with exacerbations and remissions. About one-sixth of these patients recover completely and one-sixth remain totally disabled. The intermediate two-thirds are variously symptomatic or disabled.[70] Clinical findings are not reliable as prognosticators.

**Laboratory findings**

There is no characteristic electrocardiographic abnormality.[61] Some of the symptoms, for example, palpitation, can be aggravated by isoproterenol and blocked by the beta-adrenergic blocker, propranolol.[71] Abnormalities in blood lactate,[72-74] oxygen consumption,[75] fingernail capillaries,[76] and forearm blood flow[77] have been described. In a standardized exercise test anxiety neurosis patients have a lower oxygen consumption and an excessive rise in blood lactate compared to normal individuals.[72,73] Pitts and McLure[74] were able to stimulate typical anxiety attacks in these patients, but not in controls, by giving a standard infusion of sodium lactate. Later they were able to block the onset of the symptoms produced by sodium lactate by giving doses of calcium ion. These findings have not been replicated by others.

**Treatment**

Since there are no reliable clinical signs or laboratory tests widely available to make a definitive diagnosis, anxiety neurosis is usually a diagnosis of exclusion. Other disorders that mimic it must first be ruled out—like hyperthyroidism, Meniere disease, pheochromocytoma, carcinoid syndrome, tuberculosis, brucellosis, ischemic heart disease, and multiple sclerosis. This cautious evaluation of the case is important therapeutically (as well as diagnostically) in alleviating the patient's fear of medical illness.

When the precipitating stresses are clarified, the appropriate supportive techniques and external events requiring manipulation become clearer. The opportunity to discuss anxieties with a sympathetic listener is, in itself, therapeutic and often results in anxiety reduction. However, there is no good scientific evidence that intensive psychotherapy or psychoanalysis is any more helpful for this condition than simple support, reassurance, advice on aggravating factors, environmental manipulation, and minor tranquilizers.[49]

In milder cases the relaxation techniques of meditation, hypnotherapy, behavior therapy, and biofeedback are sometimes useful for anxiety reduction. They are more likely to give lasting benefit when a behavioral model is used—when the precise antecedents and consequences of the anxiety are identified and manipulated systematically. Training the individual to use self-hypnosis can sometimes be helpful in controlling symptoms when they occur outside the physician's office. In this way it is possible to alleviate the hyperventilation episodes that aggravate and accentuate anxiety symptoms. Hypnotic suggestion and self-hypnosis may also alleviate such symptoms as chest pain and palpitations. Biofeedback, still in its infancy, has real value in reducing chronic muscle tensions and in reconditioning the autonomic nervous system via galvanic skin potential conditioning to respond less to conditioned anxiety-provoking stimuli. Because of its solid scientific base in the theory of applied operant conditioning, this technique will undoubtedly assume a more important role in our therapeutic armamentarium as its technology becomes more sophisticated and its feedback more immediately rewarding.

Drugs continue to play a role as important adjuncts in relieving anxiety. The minor tranquilizers, for example, chlordiazepoxide and diazepam, are widely prescribed for relief of mild anxiety. They are more soothing than definitively curative and their principal merit is that they are safe. However, for the cases of anxiety that are severe, chronic, and present management difficulties of the kind that usually demand psychiatric consultation, they are overrated and not nearly as effective as is generally believed. They are most effective during the first 3 weeks of their use, after which the patients may report feeling more depressed.

More effective but less widely used clinically in blocking the peripheral manifestations of anxiety is propranolol (Inderal).[69,71] The major tranquilizers, for example, phenothiazines, should not be prescribed for these patients since they may finally aggravate rather than relieve the condition and are best reserved for the anxiety of schizophrenia and other psychotic illness. Barbiturates and other sedatives, for example, bromides, should be used with caution since these patients can easily become physically dependent on them. It should, however, be pointed out that they provide at least transient symptom relief. For severe cases—especially those whose symptoms are present for over 3 weeks—two drugs are particularly effective. These are imipramine and phenelzine dihydrogen sulfate. They are both maximally effective only after the third week and then only in therapeutic doses, that is, at least 150 mg per day of imipramine or 45 mg per day of phenelzine dihydrogen sulfate. However, they usually provide lasting benefit. After 3 to 6 months of use the drug is withdrawn over a 3 week period. Although for some patients the symptoms may return when the dose is dropped below a certain threshold, others remain symptom-free. In general, patients tolerate or like imipramine less well than phenelzine dihydrogen sulfate and are more distressed by the side effects and consequently are somewhat more difficult to manage for the first 2 months. However, the necessity of a low tyramine diet and the danger of a hypertensive crisis with high tyramine foods like cheese make some physicians reluctant to prescribe them. Because of their hypochondriacal concerns, patients with anxiety neurosis are particularly cautious about the food restrictions and observe them rigorously. Imipramine and phenelzine dihydrogen sulfate are significantly superior to other drugs and treatments for severe and chronic cases of anxiety neurosis and merit more frequent trial for this condition.

**REFERENCES**

1. Agras, S., and others: The epidemiology of common fears and phobias, Compr. Psychiatry **10**:151-156, 1969.
2. Marks, I. M.: Fears and phobias, New York, 1969 Academic Press.

3. Westphal, C.: Die agoraphobie. Arch. Psychiatr. Nervenkr. **3**:138-171, 219-221, 1871-1872.

4. Freud, S.: In Stachey, J., editor: Standard edition of Freud, London, 1966, Hogarth Press and Institute of Psychoanalysis., G. W., VII, 467. S. E., IX, 250-251.

5. Roth, M.: The phobic anxiety depersonalization syndrome, Proc. R. Soc. Med. **52**(8):587, 1959.

6. Klein, D. F.: Delineation of two drug responsive anxiety syndromes, Psychopharmacologia **5**:397-408, 1964.

7. Marks, I. M.: Agoraphobic syndrome (phobic anxiety state), Arch. Gen. Psychiatry **23**:538-553, 1970.

8. Myers, A. B. R.: On the etiology and prevalence of disease of the heart among soldiers, London, 1870, J. Churchill and Sons, p. 22.

9. Da Costa, J. M.: On irritable heart: a clinical study of a functional cardiac disorder and its consequences, Am. J. Med. Sci. **61**:17, 1871.

10. Burton, R.: The anatomy of melancholy, 1621. Republished in all English text, Dell, F., and Jordan-Smith, P., editors: Tudor Publishing Co., New York, 1927, Farrar & Rinehart., Inc.

11. Lader, M. H., and Wing, L.: Physiological measures, sedative drugs and morbid anxiety, Maudsley Monograph No. 14, London, 1966, Oxford University Press.

12. Rutter, M., Tizard, J., and Whitmore, K.: Education, health and behavior, London, 1968, Longman Group Ltd, chap. 12.

13. Lader, M. H., Gelder, M. G., and Marks, I. M.: Palmar skin conductance measures as predictors of response to desensitization, J. Psychosom. Res. **11**:283-290, 1967.

14. Fenichel, O.: The psychoanalytic theory of neurosis, London, 1944, Routledge & Kegan, Paul Ltd., p. 215.

15. Paul, G. L.: Insight versus desensitization in psychotherapy: an experiment in anxiety reduction, Standford, California, 1966, Standford University Press.

16. Paul, G. L.: Outcome of systematic desensitization. In Franck, C. M. (editor): Assessment and status of behavior therapies, 1968, New York, McGraw-Hill Book Co.

17. Gelder, M. G., Marks, I. M., and Wolff, H. H.: Desensitization and psychotherapy in the treatment of phobic states: a controlled inquiry, Br. J. Psychiatry **113**:53-73, 1967.

18. Watson, J. B., and Rayner, R.: Conditioned emotional reactions, J. Exp. Psychol. **3**:1-14, 1920.

19. Wolpe, J.: Reciprocal inhibition as the main basis of psychotherapeutic effects, Arch. Gen. Psychiatry **72**:205, 1954.

20. Wolpe, J.: Psychotherapy by reciprocal inhibition, Stanford, California, 1958, Standford University Press.

21. Wolpe, J., and Lazarus, A.: behavior therapy techniques, Oxford, 1966, Pergamon Press Ltd.

22. Wolpe, J.: The practice of behavior therapy, Ed. 2, Oxford, 1973, Pergamon Press Ltd.

23. Gelder, M. G., and Marks, I. M.: Severe agoraphobia: a controlled prospective trial of behavior therapy, Br. J. Psychiatry **112**:309-319, 1966.

24. Marks, I. M., and Gelder, M. G.: A controlled retrospective study of behavior therapy in phobic patients, Br. J. Psychiatry **111**:571-573, 1965.
25. Marks, I. M., Gelder, M. G. and Edwards, J. G.: Hypnosis and desensitization for phobias: a controlled prospective trial, Br. J. Psychiatry **114**:1263-1274, 1968.
26. Gelder, M. G., and Marks, I. M.: Desensitization and phobias: a crossover study, Br. J. Psychiatry **114**:323-328, 1968.
27. Rimm, D. C., and Masters, J. D.: Behavior therapy–techniques and empirical findings, New York, 1975, Academic Press, Inc., p. 492.
28. Rachman, S.: The treatment of anxiety and phobic reactions by systematic desensitization psychotherapy, J. Clin. Soc. Psychol. **58**:259-263, 1959.
29. Lang, R. J., Lazovick, A. D., and Reynolds, D. J.: Desensitization, suggestibility and pseudotherapy, J. Abnorm. Psychol. **70**:395-402, 1965.
30. Boulougouris, J., and Marks, I. M.: Implosion (flooding): a new treatment for phobias, Br. Med. J. **2**:721-723, 1969.
31. Crowe, M. J., and others: Time limited desensitization, implosion and shaping for phobic patients: a cross-over study. Behav. Res. Ther. **10**:219-228, 1972.
32. Watson, J. P., Gaind, R., and Marks, I. M.: Prolonged exposure: a rapid treatment for phobias, Br. Med. J. **1**:13-15, 1971.
33. Stampfl, T. G.: Implosive therapy: Part I. The theory. In Armitage, S. G., editor: Behavioral modification techniques in the treatment of emotional disorders, Battle Creek, Michigan, 1967, Veteran's Administration Publication.
34. Solyom, L., and Miller, S. B.: Reciprocal inhibition by aversion relief in the treatment of phobias, Behav. Res. Ther. **5**:313-324, 1967.
35. Frankl, U.: Paradoxical intention: a logotherapeutic technique, Am. J. Psychother. **14**:520, 1960.
36. Bandura, A., and Whalen, C. K.: The influence of antecedent reinforcement and divergent modeling cues on patterns of self reward, J. Pers. Soc. Psychol. **3**:373-382, 1966.
37. Sheehan, D. V., Ballanger, J., and Jacobson, G.: The treatment of endogenous anxiety with phobic, hysterical, and hypochondriacal symptoms. In press 1978.
38. Tyrer, P., and Steinberg, D.: Symptomatic treatment of agoraphobia and social phobias: a follow up study, Br. J. Psychiatry **127**:163-168, 1975.
39. Bigger, J. T., and others: Cardiac antiarrhythmic effect of imipramine hydrochloride, N. Engl. J. Med. **296**:206-208, 1977.
40. Burrows, G. D., and others: Cardiac effects of different tricyclic antidepressant drugs, Br. J. Psychiatry **129**:335-341, 1976.
41. Jefferson, J. W.: A review of cardiovascular effects and toxicity of tricyclic antidepressants, Psychosom. Med. **37**:160-179, 1975.
42. Friedman, D.: A new technique for the systematic densensitization of phobic symptoms, Behav. Res. Ther. **4**:139-140, 1966.
43. Orwin, A.: Respiratory relief: a new and rapid method for the treatment of phobic states, Br. J. Psychiatry **119**:635-637, 1971.
44. Marks, I. M., and others: Obsessive compulsive neurosis in identical twins, Br. J. Psychiatry **115**:991-998, 1969.

45. Mowrer, O. H.: Learning theory and the symbolic processes, New York, 1960, John Wiley & Sons, Inc.
46. Nemiah, J.: Obsessive compulsive neurosis. In Freedman, A. M., Kaplan, H. I., and Sadock, B., editors: Comprehensive textbook of psychiatry, Vol. I, Baltimore, 1975, The Williams & Wilkins Co.
47. Marks, I. M., Hodgson, R., and Rachman, S.: Treatment of chronic obsessive compulsive neurosis by in vivo exposure, Br. J. Psychiatry **127:**349-364, 1975.
48. Akhtar, S., and others: A phenomenological analysis of symptoms in obsessive compulsive neurosis, Br. J. Psychiatry **127:**342-348, 1975.
49. Thorpe, J. G., Schmidt, E., Brown, P. T., and Cartell, D.: Aversion relief therapy: a new method for general application, Behav. Res. Ther. **2:**71, 1964.
50. Solyom, L.: A case of obsessive neurosis treated by aversion relief, Can. Psychiatr. Assoc. J. **14:**623, 1969.
51. Stern, R. S.: Treatment of a case of obsessional neurosis using thought stopping technique, Br. J. Psychiatry **117:**441-442, 1970.
52. Stern, R. S., and Marks I. M.: Brief and prolonged flooding: a comparison in agoraphobic patients, Arch. Gen. Psychiatry **28:**270-276, 1973.
53. Marshall, V. K., and Micev, M. D.: Clomipramine in the treatment of obsessional illnesses and phobic anxiety states, J. Int. Med. Res. **1:** 403-412, 1973.
54. Dally, P.: Chemotherapy of psychiatric disorders, London, 1967, Logos Press, pp. 27, 80, 114, 125.
55. Annesley, P. T.: Nardil response in a chronic obsessive compulsive, Br. J. Psychiatry **115:**748, 1969.
56. Jain, V. K., Swinson, R. P., and Thomas, J. G.: Phenelzine in obsessional neurosis, Br. J. Psychiatry **117:**237-238, 1970.
57. Bauer, G., and Nowak, H.: Dexepin, ein neues Antidepressivum: Wirkungsvergleich mit Amitriptylin, Arzneimittelforschung **19:**1642-1646, 1969.
58. Ananth, J.: Treatment of obsessive compulsive neurosis: pharmacological approach, Psychosomatics **17:**180-184, 1976.
59. Pippard, J.: Rostral leucotomy: a report of 240 cases personally followed 1½-5 years, J. Ment. Sci. **101:**756, 1955.
60. Hodgson, R., Rachman, S., and Marks, I. M.: The treatment of chronic obsessive compulsive neurosis: follow up, Behav. Res. Ther. **10:**181, 1972.
61. Kannel, W. B., Dawber, T. R., and Cohen, M. E.: The ECG in neurocirculatory asthenia (anxiety neurosis or neurasthenia): a study of 203 neuro-circulatory patients and 757 healthy controls in the Framingham study, Ann. Inter. Med. **49:**1351, 1958.
62. Cohen, M. E., White, P. D., and Johnson, R. E.: Neurocirculatory asthenia, anxiety neurosis or the effort syndrome, Arch. Intern. Med. **81:**260, 1948.
63. Marks, I., and Lader, M.: Anxiety states: a review, J. Nerv. Ment. Dis. **156**(1):3, 1973.
64. White, P. D., and Jones, T. D.: Heart disease and disorders in New England, Am. Heart J. **3:**302, 1928.
65. White, P. D.: Heart disease, ed. 4, New York, 1956, Macmillan, Inc., p. 582.

66. Slater, E., and Shilds, J.: Genetical aspects of anxiety. In Lader, M. H.: Studies of anxiety, London, 1969, Royal Medico-Psychological Association.
67. Shields, J.: Monozygotic twins brought up apart and brought up together, London, 1962, Oxford University Press.
68. Woods, P.: Da Costa's syndrome (or effort syndrome), Br. Med. J. **1:**756, 805-845, 1941.
69. Frolich, E. D., Tarazi, R. D., and Dustan, H. P.: Hyperdynamic beta-adrenergic circulatory state: increased beta-receptor responsiveness, Arch. Intern. Med. **123:**1, 1969.
70. Wheeler, E. O., White, P. D., Reed, E. W., and Cohen, M. E.: Neurocirculatory asthenia (anxiety neurosis, effort syndrome, neurasthenia): a twenty year follow-up study of 173 patients, J.A.M.A. **142:**878, 1950.
71. Imhof, P., Brunner, H.: The treatment of functional heart disorders with beta-adrenergic blocking agents, Postgrad. Med. **46**(Suppl.):96, 1970.
72. Jones, M., and Mellirsh, V.: A comparison of the exercise response in various groups of neurotic patients and a method of rapid determination of oxygen in expired air using a catharometer, Psychosom. Med. **1:**192, 1946.
73. Cohen, M. D., Consolzaio, R. D., and Johnson, R. E.: Blood lactate response during moderate exercise in neurocirculatory asthenia, anxiety neurosis or effort syndrome, J. Clin. Invest. **26:**339, 1947.
74. Pitts, F. M., and McClure, J. N.: Lactate metabolism in anxiety neurosis N. Engl. J. Med. **277:**1329, 1967.
75. Cohen, M. E., Johnson, R. E., Consolazio, F. C., and White, P. D.: Low oxygen consumption and low ventilatory efficiency during exhausting work in patients with neurocirculatory asthenia, effort syndrome, and anxiety neurosis, J. Clin. Invest. **25:**292, 1946.
76. Cobb, S., Cohen, M. E., Badaz, D. W.: Capillaries of the nail fold in patients with neurocirculatory asthenia (effort syndrome, anxiety neurosis), Arch. Neurol. Psychiat. **56:**643-650, 1946.
77. Kelley, D. H. W.: Measurement of anxiety by forearm blood flow, Br. J. Psychiatry **112:**789-798, 1966.

**SUGGESTED READINGS**

Carey, M. S., and others: The use of clomipramine in phobic patients: preliminary research report, Cur. Ther. Res. **17**(1):107-110, 1975.
Gorlin, R.: The hyperkinetic heart syndrome, J.A.M.A. **182:**823-829, 1962.
Marks, I. M., Birley, J. L. T., and Gelder, M. G.: Modified leucotomy in severe agoraphobia: a controlled serial inquiry, Br. J. Psychiatry **112:**757-769, 1966.

# 9

# Psychotic and borderline patients

**JAMES E. GROVES**

*"He can't stay here—he's crazy!"*
*Intern to consultant, 1973*

---

The psychotic or borderline patient with a serious physical illness can become a hospital orphan. In practice, patients with a combination of serious psychiatric and somatic illnesses tend to remain on general hospital wards because life-threatening medical or surgical conditions overrule all other considerations. Often the psychiatric consultant must coordinate the treatment and effect the behavioral management of the psychotic or disruptive patient. This chapter is a practicum for the consultant who becomes responsible for such situations. The two general areas of the consultant's work are (1) the patient and (2) the consultee and house staff. Neglect of either area rapidly undermines the other.

## THE PATIENT

Work with the patient begins with differential diagnosis; intelligent differential diagnosis begins with an awareness of the multiple manifestations and many causes of disorders of behavior and thinking. Further on, in the discussion of patient management, attention is given to the presence or absence of dependency, manipulativeness, hostility, and violence. For diagnosis, however, initial discriminations are made among conditions that manifest the following:

1. A formal disorder of thinking as shown on mental status examination
2. Acute onset, rapid deterioration, and sudden personality change without history of similar episodes
3. Impairment of consciousness, orientation, memory, perception, or intellectual function (for example, verbal, spatial, or arithmetical abilities)
4. Physical, neurological, or laboratory abnormalities

Illnesses that present symptoms in the first and second categories, but not in the third and fourth, tend to have nonorganic diagnoses, for example, schizophrenia. It is important to be aware, however, that a catastrophic deterioration of personality in persons previously functioning at a high level (category 2) often signifies an organic illness such as encephalitis. When abnormalities in intellect (category 3) are found, especially when there are also physical, neurological, or laboratory abnormalities, the clinician's suspicion of organic causes of psychosis should be increased. "Psychosis" is used here in its broadest sense as any state in which the patient is out of touch with reality. In the following box is a list of conditions in which the patient may at first appear psychotic.

### Differential diagnosis of psychotic and borderline conditions

**Schizophrenia.** The diagnosis of schizophrenia typically depends on the presence of a formal thought disorder. Kraepelin[1] pulled together several subtypes of schizophrenia under the name "dementia praecox" (after Morel). The word "praecox" connotes that most such patients are under 35 years of age at the time of diagnosis. Kraepelin described the thinking as illogical and delusional, and he described the prognosis as usually poor. A suggested criterion for the diagnosis was the absence of recovery. Bleuler[2] renamed the group of illnesses "schizophrenia" and set forth diagnostic criteria based on the presence of the "fundamental symptoms" of:

1. Loose associations—or illogical, bizarre connections in speech and thought
2. Impaired affect—or abnormal, flat, or incongruent expressions of feeling
3. Ambivalence in feelings, expression, or motivation
4. Autism—or withdrawal into peculiar, idiosyncratic frames of reference

Bleuler considered as "secondary" or "accessory" the presence of hallucinations, delusions, catatonia, and depressive symptoms. Schneider[3] searched for "first-rank" or pathognomonic symptoms unique to the illness; these, he believed were:

1. Auditory hallucinations, voices seeming to come from outside the patient's head, uttering full sentences, arguing about the patient, referring to the patient in the third person, or seeming to broadcast the patient's thoughts aloud
2. Delusions of alien experiences seemingly imposed by an external agency, such as thoughts put into or taken from the patient's mind

## DIAGNOSTIC POSSIBILITIES WHEN THE PATIENT APPEARS OUT OF TOUCH WITH REALITY

**Psychiatric**

Schizophrenia, acute or chronic[1-44]
Manic-depressive illness, manic or depressed (Chapter 10)
Personality disorders, for example, borderline[45-72]
Stress (reactive) disorders, for example, traumatic war neurosis[73-75]
Episodic dyscontrol[76-89]
Ganser syndrome

**Neurologic** (Chapter 6)[90-99]

Head trauma
Space-occupying lesions, for example, tumors, hydrocephalus
Vascular lesions, for example, infarcts, hemorrhages
Seizure disorders, especially psychomotor seizures
Degenerative diseases, for example, Alzheimer's, Pick's, and Huntington's diseases
Infections of the central nervous system

**Endocrine**

Thyroid disorders[100]
Parathyroid disorders[101]
Adrenal dysfunction
Pituitary dysfunction
Diabetes mellitus

**Metabolic**

Fluid and electrolyte imbalance
Respiratory failure
Cardiac failure
Hepatic failure
Renal failure
Hypoglycemia, hyperglycemia, ketoacidosis
Porphyria[102]
Wilson's disease[103]
Folate-responsive homocystinuria[104]
Adult phenylketonuria[105]
Periodic catatonia[106]

**Deficiency states**

Pernicious anemia
Beriberi, Wernicke-Korsakoff syndrome
Pellagra
Pyridoxine deficiency

**Postoperative states** (Chapter 5)[107-109]

Postoperative delirium
Postoperative psychosis
Postoperative depression

**Systemic illnesses**

Carcinomatosis
Infections (bacterial, fungal, parasitic)
Viral syndromes, hepatitis, mononucleosis
Starvation, dehydration, exposure, heatstroke
Collagen and autoimmune diseases

**Abstinence phenomena** (Chapters 2, 3)

Alcohol withdrawal, delirium tremens
Barbiturate withdrawal
Narcotic withdrawal

**Intoxications**

Alcohol, for example, hallucinosis, pathological intoxication[79]
Barbiturates
Hallucinogens, for example, amphetamines, LSD,
    mescaline, THC and phencyclidine
Opiates, especially cocaine[110]
Heavy metals
Bromide
Organic phosphates, (insecticides)[111]
Anticholinergic compounds[112,113]
Carbon monoxide
Carbon disulfide, other industrial agents

**Unwanted effects of medication** (Chapters 26, 27)

Antipsychotics—"psychotoxic" or "paradoxical" reactions and/or
    akathisia[114,115]
Sedative-hypnotics[116]
Antidepressants
Lithium carbonate
Disulfiram
Levodopa[117,118]
Analgesics (narcotics, pentazocine)
Anticonvulsants
Antituberculous drugs (isoniazid, cycloserine)
Antiinflammatory agents (indomethacin, phenylbutazone)
Antihypertensive agents (especially those containing reserpine and
    methyldopa)
Cardiac drugs (digitalis, procainamide, propranolol)
Idiosyncratic reactions to almost any medication

or sensations, emotions, impulses, or actions not the patient's own

3. Delusional perceptions, perceptions consensually validated by others but having for the patient a specific, personal, private meaning not validated by others

Any one of these, Schneider thought, made the diagnosis of schizophrenia certain and excluded all others. The descriptions of schizophrenia by Kraepelin, Bleuler, and Schneider, while helpful, do not reliably define an illness with high interobserver agreement or one for which the diagnosis remains stable over long periods of time. For example, many manic, depressive, and borderline patients may display Schneider's first-rank symptoms and may at first seem schizophrenic.

For research purposes many systems of criteria for the diagnosis have been proposed. The box on the opposite page presents two[4-6] such systems that are widely used. There are, of course, many others,[7-11] both for research and for clinical purposes.

As diagnostic criteria are more stringently defined, schizophrenia becomes a diagnosis of exclusion—a disorder of thinking and behavior that is not of short duration; that has no known neurological, metabolic, or toxic etiology; and that is not primarily a disturbance of mood. Clinical experience and accumulated research, such as the Feighner or WHO criteria, have caused certain long-standing assumptions to be challenged as incorrect or overly simplistic:

1. Acute and chronic, remitting and nonremitting, reactive and process types of schizophrenia are distinct from one another and are determinate from presenting symptoms; course can be predicted from presentation.
2. Affective illness and schizophrenia are two entirely separate entities; diagnosis determines prognosis in terms of remission or nonremission.
3. Schizophrenic subtypes (such as paranoid, catatonic, hebephrenic, and simple) are clearcut and have prognostic significance.
4. Organic brain disease and schizophrenia are two entirely distinct conditions.

Even Kraepelin found that a small proportion of supposedly incurable schizophrenic patients recovered from psychosis; naturally, prognosis has always been an important issue. It begins to appear, however, that diagnosis based on symptom-criteria from the initial presentation alone is a weak predictor of outcome[12] and that employment history, social competency, and duration of hospitalization are better predictors of outcome[13] than time-course of onset, presence of traumatic precipitants, or certain mental status findings, such as confusion and

---

## RESEARCH CRITERIA FOR THE DIAGNOSIS OF SCHIZOPHRENIA

**Feighner criteria, 1972[4]**
All are necessary for the diagnosis.

1. Chronic illness of at least 6 months' duration
2. Absence of depressive or manic symptoms
3. Delusions or hallucinations
4. Verbal productions that make communication difficult because of lack of logical or understandable organization
5. At least three of the following:
   a. Not married
   b. History of poor work or social adjustment
   c. Family history of schizophrenia
   d. Absence of alcoholism or drug abuse within 1 year of onset of psychosis
   e. Onset of illness before age 40

**World Health Organization (WHO) criteria, 1973[5,6]**
Twelve items especially discriminative for schizophrenia

1. Restricted affect as manifested by blank, expressionless face or absence of emotional display during discussion of material that would ordinarily elicit emotion
2. Poor insight into illness
3. Thought broadcasting or auditory hallucinations
4. Absence of early morning awakening
5. Absence of feeling of rapport with patient by examiner
6. Absence of sad, depressed facial expression
7. Absence of manifestations of elated, joyous mood
8. Widespread delusions, with several areas of patient's life being interpreted delusionally
9. Free and spontaneous flow of incoherent speech
10. Lack of credibility of information obtained in the examination
11. Incomprehensible, bizarre delusions
12. Presence of nihilistic body delusions, such as missing body parts or deadness and dissolution

---

depression.[14,15] In general, only long-term follow-up with established remission is a strong predictor of good outcome. Attempts to correlate traumatic precipitant and presence of affective symptoms with good outcome, in the absence of prolonged observation, almost always fail. While there appears to be some correlation between good outcome and the presence of depressive symptomatology[16-18] or with reactivity to trauma ("reactive psychosis"),[16,19,20] lively debate continues about whether the "schizoaffective" and related psychoses are variants of schizophrenia, variants of affective illness, or a third psychosis distinct from both.[21] The presence of a thought disorder—even with a diagnosis of affective illness—seems to be associated with a nonremitting course for a majority of patients.[22] Similarly, the distinct subtypes schizophrenia of Kraepelin and Bleuler are neither clearcut nor prognostically useful,[15,23] even in the presence of such seemingly distinctive signs as those of catatonia.[24]

Even neurological signs of "organicity" do not exclude a diagnosis of schizophrenia; at some level of organization of the central nervous system (CNS), it is an organic disease of the brain[11] with some as yet unknown basis in disordered biogenic amine metabolism, possibly that regulating "gating" by the "striatal filter" of the limbic system.[25] Clearly, genetic predisposition plays a role in pathogenesis[26] and perhaps interacts with environment by lowering the threshold to external stressors, such as those inherent in the parent-child relationship.[27] There is some evidence that schizophrenic patients have disturbed perceptual-integrative functions, that they may abnormally process incoming information[28-32] (perhaps through a disordered limbic "striatal filter"[25]). The impairment of these functions possibly finds its expression in abnormal size-constancy tests[33,34] or in abnormal critical flicker fusion frequencies.[9] Information processing and perceptual abnormalities in schizophrenic individuals are still elusive, however, and there is good reason to doubt many studies on methodological grounds[35]; at basic levels of organization of the CNS, thinking, perception, and attention are difficult to separate.[36] It is difficult to know how to explain or what importance to attach to such findings as impairment of smooth-pursuit eye movements in schizophrenic patients and their relatives[37,38]; schizophrenic patients frequently have "soft neurological signs," such as mild cranial nerve abnormalities, incoordination, abnormal reflexes, impaired mechanics of speech, dystonic posturing, choreiform movements,[39-41] or even certain types of electroencephalographic abnormalities.[11,42] One of the not uncommon late sequelae of epilepsy is a schizophrenia-like psychosis.[11,43,44] Rather than showing that schizophrenia is actually epilepsy or that epilepsy leads to schizophrenia, overlap between conditions usually termed "functional" and those commonly called "organic" suggests their common basis in neurochemical abnormalities in limbic structures.

Manic-depressive illness presenting with either depression or mania may resemble schizophrenia. Dysphoric mood, vegetative signs and symptoms of depression—such as weight loss, early morning awakening, loss of libido, and diurnal mood variation—along with guilt, rumination, agitation, or psychomotor retardation, all strongly indicate a diagnosis of affective illness. Sometimes paranoid thinking is associated with depressive illness and there may be hallucinations and delusions; usually, however, there is a tinge of guilt or self-reproach with these. The patient will be convinced of wrongdoing, bodily damage, or a terminal condition, such as cancer. In manic psychosis, there is usually paranoia and almost always elation or irritation. The affect is labile and sometimes inappropriate. Speech displays flight of ideas—rapid jumping from topic to topic so that connections are usually apparent and sometimes related to external stimuli—unlike loose associations, in which connections are illogical or bizarre. The manic patient is frequently amusing, charming, or touching, and does not seem as alien to the examiner as the schizophrenic patient.

"**Borderline personality organization.**" This term connotes a severe disorder of character with features so vague that the disorder may be called "pseudoneurotic schizophrenia" in one hospital or clinic and "primary affective disorder" in another. The term is often more an epithet than a diagnosis; it implies about as much for etiology in psychiatry as "fever" does in medicine. The diagnosis is not recognized in current official psychiatric nomenclature, and, as Guze points out,[45] many patients called "borderline" actually satisfy the criteria of Feighner and colleagues[4] for sociopathy, alcoholism, drug dependence, hysteria, primary or secondary affective illness, or schizophreniform illness. While the term lacks reliability [45,46] (much less, validity), it is only fair to point out that such terms as "personality disorder" similarly lack diagnostic precision. Welner, Liss, and Robins [47] found that a cohort of patients initially given a diagnosis of "personality disorder" received a plethora of diagnoses on follow-up 1 to 2 years later: 26% received a diagnosis of affective illness; 22%, drug dependence; 13%, antisocial personality; 28%, undiagnosed; and the remainder, half a dozen other diagnoses. The point is that there is a group of patients who are neither clearly psychotic nor clearly neurotic; given sufficiently refined diagnostic criteria and observation over adequate periods of time, they can be given a variety of more precise diagnoses. At present, many such patients are initially called "borderline," an umbrella term that continues to be used and refined in the United States. In a review of the literature Gunderson and

---

**BORDERLINE PERSONALITY ORGANIZATION***
**Gunderson and Singer Criteria**

1. Presence of intense affect—usually of a strongly hostile or depressed nature—not flat, as in schizophrenia, but depersonalized, as in neurosis.
2. History of impulsive behavior—both episodic acts, such as self-mutilation and overdosage, and more chronic behavior patterns, such as drug dependency and promiscuity—resulting in self-destructiveness even if the intent is not self-destructive.
3. Social adaptiveness—manifested as good achievement in school, job, appropriate appearance and manners, and strong social awareness. Apparent strength, however, may reflect a disturbed identity masked by rapid and superficial identification with others.
4. Brief psychotic experiences—of a paranoid quality; this potential is believed to be present even in the absence of a history of such experiences. Such episodes tend to become evident during drug use or in unstructured situations and relationships.
5. Psychological testing performance—giving bizarre, dereistic, illogical, or primitive responses on unstructured tests such as the Rorschach but not on more structured tests such as the Wechsler Adult Intelligence Scale.
6. Interpersonal relationships—which characteristically vacillate between transient, superficial ones and intense, dependent relationships marred by devaluation, manipulation, and demandingness.

*Adapted from Gunderson, J. G., and Singer, M. T.: Defining borderline patients, Am. J. Psychiatry **132:**1-10, 1975. Copyright 1975, the American Psychiatric Association.

---

Singer[48] found that six features are typically present in an initial interview of the so-called borderline patient. The psychoanalyst Kernberg lists six "presumptive diagnostic elements," any two or three of which suggest the diagnosis.[49,50]

Borderline personality is seen as a severe, stable disorder of personality "lying between" the psychoses and the neuroses.[51,52] Grinker, Werble, and Drye[53] find borderline patients generally have defects in relationships, angry explosions, poor impulse control, lack of consistent self-identity, and depression characterized by loneliness rather than guilt. The presentation of the borderline patient may range, in Grinker's terms, from the "border with the psychoses"—in which the patient is chaotic, explosive, and impaired in reality testing,

---

**BORDERLINE PERSONALITY ORGANIZATION\***
**Kernberg's "Presumptive Diagnostic Elements"**

1. Chronic, diffuse, free-floating anxiety.
2. Polysymptomatic neurosis—multiple phobias, multiple personality, bizarre conversion symptoms, or obsessive-compulsive behaviors of a rigid, unshakable, ego-syntonic sort.
3. Polymorphous perverse sexual trends, such as are seen with multiple, indiscriminate, compulsive sexual liaisons with persons of either sex without any regard for long-term or personal relationships.
4. The " 'classical' prepsychotic" personality disorders—cyclothymic, hypomanic, paranoid, schizoid—once felt to progress to manic and schizophrenic psychoses.
5. Impulse neuroses and the addictions.
6. "Lower level" character disorders—hysterical, infantile, narcissistic, or depressive-masochistic characters.

\*Adapted from Kernberg, O.: Borderline personality organization, J. Am. Psychoanal. Assoc. **15**:641-685, 1967: and, Kernberg, O.: Borderline conditions and pathological narcissism, New York, 1975, Jason Aronson, Inc.

---

and yet, without a formal thought disorder—to the "border with the neuroses"—in which the patient is a depressed, empty, clinging individual with an inordinate need for companionship, tribute, and reassurance. Also, borderline individuals may appear to lack a coherent sense of self and adapt, chameleon-like, to their environment of the moment (like Deutsch's "as-if" personality[54]). Grinker's "core borderline" person is the superficially normal individual who has interpersonal relationships that range from transient and shallow to intensely dependent, punctuated by demandingness, manipulation, envy, and rage. Long-term follow-up studies are few,[55-57] but seem to suggest that the borderline patient's symptomatology is stable and does not progress to symptoms of chronic psychosis nor remit to symptoms of neurosis.

The psychoanalytic view of pathogenesis sees the borderline personality as arising from failure by the patient's parent to engender stable, coherent self-object differentiation and identity in the pre-oedipal period.[49-51,58-61] Whereas in normal development the child learns to separate from important objects with sadness and anger rather than with despair and rage, the borderline patient has not learned to tolerate negative affects associated with separation [62,63] and continues into adulthood the preoedipal child's clinging, as if others were desperately needed parts of the self rather than separate persons.[64,65] The boundaries between the self and others are blurred to such an extent that closeness seems to threaten self-loss by fusion and separation seems to threaten self-loss by emotional starvation. Because the patient's stance toward others is both too close and too distant, the sense of self becomes fragmented. Sexuality and dependency are confused with aggression; needs are felt as rage; there is little sense of ability to master painful feelings or to channel needs or aggression into creative achievement. Such a person feels so empty and so fragile that ambivalence is ill-tolerated and impulse control is poor. The borderline patient has a split representation of the self as simultaneously all bad and all powerful; the self-view is a chaotic mixture of frightened, shameful, and grandiose images.[49,50,61]

Important for patient management are the "primitive ego mechanisms of defense" of the borderline patient.[49,50] These maladaptive cognitive operations can be highly visible during inpatient work with the borderline patient.[66]

1. *Splitting* refers to a seemingly active process of keeping apart perceptions and feelings of opposite quality. Staff members are divided into "all good" and "all bad" ones, as if the patient cannot tolerate the anxiety-producing idea that caregivers are both "good" and "bad" at the same time.

2. *Primitive idealization* is the tendency to see some staff as totally "good" in order to protect the patient from "bad" staff and painful experiences.

3. *Projective identification* is a tendency to see some staff members as "bad" as the felt self. This gets translated into behavior based on the following kind of "logic": "I'm bad and you take care of me. That means you're rotten and dangerous as I am or otherwise you wouldn't have any dealings with me."

4. *Primitive denial* is an alternating expungement from consciousness of first one and then another perception of opposite quality or a wish so powerful that it obliterates crucial aspects of reality contradicting it. For instance, fear may cause the patient to deny a serious medical illness and flee the hospital where it could be treated.

5. *Omnipotence and devaluation* represent a shift between the need to establish a relationship with a magically powerful staff and a conviction of omnipotence in the self that makes all others impotent by comparison. The omnipotent caregivers are supposed to deliver the borderline patient from all evil; when this does not happen, the staff becomes impotent and hateful.

From the psychoanalytic point of view, these are characteristic of borderline personality organization but, in fact, the behaviors that reflect such mental operations may also be seen in psychotic patients and in some neurotic patients. An attempt at differentiation of borderline personality from schizophrenia[57] is shown in Fig. 9-1, in which results based on the 360-item Present State Examination of the World Health Organization show that the borderline personality seems to be characterized by the absence of a definite or prolonged psychotic episode, by the relative severity of dissociative experiences, by more severe anger, and by less anxiety, restlessness, withdrawal, and inappropriate affect.

While developmental factors may play a large role, the influence of heredity in the psychopathogenesis of borderline personality may be equally important. Certain aspects of the personality (for example, splitting) are seen in sociopathy.[67] Also alcoholism, poor impulse control, criminality, and poor object relationships may have large genetic determinants.[68-72]

In the differential diagnosis of borderline personality, several other diagnostic entities deserve consideration. Traumatic war neurosis[73-75] may present similar symptoms, but it occurs in combat veterans and, in its classical presentation, the patient's prewar adjustment is said to have been good. In contrast, the borderline patient's history of maladjustment goes back to childhood or early adolescence. The episodic dyscontrol syndrome, which is usually synonymous with "explosive personality," is also similar to borderline personality.[11,72,76-79] Such individuals, usually male, come to attention because of gross outbursts of rage and verbal or physical abusiveness. These outbursts are sudden, intense, and in response to various gradations of provocation ranging from minimal to massive. Between episodes, the individual may exhibit some social maladjustment but sometimes exhibits quite ordinary behavior or is even deeply repentant at these losses of control. Clearly, dyscontrol is multietiological. When large cohorts of nonpsychotic violent patients are studied,[80] a small percentage is found to have temporal lobe epilepsy, a larger percentage has "seizure-like" episodes, and a large percentage has pathological intoxications with alcohol.[79] About half of these patients, however, have no such obvious explanation and fall into a mixed group that may contain persons with psychosis or seizures or persons with borderline or antisocial personality. Monroe's schema[76] for classifying episodic behavioral disorders has great appeal because such conditions are arranged along a continuum ranging from disorganized, amorphous,

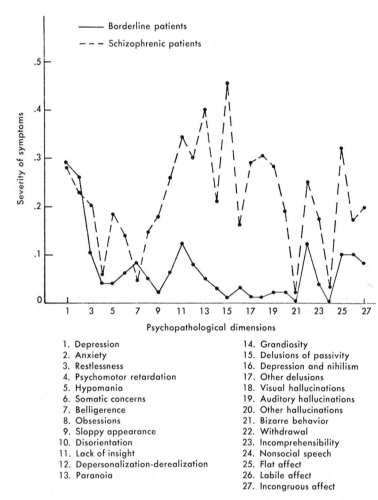

1. Depression
2. Anxiety
3. Restlessness
4. Psychomotor retardation
5. Hypomania
6. Somatic concerns
7. Belligerence
8. Obsessions
9. Sloppy appearance
10. Disorientation
11. Lack of insight
12. Depersonalization-derealization
13. Paranoia

14. Grandiosity
15. Delusions of passivity
16. Depression and nihilism
17. Other delusions
18. Visual hallucinations
19. Auditory hallucinations
20. Other hallucinations
21. Bizarre behavior
22. Withdrawal
23. Incomprehensibility
24. Nonsocial speech
25. Flat affect
26. Labile affect
27. Incongruous affect

**Fig. 9-1.** Comparison of present state examination profiles of borderline and schizophrenic patients. (From Gunderson, J. G., Carpenter, W. T., and Strauss, J. S.: Am. J. Psychiatry **132**:1262, 1975. Copyright 1975, the American Psychiatric Association. Reprinted by permission.

uncoordinated attacks on the nearest object at hand (ictal), through conditions in which there is a period of increasing tension and internal struggle preceding the explosive attack, after which an enormous sense of relief supervenes (impulse dyscontrol), to conditions in which there is unconscious conflict and considerable neutralization of the aggressive act by ego defense mechanisms (acting-out). Depending on where along the continuum the dyscontrolled acts fall, Monroe recommends pharmacological treatment with anticonvulsants, benzodiazepines, or a combination of the two.[76]

There is a body of evidence that implicates hereditary factors and organic brain disorders in the etiology of impulsive and dyscontrolled behavior. For instance, adoption studies suggest that a criminal biological father's offspring who are reared by a noncriminal adoptive father are more likely to become criminal than those of a noncriminal biological father whose offspring are reared by a criminal adoptive father.[69,70] Persons with antisocial behavior have a high prevalence of abnormal electroencephalographic findings and of "soft neurological signs" similar to those accompanying "minimal brain damage."[78] Finally, there is evidence suggesting that the hyperkinetic syndrome of childhood, which is often part of the family history,[81-83] may go on to be associated with delinquency and episodic dyscontrol in adulthood.[84-86] Moreover, amphetamines or tricyclic antidepressants not only benefit hyperactive children, but may also ameliorate impulsive and dyscontrolled behavior in adults.[87-89]

In the differential diagnosis of psychotic disorders, it is important to consider neurological conditions,[90] especially disorders of the temporal lobe and limbic system,[91-99] that may give a picture of "classical" schizophrenia. Also, endocrine[100-101] metabolic,[102-106] or deficiency diseases may present as psychosis without other findings. Postoperative syndromes,[107-109] abstinence phenomena, intoxications with drugs of abuse[110] or industrial compounds,[111] and unwanted effects of medication[112-118] may all be mistakenly diagnosed as schizophrenia.

**Psychopharmacological management**

Although psychopharmacology is discussed in more detail in Chapters 26 and 27, a few basic points are worth attention here:

    1. The consultant should be knowledgeable about one or two drugs from each class—the sedative hypnotics, the antipsychotics, the antidepressants, lithium, and the antiparkinson drugs—rather than lightly conversant with myriad drugs.

    2. Pharmacological control, if indicated, of disruptive behavior is

crucial for the safety of the patient, of fellow patients, and of the staff. Undermedication—especially with inadequate supervision of the patient—is typically far more hazardous than the commonly feared "overdosing" of a patient.

3. Drug interactions are to be avoided whenever possible. A common hazard for psychotic patients on pressors is epinephrine reversal with phenothiazines. Another, for patients taking antihypertensive medication, is hypotension or hypertension with antidepressants.

4. Route of administration deserves attention: benzodiazepines are absorbed much better orally than intramuscularly, unlike most other psychoactive drugs.

5. Illness-drug interactions require forethought. Antidepressants are particularly taxing to the cardiovascular system and often require so long for effect that electroconvulsive therapy should be considered as a safer alternative for consenting severely depressed individuals (and even some with other psychotic illnesses), provided the patient is free of CNS pathology. The serum half-life of tranquilizers is prolonged in patients with liver disease. Especially troublesome are the benzodiazepines because they are often given "routinely" and signs of overdose may not become apparent until several days after the first administration.

6. Careful attention to the dose of antipsychotic medications is necessary because clinical response (and probably serum levels[119]) vary widely from patient to patient and from dose to dose.

7. Whenever a psychotic illness is thought to be caused by a neurological, toxic, metabolic, or endocrine condition, treatment of the underlying condition should—if at all possible—be carried out without resort to psychopharmacological controls in order not to confuse the clinical picture.

Finally, the psychopharmacological management of the nonpsychotic disruptive or borderline patient deserves separate consideration, not only because psychiatric nosology is so confused in this area but also because such patients are prone to impulsivity, fragile reality-testing, and self-destructiveness. Klein's brief review[46] of this area suggests that tricyclic antidepressants are of value for patients who resemble neurotic depressive patients, phobic-anxious patients, and withdrawn, obsessional patients, if they appear to have a phasic depression but are otherwise well integrated. At the other end of the spectrum lie the chaotic, inappropriate, negative, and hostile patients (near the psychotic "border") and the extremely labile, vacillating patients who resemble patients with unstable character disorders (Grinker's "core borderlines"); for such patients "phenothiazine medication is distinctly valuable." Klein also reviews evidence that suggests lithium carbonate is of value in dampening mood swings in such patients and evidence that suggests monoamine oxidase inhibitors are useful in the treatment of "hysteroid dysphoric" patients.[46]

The house staff on a medical or surgical ward tends to begin therapy for nonpsychotic disruptive patients with sedative-hypnotics. If such a regimen is not effective—and often it is not—this tends to tantalize or anger the patient and staff. The result of such a trial may be a patient who is more out of control on than off medication, or a patient who is moving toward addictive doses of sedative-hypnotics. If a patient is not responding well to the antianxiety effects of sedative-hypnotics—and especially if the patient's reality-testing or impulse control is marginal—an antipsychotic medication in adequate doses is indicated and should be prescribed without delay. Haloperidol is generally fairly trouble-free for psychotic[120] and disruptive individuals with coexisting medical and surgical problems, except for frequent extrapyramidal side effects, especially akathisia and dystonia.

**THE CONSULTEE AND HOUSE STAFF**

The 4 year experience of Reding and Maguire[121] in managing acute psychiatric admissions to a general hospital in which psychiatric patients were not segregated from medical and surgical patients demonstrates the utter necessity for the intensive collaboration of the psychiatric consultant and the attending physician and nursing staff. The consultant in their hospital was not only readily available to the consultee but also gave particular attention to the nursing staff's education in the psychological management of the patient and to apprehensions regarding the potentially disruptive patient. The study reported on 344 admissions for acute psychiatric disorders spanning more than 4,000 patient-in-hospital days; 40% of these patients were acutely schizophrenic or paranoid and 25% were psychotically depressed or suicidal. During this time not one homicidal or suicidal attempt was made and only seven patients had to be transferred to a psychiatric hospital.

The 7 year experience of Reich and Kelly[122] showed that suicide attempts on medical and surgical wards correlated not so much with depression in serious medical illness such as cancer, but rather, with anger over loss of social supports in patients with personality disorders and psychosis. Of seventeen suicide attempts, fifteen occurred in a clinical setting in which the patient's experience was of being abandoned—during failing treatment, imminent discharge, dispute with the staff, or staff holiday (see Chapter 13).

The consultant can conceptualize the psychiatric consultation in several different ways. Meyer and Mendelson[123] see consultations as issuing from a feeling of uncertainty in the consultee, coupled with a sense of responsibility. If a patient throws a drinking glass while experiencing delirium tremens, the consultee has the sense of responsibility but not the uncertainty; the patient is exhibiting common behavior for a common condition. Identical behavior by a patient who has an undiagnosed illness is much more likely to precipitate a high anxiety request for consultation. Caplan[124] sees as determinants for consultation requests in community health centers feelings in the consultee of "(a) lack of knowledge, (b) lack of skill, (c) lack of self-confidence, or (d) lack of professional objectivity." Something about the patient's illness or behavior causes the consultee to feel inadequate to the situation. Lipowski[125] finds that psychiatric consultation requests occur (1) when no convincing organic cause can be found for somatic complaints, (2) when there is a change in the patient's habitual behavior, (3) when the patient has a recognizable psychiatric illness for which the consultee seeks management recommendations, and (4) when the patient displays "deviant illness behavior, such as self-destructive noncompliance with medical advice, excessive dependence, gross denial of illness, a given-up attitude, factitial illness, or suicidal threats or attempts."[125]

Bibring[126] has noted that when problems occur between physicians and patients it is not so much that physicians may not understand the patients but that the physicians may not understand their own reactions to the patients. Bibring and Kahana[127,128] discuss several personality types and the typical reactions of each to the stress of illness: the dependent patient asks for unlimited attention; the over-orderly patient obsesses about details; the overanxious, overinvolved patient is intense and dramatic; the long-suffering, martyr-like patient rejects comforting; guarded and aggrieved, overindependent, and aloof, fearful patients appear quarrelsome, hostile, or disdainful. For Bibring and Kahana, the work of the consultant is to recognize the wishes and fears that underlie such behaviors and to advise the staff about coping with them.

These several conceptual schemata treat the physician-patient-staff relationship as a system into which the psychiatrist is summoned for information or expertise. They acknowledge that the consultant's best work with the patient may be in vain without equally careful work with the staff. They imply the presence of dysfunction in consultee and staff that sunders them from customary effective functioning. They do not, however, systematically explore how the patient's behavior may be seen by the consultant as a source of staff dysfunction. The approach to consultation described in this chapter is based on an examination of behavior rather than personality because it is not the personality of the patient that is bothersome to the staff. It is the *behavior.* Moreover, the simplest possible approach is preferable when the consultant is summoned to see the psychotic or borderline patient.

**Consultee and staff reactions to disturbing behaviors**

A medical or surgical ward is a somewhat rigid social system with its own history, boundaries, hierarchy, customs, taboos, and aspirations. The introduction into this system of a psychotic or borderline patient—especially the violent or covertly destructive patient—sometimes places sufficient stress on the system to cause malfunction in caregiving or extrusion of the patient from the ward. Psychotic patients and especially those patients with borderline personality are exquisitely vulnerable to caregivers' (human) failures in communication, constancy of care, and uniformity of limit-setting. They are also remarkably attuned to their caregivers' negative feelings, such as anxiety, shame, anger, and depression. Similarly, the orderly, logical medical or surgical ward is exquisitely sensitive to forces that go against its rhythm, style, and direction. After diagnosis and treatment of the patient, the consultant's first priority should be to assess the amount of stress the patient is causing the staff.

Psychiatric patients may cause a state of "regression" in the medical or surgical house staff.[66] Regression may emerge as anger and disagreement among staff,[129,130] as inappropriate confrontation or rejection of the patient,[131-133] or as deterioration in the patient's behavior.[134-138] Regression on a ward seems to occur when there exists a noticeable disparity between what is expected and what is found. Troublesome dissonance between patient and staff may generally occur in any or all of the three dimensions of (1) perception of reality, (2) values governing control and aggression, and (3) rules about interpersonal closeness. The alliance between the consultant and the consultee is never firm until the consultant addresses these types of dissonance between the staff and the psychotic or borderline patient. The earliest, and often best, clue to the nature of the dissonance is in the consultation request. Its wording, tone, covert and overt messages, intensity, timing in the hospitalization, and the route over which it reaches the consultant all reflect the dissonance between patient and staff expectations.

**Consultation is sought when the patient is out of touch with the staff's perception of reality.** Such dissonance may range from mild—as when the patient is from a different class or value system—to moderate—as when the patient disagrees about the nature and treatment of the illness—to severe—as when the patient is psychotic. When something about the patient's view of reality strikes the consultee as strange, a consultation request ensues. Such requests mirror the degree of consultee stress. When the patient is psychotic but docile, tractable, and sexually well behaved, the consultation request is typically factual, lacks covert content, and reaches the consultant via a slow route, such as a note in the chart or a telephone call from the ward secretary. When, however, a psychosis is atypical or of unknown origin or when the patient exhibits grotesquely sexual or eerie behavior, the request may be intense and full of covert messages.

**Consultation is sought when the patient's aggression violates staff expectations.** The staff expects to be in control of the patient's regimen. It expects the patient to be grateful, obedient, and nonviolent. Patient-staff dissonance may range from mild—as when the patient sulks—to severe—as when the patient is violent or suicidal. The tone of the consultation request ranges from controlled and controlling irritation all the way to outright fear, depending on the behavior the patient is displaying toward the staff.

**Consultation is sought when the patient's need for closeness differs with what the staff deems appropriate.** The staff expects the patient to be involved with the caregivers; when a patient withdraws, dissonance is felt by the staff. Likewise, the staff expects the patient to keep a certain distance, and when the patient asks for too much, dissonance also occurs. It may range from mild—as when the patient is overanxious and asks for repeated reassurance—to severe—as when the patient makes inexhaustable, contradictory, or manipulative demands of the staff. Dissonance of this sort often comes to the consultant in the form of requests that reflect varying degrees of anger and depression in the staff. Arrogant, peremptory requests, sometimes concerning transfer or discharge of the patient, often signify a hostile, dependent, manipulative patient; depressed, tired requests may mean a clinging, empty patient.

### The approach to the consultation with psychotic and borderline patients

An orderly approach to consultations on medical and surgical wards saves time, reduces difficulty in diagnosis, and prevents oversight.

Generally the path the consultant takes should first lead directly to the consultee. The request and the history and hospital course of the patient should be elicited in person (or at least on the telephone) because the medical record does not commonly reveal all the problems in the management of a patient. Next, the consultant should go to the head nurse to get additional information about the patient's response to ward routine. Then, the consultant should read the chart in detail, review medication and management orders, and compare the orders with the nurses' record of medications given the patient, including scheduled doses and medication requested by the patient. After these steps the consultant will have some hypotheses about the roots of the problems for which consultation is requested and is now ready to test them in the clinical examination of the patient. Last, the consultant may need to speak with family, friends, or other hospital staff, such as the social worker, physiotherapist, or chaplain.

As the consultant goes through these steps, an orderly treatment plan emerges:

1. Physical or social restraints in emergencies—whenever the patient appears in danger of losing control of violent, disruptive, or self-destructive impulses
2. Differential diagnosis of the patient's condition
3. Identification of any staff-patient dissonance
4. Treatment recommendations—psychological and pharmacological, short- and long-term—taking into account the ongoing medical or surgical treatment and addressing staff-patient dissonance as well as the patient's illness
5. Education of the consultee and staff, not only to reduce dissonance and formulate contingency plans for changes in the patient's course, but also to form a conceptual framework for dealing with similar patients in the future
6. Follow-up and disposition planning adequate for the medical and psychiatric needs of the patient

The consultant's note in the medical record—by its tone, helpful information, and description of a patient that the staff can immediately recognize—is a part of the alliance with the staff; it remains at all hours as a tangible symbol of the consultant's helping presence. It should briefly outline the precipitant and history of the present illness, the patient's mental status at the time of the examination, the patient's previous psychiatric history, and previous behavior in ward situations. It should be explicit about medications, any suicide potential, and specific management recommendations, as in this excerpt from a note about a borderline patient:

*Impression:* Ms. B. is thought to have a chronic, severe character disorder sometimes called "borderline personality," meaning that she lies somewhere between neurosis and psychosis diagnostically and has only marginal social adjustment.

*Recommendations:* 1. Continue haloperidol, 2 to 10 mg orally twice a day or as needed. 2. Have brief, daily staff conferences to compare notes and reach a consensus about Ms. B's treatment plan. 3. Try to have the same staff members work with Ms. B. each day; bear in mind that she tends to panic at each change of shift. 4. Set firm limits on her multiple and contradictory demands; she is quick to rage when her demands are not met and may threaten suicide. Do not imply that Ms. B. does not deserve the things she demands, but rather say over and over again that you understand what she is asking but because you feel she *deserves* the best possible care, you are going to continue to follow the course dictated by your experience and judgment. If she continues spitting in her hyperalimentation line, assure her that physical restraint will ensue. (These limits do not mean that she should not be allowed to complain but do mean that you needn't tolerate more than twice as much as you would from the average patient.) 5. Suicide precautions; search her luggage.

The consultant has addressed dissonances arising from the patient's compromised ability to test reality, her tendency to act out self-destructively or violently, and her demandingness, entitlement, and manipulativeness. The consultant has given a mandate for open communication and daily staff conferences to prevent staff splitting; constant personnel and supportive environment are recommended; and firm limits without challenging the patient's sense of entitlement are explicitly set forth. The task now becomes that of seeing that treatment recommendations are carried out.

**Effecting the treatment recommendations**

There is nothing more frustrating than to labor to devise a treatment plan and then find that it is not being carried out. When this happens, the consultant typically finds that the source of resistance is unresolved staff-patient dissonance. Diagnosis, treatment, and staff education are intertwined. The consultant can "think aloud" about the patient with the staff to add credibility to treatment recommendations so that they are instituted intelligently. But principally the consultant ensures that recommendations are followed by systematically reducing dissonances that baffle effective staff functioning.

*Dissonance arising when the patient is out of touch with the staff's reality* is in many ways the easiest to reduce. Generally a simple statement to the effect that the patient is of a different culture, has a different attribution of illness, or is psychotic will suffice to give staff enough distance from their conflicts to restore effective functioning.

Educating the staff about psychosis or lesser degrees of difference between their reality and the patient's can help the staff know when to challenge the patient's view. When the staff gains a sense of mastery in psychological management, anxiety is reduced. The major lesson the consultant has for the staff is that the environment of the psychotic patient should be highly structured. Structuring maneuvers range from scheduling tasks on the ward to reality-testing for the psychotic patient.

The term "reality-testing" is much bandied about, but staff may nonetheless try to humor the patient owing to fear that challenging paranoid thinking or delusional thoughts will somehow make the patient worse. The consultant may need to model reality-testing for the staff:

> *Patient:* I don't trust you.
> *Consultant:* Why should you—you've never seen me before. I'm Dr. Smith. Dr. Jones asked me to help you with your anxiety.
> *Patient:* Dr. Jones hates me.
> *Consultant:* Dr. Jones is irritated with your pulling out your intervenous tubing, but he isn't going to harm you.
> *Patient:* You're like all of them—want to kill a guy.
> *Consultant:* You're wrong about that. We want to help you get over this infection.
> *Patient:* Bullshit!
> *Consultant:* No bullshit.

*Dissonance arising when the patient has different values governing control and aggression* is typically reduced when the consultant defines the range of appropriate responses to patient anger; such responses range from supporting the angry, dissatisfied patient or giving in to a mildly demanding patient all the way to setting absolute limits on violence or self-destructive behavior. The staff may not know what to do about anger in the patient and fear underreacting or overreacting. The consultant reduces this anxiety by explaining the nature and management of varying degrees of aggression. Control of violent, assaultive behavior is an issue in treating only a small minority of patients in the general hospital. Disruptions usually result from maladaptive defense and flight impulses in the confused or delirious patient. Rarely, however, a patient will become dangerous to staff or other patients. In these rare instances, the most common warning is fear; someone becomes scared of the patient. Staff members almost never become frightened by delirious behavior, controllable anger in the patient, or senile pique, but they do tend to become edgy, then wary, then scared of impending violence. The consultant must heed the presence of this fear; the intuition of the caregivers is often the only warning before an explosion. Ominous signs in the patient are (1) rapidly increasing demands, (2) more frequent and intense anger, especially with abusive language, (3) mounting agitation and paranoia, and (4) an implacable crescendo of menace.

Before any decision about physical restraint of a potentially violent patient is made, hospital police or security guards—four to six experienced persons—should be standing by on the ward. This is a *first* step in the decision; security can always be dismissed with thanks after standing by, but to delay summoning help until after such a decision is to risk provoking the patient: paranoid patients are notoriously sensitive to minute changes in the rhythm and atmosphere of a ward. If several security personnel are not available, understatement is best and behavioral control should be managed by the calmest, least-ruffled, staff person available. This person should gently try to convince the patient of the security and safety of restraints. (Force is much safer, however, with violent patients.)

*Dissonance arising when the patient's need for closeness seems inappropriate to the staff* is often effectively reduced when the consultant gives the staff permission to give a withdrawn patient some distance and when the consultant encourages staff to say "no" to the patient who demands too much. Giving is a familiar and valued role for caregivers but they may feel guilt or failure when they cannot satisfy all of the patient's needs. Much dissonance occurs when the staff is angry and feeling trapped between the obligation to give and the desire to withold.

Pathological dependency presents most infuriatingly as manipulativeness—as intense, covert, contradictory, and self-defeating attempts to get needs met. Manipulativeness is the behavioral manifestation of a need by the patient to be very close to, but at the same time very distant from, sources of emotional support. Borderline patients especially are famished for closeness; at the same time, their sense of self is so poor that feelings of being close cause them to feel engulfed, overpowered, or not really alive. A manipulative patient can wreak havoc on a medical or surgical ward, especially if the staff is unaware of the communication problems the patient can create by using splitting.[66] Ever since the Stanton-Schwartz phenomenon was described,[134] it has been recognized that *covert* staff disagreement may exacerbate disruptive behavior by mental patients. Burnham[130] expanded the idea of patient-as-victim-of-conflict to include patient-as-cause-of-conflict as well. According to dynamic theories, the borderline patient, in order to cope with deep self-loathing, may see the staff as loathsome—otherwise why would they take care of such a person? (projective identification). Or the patient may see the staff as magically all good, to keep all the badness in the world away (primitive idealization). In order to cope with the anxiety of ambivalent feelings, psychotic and borderline patients may choose some people on the staff to be "all good" and some to be "all bad" (splitting). When the patient views a staff through this sort of cognitive model, the patient may eventually split the staff. The patient will tell a designated "all good" staff member what terrible things an "all bad" staff member has done or said or thought—and then swear the "good" one to secrecy. The "good" staff member, flattered by the confidence, will keep it secret. Meanwhile, the patient is provocative toward the designated "bad" staff member. There is less and less communication about the patient because of an accumulation of confidences by "good" staff and of contempt and withdrawal by "bad" staff. Eventually the two segments of the staff, each with a stereotyped view of the patient, come into conflict over the management of the patient. "Good" staff vote for more privileges and nurturance for the patient; "bad" want more limitation and punishment for the patient. The remedy for such staff conflict is the reestablishment of open communication, even if it is hostile, so the staff can come together in a more realistic, if ambivalent, view of the patient.

Although splitting and manipulativeness may be seen in many psychotic, anxious, or depressed patients, they are most stunningly demonstrated by the borderline patient. Such a patient necessitates the setting of firm limits on maladaptive behaviors. Adler[131] discusses firm, nonpunitive limit-setting as crucial for inpatient treatment of borderline patients because these patients need the security of knowing that they cannot destroy the caregiving system nor be destroyed by it, no matter how much they may wish this or fear it. It is a natural human impulse to confront such patients angrily, but Adler and Buie[132] offer a useful set of precautions for confrontations with borderline patients:

1. Acknowledge the real stresses in the patient's situation.
2. Avoid breaking down needed defenses.
3. Avoid overstimulation of the patient's wish for closeness.

4. Avoid overstimulation of the patient's rage.
5. Avoid confrontation of narcissistic entitlement.

This last precaution is as important as it is difficult to follow. Some patients exude a repugnant sense of innate deservedness so foul and palpable that angry or overworked staff members are tempted to confront it suddenly and devastatingly. But the point is, this sense of deservedness and specialness—magical as it may be—is sometimes the only defense the patient has to prevent being overwhelmed with panic, especially during the multiple stresses of a medical or surgical hospitalization. In limit-setting confrontations with manipulative, acting-out patients, firmness, repetition, and an appeal to the patient's sense of entitlement (rather than an assault on it) will need to be modeled for the caregiving staff:

*Consultant:* . . . Now what is this about your not taking the antibiotics that Dr. Black has prescribed?

*Patient:* I am not gonna talk especially with *that* one here. Listen, I don't like her face and you can't force me, force this crap down my throat!

*Consultant:* Well, you don't have to like this lady here, and there's no particular reason why you should have to like *me* either, but there are several very good reasons why you should take your antibiotics that Dr. Black has prescribed for you.

*Patient:* Yeah, well, I'm not going to talk with her here. I know my rights. And I'm not going to take that damn stuff. Get me a lawyer! I know my rights!

*Consultant:* You have every right to the very best medical care we can give you. Why is it that you feel so strongly against the antibiotics that Dr. Black has prescribed for you?

*Patient:* It's no good and, besides, Dr. Green said I oughtn't ever take antibiotics.

*Consultant:* Dr. Green said you should *never* take antibiotics? *Really?*

*Patient:* He said they'd kill me.

*Consultant:* Really? How come?

*Patient:* ARE YOU SAYING THAT DR. GREEN IS A LIAR?

(Here the consultant realizes that he is overstimulating the rage of the patient and allowing himself to be split against Dr. Green. He decides to lead back to an appeal to the patient's sense of entitlement.)

*Consultant:* Dr. Green . . . was he your doctor from before?

*Patient:* Best damn doctor I ever had and one million times better than the rest of you put together!

*Consultant:* Sounds like you like him a lot. He saw you through that other time you were in hospital?

*Patient:* Yes.

*Consultant:* And at that time you didn't need antibiotics.

*Patient:* Listen, goddammit, I am not going to take that crap!

*Consultant:* Well, the reason I ask is that you now have a fever from this infection and we on the staff feel that you deserve to have it treated in the best way possible.

*Patient:* Dr. Black, what does she know?

*Consultant:* Well, we *all* feel—

*Patient:* I am not . . . look, Dr. Green said that I shouldn't take antibiotics.

*Consultant:* —that you deserve the best possible treatment of this infection. I'm sure that if Dr. Green were here now he would *want* you to have the very best possible treatment of this infection, that he would agree that you deserve—

*Patient:* Well get him here. Get him on the phone.

*Consultant:* —would agree that you deserve—

*Patient:* Well, call him up. Get him on the phone.

*Consultant:* I can't. (Pauses.) Don't you think that if Dr. Green knew you were suffering from an infection that he would want you to have antibiotics, that he would want you to get the very best treatment, which you deserve.

*Patient:* No.

*Consultant:* You don't feel you deserve the best possible care of this infection?

*Patient:* Get her out of here! I don't like her face.

*Consultant:* We're going to leave you now for a little while and I hope that you'll think it over and allow yourself to have the kind of good medical care you're entitled to.

The consultant has to keep uppermost in mind the appeal to the patient's entitlement and not be sidetracked by attempts to split nor drawn into logical or illogical arguments. Repetition is crucial; this confrontation had to be repeated three times at 10 minute intervals before the patient agreed to take the medication.

*Dependent, manipulative patients stir up sadism in the caregivers that inhibits them from setting firm, effective limits.* Day in and day out the consultee and staff on a medical or surgical ward routinely and effectively help most patients establish better contact with reality, aid them in finding appropriate interpersonal distance, and suffer with and support them when they are angry and sad. What is it about the borderline patient that so compromises these intuitive functions in the staff? Regression in the staff under the pressures of the patient's character pathology is probably at least partially due to the subtlety of the patient's distortions of reality and the grossness of the patient's dependency and rage. The caregiver's ideal is "to know all, to love all, to heal all,"[133] to give perfect care. Especially alien to the staff's ideal is malice and aversion—hatred—for sick people; but the patient can at times generate a lively sense of hatred and sadism because the patient's unceasing demands make the staff feel devalued and unremitting anger makes them feel frightened and depressed. It is probably the additional heavy burden of having to deny or disown from the self such unwanted hateful feelings that most compromises the staff's effective functioning. Thus the consultant's main task is to create a relationship with the consultee and staff in which such negative feelings can be owned and dealt with.

The consultant does this by supporting the staff's collective self-esteem, reinforcing strengths rather than pointing out weaknesses, teaching and lending a conceptual framework to support their anxiety, modeling interactions, helping them to identify with an effective clinician, and, most of all, by matter-of-factly stating that such patients stir up hatred, even in the best of caregivers:

> *Consultant:* Now let me see if I understand . . . you don't feel you're getting anywhere with her because—because why?
>
> *Staff A:* Well, it's just that—oh heck—all the things we've just talked about. She's bitchy, she's a liar. She's manipulative. She doesn't listen. She tells lies about us.
>
> *Consultant:* And the team meetings?
>
> *Staff A:* Well they've helped a certain extent . . . at least we're not at each other's throats. At least we can compare notes and sort out the lies . . . but we . . . or at least *I* can't get anywhere.
>
> *Consultant:* Even though the meetings have helped and her behavior has settled down, you don't *feel* like you're getting anywhere.
>
> *Staff A:* I can't do it . . . I mean, can't get her to do what's best for her, can't get her to listen to me—I mean, it's not like I'm wanting to punish her, not like I *want* her to suffer with the dressing changes and so on—but like she won't mind me and acts like I'm *trying* to hurt her—
>
> *Staff B:* She's just the same with me! I mean, like you go near her and she yells the roof down. I can't stand it any more. I just don't go near her any more because I don't like being accused of deliberately hurting her.
>
> *Consultant:* So everybody feels the same way—she won't listen, she lies, and she makes us feel like we're deliberately hurting her. (Pause.) Sounds like she needs a *spanking* . . .
>
> (Pause, then A and B laugh explosively.)
>
> *Staff A:* I'm glad *you* said that, not me!
>
> *Staff B:* I've thought that myself!
>
> *Consultant:* Well, we've all thought it. She makes me mad as hell. You folks work your guts out but she makes you feel like you're sadists or something. She's the kind of patient who makes us *wish* something bad would happen to her—or makes us stay away from her, as you have (nods to Staff B).
>
> *Staff A:* You know, if she didn't make me so mad at her, I think I wouldn't mind so much that she doesn't listen or tells lies.
>
> *Consultant:* Exactly! She makes us mad and stirs up rejecting feelings—feelings of hate that are perfectly normal in dealing with

this type of patient—and as a consequence, we feel guilty, feel like we are bad somehow for having these normal feelings of anger.

*Staff B:* But what do we do to get rid of the angry feelings?

*Consultant:* I'm not sure we *can* "get rid" of the hate she causes us to feel—all we can do is not let it interfere with our job with her . . . you know, she's pulling what I like to call the "skunk maneuver." (A and B laugh.) You know what I mean: Her behavior makes us so mad that she "stinks" us away—I try *not* to deny the bad smell but, even knowing that I'm very angry, keep on trying to do my job, keep on setting firm, consistent limits.

Whenever the staff brings even a hint of negative reference about the patient, the consultant can recognize it by saying something like, "Yeah, these patients *are* manipulative—and irritating as hell!" Or, "Everybody dislikes dealing with this kind of patient—I know *I* do." This legitimizes hostility toward the patient but brings it to the consultant rather than to the patient.

*Termination* of the hospital stay of the manipulative and dependent psychotic or borderline patient is fraught with hazard. The consultant should ensure an adequate disposition for the patient. Also, the staff should be warned that the patient may not only intensify disruptive behavior as it becomes time for discharge but, simultaneously, may try to prolong the hospital stay. For instance, a borderline patient may secretly infect dressings or intravenous lines with saliva or feces and develop a fever—while simultaneously threatening to leave the hospital against advice. Or the patient may increase suicidal gestures, such as wrist-slashing,[139] in order to manipulate the staff. Firm limits and contingency plans for sabotage and premature leaving should be discussed with the staff. As the patient's discharge date approaches, the staff should be more observant of the patient and more visible and available to the patient. A definite discharge date should be set and firmly adhered to despite the predictable worsening in the patient's psychological status.[139]

After the patient has left, it is well for the consultant to return to the ward to review the treatment of the patient and to share some of the consultant's own feelings during the hospitalization. In this way, the consultant not only "terminates" with the staff but prepares the way for future work with the next psychotic or borderline patient who comes to the medical or surgical ward.

**REFERENCES**

1. Kraepelin, E.: Clinical psychiatry, New York, 1912, Macmillan Inc.
2. Bleuler E.: Dementia praecox or the group of schizophrenias, translated by J. Zinkin, New York, 1950, International Universities Press.

3. Schneider, K.: Clinical psychopathology, translated by M. W. Hamilton, New York, 1959, Grune & Stratton, Inc.
4. Feighner, J. P., and others: Diagnostic criteria for use in psychiatric research, Arch. Gen. Psychiatry **26:**57-63, 1972. Copyright 1972, American Medical Association.
5. Carpenter, W. T., Strauss, J. S., and Bartko, J. J.: Flexible system for the diagnosis of schizophrenia: report from the WHO international pilot study of schizophrenia, Science **182:**1275-1278, 1973.
6. World Health Organization: Report of the international pilot study of schizophrenia, Geneva, 1973, World Health Organization.
7. Astrachan, B. M., and others: Checklist for the diagnosis of schizophrenia, Br. J. Psychiatry **121:**529-539, 1972.
8. Yusin, A., Nihira, K., and Mortashed, C.: Major and minor criteria in schizophrenia, Am. J. Psychiatry **131:**688-692, 1974.
9. Lehmann, H. E.: Schizophrenia: clinical features. In Freedman, A. M. Kaplan, H. I., and Sadock, B. J., editors: Comprehensive textbook of psychiatry, ed. 2, Baltimore, 1975, The Williams & Wilkins Co., pp. 890-923.
10. Slater, E., and Roth, M., editors: Mayer-Gross, Slater and Roth, clinical psychiatry, ed. 3, London, 1969, Baillère Tindall, chaps. 5, 6.
11. Pincus, J. H., and Tucker, G. J.: Behavioral neurology, London, 1974, Oxford University Press, chaps. 1-4.
12. Strauss, J. S., and Carpenter, W. T.: Characteristic symptoms and outcome in schizophrenia, Arch. Gen. Psychiatry **30:**429-434, 1974.
13. Strauss, J. S., and Carpenter, W. T.: The prediction of outcome in schizophrenia. II. Relationships between predictor and outcome variables, Arch. Gen. Psychiatry **31:**37-42, 1974.
14. Serban, G., and Gidynski, G. B.: Differentiating criteria for acute-chronic distinction in schizophrenia, Arch. Gen. Psychiatry **32:**705-712, 1975.
15. Hawk, A. B., Carpenter, W. T., and Strauss, J. S.: Diagnostic criteria and five-year outcome, Arch. Gen. Psychiatry **32:**343-347, 1975.
16. Kasanin, J.: The acute schizoaffective psychoses, Am. J. Psychiatry **13:**97-126, 1933.
17. Vaillant, G. E.: The natural history of the remitting schizophrenias, Am. J. Psychiatry **120:**367-376, 1963-1964.
18. Fowler, R. C., and others: The validity of good prognosis schizophrenia, Arch. Gen. Psychiatry **26:**182-185, 1972.
19. McCabe, M. S.: Reactive psychoses and schizophrenia with good prognosis, Arch. Gen. Psychiatry **33:**571-576, 1976.
20. McCabe, M. S., and Strömgren, E.: Reactive psychosis: a family study, Arch. Gen. Psychiatry **32:**447-454, 1975.
21. Welner, A., Croghan, J. L., and Robins, E.: The group of schizoaffective and related psychoses—critique, record, follow-up, and family studies. I. A persistent enigma, Arch. Gen. Psychiatry **31:**628-631, 1974.
22. Croghan, J. L., Welner, A., and Robins, E.: The group of schizoaffective and related psychoses—critique, record, follow-up, and family studies. II. Record studies, Arch. Gen. Psychiatry **31:**632-637, 1974.
23. Carpenter, W. J., and others: Another view of schizophrenia subtypes, Arch. Gen. Psychiatry **33:**508-516, 1976.
24. Abrams, R., and Taylor, M. A.: Catatonia, a prospective clinical study, Arch. Gen. Psychiatry **33:**579-581, 1976.

25. Stevens, J. R.: An anatomy of schizophrenia? Arch. Gen. Psychiatry **29:**177-189, 1973.
26. Kety, S., and others: Mental illness in the biological and adoptive families of adopted schizophrenics, Am. J. Psychiatry **128:**302-306, 1971.
27. Rosenthal, D., and others: Parent-child relationships and psychopathological disorder in the child, Arch. Gen. Psychiatry **32:**466-476, 1975.
28. Buchsbaum, M., and Silverman, J.: Stimulus intensity control and cortical evoked response. Psychosom. Med. **30:**12-22, 1968.
29. Tucker, G. J., and others: Perceptual experiences in schizophrenic and nonschizophrenic patients, Arch. Gen. Psychiatry **20:**159-166, 1969.
30. Harrow, M., Tucker, G. J., and Shield, P.: Stimulus overinclusion in schizophrenic disorders, Arch. Gen. Psychiatry **27:**40-45, 1972.
31. Houpt, J. L., Tucker, G. J., and Harrow, M.: Disordered cognition and stimulus processing, Am. J. Psychiatry **128:**1505-1510, 1972.
32. Broen, W. E., and Nakamura, C. Y.: Reduced range of sensory sensitivity in chronic nonparanoid schizophrenics, J. Abnorm. Psychol. **79:**106-111, 1972.
33. Weckowicz, T. E., and Blewett, D. B.: Size constancy and abstract thinking in schizophrenic patients, J. Ment. Sci **105:**909-934, 1959.
34. Hamilton, V.: The size constancy problem in schizophrenia: a cognitive skill analysis, Br. J. Psychol. **63:**73-84, 1972.
35. Sutton, S.: Fact and artifact in the psychology of schizophrenia. In Hammer, M., Salzinger, K., and Sutton, S., editors: Psychopathology: contributions from the social, behavioral, and biological sciences, New York, 1972, John Wiley & Sons, Inc., pp. 197-213.
36. Luria, A. R.: The working brain: an introduction to neuropsychology, translated by B. Haigh, New York, 1974, Basic Books, Inc., Publishers.
37. Holzman, P. S., Proctor, L. R., and Hughes, D. W.: Eye-tracking patterns in schizophrenia, Science **181:**179-181, 1973.
38. Holzman, P. S., and others: Eye-tracking dysfunctions in schizophrenic patients and their relatives, Arch. Gen. Psychiatry **31:**143-151, 1974.
39. Pollin, W., and Stabenau, J.: Biological, psychological, and historical differences in a series of monozygotic twins discordant for schizophrenia. In Rosenthal, D., and Kety, S., editors: Transmission of schizophrenia, London, 1968, Pergammon Press Ltd.
40. Rochford, J. M., and others: Neuropsychological impairments in functional psychiatric diseases, Arch. Gen. Psychiatry **22:**114-119, 1970.
41. Quitkin, F., Rifkin, A., and Klein, D. F.: Neurologic soft signs in schizophrenia and character disorders, Arch. Gen. Psychiatry **33:**845-853, 1976.
42. Tucker, G. J., and others: Behavior and symptoms of psychiatric patients and the electroencephalogram, Arch. Gen. Psychiatry **12:**278-286, 1965.
43. Guerrant, J., and others: Personality in epilepsy, Springfield, Illinois, 1962, Charles C Thomas, Publisher.
44. Slater, E., Beard, A. W., and Glithero, E.: The schizophrenia-like psychosis of epilepsy, Br. J. Psychiatry **109:**95-150, 1963.
45. Guze, S. B.: Differential diagnosis of the borderline personality syndrome. In Mack, J. E., editor: Borderline states in psychiatry, New York, 1975, Grune & Stratton, Inc., pp. 69-74.
46. Klein, D. F.: Psychopharmacology and the borderline patient, In Mack, J.

E., editor: Borderline states in psychiatry, New York, 1975, Grune & Stratton, Inc. pp. 75-91.

47. Welner, A., Liss, J. L., and Robins, E.: Personality disorder. II. Follow-up, Br. J. Psychiatry **124**:359-366, 1974.
48. Gunderson, J. G., and Singer, M. T.: Defining borderline patients, Am. J. Psychiatry **132**:1-10, 1975.
49. Kernberg, O.: Borderline personality organization, J. Am. Psychoanal. Assoc. **15**:641-685, 1967.
50. Kernberg, O.: Borderline conditions and pathological narcissism, New York, 1975, Jason Aronson, Inc.
51. Knight, R. P.: Borderline states, Bull. Menninger Clin. **17**:1-12, 1953.
52. Grinker, R. R.: Neurosis, psychosis, and the borderline states. In Freedman, A. M., Kaplan, H. I., and Sadock, B. J., editors: Comprehensive textbook of psychiatry, ed. 2, Baltimore, 1975, The Williams & Wilkins Co., pp. 845-850.
53. Grinker, R. R., Werble, B., and Drye, R.: The borderline syndrome, a behavioral study of ego-functions, New York, 1968, Basic Books, Inc., Publishers.
54. Deutsch, H.: Some forms of emotional disturbance and their relationship to schizophrenia, Psychoanal. Q. **11**:301-321, 1942.
55. Werble, B.: Second follow-up study of borderline patients, Arch. Gen. Psychiatry **23**:3-7, 1970.
56. Small, I. F., and others: Passive-aggressive personality disorder: a search for a syndrome, Am. J. Psychiatry **126**:973-983, 1970.
57. Gunderson, J. G., Carpenter, W. T., and Strauss, J. S.: Borderline and schizophrenic patients: a comparative study, Am. J. Psychiatry **132**:1257-1264, 1975.
58. Zetzel, E.: The so-called good hysteric, Int. J. Psychoanal. **49**:256-260, 1968.
59. Zetzel, E.: A developmental approach to the borderline patient, Am. J. Psychiatry **127**:867-871, 1971.
60. Kernberg, O.: Structural derivatives of object relationships, Int. J. Psychoanal. **47**:236-253, 1966.
61. Kernberg, O.: The treatment of patients with borderline personality organization, Int. J. Psychoanal. **49**:600-619, 1968.
62. Zetzel (Rosenberg), E.: Anxiety and the capacity to bear it, Int. J. Psychoanal. **30**:1-12, 1949.
63. Winnicott, D. W.: The capacity to be alone, Int. J. Psychoanal. **39**:416-420, 1958.
64. Winnicott, D. W.: Transitional objects and transitional phenomena, Int. J. Psychoanal. **34**:89-97, 1953.
65. Modell, A.: Primitive object relationships and the predisposition to schizophrenia, Int. J. Psychoanal. **44**:282-292, 1963.
66. Groves, J. E.: Management of the borderline patient on a medical or surgical ward: the psychiatric consultant's role, Int. J. Psychiatry Med. **6**:337-348, 1975.
67. Vaillant, G. E.: Sociopathy as a human process, Arch. Gen. Psychiatry **32**:178-183, 1975.
68. Miner, G. D.: The evidence for genetic components in the neuroses, Arch. Gen. Psychiatry **29**:111-118, 1973.

69. Crowe, R. R.: An adoption study of antisocial personality, Arch. Gen. Psychiatry **31**:785-791, 1974.
70. Hutchings, B., and Mednick, S. A.: Registered criminality in the adoptive and biological parents of registered male adoptees. In Fieve, R. R., Brill, H., and Rosenthal, D., editors: Genetic research in psychiatry, New York, 1974, New York University Press.
71. Goodwin, D. W., and others: Drinking problems in adopted and non-adopted sons of alcoholics, Arch. Gen. Psychiatry **31**:164-169, 1974.
72. Winokur, G., and Crowe, R. R.: Personality disorders. In Freedman, A. M., Kaplan, H. I., and Sadock, B. J., editors: Comprehensive textbook of psychiatry, ed. 2, Baltimore, 1975, The Williams & Wilkins Co., pp. 1279-1297.
73. Van Putten, T., and Emory, W. H.: Traumatic neuroses in Vietnam returnees—a forgotten diagnosis? Arch. Gen. Psychiatry **29**:695-698, 1973.
74. Haley, S. A.: When the patient reports atrocities, Arch. Gen. Psychiatry **30**:191-196, 1974.
75. Fox, R. P.: Narcissistic rage and the problem of combat aggression, Arch. Gen. Psychiatry **31**:807-811, 1974.
76. Monroe, R. R.: Episodic behavioral disorders, a psychodynamic and neurophysiologic analysis, Cambridge, 1970, Harvard University Press.
77. Robins, L. N.: Deviant children grown up: sociologic and psychiatric study of sociopathic personality, Baltimore, 1966, The Williams & Wilkins Co.
78. Mark, V. H., and Ervin, F. R.: Violence and the brain, New York, 1970, Harper & Row, Publishers.
79. Detre, T. P., and Jarecki, H. G.: Modern psychiatric treatment, Philadelphia, 1971, J. B. Lippincott Co.
80. Bach-y-Rita, G., and others: Episodic dyscontrol: a study of 130 violent patients, Am. J. Psychiatry **127**:1473-1478, 1971.
81. Cantwell, D. P.: Psychiatric illness in families of hyperactive children, Arch. Gen. Psychiatry **27**:414-417, 1972.
82. Morrison, J. R., and Stewart, M. A.: A family study of the hyperactive child syndrome, Biol. Psychiatry **3**:189-195, 1971.
83. Morrison, J. R., and Stewart, M. A.: The psychiatric status of the legal families of adopted hyperactive children, Arch. Gen. Psychiatry **28**:888-891, 1973.
84. Mann, H. B., and Greenspan, S. I.: The identification and treatment of adult brain dysfunction, Am. J. Psychiatry **133**:1013-1017, 1976.
85. Quitkin, F. M., and Klein, D. F.: Two behavioral syndromes in young adults related to possible minimal brain dysfunction, J. Psychiatr. Res. **7**:131-142, 1969.
86. Mendelson, W., Johnson, N., and Stewart, M. A.: Hyperactive children as teenagers: a follow-up study, J. Nerv. Ment. Dis. **153**:273-279, 1971.
87. Richmond, J. S., Young, J. R., and Groves, J. E.: Violent dyscontrol responsive to *d*-amphetamine, Am. J. Psychiatry **135**:365-366, 1978.
88. Wood, D. R., and others: Minimal brain dysfunction in adults, Arch. Gen. Psychiatry **33**:1453-1460, 1976.
89. Morrison, J. R., and Minkhoft, K.: Explosive personality as a sequel to the hyperactive-child syndrome, Compr. Psychiatry **16**:343-348, 1975.
90. Davison, K., and Bagley, C. R.: Schizophrenia-like psychoses associated

with organic disorders of the central nervous system: a review of the literature. In Herrington, R. N., editor: Current problems in neuropsychiatry, British Journal of Psychiatry Special Publication no. 4, Ashford, Kent, 1969, Headley Bros.

91. Malamud, N.: Psychiatric disorder with intracranial tumors of the limbic system, Arch. Neurol. **17**:113-123, 1967.

92. Falconer, M. A.: Reversibility by temporal-lobe resection of the behavioral abnormalities of temporal-lobe epilepsy, N. Engl. J. Med. **289**:451-455, 1973.

93. Wells, C. E.: Transient ictal psychosis, Arch. Gen. Psychiatry **32**:1201-1203, 1975.

94. Waxman, S. G., and Geschwind, N.: The interictal behavior syndrome of temporal lobe epilepsy, Arch. Gen. Psychiatry **32**:1580-1586, 1975.

95. Glaser, G. H., and Pincus, J. H.: Limbic encephalitis, J. Nerv. Ment. Dis. **149**:59-67, 1969.

96. Himmelhoch, J., and others: Subacute encephalitis: behavioral and neurological aspects, Br. J. Psychiatry **116**:531-538, 1970.

97. Raskin, D. E., and Frank, S. W.: Herpes encephalitis with catatonic stupor, Arch. Gen. Psychiatry **31**:544-546, 1974.

98. Wilson, L. G.: Viral encephalopathy mimicking functional psychosis, Am. J. Psychiatry **133**:165-170, 1976.

99. Stewart, R. M., and Baldessarini, R. J.: Viral encephalopathy and psychosis, Am. J. Psychiatry **133**:717, 1976.

100. Davis, P. J., and others: Three thyrotoxic criminals, Ann. Intern. Med. **74**:743-745, 1971.

101. Gatewood, J. W., Organ, C. H., and Mead, B. T.: Mental changes associated with hyperparathyroidism, Am. J. Psychiatry **132**:129-132, 1975.

102. Tschudy, D. P., Valsamis, M., and Magnussen, C. R.: Acute intermittent porphyria: clinical and selected research aspects, Ann. Intern. Med. **83**:851-864, 1975.

103. Strickland, G. T., and Leu, M.: Wilson's disease: clinical and laboratory manifestations in 40 patients, Medicine **54**:113-137, 1975.

104. Freeman, J. M., Finkelstein, J. D., and Mudd, S. H.: Folate-responsive homocystinuria and "schizophrenia," a defect in methylation due to deficient 5, 10-methylenetetrahydrafolate reductase activity, N. Engl. J. Med. **292**:491-496, 1975.

105. Perry, T. L., and others: Unrecognized adult phenylketonuria: implications for obstetrics and psychiatry, N. Engl. J. Med. **289**:395-398, 1973.

106. Takahashi, S., and Gjessing, L. R.: Studies of periodic catatonia: IV. Longitudinal study of catecholamine metabolism, with and without drugs, J. Psychiatr. Res. **9**:293-314, 1972.

107. Layne, O. L., and Yudofsky, S. C.: Postoperative psychosis in cardiotomy patients, the role of organic and psychiatric factors, N. Engl. J. Med. **284**:518-520, 1971.

108. Hackett, T. P., and Weisman, A. D.: Psychiatric management of operative syndromes: I. The therapeutic consultation and the effect of noninterpretive intervention, Psychosom. Med. **22**:267-282, 1960.

109. Hackett, T. P., and Weisman, A. D.: Psychiatric management of operative

syndromes: II. Psychodynamic factors in formulation and management, Psychosom. Med. **22:**356-372, 1960.
110. Post, R. M.: Cocaine psychoses: a continuum model, Am. J. Psychiatry **132:**225-231, 1975.
111. Levin, H. S., Rodnitzky, R. L., and Mick, D. L.: Anxiety associated with exposure to organophosphate compounds, Arch. Gen. Psychiatry **33:** 225-228, 1976.
112. Greenblatt, D. J., and Shader, R. I.: Anticholinergics, N. Engl. J. Med. **288:**1215-1219, 1973.
113. Granacher, R. P., and Baldessarini, R. J.: Physostigmine, Arch. Gen. Psychiatry **32:**375-380, 1975.
114. Van Putten, T., Mutalipassi, L. R., and Malkin, M. D.: Phenothiazine-induced decompensation, Arch. Gen. Psychiatry **30:**102-105, 1974.
115. Groves, J. E., and Mandel, M. R.: The long-acting phenothiazines, Arch. Gen. Psychiatry **32:**893-900, 1975.
116. Greenblatt, D. J., and Shader, R. I.: Benzodiazepines, N. Engl. J. Med. **291:**1011-1015, 1239-1243, 1974.
117. Ryback, R. S., and Schwab, R. S.: Manic response to levodopa therapy, report of a case, N. Engl. J. Med. **285:**788-789, 1971.
118. Yahr, M. D.: Levodopa, Ann. Intern. Med. **83:**677-682, 1975.
119. Rivera-Calimlim, L., and others: Clinical response and plasma levels: effect of dose, dosage schedules, and drug interaction on plasma chlorpromazine, Am. J. Psychiatry **133:**646-652, 1976.
120. Anderson, W. H., and Kuehnle, J. C.: Strategies for the treatment of acute psychosis, J.A.M.A. **229:**1884-1889, 1974.
121. Reding, G. R., and Maguire, B.: Nonsegregated acute psychiatric admissions to general hospitals—continuity of care within the community hospital, N. Engl. J. Med. **289:**185-189, 1973.
122. Reich, P., and Kelly, M. J.: Suicide attempts by hospitalized medical and surgical patients, N. Engl. J. Med. **294:**298-301, 1976.
123. Meyer, E., and Mendelson, M.: Psychiatric consultation with patients on medical and surgical wards: patterns and processes, Psychiatry **24:** 197-220, 1961.
124. Caplan, G.: The theory and practice of mental health consultation, New York, 1970, Basic Books, Inc., Publishers.
125. Lipowski, Z. J.: Consultation-liaison psychiatry: an overview, Am. J. Psychiatry **131:**623-630, 1974.
126. Bibring, G. L.: Psychiatry and medical practice in a general hospital, N. Engl. J. Med. **254:**366-372, 1956.
127. Bibring, G. L., and Kahana, R. J.: Lectures in medical psychology, New York, 1968, International Universities Press.
128. Kahana, R. J., and Bibring, G. L.: Personality types in medical management. In Zinberg, N. E., editor: Psychiatry and medical practice in a general hospital, New York, 1964, International Universities Press.
129. Main, T. F.: The ailment, Br. J. Med. Psychol. **30:**129-145, 1957.
130. Burnham, D. L.: The special-problem patient: victim or agent of splitting? Psychiatry **29:**105-122, 1966.
131. Adler, G.: Hospital treatment of borderline patients, Am. J. Psychiatry **130:**32-35, 1973.

132. Adler, G., and Buie, D. H.: The misuses of confrontation with borderline patients, Int. J. Psychoanal. Psychother. **1:**109-120, 1972.
133. Maltsberger, J. T., and Buie, D. H.: Countertransference hate in the treatment of suicidal patients, Arch. Gen. Psychiatry **30:**625-633, 1974.
134. Stanton, A. H., and Schwartz, M. S.: The mental hospital, New York, 1954, Basic Books, Inc., Publishers.
135. Quitkin, F. M., and Klein, D. F.: Follow-up of treatment failure: psychosis and character disorder, Am. J. Psychiatry **124:**499-505, 1967.
136. Friedman, H. J.: Psychotherapy of borderline patients: the influence of theory on technique, Am. J. Psychiatry **132:**1048-1052, 1975.
137. Friedman, H. J.: Some problems of inpatient management with borderline patients, Am. J. Psychiatry **126:**299-304, 1969.
138. Pardes, H., and others: Failures on a therapeutic milieu, Psychiatr. Q. **46:**29-48, 1972.
139. Grunebaum, H. U., and Klerman, G. L.: Wrist slashing, Am. J. Psychiatry **124:**527-534, 1967.

# 10

# Depression

**NED H. CASSEM**

Commonest among psychiatric disorders, depression sufficient to warrant professional care affects from 2% to 4% of the general population.[1] Although this condition ranks first among reasons for psychiatric hospitalization (23.3% of the total hospitalizations), it has been estimated that 92% of all persons suffering from it are either treated by nonpsychiatric personnel or are not treated at all.

Depression is often seen in general medical practice and one British study estimates that of all medical inpatients 24% show at least mild depression.[2] In about 30% of the consultation requests to see medical patients with life-threatening illnesses depression will be identified.[3] In practical terms the consultant's task becomes sorting out from the despondency normal in any serious illness the bona fide depression likely to respond to somatic therapies. Both the normal despondency and depression merit and generally respond well to therapeutic attention.

## DESPONDENCY CONSEQUENT TO SERIOUS ILLNESS

Despondency in serious illness appears to be a natural response and is here regarded as the psychic damage done by the disease to the patient's self-esteem. Bibring's definition of depression is a "response to narcissistic injury."[4] The response is here called "despondency" and not "depression" because "depression" is reserved for those conditions that meet the research criteria of primary or secondary affective disease. In any serious illness, then, the mind sustains an injury of its own, as though the illness, for example, myocardial infarction, produced an ego infarction. Even when recovery of the diseased organ is complete, recovery of self-esteem appears to take somewhat longer. In myocardial infarction patients, for example, while the myocardial scar has fully formed in 5 to 6 weeks, recovery of the sense of psychological well-being seems to require 2 to 3 months.

## Management of the acute phase of despondency

A mixture of dread, bitterness, and despair, despondency presents the self as broken, scarred, ruined. Work and relationships seem jeopardized. Now it seems to the patient too late to realize career or personal aspirations. Disappointment with both what has and has not been accomplished haunts the individual, who may now feel old and a failure. Concerns of this kind become conscious very early in acute illness and their expression may prompt consultation requests as early as the second or third day of hospitalization.[3]

Management of these illness-induced despondencies is divided into acute and long-term phases. In the acute phase, the patient is allowed, but never forced, to express such concerns. The extent and detail are determined by the individual's need to recount them. Many patients are upset to find such depressive concerns in consciousness and even worry that this signals a "nervous breakdown." It is therefore essential to let patients know that such concerns are the normal emotional counterpart of being sick, and that even though there will be "ups and downs" in their intensity, these concerns will probably disappear gradually as health returns. It is also helpful for the consultant to be familiar with the rehabilitation plans common to various illnesses, so that patients can also be reminded, while still in the acute phase of recovery, that plans for restoring function are being activated.

Paradoxically, many of the issues discussed in the care of the dying person (Chapter 16) are relevant here. Heavy emphasis is placed on maintaining the person's sense of self-esteem. Self-esteem often falters in seriously ill persons even though they have good recovery potential. Hence, efforts to learn what the sick person is like can help the consultant alleviate the acute distress of a damaged self-image. The consultant should learn any "defining" traits, interests, and accomplishments of the patient so that the nurses and physicians can be informed of them. For example, after learning that a woman patient had been a star sprinter on the national Polish track team preparing for the 1940 Olympics, the consultant relayed this both in the consultation note and by word of mouth to her caregivers. "What's this I hear about your having been a champion sprinter?" became a common question that made her feel not only unique, but appreciated. The objective is to restore to life the real person within the patient who has serious organic injuries or impairment.

Few things are more discouraging for the patient, staff, or consultant than no noticeable sign of improvement. When there is no real progress, all the interventions discussed in Chapter 16 are necessary.

At other times progress is occurring but so slowly that the patient cannot feel it in any tangible way. By using ingenuity the consultant may find a way to alter this. Many of the suggestions of the next section apply, and a knowledge of the physiology of the illness is essential. However, psychological interventions can also be helpful. For example, getting a patient with severe congestive heart failure out of bed and into a reclining chair (known for 25 years to produce even less cardiovascular strain than the supine position[5]) can provide reassurance and boost confidence. For some patients with severe ventilatory impairments and difficulty weaning from the respirator, a wall chart depicting graphically the time spent off the ventilator each day (one gold star for each 5 minute period) is encouraging. Even if the patient's progress is slow, the chart documents and dramatizes each progressive step. Of course, personal investment in very ill persons may be far more therapeutic in itself than any gimmick, but such simple interventions have a way of focusing new effort and enthusiasm on each improvement.

### Management of postacute despondencies: planning for discharge and after

Even when the patients are confident their illness is not fatal, they usually become concerned that it will cripple them. As noted, psychological "crippling" is a normal hazard with organic injury. Whether the patient is an employable uncomplicated myocardial infarction patient or a chronic emphysematous "panter" with a carbon dioxide tension of 60, only restoration of self-esteem can protect from emotional incapacitation. Even when the body has no room for improvement, the mind can usually be rehabilitated.

Arrival home from the hospital often proves to be a vast disappointment. The damage due to illness has been done, acute treatment is completed, and health professionals are far away. Weak, anxious, and demoralized, the patient experiences, in Hackett's words, a "homecoming depression."[6] Weakness is a universal problem for any individuals whose hospitalization required extensive bedrest; in fact, it was the symptom most complained of by one group of postmyocardial infarction patients visited in their homes.[6] Invariably the individuals attribute this weakness to the damage caused by the disease (to heart, lungs, liver, etc.). However, a large part of this weakness is due to muscle atrophy and the systemic effects of immobilization. Bedrest, a disease in itself, includes among its ill effects venous stasis with threat of phlebitis, embolism, orthostatic hypotension, a progressive increase in resting heart rate, loss of about 10% to 15% of muscle strength per week (due to atrophy), and reduction of about 20% to 25% in maximal oxygen uptake capacity in a 3 week period. This was dramatically illustrated by the Dallas study[7] of five healthy college students who, after being tested in the laboratory, were placed on 3 weeks' bedrest. Three of the men were sedentary and two were trained athletes. As shown in Fig. 10-1, after the period of bedrest, it took the three sedentary men 8, 10, and 13 days to regain their prebedrest maximal oxygen uptake levels, whereas it took the two athletes 28 and 43 days to reach their initial values. The better the patient's condition, the longer the recovery of strength takes. Entirely unaware of the physiology of muscle atrophy, patients mistakenly believe that exercise, the only treatment of atrophy, is dangerous or impossible.

Fear can be omnipresent following discharge from the hospital. Every least bodily sensation, particularly in the location of the affected organ, looms as an ominous usher of the worst—recurrence (myocardial infarction, malignancy, gastrointestinal bleeding, perforation, or

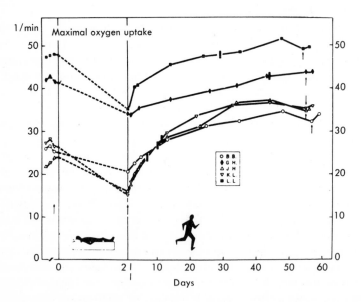

**Fig. 10-1.** Maximal oxygen uptake before and after 3 weeks of bed rest in five healthy college students. (From Saltin, B., and others: Response to exercise after bed rest and after training, Circulation **38**(7):1, 1968. By permission of the American Heart Association, Inc.)

other), metastatic spread, (another) infection, or some new disaster that will cripple the individual even further. Most of the alarming symptoms felt in the early posthospital days are so trivial that they would never have been noticed before, but the threshold is far lower now and patients may find any unusual sensation a threat. When the alarm has passed, they may then feel foolish or even disgusted with themselves for being hypochondriacs. It helps to know in advance that such hypersensitivity to bodily sensations commonly occurs, that it is normal, and that it is time-limited. Though there are wide ranges in the time it takes for this problem to disappear, a well-adjusted patient who has an uncomplicated myocardial infarction requires from 2 to 6 months for these fears to resolve (far more time than the recovery of the myocardium). With specific measures, this time may be shortened.

Whether the person can improve a physical function like oxygen consumption (for example, patients with myocardial infarction or gastrointestinal bleeding) or cannot do so at all (for example, a person with chronic obstructive lung disease), the mental state is basically the same—a sense of imprisonment in a damaged body, unable to sustain the everyday activities of a reasonable life. The illness has mentally crippled the individual. Horizons have shrunk drastically, so that the person may feel literally unable or afraid to leave the house, to walk across a room, or to stray far from the phone. Moreover, such people are likely to regard routine activities like walking, riding a bike, or raking leaves as too exhausting or dangerous. For some individuals, life comes to a near standstill.

The best therapy for such psychological constriction is a program that emphasizes early and progressive mobilization in the hospital and exercise after discharge. A physician might naturally be wary of prescribing this for a person with severe chronic obstructive pulmonary disease who is dyspneic while walking at an ordinary pace. However, Alpert and others[8] studied five such individuals, measuring pulmonary function and performing catheterization of the right side of the heart before and after an 18 week physical training program. Even though the investigators found that cardiopulmonary functions were essentially unaltered by physical conditioning, these patients reported great improvement in subjective exercise tolerance. Objective bicycle exercise tolerance increased as much as 1,000% in all five persons examined. The self-imposed restriction (for example, never being far from an oxygen tank) was dramatically relieved.

Progress in writing exercise regimens for the recuperation period has been greatly helped by the definition and use of the metabolic equivalent (MET). One MET is defined as the energy expenditure per kilogram per minute of the average 70 kg person sitting quietly in a chair. This amounts to about 1.4 calories per minute or 3.5 to 4.0 ml of oxygen consumed per minute. Table 10-1 lists activities for which measurements in METS have been determined.[9] For example, after recovery from uncomplicated myocardial infarction average middle-aged people are capable of performing at a level of 8 to 9 METS. This includes running at 5.5 miles per hour (jogging slightly faster than 11 minute miles), cycling at 13 miles per hour, skiing at 4 miles per hour, noncompetitive squash and handball, fencing, and vigorous basketball. If, however, less than ordinary activity produces symptoms, then the capacity of the postcoronary patient is nearer 4 METS. Despite obvious impairment, this level of capacity includes swimming the breast stroke at 20 yards per minute, cycling at 5.5 miles per hour, walking up a 5% incline at 3 miles per hour, playing ping-pong, golf (carrying clubs), badminton, tennis doubles, and raking leaves. For the patient these are carefully computed, quantitated capacities. A list of activities quantified in METS is far more concrete and specific than statements such as, "Use your own judgment," or, "Do it in moderation." Instead, the patient can be given a list and told to select activities up to a specific level of METS. The physician who wishes to determine a tolerable level can use such devices as step test, treadmill, and bicycle ergometer for which energy demand in METS at different levels has already been determined. Handy charts can be obtained in the American Heart Association manual.[10]

Activity levels can be gradually increased if appropriate, and patients should take responsibility for extra costs that emotional involvement may require. For example, they could be told, "I now move you to a level of activity of 5 METS. You will find at this level all the activities that your heart (or lungs or body) are physically capable of performing. Activities you enjoy are the best. Remember that getting emotionally upset or very competitive during activity greatly increases the energy cost to your heart (lungs, body, etc.). If you cannot do some of these things without getting all worked up, you will have to ease off; only you can judge that. But you now know that you are physically capable of performing at 5 METS." In this statement vagueness remains, but only in the area of subjective emotions. Patients not only experience their emotions physically and mentally but also should be aware of them, whereas they cannot detect changes in their left ventricular end diastolic pressure or arterial oxygen saturation. Moreover, emotional self-control is a fair request to make

**Table 10-1.** Energy expenditure per kg per min (METS) in the average 70 kg individual*

| Activity | METS | Activity | METS |
|---|---|---|---|
| **Self-care** | | **Housework activities** | |
| Rest, supine | 1 | Hand sewing | 1 |
| Sitting | 1 | Sweeping floor | 1.5 |
| Standing, relaxed | 1 | Machine sewing | 1.5 |
| Eating | 1 | Polishing furniture | 2 |
| Conversation | 1 | Peeling potatoes | 2.5 |
| Dressing, undressing | 2 | Scrubbing, standing | 2.5 |
| Washing hands, face | 2 | Washing small clothes | 2.5 |
| Bedside commode | 3 | Kneading dough | 2.5 |
| Walking, 2.5 mph | 3 | Scrubbing floors | 3 |
| Showering | 3.5 | Cleaning windows | 3 |
| Using bedpan | 4 | Making beds | 3 |
| Walking downstairs | 4.5 | Ironing, standing | 3.5 |
| Walking, 3.5 mph | 5.5 | Mopping | 3.5 |
| Propulsion, wheelchair | 2 | Wringing by hand | 3.5 |
| Ambulation with braces and | | Hanging wash | 3.5 |
| crutches | 6.5 | Beating carpets | 4 |
| **Industrial activities** | | **Recreational activities** | |
| Watch repairing | 1.5 | Painting, sitting | 1.5 |
| Armature winding | 2.0 | Playing piano | 2 |
| Radio assembly | 2.5 | Driving car | 2 |
| Sewing at machine | 2.5 | Canoeing, 2.5 mph | 2.5 |
| Bricklaying | 3.5 | Horseback riding, slow | 2.5 |
| Plastering | 3.5 | Volley ball | 2.5 |
| Tractor ploughing | 3.5 | Bowling | 3.5 |
| Wheeling barrow, 115 lb, 2.5 | | Cycling, 5.5 mph | 3.5 |
| mph | 4.0 | Golfing | 4 |
| Horse ploughing | 5.0 | Swimming, 20 yards per | |
| Carpentry | 5.5 | minute | 4 |
| Mowing lawn by hand | 6.5 | Dancing | 4.5 |
| Felling tree | 6.5 | Gardening | 4.5 |
| Shoveling | 7.0 | Tennis | 6 |
| Ascending stairs, 17 lb load. | | Trotting horse | 6.5 |
| 27 feet per minute | 7.5 | Spading | 7 |
| Planing | 7.5 | Skiing | 8 |
| Tending furnace | 8.5 | Squash | 8.5 |
| Ascending stairs. 22 lb load. | | Cycling, 13 mph | 9 |
| 54 feet per minute | 13.5 | | |

*From Cassem, N. H., and Hackett, T. P.: Psychological aspects of myocardial infarction, Med. Clin. North. Am. **61:**711-721, 1977.

of patients who, although not responsible for detecting rising wedge pressure on the tennis court, must control rising killer instincts.

In any serious illness where there are likely to be so many "don't's" constricting the patient's world, an exercise regimen provides something to do that widens the space of existence. If a patient were limited by a maximum tidal volume of 13 liters per minute, an exercise program could not increase it, but would help him see that even within those limits he can increase (at least) subjective exercise tolerance, venture farther (for example, away from oxygen), and hopefully experience increased freedom. Some patients suffer illnesses in which reserves wax and wane (the cancer patient with remissions and exacerbations, aplastic anemia patients between transfusions). They may view life energy as a fixed quantity that is used up by activity little by little; thus, they fear activity. The psychological benefits of exercise are such that activities should bring some sense of renewed vitality (improved sleep and appetite are common effects) rather than a sense of depletion or exhaustion. As hematocrit decreases (or blood urea nitrogen increases), capacity for exercise decreases. To continue exercising, such a person could set as a target heart rate that which was commonly experienced while exercising at his prescribed level of METS, or time and distance could be decreased accordingly. When his chronic congestive heart failure worsened, one man simply returned to the scene of his exercising, changed into his exercise gear, and sat talking with the "regulars" before returning home.

Just as getting sick is depressing, so is lack of progress in getting well. This normal despondency can further retard recovery. Self-esteem is restored by the methods described in Chapter 16. Yet it is also restored by recovery of the body. The consultant who continuously studies the iatrogenic and reversible aspects of physical abnormality and mythical obstacles to recovery can more effectively contribute to the shortening of convalescence and the rehabilitation of self-esteem.

## DEPRESSION
### Identification of treatable depression

Up to this point, no mention of somatic treatment (antidepressant medication or electroconvulsive therapy) has been made. One of the first problems in the consultant's mind is the identification of the patient for whom these therapies should be prescribed. "Depression" has been reserved for such conditions—as opposed to "despondency," which refers to the more general category of narcissistic injury. Moreover, it is assumed that (1) this depression shares the pathophysiology of unipolar affective disease, and (2) the most rational and efficient diagnosis is made by applying the criteria for unipolar affective disease.

Efforts to distinguish various types of depression—for example, endogenous-reactive, neurotic-psychotic, post partum, and involutional—provide no practical help in determining whether to use an antidepressant medication and are unnecessary. One useful distinction still retained is that between primary and secondary affective illness. The key to differentiating the two is the timing of the depressive event. The depressive event is called primary if it precedes any other psychiatric or serious medical diagnosis, or if the only preceding episodes of psychiatric illness were also affective (depressive or manic). The depressive episode is called secondary when there is a preexisting psychiatric diagnosis (alcoholism, schizophrenia, etc.) or a preexisting medical illness that changes life-style or threatens life itself. The only other distinction made is whether the illness is bipolar, that is, includes episodes of depression and mania, or unipolar, presents depression only. Fig. 10-2 diagrams the classification of clinical states of depression.

What then qualifies as a bona fide episode of depression? To determine whether patients should be given medication, the con-

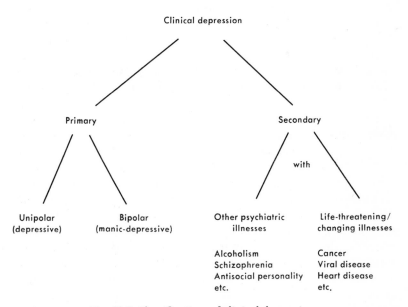

**Fig. 10-2.** Classifications of clinical depression.

sultant should methodically examine them for the presence of the Washington University research criteria for depression[11]:

1. Poor appetite or weight loss
2. Sleep disturbance, including any type of insomnia or hypersomnia
3. Fatigue, loss of energy, tiredness
4. Agitation or retardation
5. Loss of interest in usually stimulating activities—job, hobbies, social activities, decreased sexual drive
6. Decreased ability to think or concentrate; slow or mixed-up thinking
7. Feelings of self-reproach or guilt
8. Recurrent thoughts of death or suicide, including the wish to be dead

A patient who has five of the eight criteria is definitely depressed; four, probably so. The presence of a distinguishable loss or life event is not necessary for the diagnosis but is present in about 25% of the cases. The dysphoric emotional state should be present for at least 1 month, but the patient may actually deny being depressed. Although acknowledging not being up to par, medical patients sometimes have difficulty finding words for feelings. Also, the practitioner will readily see that persons with serious illness may automatically show criteria 1 and 3. Nevertheless, provided the medical illness has already been treated, the diagnosis of depression should still be made when the criteria are met. The follow-up experience of the Washington University group in diagnosing depression in medically ill patients is that the accuracy of the diagnosis, when these uncertainties arise, decreases from almost 100% to around 80%[12]—a statistic that fully supports the usefulness of these criteria.

The consultant must be vigilant for the presenting symptoms of medical illness in which depressive features may play a prominent but misleading part. Neurological (as multiple sclerosis), systemic, infectious (especially viral), endocrine (adrenal, thyroid, parathyroid), hematological (vitamin $B_{12}$ deficiency, anemia), malignant (pancreatic carcinoma), traumatic (subdural hematoma), and cardiovascular (thrombosis, stenosis, sick sinus syndrome) diseases occasionally present nonspecific symptoms of dysphoria resembling depression. Then, of course, the treatment required is that of the primary illness. The diagnosis of secondary depression cannot be made until such treatment has been continued long enough to reverse or control the primary illness.

Medications associated with depression include reserpine, levodopa, propranolol, methyldopa, steroids, adrenocorticotropic hormone, barbiturates, oral contraceptives, amphetamines, spironolactone, diazepam, and chlordiazepoxide. Most of these drugs, except for reserpine, methyldopa, and possibly oral contraceptives, will not produce a syndrome that qualifies as depression according to the research criteria. The other drugs produce polysymptomatic abnormalities of affect and cognition. Chlordiazepoxide, for example, can produce episodic uncontrolled weeping, but the patient usually reports that these spells are embarrassing and inappropriate. Diazepam may contribute to an overall sense of mental slowing, while some patients on propranolol report loss of a sense of excitement and zest (perhaps secondary to the blockade of sympathetic arousal). These are likely to be idiosyncratic reactions and the consultant's best clue to a drug effect is usually the patient's ability to relate the onset of dysphoria to the time when the medication was first administered. Steroids and adrenocorticotropic hormone (ACTH) produce a wide spectrum of mental disturbances, including depressive changes. Since individuals taking steroids often already have organic brain disease (systemic lupus erythematosus [SLE], cerebral metastasis, multiple sclerosis), diagnosing drug effects can be very difficult. Stopping the administration of a drug is the simplest way to test its role in producing mental changes, but if dexamethasone is being given to reduce brain swelling, the physician may be very reluctant to discontinue use of it. Management of symptoms with haloperidol can be helpful while steroids are continued, but it is usually necessary to hold, taper, or stop the use of them.

When should the physician suspect that depression is present but masked or missed in a patient? In general, any complaints for which no organic basis can be discovered, particularly where chronic pain is a component, should alert the physician to the possibility of depressive illness. Lesse[13] suggests that displays of irritability, antisocial acts, impulsive sexual behavior, sadomasochistic acts, compulsive work or behavior patterns, new or increased drug or alcohol use, and accident proneness can all hide a depressive core. However complex these issues may be, diagnosis of depression is best decided by application of the Washington University diagnostic criteria, once the suspicion has arisen.

## Pathophysiology of depressive illness

As a diagnosis, depression implies an underlying biochemical derangement of the central nervous system (CNS). The current accepted hypothesis is that a functional deficiency of two central neurotransmitters (both monoamines—norepinephrine and serotonin) is important in depressive illness. Contained in vesicles and stored in the presynaptic neuron, these monoamines are discharged by exocytosis into the interneuronal space and become molecular carriers of impulse transmission to the postsynaptic neuron. Transmission occurs when the discharged neurotransmitter binds to the postsynaptic neuron. The binding is brief and the molecule is released back into the cleft to be degraded or reabsorbed. The amount of neurotransmitter stored in presynaptic neurons is a function of (1) synthesis within the neuron and (2) reuptake from the extracellular fluid, that is, from the synaptic cleft. For norepinephrine about 80% of that stored comes from reuptake. Destruction of the unstored monoamine occurs within the cell by the monoamine oxidase (MAO) enzymes and in the extracellular space by the enzymes called O-methyl-transferases.

Current single amine theories simply cannot account for the clinical diversity of depression.[14] There do, however, appear to be two sets of promising evidence suggesting that norepinephrine-deficient and se-rotonin-deficient states of the CNS can be associated with two clinical subgroups of depressed patients. One group, with hypothesized inadequate CNS catecholamine function,[15,16] is characterized by low urinary levels of a norepinephrine metabolite, 3-methoxy-4-hydroxy-phenylglycol (MHPG), and respond to imipramine, but not to ami-triptyline. The other group, recently differentiated by Swedish investigators,[17] is characterized by normal levels of MHPG and low levels of cerebrospinal fluid 5-hydroxyindoleacetic acid (5-HIAA, a serotonin metabolite), and is presumed to represent a CNS serotonin-deficient depression. It might be assumed that the depressed patients with normal MHPG levels who respond to amitriptyline but not to imipra-mine are included partly or completely in the low 5-HIAA group. These theories are relevant to the choice of antidepressant medication.

**Choice of appropriate treatment**

Antidepressant medications act by increasing the amount of available neurotransmitter substances in the CNS. Tricyclic antidepressants do so by blocking reuptake of the neurotransmitter from the synaptic cleft, while MAO inhibitors increase the concentration of transmitter by interfering with the enzyme that destroys it within the presynaptic neuron.

In Chapters 26 and 27 the properties, side effects, dosages, and drug interactions of antidepressant medications are discussed in detail. For the specific setting of consultation the general principles remain the same. Tricyclic antidepressants are the first drugs usually tried and choice of the specific agent is often based on the drug's side effects.

About one-third of patients correctly diagnosed for depressive illness will not respond to tricyclic antidepressants. Many of these individuals will show improvement with MAO inhibitors, which are discussed in Chapter 26.

Electroconvulsive therapy (ECT) remains the single most effective somatic treatment of depression. Recent nationwide review of its use has not altered respect for its effectiveness. Indications for its use are discussed in Chapter 11.

### Prescribing antidepressants for the cardiac patient

Since the cardiac patient generates most concern in the use of tricyclic antidepressants, a specific approach to prescribing for this patient is emphasized. In general, the physician tends to select a sedating agent (amitriptyline or doxepin) for an agitated patient or a nonsedative agent (such as imipramine, protriptyline) for a retarded patient.[18]

Ever since sudden death in cardiac patients was first associated with amitriptyline,[19,20] physicians feared use of tricyclic antidepressants when cardiac disease is present. Fowler and others[21] recently emphasized that life-threatening arrhythmias can occur in patients without cardiac disease. How, then, can a physician prescribe an anitdepressant for a depressed cardiac patient?

Depression itself is a life-threatening disease and should be treated. Cardiac patients are not spared this distressing state and, when depressed, merit somatic treatment. Choice of the agent can be made

**Table 10-2.** Properties of tricyclic antidepressants

| Drug | Biogenic amine affected* | | Sedative potency‡ | Relative anticholinergic potency† |
|---|---|---|---|---|
| | **5-HT** | **NE** | | |
| Amitriptyline | ++++ | 0 | High | 8 |
| Nortriptyline | ++ | ++ | Moderate | 2 |
| Imipramine | +++ | ++ | Low | 2 |
| Desipramine | 0 | ++++ | Low | 1 |
| Protriptyline | ? | ? | O | (2)? |
| Doxepin | ? | ? | High | 2 |

*Adapted from Maas.[16]
†Adapted from Snyder and Yamamura.[22]
‡Adapted from U'Pritchard and others.[23]

methodically, keeping in mind the basic beneficial and toxic effects of the drugs. Table 10-2 lists the properties of the six tricyclic antidepressants. Tabulated effects for each are based on adaptations from Maas,[16] Snyder and Yamamura,[22] and U'Pritchard and others.[23] These agents have measurable neurochemical effects:

1. They show affinity for alpha adrenergic receptors[22] and, thus, are alpha adrenergic blockers. The tertiary amines (imipramine) are the more potent than secondary (desipramine) as alpha adrenergic blockers.

2. They block monoamine reuptake, either of serotonin, which is thought to be related to a sedative effect (tertiary are more potent than secondary), or of norepinephrine, which is thought to be related to activating properties of the drug (secondary more potent than tertiary).

3. They show anticholinergic properties, both centrally and peripherally.

In cardiac patients side effects of these agents can be viewed quite specifically.

1. Anticholinergic effects account for many more dangerous side effects in cardiac patients than all others combined. The sinus tachycardia that can result, particularly from use of amitriptyline, is the most common and potentially disastrous in these patients. In fact, 30% of a group of normal individuals will respond with tachycardia to amitriptyline[24] and cardiac patients are much more sensitive, as are elderly patients. As Table 10-2 shows, all tricyclic antidepressants are about equipotential as anticholinergic agents (2+) except for amitriptyline's extreme potency (8+) and desipramine's lower potency (1+). Therefore, if the physician seeks an agent with the lowest anticholinergic potency, for example, for a patient with congestive heart failure, desipramine is a logical choice.

2. Conduction defects, while more feared, are actually less common than anticholinergic effects. Moreover, they are quite specific. Bigger and others[25] commented on the similarity of imipramine to Group I antiarrhythmic agents like quinidine and procaine amide. Electrocardiograms (ECGs) of persons taking tricyclic antidepressants have shown increased duration of PR, QRS, and $QT_C$ intervals (the last corrected for heart rate).[25] Tricyclic antidepressants appear to slow both atrial and ventricular depolarization. Burrows and others[26] recording

His's bundle ECGs of patients taking various antidepressants, found that the major effect of the drugs was on the distal portion of the His-Purkinje system. These distal defects were present for amitriptyline, nortriptyline, and imipramine, but not for doxepin. Patients showing the effects were both overdose victims and persons taking therapeutic doses. Patients with doxepin overdose did not show the defect. It is safe to assume that all tricyclic antidepressants used currently in the United States except doxepin can produce these effects. Practically speaking, a patient with premature ventricular contractions could be helped by the quinidine effects of a tricyclic antidepressant, and if an antiarrhythmic drug were already prescribed, its dose might have to be reduced somewhat. If the patient shows bundle branch block, anterior hemiblock, or other conduction defect, doxepin may be the drug of choice. Even if another agent seemed preferable to doxepin, its effects could be measured by ECG. This effect does not always occur with therapeutic doses.

3. Does a tricyclic antidepressant depress the myocardium itself? This is the rarest of the three categories of dangerous side effects and is relevant only in patients whose ventricular function is marginal, as with patients in congestive failure or low output states. Nevertheless, in vitro[27] evidence for negative chronotropic and inotropic effects exists. Burckhardt[28] demonstrated decreased left ventricular ejection times (and therefore decreased contractility) in patients taking therapeutic doses of imipramine and amitriptyline. This is probably an effect of blocked norepinephrine reuptake, demonstrated in isolated rat hearts.[29] It is an effect that would require at least 3 weeks to develop and could therefore be insidious. However, as mentioned, only patients with borderline ventricular function are likely to develop this difficulty.

Orthostatic hypotension is clearly a common effect of tricyclic antidepressants in patients with cardiac disease.[24] Ideally its frequency should be predicted by the alpha adrenergic blocking properties of each drug. That is, tertiary amines should be more potent in this regard than their derivative secondary amines. Since cardiac patients in a hospital are often in bed they may not test the postural effects of drugs often. Caution is common sense. Cardiac patients are less likely to stop taking a tricyclic antidepressant for hypotensive effects than for anticholinergic effects.

Selection of a tricyclic antidepressant, then, can follow a clear rationale. If the patient is agitated, a tertiary amine or doxepin is preferable. One then makes the specific selection according to side effects that should be most avoided. A retarded depressed patient with normal conduction and PVC'S should be started on imipramine. An agitated, depressed patient with left bundle branch block would be safest on doxepin. A retarded depressed patient with congestive heart failure could be treated with desipramine.

A suggested dose regimen is to give the patient a single unit dose (25 mg for all tricyclic antidepressants except protriptyline, which is 5 mg) the first day. The dose is then increased slowly as clinical monitoring proceeds, particularly of heart rate and subjective reports. Tachycardia, excessive sedation, and orthostatic hypotension are the symptoms most likely to require slowing of the dosage increase. Sedative drugs can be given in a single bedtime dose as usual. Propranolol may be used to guard against the vagolytic tachycardia of these agents, but many cardiac patients either already receive it, have respiratory disease, or may not tolerate its negative inotropic effects.

Depression can be life-threatening and more damaging to cardiac function than a drug. It must be treated.

**REFERENCES**

1. Williams, T. A., and others: Special report on the depressive illnesses, Washington, D.C., November, 1970, U.S. Dept. of Health, Education and Welfare.
2. Moffic, H. S., and Paykel, E. S.: Depression in medical inpatients, Br. J. Psychiatry **126**:346, 1975.
3. Cassem, N. H., and Hackett, T. P.: Psychiatric consultation in a coronary care unit, Ann. Intern. Med. **75**:9-14, 1971.
4. Bibring, E.: The mechanism of depression. In Greenacre, P., editor: Affective disorders: psychoanalytic contributions to their study, New York, 1953, International Universities Press, pp. 13-48.
5. Levine, S. A., and Lown, B.: "Armchair" treatment of acute coronary thrombosis, J.A.M.A. **148**:1365, 1952.
6. Wishnie, H. A., Hackett, T. P., and Cassem, N. H.: Psychologic hazards of convalescence following myocardial infarction, J.A.M.A. **215**:1292-1296, 1971.
7. Saltin, B., and others: Response to exercise after bed rest and after training, Circulation **38**(Suppl. 7):1, 1968.
8. Alpert, J. S., and others: Effects of physical training on hemodynamics and pulmonary function at rest and during exercise in patients with chronic obstructive pulmonary disease, Chest **66**:647-651, 1974.
9. Cassem, N. H., and Hackett, T. P. Psychological aspects of myocardial infarction, Med. Clin. North Am. **61**:711-721, 1977.
10. Exercise testing and training of individuals with heart disease or at high risk for its development, Dallas, 1975, American Heart Association.

11. Feighner, J. P., and others: Diagnostic criteria for use in psychiatric research, Arch. Gen. Psychiatry **26**:57-63, 1972.
12. Robins, E., Gentry, K. A., Munoz, R. A.., and Marten, S.: A contrast of the three more common illnesses with the ten less common in a study and eighteen-month follow-up of 314 psychiatric emergency room patients: III. Findings at follow-up, Arch. Gen. Psychiatry **34**:285-196, 1977.
13. Lesse, S., editor: Masked depression, New York, 1974, Jason Aronson, Inc.
14. Baldessarini, R. J.: Biogenic amine hypotheses in affective disorders, Arch. Gen. Psychiatry **32**:1087-1093, 1975.
15. Schildkraut, J. J.: Neuropsychopharmacology and the affective disorders, Boston, 1970, Little, Brown and Co.
16. Maas, J. W.: Biogenic amines and depression: biochemical and pharmacological separation of two types of depression, Arch. Gen. Psychiatry **32**:1357-1361, 1975.
17. Åsberg, M., and others: Serotonin depression—a biochemical subgroup within the affective disorders? Science **191**:478-480, 1976.
18. Beckmann, H., and Goodwin, F. K.: Antidepressant response to tricyclics and urinary MHPG in unipolar patients, Arch. Gen. Psychiatry **32**:17-21, 1975.
19. Coull, D. C., and others: Amitriptyline and cardiac disease: risk of sudden death identified by monitoring system, Lancet **2**:590-591, 1970.
20. Robinson, D. S., and Barker, E.: Tricyclic antidepressant cardiotoxicity, J. A. M. A. **236**:1089-2090, 1976.
21. Fowler, N. O., and others: Electrocardiographic changes and cardiac arrythmias in patients receiving psychotropic drugs, Am. J. Cardiol. **37**:223-230, 1976.
22. Snyder, S. H., and Yamamura, H. I.: Antidepressants and the muscarinic acetylcholine receptor, Arch. Gen. Psychiatry **34**:236-239, 1977.
23. U'Prichard, D. C., Greenberg, D. A., Sheehan, P. P., and Snyder, S. H.: Tricyclic antidepressants: therapeutic properties and affinity for noradrenergic receptor binding sites in the brain, Science **199**:197-198, 1978.
24. Jefferson, J. W.: A review of the cardiovascular effects and toxicity of tricyclic antidepressants, Psychosom. Med. **37**:160-179, 1975.
25. Bigger, J. T., and others: Cardiac antiarrhythmic effect of imipramine hydrochloride, N. Engl. J. Med. **296**:206-208, 1977.
26. Burrows, G. D., and others: Cardiac effects of different tricyclic antidepressant drugs, Br. J. Psychiatry **129**:335-341, 1976.
27. Sigg, E. G., Osborne, M., and Porol, B.: Cardiovascular effects of imipramine, J. Pharmacol. Exp. Ther, **141**:237-243, 1963.
28. Burckhardt, D., and others: Cardiovascular effects of tricyclic and tetracyclic antidepressants, J.A.M.A. **239**:213-216, 1978.
29. Axelrod, J., Hertting, G., and Potter, L.: Effect of drugs on the uptake and release of tritiated norepinephrine in the rat heart, Nature **194**:297, 1962.

# 11

# Indications for electroconvulsive therapy in treatment of depression

MICHEL R. MANDEL

Depression is a disease of protean manifestations. Clinicians charged with its management strive for accurate assessment of its severity and proper treatment. Once the decision is made that somatic therapy is indicated, should a tricyclic antidepressant be used? When is electroconvulsive therapy (ECT) more likely to reverse the patient's condition?

Following its introduction in the late 1930s, ECT soon became the treatment of choice for severe depressive illness. During the 1950s and 1960s, the monoamine oxidase (MAO) inhibitors and tricyclic antidepressants (TCA) were introduced, and the efficacy of these drugs, plus their ease of administration by any physician and their relatively low cost, accounted for their rapid acceptance and the reduced popularity of ECT.[1] Some recent studies have emphasized that, in appropriate dosage, tricyclic antidepressants may be as effective as ECT in primary affective disease.[2] Other authors have stressed that ECT has unique beneficial effects over antidepressants when delusions are manifested in the course of a depression.[3] It has also been reported that some patients have been unable to tolerate the side effects of tricyclics or fail to demonstrate an antidepressant response even in adequate dosage.[4] Although a British Medical Research Council group found that roughly 50% of a group of tricyclic antidepressant–resistant depressed patients will respond to ECT,[5] no precise method has been described for the prediction of ECT response in a group of patients specifically defined as medication-intolerant or medication-resistant. This chapter offers some clinical guidelines to physicians who seek answers to these problems.

□This chapter, including Tables 11-1 and 11-2, contain extensive quotes from Mandel, M. R., Welch, C. A., Mieske, M., and McCormick, M.: Prediction of repsonse to ECT in tricyclic-intolerant or tricyclic-resistant depressed patients, McLean Hosp. J. **2:**203-209, 1977.

Previous researchers in this area developed predictive indices based on features of the history and clinical state of their patients.[6-8] Examination of their data, however, reveals that the samples in these earlier studies were quite different than those reported more recently. For instance, in recent research patients are more likely to be older and are selected for ECT at least partially because of their resistance of drug therapy.[4] Moreover, the evidence now strongly suggests that no correlation exists between any of these previous indices and posttreatment clinical rating scores, when applied to a modern sample of depressed patients.[9]

The consultant seeks the most appropriate somatic treatment for the individual depressed patient. At Massachusetts General Hospital a study was conducted by the Somatic Therapies Unit of those patients who had been treated with tricyclic antidepressants (200 mg/day of imipramine or the equivalent for at least 3 weeks), but for whom the drug treatment failed to reverse the depression.[10] Thus these patients were already treatment failures on medication. Is it possible to tell which patients will not respond to a drug trial but will respond to ECT?

Among depressed patients at MGH who did not improve with drug therapy, 71% did respond to ECT. The clinical features that differentiated ECT responders from ECT nonresponders are listed in Table 11-1. A larger percentage of ECT responders had sudden onset, guilt, somatic and paranoid delusions, a fluctuating course, and labile mood than ECT nonresponders. More nonresponders had medical illness and pain. The nonresponders represented failure of two treatments, first drugs, and then ECT. Previous ECT prediction studies[6-8] also indicated that sudden onset, guilt, and delusions are associated with a successful outcome.

What basis exists for clinical choice of ECT or antidepressant for a depressed patient? Bielski and Friedel[11] have made similar studies of depressed patients to predict response to tricyclic antidepressants. Clinical features associated with a favorable response to these drugs included: psychomotor retardation, weight loss, early and mid insomnia, diurnal variation, and poor appetite. If, on the other hand, the patient showed neurotic traits, including hysteria and hypochondriasis, or was delusional, an unfavorable outcome was likely.

The predictive traits for response to tricyclic antidepressants and ECT are arranged in Table 11-2 for comparison and contrast. While these data are taken from studies utilizing different designs and will require further confirmation and study, some rough guides for the

**Table 11-1.** Clinical traits of ECT responders and nonresponders

|  | N | Percentage with trait | | p |
|---|---|---|---|---|
|  |  | r | n |  |
| Pain | 76 | 16.7 | 50.0 | .01 |
| Impaired concentration | 57 | 80.5 | 50.0 | .02 |
| Severe depressed mood | 73 | 57.7 | 28.6 | .02 |
| Paranoid delusions | 65 | 41.7 | 11.8 | .03 |
| Self-pity | 49 | 76.5 | 100.0 | .04 |
| Sudden onset | 72 | 49.0 | 23.8 | .05 |
| Medical illness | 76 | 53.7 | 77.3 | .06 |
| Guilt | 46 | 75.8 | 46.2 | .06 |
| Mania | 66 | 16.7 | 0.0 | .07 |
| Somatic delusions | 62 | 31.8 | 11.1 | .09 |
| Inadequate personality | 44 | 63.6 | 90.9 | .09 |
| Fluctuating course | 70 | 44.9 | 23.8 | .10 |
| Lability of mood | 55 | 47.4 | 23.5 | .10 |

N, number of patients in series (total N is 76).
r, ECT responders.
n, ECT nonresponders.
p, Significance of the difference between independent proportions.

clinician appear to emerge. The presence of classical symptoms of endogenous depression, with insomnia, anorexia, weight loss, psychomotor retardation, and diurnal mood variation, strongly suggests a successful outcome for tricyclic antidepressant therapy. The data also suggest that delusions, particularly of the paranoid type, predict failure for tricyclic antidepressant therapy and a favorable response to ECT or perhaps a combination of tricyclics and antipsychotic medications. Persons with neurotic traits or styles (hysterical, hypochondriacal, inadequate) are not likely to do well with either form of treatment. It is also clear that many patients who respond well to tricyclics would also improve with ECT.

Even when both drugs and ECT are likely to succeed, ECT may be the therapy of choice, as when the severity of the depression warrants the most rapid and effective treatment. A serious risk of suicide in an endogenously depressed person is one such instance.

The pre-ECT evaluation should routinely include a complete history and physical examination, complete blood count, urinalysis, fasting blood sugar, blood urea nitrogen, chest and spine x-rays, serologic tests for syphilis, SGOT, and electrocardiogram. Other additional tests and

**Table 11-2.** Factors correlating with response to ECT and tricyclic antidepressants—depressed patients

| Favorable | TCA | ECT |
|---|---|---|
| Insidious onset | X | |
| Sudden onset | | X |
| Guilt | | X |
| Psychomotor retarda-tion | X | |
| Insomnia—late | X | |
| Weight loss | X | |
| Delusions—somatic | | X |
| Fluctuating course | | X |
| Delusions—paranoid | | X |
| Impaired concentra-tion | | X |
| Poor appetite | X | |
| Insomnia—mid | X | |
| Diurnal variation | X | |
| Mania | | X |
| Severe depression | | X |
| Lability of mood | | X |

TCA, Tricyclic antidepressants.[11]
ECT, Electroconvulsive therapy.[10]

consultations should be accomplished according to the individual patient's needs.

Few patients require less than four or more than twelve ECTs in a treatment program (the MGH average is six). Unilateral techniques that spare the verbal short-term memory areas of the dominant hemisphere should be used de rigeur. Much attention has also been recently directed to the use of low energy stimulus generators that may reduce adverse memory effects of ECT. Even for depressed patients who do not respond to antidepressant drugs, a 50% to 80% success rate is likely with ECT. This treatment modality can be invaluable to the consultant.

**REFERENCES**

1. Klein, D. F., and Davis, J. M.: Diagnosis and treatment of psychiatric disorders, Baltimore, 1969, The Williams & Wilkins Co., pp. 187-298.
2. Simpson, G. M., and others: Two dosages of imipramine in hospitalized endogenous and neurotic depressives, Arch. Gen. Psychiatry 33:1093-1102, 1976.

3. Glassman, A. H., Kantor, S. J., and Shostak, M.: Depression, delusions, and drug response, Am. J. Psychiatry **132**:716-719, 1975.

4. Hamilton, M.: Prediction of resonse of ECT in depressive illness. In Angst, J., editors: Classification and prediction of outcome in depression, Stuttgart, West Germany, 1974, F. K. Schattauer Verlag Gmbh, p. 275.

5. Medical Research Council: Clinical trial of the treatment of depressive illness, Br. Med. J. **5439**:881-886, 1965.

6. Hobson, R. F.: Prognostic features in electric convulsive therapy, J. Neurol. Neurosurg. Psychiatry **16**:275-281, 1953.

7. Carney, M. W. P., Roth, M., and Garside, M.: The diagnosis of depressive syndromes and the prediction of ECT response, Br. J. Psychiatry **111**:659-674, 1965.

8. Mendels, J.: Electroconvulsive therapy and depression: I. The prognostic significance of clinical factors, Br. J. Psychiatry **111**:675-686, 1965.

9. Abrams, R., Fink, M., and Feldstein, S.: Prediction of clinical response to ECT, Br. J. Psychiatry **122**:457-460, 1973.

10. Mandel, M. R., Welch, C. A., Mieske, M., and McCormick, M.: Prediction of response to ECT in tricyclic-intolerant or tricyclic-resistant depressed patients, McLean Hosp. J. **2**:203-209, 1977.

11. Bielski, R. J., and Friedel, R. O.: Prediction of tricyclic antidepressant response, Arch. Gen. Psychiatry **33**:1479-1489, 1976.

# 12

# Disruptive states

**THOMAS P. HACKETT**

---

A number of emotionally charged situations occur regularly in a general hospital. Although they often defy standard diagnostic classification, they usually become the responsibility of the psychiatrist. Many of these situations are dealt with in individual chapters but a mixed bag remains. Those here described by no means constitute the complete repertoire, but they do represent the more commonplace disruptive states.

## THE PATIENT WHO THREATENS TO SIGN OUT AGAINST MEDICAL ADVICE

Each year on the consultation service at Massachusetts General Hospital (MGH) there are five to ten occasions when the issues of signing out against medical advice poses a serious, life-threatening problem to a patient. At such a time, the confidence of the primary physician is shaken and the hospital's reputation endangered. These situations reach the liaison man at the eleventh hour. For each serious threat there are perhaps twenty manipulative threats that fall short of emergencies.

A careful study of the premature sign-out process over the last 3 years reveals that it is, in nearly all instances, a two-way transaction. The patient threatens to sign out because in his eyes he has been mistreated, misunderstood, misinformed, or in some way mismanaged. While this is not always an accurate observation since the misunderstanding may well be the fault of the patient, it is crucial to realize that the serious threat to leave the hospital is rarely a sudden act of rash bravado. Most often it is the result of a series of transactions between patient and staff that progressively set the points of the patient's compass toward the front door.

Since most patients who threaten to leave have a grievance against the staff, the liaison psychiatrist's best tack is to ally himself with the patient, even if this requires an agreement that a wrong has been done.

Once the patient feels he has an ally, he is usually willing to delay his sign-out long enough to have the problem aired to the concerned parties. This generally effects a resolution. Patients are usually relieved at the chance to remain—especially if a concession is made to them. For most patients the sign-out is a desperate act, one they are forced into by what they believe is an immutable pattern of behavior on the part of the staff.

There are exceptions to this rule. Perhaps the most common is the individual with organic brain disease. His difficulty with memory and orientation and his low tolerance for anxiety leave him ill-equipped to cope with the strangeness of the hospital setting and primed for panic. An impatient nurse or an abrupt physician may induce an alarm response and a threatened sign-out. Careful explanations, round-the-clock visitation by trusted family members, and patience are usually the answer to such problems.

Although psychotropic medications are useful with psychotic patients who threaten to sign out as a result of delusions of hallucinations, the last thing one should do in facing the nonpsychotic threatened sign-out is to "snow" him with drugs. Such an attempt is often times regarded as "the last straw." It may well confirm the patient's fear of coercive betrayal. Furthermore, heavy doses of medication are contraindicated when the underlying pathology is organic brain syndrome.

As a rule of thumb it is well to remember that most patients who threaten to sign out do not do so when they speak with a reasonable physician who takes their side and acts as an advocate. Since this physician is usually the liaison psychiatrist, it will also be his job to ask the other parties involved—physician or nurse—to take a more objective view of their role and to see themselves through the patient's eyes. Sometimes the situation can be detoxified by pointing out that the staff members are symbols of a patient's frustration and rage based on transference feelings.

As a final strategy, it often helps to suggest that the patient leave the hospital on an overnight pass if this is compatible with good medical management. A sense of autonomy is restored by giving him the option of leaving the hospital with the understanding that he can return. So often it is the unfortunate decision, wrought in anger, usually by a young staff physician or house officer, that the patient who leaves is no longer entitled to return. In the opinion of Albert and Kornfeld this attitude "rarely dissuades the patient from leaving, but it may make continuing outpatient treatment less likely."[2]

M. P. was a friendly, 72-year-old pharmacist who had undergone an open heart procedure 5 years earlier. He had unpleasant memories of the postoperative period when he had been delirious for 5 successive days. It had been a frightening time and he held his surgeon accountable for not providing proper medication for sleep. The only hypnotic in which the patient had any faith was phenobarbital. His surgeon had given him one of the newer sedatives and it hadn't worked. This time he wanted to make certain he would get phenobarbital for sleep. Everyone assured him that he would. He was amiable and good-natured and did not strongly press this demand. As a consequence, his request was forgotten until after his subtotal gastrectomy. On his first postoperative day he moaned incessantly, asking for phenobarbital. Instead he was given small doses of diazepam (Valium). Throughout the night he continued to whine and moan piteously, reminding everyone that he had been promised a barbiturate. Actually no promise had been made and the recovery room people who were now responsible for his care had never met him before. The following day he howled in a loud voice that unless he saw his physician by midday and was given something to help him sleep, he was going to remove his tubes and walk out. Although his physician did his best to meet the deadline, he was late by 10 minutes, during which time the patient had removed a catheter and an intravenous tube. The physician immediately ordered phenobarbital and the patient went into a relaxed sleep. Medication was continued until the patient's discharge.

The smoke signals in this case were the patient's reasonable request for a specific hypnotic and his past history of postoperative delirium. His easygoing manner and confidence that his request would be carried out worked against him. Furthermore, he had no idea that barbiturates are thought by some to contribute to the incidence of postoperative delirium and, therefore, are seldom used. Requests for specific medication should always be heeded, especially when they come from people with a medical background. A promise made to use a drug should certainly be carried out or a reasonable explanation for the drug's omission or substitution must be given.

Mr. J. was a valued hospital employee who had worked in the engineering shop for 20 years. He was admitted to the Coronary Care Unit with an acute myocardial infarction. Popular with the nurses, he was usually gregarious, but after 3 days he became visibly apprehensive. A snowstorm had moved in and winds from the Atlantic had whipped the snow into blinding flurries that rendered driving hazardous from Maine to New Jersey. The patient's frequent requests to use the telephone meant moving it into his room and then returning it to its stand. No one had time to wonder why Mr. J. needed to make these calls. At midday two persons were admitted and the patient's request for the telephone could not be honored for about 3 hours. When the nurse finally agreed to bring him the telephone, she did so with a trace of anger. She was delayed in bringing the phone and by the time she returned, the patient had removed his monitoring leads, taken out his intravenous tubing and was in the midst of putting on his clothes. The nurse was stunned by this unexpected spectacle and angry at herself for being the probable cause. He refused to speak, just shook his head sadly, and continued tying his shoestring. The house officer on duty approached the patient quietly and gently inquired what we had done to make him want to leave. Mr. J. continued to shake his head and tie his shoe. Finally, in response to the repeated urgings of the house officer, Mr. J. said that his son was driving up from New Jersey and that he had been calling home hourly to make sure everything was alright. The telephone was his lifeline. Without it he felt powerless. Leaving the hospital seemed his only alternative. The house officer immediately apologized for the lack of a telephone and instantly called the patient's home to check on his son. He then got a telephone from another floor for the patient. Mr. J. agreed to return to bed as long as he could keep the phone in his room. This request was immediately granted.

In retrospect it is easy to see that someone should have asked Mr. J. why he needed the telephone so frequently and so urgently. However, the lesson of this case is taught by the intern. His immediate response was not to blame the patient for acting foolishly, but to assume that the unit was at fault. This is an ideal tactic when the physician faces a prospective sign-out patient whose motive is not immediately discernible. It allows the patient a chance to explain without being defensive. Rightly or wrongly, the patient usually feels aggrieved and angry. The medical caregiver should be prepared to be scapegoated either directly or symbolically. If an error has been made, it is imperative that the individual involved acknowledge the mistake.[2,3]

## THE SEDUCTIVE FEMALE

When a male physician thinks of a sexually provocative patient the usual image brought to mind is that of a young, partially clad, attractive woman whose working diagnosis is hysteria. The scenario would then call for a young, earnest, but inexperienced physician to take charge of the patient and be seduced into making a fool of himself. This seldom occurs. Physicians are possibly less sexually naive than was the case a decade ago. They seem less susceptible to coercion through overt seduction. However, a more subtle type of seduction sometimes occurs, usually directed by an attractive woman who is not necessarily hysteric. She finds in the physician someone who is patient, kind, and, perhaps, aware of her charms. Generally a marital problem is part of her clinical picture. She had a husband who, for one reason or another, does not understand her. During a period of turning to the physician for comfort, she develops a warm, compassionate, platonically romantic attachment to him. It is my experience that such a physician is usually naive, gullible, and insecure with women. A relationship then develops that sometimes includes minor transgressions. More often than not, the physician is unaware of the romantic fantasies of his patient.

> Mrs. C. L. was an attractive brunette who, at age 38, looked 10 years younger, and had a good sense of humor. She was married to a physician who spent most of his time attending to his practice. They had been married for almost 20 years and over the last 15 years he had been slowly losing interest in her. Nonetheless, he was a loyal husband who had developed no liaisons and was essentially married to her for life.
>
> The patient developed a recurrent back syndrome. The neurosurgeon who attended her was married and well-respected by his colleagues. He kept his patient in the hospital for 2 months, during which he saw her daily. In the course of his visits the patient told him how she had been neglected for years. She also greatly exaggerated the amount of alcohol her husband consumed. A psychiatric consultant was called in to advise the patient about her husband's drinking problem. When the psychiatrist asked the neurosurgeon if he had spoken to the patient's husband, he found that no contact had been made. The psychiatrist pointed out that the neurosurgeon had in fact accused a colleague on circumstantial evidence and had entered this in the patient's chart without ever having confirmed the story. The surgeon quickly saw the need to see his patient's husband, but was unwilling to do so himself. An interview between the husband and the psychiatrist and phone calls to medical colleagues of the husband revealed that the problem was in the marriage and not in alcohol.
>
> The referring neurosurgeon was infuriated with himself, but quickly turned this anger toward the patient. The psychiatric consultant pointed out that both patient and surgeon were culpable and encouraged him to discuss the situation with his patient. The woman felt betrayed and forsaken by her physician. Her marriage ultimately ended also. Much, if not all, of this unpleasantness could have been averted if the neurosurgeon had been less naive.

When sex is used, either actually or symbolically, between patient and doctor in a manipulative way, look for a mantrap. The entrapment may not be deliberate, but the net result is the same. The storm warning should be out when one senses a seduction. It might also be valuable to warn one's colleagues when one sees it.

## THE MALE SEXUAL PROVACATEUR

The male sexual provocateur has an altogether different approach and his disruptive effect is far more immediate and intense. There are roughly three varieties of male sexual disturbance commonly seen in a general hospital. They represent degrees on a sliding scale of indescretion. The mildest indiscretion is the flirt. He is constantly making excessive references to the physical attributes of those who care for him, using pet names, and sometimes suggesting sexual activities, but never offering a serious proposition. Generally he embarrasses the nursing personnel more than he angers or frightens them. Next is the obscene seducer. His idea of seduction is to tell dirty jokes or to make lewd comments about the anatomical parts of the nurses. His coarseness and vulgarity are offensive and sometimes he does make serious advances. The obscene seducer usually induces reactions of revulsion and anger from the nursing staff. The most indiscreet is the exhibitionist who exposes himself either passively by letting the sheet fall away from his genitals or actively by openly masturbating in the presence of the nurse. The exhibitionist causes the same response as the obscene seducer but combined with a fear that something is so unbalanced in the patient that a more serious assault might occur.

To understand these three degrees of maladaptive behavior one must recognize that serious illness, such as a myocardial infarction, even when its full impact is denied, is a major threat to the masculine ego. The fear of functional castration is apt to be more pronounced in individuals who value their sexual ability above other personal attributes. It is also found in individuals who have had problems with sexual adequacy before their illness. In any event, attempting to arouse a show of interest from the nurses by flirting is often no more than a man's harmless method of testing sexual viability. Engaging in sexual banter with nurses may also be an attempt to prove potency by evoking an erection. Usually the perpetrator is unaware of his motive, just as he is blind to the impact of his behavior on others.

> C. G. was a 42-year-old maritime pilot whose myocardial infarction occurred 3 months after his wife divorced him. He was tall, thin, somber, and solemn. The second day in the unit he began addressing the nurses as "gorgeous," "hot lips," "luscious," and "sex pot." He also managed to pat the posterior of the charge nurse and tried to kiss another when she was taking his temperature. It was done in a humorless and mechanical way as though he were a wind-up doll programmed to make advances. By the third day his advances

increased in frequency. Any dialogue with a nurse was embellished with amorous epithets and archly suggestive allusions.

A psychiatric consultant was asked to speak to the patient. During this conversation the patient appeared likable but quite despondent about his recent divorce. His wife was the only woman he had ever known well. He had spent most of his life on the oceans of the world and had had such little contact with women that he behaved toward them in a stereotyped way. He said that he had always called women "dear" or "sweetie" instead of using proper names. When confronted with the fact that he had tried to kiss one of the nurses and given another a friendly pat, he said that he thought this would make them like him more and it would given them "encouragement." "I lost one wife because I wasn't a ladies' man. Now with my ticker on the fritz I'm even less a ladies' man." The psychiatrist suggested he stop trying to give the girls "encouragement" and try to treat them like shipmates. (He got along beautifully with men.) The nurses warmed to him as soon as the phony flirting stopped. Their changed attitude reinforced his altered patterns of behavior, and by the time he left the hospital he was communicating with women more naturally.

It was apparent that this man was quite innocent in his attempts at flirting. He had no idea that his efforts were as clumsy and awkward as they were. His self-esteem with regard to women had always been low and assumed a new depth now that his "ticker was on the fritz." The term "encouragement" seemed a projection of his own need. When the psychiatrist told him literally how to behave, he did so and received immediate encouragement. The nurses, had they been advised, might have done the same for him from the start.

Q. B., a paunchy, 62-year-old educator with thickset facial features cast in a dour expression, was admitted with his second myocardial infarction in 7 years. His cardiac condition had stabilized by the second day. While bathing the patient that morning the nurse observed him fondling his penis into semierection. Every time she drew the sheet over his hips, he removed it. She left the room. When she returned, he had finished bathing and said nothing to her. Throughout the rest of the day the nurses noted that he lay in bed fully exposed. This was disconcerting to them. With considerable tact the head nurse confronted him about his exhibitionism. Contending that his sheet had merely slipped down, Q. B. denied intent. The next day another nurse who bathed him had the same experience. His physician was asked to help him curb his exposing, but the patient simply assumed an air of injured innocence. At this point the psychiatrist was called. The patient again denied any wrongdoing just as he did not acknowledge any fear of impaired sexuality. His mental status was quite normal. He showed no evidence of psychosis and was not delirious. Because no individual had been able to halt this man's denial, a more imposing confrontation was thought to be called for.

After consulting his physician and gaining permission, the nursing staff of the afternoon and evening shifts, accompanied by the psychiatrist entered the patient's room. The chief nurse took on the role of spokesperson. Pleasantly, with even-toned assurance, she told the patient that his behavior had worried all of the nurses. They wondered whether or not he knew what he was doing and, more importantly, the effect that it was having on them. She assured him that the staff liked him and regretted his misfortune. However, they were sufficiently distressed by his behavior that some were reluctant to help him bathe. She went on to explain that they had come in a group to make sure he knew that they all felt the same way. Surveying them with a visage that displayed neither alarm nor embarrassment, he denied any notion of what they were talking about. The nurses responded almost in chorus that they knew he did. They expressed a desire to help him. He made no effort to respond. The meeting ended, and the nurses felt even more frustrated and powerless. However, at the next bath he behaved in a sullen but modest manner, a pattern that continued throughout hospitalization.

It is difficult to imagine what went on in this man's mind to change his behavior. There had been no threat offered, nor had there been any display of vindictive animosity. The reason may have been the size of the assemblage and the unity in expressing opposition. This type of confrontation has been successful in similar cases. It is harsh treatment and requires the presence of a psychiatrist skilled in group techniques to ensure that the situation does not get out of hand. There is always the danger that the stress incurred may adversely affect the patient's heart, but this must be weighed against the toll such behavior takes from the nursing staff.

**THE MALINGERER**

Malingering is the conscious simulation of an illness or of symptom. Illness is feigned by the patient in order to accomplish a particular goal. This goal may be a financial reward, the avoidance of an unpopular duty, or the creation of guilt in the minds of involved friends or family. Whatever the motive, the modus operandi is the same: faking for gain. Hypochondriasis, compensation neurosis, and Münchausen's syndrome are sometimes confused with malingering.[4-6] Because it is difficult to spot the malingerer, we should keep him in mind when dealing with the symptoms where the elements of secondary gain are prominent. Usually malingerers are found in armed service medical facilities or Veteran's Adminstration hospitals rather than in general hospitals. Aside from the prominence of secondary gain, they usually have a past history of malingering, or "goldbrick-

ing," that can be unearthed from old records. An important characteristic of the malingerer is that he often has a record of antisocial acts.
Although he manages to avoid jail he may have a bad conduct
discharge from the armed forces and a history of being expelled from
school and fired from jobs. The tracks of his misbehavior meander
back through early adolescence.

The most dramatic of the malingerers to have come our way was a
prototypical charlatan. Some years ago a young man from the
Himalayas came to MGH for an examination of his blindness. He was
well over 6 feet tall and had the finely chiseled handsomeness of a
mountain prince. He wore a turban and long white cape. Allegedly he
had been kicked by a horse. Although his face bore no scar and his eyes
were the best feature of his impressive face, he nonetheless had x-ray
evidence of an old fracture over the occipital area. In his country, due
to political connections and personal magnetism, he had formed a
school for the blind and infirm. In order to subsidize it he took lecture
tours around the world. That was his reason for being in the United
States. He spoke excellent English. His tour through the United States
had been very successful and was ending in New England. It was
because he had attracted so much attention and won so many friends
that he found himself on the neurological service of MGH. His friends
had literally forced him to become a patient in order to afford him the
best appraisal modern medicine could offer on the faint chance that
something could be done to help his blindness.

It soon became apparent by all tests that he had excellent visual
acuity. Although he was highly skilled in behaving as a totally
sightless person, he was unable to outwit the various neuro-oph-
thalmologic tests. After these tests had exhaustively demonstrated the
soundness of his optic system, we were faced with the dilemma of
having to deal with a fraud who was in the United States at the
invitation of our government. In addition, he enjoyed the friendship of
many individuals in high places, including benefactors of the hospital.

It was decided to give him the opportunity of bowing out gracefully. He would be told that all of the tests had been performed and
the results were excellent. His prognosis was far better than anyone
could have imagined at the time of his admission. He had a type of
blindness that could be cured. A treatment had recently been devised
at the hospital wherein, employing combination of eyewashings and
certain injections, he would begin to regain light perception within as
little time as a day. He was then instructed in the following manner.
"When you begin to see light, as we know you will, the following will
happen. You will begin to feel immensely better by the third
treatment. The following day you will begin to see forms and
movement. This will increase your mood to a higher form of happiness. The following morning you will begin to see faces, and by that
afternoon you will be able to perceive the visual world as you did

before the horse kicked you. One of your first acts after full restoration of your vision will be to obtain air transportation to your homeland. That being done, your case will be closed at the hospital, and no follow-up will be done. However, if you fail for some reason to depart the country and return to your sanitorium, where you are badly needed, additional follow-up investigations might have to be done and disclosures of a painful nature made." He was quick to get the point, smiled faintly as the instructions were given him, nodded his head, and said, "I understand and I thank you." He performed his part of the bargain, and we kept our word.

The malingerer is often a charming person. Unlike the hypochondriac, he is not querulous and demanding. While willing to have some diagnostic tests, he is unlikely to submit to painful procedures or surgery that patients with Münchausen's syndrome commonly undergo. The review of symptoms and past history is atypical for hysteria, and generally he does not have a lawyer or the history of litigation with industrial accident boards that is true of the compensation neurotic. However, there are no criteria by which the diagnosis can be made except by: (1) ruling out the other diagnoses already mentioned, (2) noting a large element of secondary gain, and (3) noting a past history of mild to moderate sociopathy and previous instances in which physical illness or symptoms have been put to use in the patient's behalf.

## THE DEMANDING PATIENT

The demanding patient is a person who requests more service than the staff believes he is entitled to. There are, however, wide variations in the tolerance of individual caregivers. What is demanding to one nurse or physician may not be to another. Also, there are levels of subtlety in the way demands are voiced such that some caregivers, rather than feeling used, are only aware of a growing antagonism toward a patient.

Liaison psychiatrists are perhaps overly sensitive to the demanding patient. Oftentimes they misconstrue perfectly legitimate requests as evidence of demanding behavior. For example, someone immobilized by a cast often asks a visitor to perform such tasks as lighting a cigarette, handing water cups, or cranking the bed. Frequently a rash of these requests will be made as soon as the physician enters the room. This may be less the sign of a demanding nature than evidence of an overburdened nursing staff. It is important that a diagnosis of demanding behavior be based not on one but many such instances. There are a number of types of demanding behavior, some examples of which are the following:

## The perfectionist

Perfectionism is perhaps the most frequently encountered type of demanding behavior. The perfectionist is usually obsessive-compulsive by nature. He knows the room rate and his rights. Punctuality is expected. Meals are to be given at a certain time, pills and shots at another. Complaints are issued when service lags. When criticism is accompanied by a sense of humor little difficulty arises, but the same complaint offered sullenly will earn short shrift for the patient. The perfectionist is not so apt to ask for special favors as he is to insist on being given what is due him at the time it is due. Individuals of this sort are seldom referred to a psychiatrist unless they are in the hospital for a period of months. If this happens, their sense of entitlement may expand to regal proportions and alienate nurses and physicians to the point where they believe something must be done.

The most effective type of intervention for perfectionism is confrontation. One may begin by agreeing that the patient has certain rights as a paying guest at a medical hostelry. However, because it is medical there are apt to be emergencies and unforeseen incidences that make it impossible for the staff to serve patients in a fashion they might expect aboard a luxury liner. Perfectionists, the patient can be told, unless they are critically ill, tend to be served last. Sometimes this message is written in a letter and handed out like a business card to appropriate patients. The staff often has its own way of reacting to the person who demands too much.

## The reactive demander

Demandingness of the reactive type is a form of hospital regressive behavior. The hospital environment tends to favor regressive behavior and the more severe or chronic the illness, the more regressed the individual. Demandingness of this type is apt to occur in compensation for the sense of impairment or the helplessness that a patient feels. One phase of the adaptation to quadriplegia is demandingness. As a phase, it eventually passes. Similarly, patients with severe burns, multiple fractures, or any other injury or surgical illness that necessitates long hospitalization and dependency will demonstrate demanding behavior.

> A 32-year-old woman was hospitalized to have an ileostomy for severe ulcerative colitis. She had had many previous hospitalizations, all in an effort to avoid the ileostomy, but now her condition necessitated surgery. After the ileostomy she refused to take care of the stoma. She only halfheartedly cooperated with those who taught her how to adjust the bag. Before long, a series of stomal abscesses

formed. These were suppurative, ugly, and malodorous. Feces stained her fingers and her bed. She began to talk in a lispy, whiney tone, and to request all types of service from having her hands and face washed to back rubs at all hours. Nurses began to avoid her room and refer to her as "psychotic." Her physician had lost patience with her when she refused to cooperate with the nurse who taught care of the stoma. He rarely visited her for more than 2 minutes at a time and the floor nurses could not depend on him to establish any discipline with her. With reluctance he agreed to make a request for a psychiatric consultation.

The psychiatrist was appalled by the condition of the room and the patient. Her first comment was, "I want the nurse and my cigarettes." Although she answered questions in monosyllables, she paid little attention to the examiner and seemed entirely unaware of her unwholesome surroundings. While there was no evidence of psychosis, it was clear that she was living in a world whose unnaturalness verged on the insane.

After a consultation with the nurses and her physician about his strategy, the psychiatrist again approached the patient. She was told that one reason the nurses and her physician did not visit her was the stench—for which she seemed to accept no responsibility. Like a child, she had turned over her personal hygiene to others. She broke into tears and replied, "Well, how do you think I feel?" The consultant acknowledged that she must feel dreadful, but also explained that if she continued to let herself go, the result could be serious and possibly fatal. To assist her in mending her relationships with her caregivers, a list of rules was prescribed including cooperation with the nurse who taught her stomal care, improved personal hygiene, friendliness to the nursing staff, and ambulation. In return she would be moved to a new room with a much better view (the current room faced an air shaft), be provided with a new television set, and receive daily visits from the psychiatrist. The alternative would mean continued poor nursing care, loneliness, and eventually transfer to a psychiatric facility. The psychiatrist knew that she was depressed. She had told him so. Her situation was evidence of passive neglect by the medical community—an unconscious or indeliberate manifestation of their anger. The anger of the psychiatric consultant at this demanding infantile patient, though felt, was not expressed until he had spoken with the nurses and had examined the patient to reassure himself that she was not psychotic. He then used his anger to call the patient's attention vividly to the circumstances of her condition. Next came the setting of limits, followed by the alternative reward or punishments. This program could only be carried out with the understanding, agreement, and cooperation of the nurses.

This case points out three principles for management of the demanding patient:

**Self-awareness.** Be aware of the response the patient arouses in you.

If it is anger, acknowledge it as such. Some individuals act out their anger covertly by avoiding the person who causes it. Avoidance had been one of the major responses to this patient. Anger at someone who is desperately ill is hard to countenance, yet it is human and must be contended with.

**Limit-setting.** It is important to list the things one wants to accomplish. Talk them over with the patient, see what is reasonable and what is not until both parties—caregiver and patient—can arrive at a suitable compromise. The rewards and punishments of the system should be made clear.

**Confrontation.** It is always better to confront patients with their demanding behavior rather than to let the demands continue uncontested. The confrontation should be made before the staff has become so angry that the message contains unnecessary belligerence. The confrontation should be firm but gentle; for example, "Do you realize that you are only commenting on things we do wrong? You never say a word when we do something right. You comment when the pill is 5 minutes late, the same way you do when it is half an hour late. You leave us no latitude."

## The demanding hypomanic patient

Many individuals are not so demanding as they are hyperactive. These are people who resist being sick because they cannot stand to be inactive. The tendency to activity stands them in good stead if they are undergoing a course of rehabilitation that requires full cooperation. However, it is apt to become a problem when they are forced into the passive role. In this situation the hospital staff must realize how inflexible hospital routines are apt to be. Sometimes the answer is to loosen these routines if it can be done with no inconvenience to other patients and no harm to the hyperactive patient.

> Mr. A. J., a 49-year-old silk importer, was basically well-intentioned and courteous, but he was accustomed to giving orders like a drill instructor. As soon as the nursing staff reminded him that this was not Parris Island, he apologized and phrased his requests more politely. The main problem, however, was not the manner of his requests, but the content. He insisted on having two telephones—one line directly to his office, the other for outside calls. He also wanted a small bar in his room for the busineess meetings that he began scheduling. He had just entered the Coronary Care Unit (CCU) with what appeared to be a septal infarction. At first the nurses thought his requests were the result of morphine-induced euphoria. As a consequence morphine was withheld and the patient experienced a return

of chest pain. This was enough to quiet him for a while. He was given a large oral dose of a hypnotic for sleep, which carried him through the night.

The next day he awoke pain free and in excellent spirits. His energy had returned and he was about to leave his room when he was halted by a team of nurses who rushed in because his action had dislodged one of the monitoring electrodes and set off an alarm. He returned to bed without protest, but once again asked for telephones and a bar. On morning rounds his physician told him that alcohol in any form was prohibited in the hospital. This he accepted gracefully, but he told the physician that the telephones were a necessity. The physician said that he would consider it, but increased his tranquilizer instead. This produced an outburst of anger from Mr. A. J. He felt "patronized" and "ignored." He declared, "My doctor gave me the medicinal brush-off." He once again left his bed and paced the floor, tripping the alarm and triggering a series of premature ventricular contractions. His physician was summoned and spent 20 minutes talking with him about the need for absolute bedrest and avoidance of excitement. The patient pointed out that he could not control his nerves, that he was used to being active during the day, that several things were happening in his business requiring immediate attention, and that no amount of sedation was going to soothe his nerves while his business was about to be dismantled in his absence.

He was a man who had never been ill before in his life. He had made no provision for illness, never having even considered the possibility. He still refused to admit that he was as sick as his electrocardiograms and enzymes indicated. Part of his desire for telephone contact with the outside world was interpreted by the physician as an attempt to deny the seriousness of his plight. This was pointed out to him, but had no effect whatever. As midafternoon approached, his agitation seemed to mount and he refused to take any more tranquilizers. He was so restless in bed that his nurse made the comment, "If anybody could pace the floor while remaining in bed, Mr. A. J. would be the man to do it." By late afternoon his physician thought it wise to meet him halfway by putting in one telephone that he could use without restrictions. The result was immediate. The patient called his secretary and began lining up telephone calls and scheduling activities. There was an immediate change in his manner. He became much more himself and had a notable decrease in ventricular irritability in the next 48 hours. An agreement was reached with the physician that there would be no business meetings until he left the Coronary Care Unit, but that two telephones would be installed as long as his secretary could help him with business. Although the telephones were in constant use from dawn until dusk, he did agree to take three 1 hour rest periods during the day, at which time the phones were unplugged. The remainder of his stay was altogether uncomplicated in the CCU. When Mr. A. J. left the unit, his physician allowed him to have daily business meetings. He was monitored for the first 2 days, but the meetings were quiet and produced no disturbance in mood or myocardium.

Clearly in this instance, physical and mental inactivity were more stressful than "business as usual." Medical caregivers must be prepared to recognize individuals whose mental well-being depends on activity and to shape their therapeutic program to reduce emotional wear. Although some activities may violate the policy of a unit, enough latitutde should be available to accommodate the exceptional person. Furthermore, in an instance such as the one described, the patient was under constant monitoring. If conducting business increased myocardial irritability, an alternative activity could be found. Bargains can always be made with the movers and shakers. They are usually practical individuals, more inclined toward self-preservation than reckless misbehavior. If a program of physical conditioning is available in the hospital, these individuals are likely to enjoy participating, since it gives them something to do. Also, having a business partner visit a patient regularly can be of value. Whether or not these devices— telephones, business partner, secretary—support the patient's denial is incidental to the fact that they usually improve his state of mind and modify his behavior favorably. These goals are worth accomplishing even if the psychodynamics of the disruptive behavior are unknown.

**The passive-aggressive individual with demanding behavior**

There are a number of individuals whose demands are a form of hostility. At times of stress this tendency may be more apparent. Usually these people have a long history of personality malfunction studded with incidents in which they have alienated people or caused rows of various sorts. Often they can be immediately identified by a sense of entitlement so ingrained that they feel no need to acknowledge a service rendered. The pleasantry "thank you" may not be in their vocabulary.

M. G., a 57-year-old accountant, was such an individual. He occupied a bed on the convalescence floor of a coronary unit where he had gained the title, "Mr. Coffee Nerves." Every time one of his fellow patients turned a radio up, "Mr. Coffee Nerves" would shout across, "Turn that God-damn thing down!" Whenever the nurse was delayed in bringing a medication he would shout at her, "Get your sweet little ass over here, Honey!" On rounds he would address the medical students and interns as "Boy." "Boy, hand me that paper before you leave" was said to an intern on rounds; or, "Sonny, you come back when I'm feeling better before you listen to my chest. I'm tired of being a pincushion for you kids." The second week there he insisted on smoking on the ward, which was against rules, and threatened to sign out unless they allowed him this privilege. The resident in charge said he would not allow him to smoke and if he wanted to sign out against advice he not only would allow him to do so, but would open the door for him. This in fact is what happened. The patient walked out, went home, and, shortly afterwards, died.

It is difficult to know how this individual could have been managed to everyone's satisfaction. The likelihood is that any attempt would have been met with a hostile, negative rebuff. However, a psychiatrist should have been called in as was agreed on during the postmortem discussion. Confrontation and limit-setting also ought to have been the order of the day as soon as the early signs of this type of behavior began to occur.

A variant on the theme is found in the case of Dr. R. R., 55, who acted as though all of the house officers were servants; only the chiefs of service were considered equals. A psychiatric consultant was asked to see him to help alleviate his chronic pain. The first thing the physician did when the psychiatrist entered was to ask him to move a filled bedpan from his bedside to a distant part of the room. The psychiatrist did this. Then the telephone rang and the patient asked the consultant to step out and kept him waiting for 20 minutes. He then requested a cigarette and a light. Once the interview began he interrupted the questioning to urge the consultant to find out why the nurse had not come with his pain medication. He was turning the consultant's role into that of an unwilling and increasingly angry Ganymede. At the end of the interview, the psychiatrist noted that he had been asked to do ten jobs, only one of which he considered a reasonable request. Armed with these examples, he revisited the patient the following day and once again was asked to move the bedpan. The psychiatrist instantly sat down and pointed out the unpleasant tasks the patient had asked him to perform. The psychiatrist ended his comments by observing, "If this is the way you deal with your colleagues, it is no wonder you have so few visitors." The patient was infuriated and terminated the interview on the spot. He sent a formal letter of complaint to the psychiatrist's Chief of Service, but nothing came of it. The only satisfaction was to the psychiatrist, who had aired his complaint. It may have done the patient some good. The next psychiatrist to see him was treated with much more consideration and judged his pain to be emotional in origin.

## THE ASSAULTIVE PATIENT

Patients who are physically combative or dangerously assaultive are rare in liaison practice. Far more common is the disruptive, disoriented, delirious individual, someone with strength enough to harm himself, but with neither the intention nor the wherewithal for injuring another. However, occasionally delirious patients, such as individuals in withdrawal states, can pose a problem on the ward as can the psychotic in catatonic furor or the epileptic in epileptic furor.[7] Prevention is the best type of management. Individuals with a potential for dangerous assault who can be identified by virtue of their previous performance or past history elsewhere should be covered with an appropriate medication. In addition a special attendant should be available along with a trusted friend or relative. The latter are often the most effective instruments available to avert violence. Room confinement or body restraint is at times necessary. It must be cautioned, however, that physical restraint in the odd case can serve as a precipitant to increased truculence rather than to submissiveness.

When a patient becomes unexpectedly obstreperous, seeks exit from the ward, and threatens to dispose of anybody who obstructs his way, quick action is called for. Most often the psychiatrist is the one who is expected to interpose some form of barricade between the patient and the door. Most psychiatrists have enough sense to resist the role of David without a sling. A very quick survey of the situation is usually enough to determine whether or not the patient is amenable to conversation. Is the patient, for example, willing to accept medication as long as he is not asked to return to bed? Before an interview is conducted, however, the psychiatrist should make sure that the security forces are alerted and several male attendants are on their way to the location where they should remain out of sight unless needed. If the individual will take medication, it should be given. The security force should remain in the area until the patient is fully sedated. An effective dose is one that leaves the individual asleep or semistuporous. If, on the other hand, the individual is not amenable to conversation (generally they are not because persuasive methods have been attempted long before the psychiatrist is called), then the psychiatrist should follow one cardinal rule of conduct—never move in on a violent assaultive patient without at least four assistants. The rule of thumb is one helper for each extremity. Hopefully, there will be an extra for good measure. The bigger they are, the better. It is better to have ten than five, better to have fifteen than ten, and the progression is linear in direct proportion to the patient's size and pugilistic talent. A show of force of this kind is often enough in itself to stop the individual from acting out. A smaller number might serve as a challenge to the patient's sense of machismo or the patient might have sufficient martial skills to believe that he can handle himself against any but a mob.

During my service as a Public Health Officer at a United States reformatory I had an experience that serves as my model for handling a violent patient.

A 6 foot, 7 inch, 260 pound inmate was admitted to the reformatory hospital on his way to the federal hospital at Springfield, Missouri. He was diagnosed as having paranoid schizophrenia. I have never seen a larger or more heavily muscled man. After being unshackled he was placed in a security room within the neuropsychiatric section of the hospital. Shortly thereafter, for reasons that are unknown, he tore the iron gate from the wall of his cell and within minutes dislodged the entire cell door. Using this as a flail, he was terrifying the other inmates who screamed for help. When I arrived I foolishly walked toward him asking him to sit down with me and talk. Instead he flung the door at me, a distance of some 20 feet. Fortunately he missed. I realized if I tried to subdue him with the five or six orderlies on duty I would have been faced with a Donnybrook. I evacuated the ward of everyone but the patient and asked the warden to send over the riot squad along with a riot truck. The warden questioned my judgement, but was eventually persuaded. With a squadron of thirty guards at my back and a riot truck bearing teargas canisters and a riot hose positioned at a window facing him, I advanced with a syringe containing a sedative. I told him that he could have it his way or my way, but in any event he was going to be sedated. One way he would get hurt, as would we; the other way, no one would be harmed. For a moment he paused, looking at the phalanx in a menacing way, and then simply said, "Aw, shit, go ahead," dropped his pants, and turned around so that I had easy access to an injection in his buttock.

This example illustrates the principle of force. The greater the force, the less apt there is to be bloodshed or fracture.

The intervention strategies in the examples mainly demonstrate the practice of common sense. Interwoven with common sense are a few psychological principles that are important. Hopefully the case examples are vivid enough to serve as a linchpin for memory.

**REFERENCES**

1. Albert, H. D., and Kornfeld, D. S.: The threat to sign out against medical advice, Ann. Intern. Med. **79:**888-891, 1973.
2. Hackett, T. P.: Management of the disruptive patient in the intensive care setting, Cardiovasc. Nurs. **2:**45-50, 1975.
3. Koumans, A.: Psychiatric consultation in an intensive care unit, J.A.M.A. **194:**163-167, 1965.
4. Cramer, B., Gershberg, M. R., and Stern, M.: Münchausen syndrome: its

relationship to malingering, hysteria, and the physician-patient relationship, Arch. Gen. Psychiatry **24:**573-578, 1971.
5. Hackett, T. P., and Weisman, A. D.: Psychiatric management of operative syndromes I, Psychosom. Med. **22:**267, 1960.
6. Hackett, T. P., and Weisman, A. D.: Psychiatric management of operative syndromes II, Psychosom. Med. **22:**356, 1960.
7. Tupin, J. P.: Management of violent patients. In Shader, R. I., editor: Manual of psychiatric therapeutics, Boston, 1976, Little, Brown and Co., chap. 7.

# 13

# Suicide

**FREDERICK G. GUGGENHEIM**

---

In the general hospital, the psychiatric consultant may be called on to evaluate and to initiate treatment of suicidal patients in the emergency ward and on medical and surgical floors. Since some of the issues encountered differ considerably in each setting, the problems are discussed separately.

## THE SUICIDAL PATIENT ADMITTED TO THE EMERGENCY WARD

Once a person identified as a potentially active suicide arrives in the emergency ward, the consultant's first task is to take responsibility for the management of the patient's physical safety to prevent further self-damage. Then the consultant must gather relevant data about the degree of suicidal intent. Finally, the consultant will have to make decisions about, and often assist in, the patient's transfer to other facilities or his discharge home.

When consultants are called to the emergency ward, they may be tempted to assume that their patient will not manifest further suicidal behavior while in a hospital setting. While this is generally true, it is nonetheless imprudent to expect that any place is free of self-destructive opportunities. An intravenous bottle can be smashed and used to inflict lacerating wounds; a needle can be swallowed; scissors or other surgical instruments can produce penetrating wounds. Also, the unattended patient may make use of a concealed weapon or poison.

### Suicide precautions

Of all the antisuicide devices and strategies available, the best is constant vigilant accompaniment by an appropriate caregiver. This approach is labeled "intensive, strict suicide precautions" or "one-to-one." Depending on the perturbation of the patient and the resources of the hospital, the caregivers may be aides, nurses, security guards, or even family members, if they calm rather than agitate the patient. In all instances back-up staff must be close at hand. The consultant may need to stay with the patient until physical, chemical, and interpersonal restraints have secured the situation. In far too many instances recently admitted patients have eloped or plunged out of a window while the consultant was momentarily away telling the nursing staff of the patient's dangerously suicidal tendencies.

Intensive, strict suicide precautions need not always be instituted. Sometimes, after a suicide gesture with high manipulative intent (especially if low risk to life was involved), the patient may have achieved considerable secondary gain from the behavior and precautions other than basic suicide precautions may not be necessary.

## Collating and exchanging information

After the patient's physical safety has been assured, the consultant's task is to take a history. In obtaining information from the medical or surgical staff, the consultant may notice a particularly negativistic staff attitude that can even approach malice.[2] "Here are all these other patients with legitimate illnesses, and then this clown goes and makes himself sick!" It does little good for the consultant to point out the inappropriateness of this attitude, especially if the patient was admitted at 3:00 A.M. At a more tranquil time it is often useful to provide the consultee with more details of the history, explaining the patient's misery prior to the attempt. An understanding of the dilemma of the suicidal patient helps the medical staff to see the nontrivial nature of the patient's predicament.

## Medication

While exchanging information about the patient's history and the type of suicide precautions needed, the consultee may ask about the necessity for further psychoactive medication. The patient who has overdosed rarely needs medication until delirium and lethargy have cleared. However, if the patient has overdosed with a tricyclic antidepressant,[3] 1 to 2 mg. of physostigmine may reverse the catatonic atropine psychosis for up to 4 hours. In situations where agitation is life-threatening 5 to 20 mg of diazepam may be given intravenously. Careful attention must be given to respiratory rate because sudden respiratory arrest can occur.

The suicidal patient who has incurred some type of traumatic bodily injury usually does not manifest extreme agitation, but should this occur, 50 to 100 mg of chlorpromazine given intramusculary every

1 to 3 hours or 5 mg haloperidol every 1 to 3 hours will usually suffice. Many times patients with psychiatric histories will be able to tell the consultant what their usual effective maintenance dosage schedule is.

The compliance of most suicidal patients while receiving medical or surgical care is striking, bringing to mind Louis Dublin's observation that patients often want to die in a very specific way.[4] For example, the person who is trying to drown will swim to shore rather than be shot. The patient who has recently tried to overdose does not usually pull out intravenous tubing or a central line. Nonetheless, the medical staff should not allow the suicidal patient easy access to potentially lethal medical support apparatus.

### Communication with the patient

Retrieving information from the patient may become a time-consuming matter because of factors such as drug-induced somnolence, hoarseness from an endotracheal tube, or the generalized debility associated with life-threatening conditions. Symptoms of the devastating mental illness such as psychomotor retardation, persecutory delusions, or distractability may also make it difficult to establish adequate rapport to gain a clear account from the patient of the events leading to hospitalization.

Despite these barriers, most patients will divulge to a kind, interested person whether they wish to live or to die. Many will spontaneously confess their lethal desires to the consultant. Others will reveal such wishes only to a particular staff or family member.

However, there are patients who reject all help and purposely conceal their disappointment at survival. The consultant is often served best in dealing with such patients by using indirect questioning to estimate potential for further life-threatening behavior. One very useful indirect question is: "Were you surprised to survive the attempt?" This simple question taps straight into the dimension of gesture-for-attention. It can help to separate such a gesture from a serious attempt at dying that proved ineffective.

### Risk-rescue ratio scale

Another method the consultant may use is the determination of the ratio of risk factors to rescue factors.[5] Although it is indirect and primarily a research tool, the risk-rescue ratio scale embodies in a standardized, numerical fashion what astute clinicians have done empirically on an ad hoc basis. It determines the seriousness of the attempt and the hope for rescue from the facts of the attempt rather than from what the patient says about it. Many data are found in the emergency room chart—the number of pills taken, the time they were ingested, the approximate hours the individual was unconscious before arriving at the hospital, previous maintenance dosage of the medication, whether or not alcohol was used in addition. The magnitude of self-induced lesion is also pertinent. For example, 3.2% of patients making a nonserious suicide attempt will commit suicide sometime within the following 5 years while 6.4% of those patients making a serious suicide attempt will be dead within the same time span.[6] Hence, the consultant might be tempted to undertake a more intensive treatment program with patients who have seriously attempted suicide.

Understanding the factors that led to rescue rather than completed suicide contribute to accurate assessment. Surprisingly, these data are generally not readily found in medical charts although they are usually easily determined from the patient or from the rescuer. Often the patient will give several clues and cues about this. Was the patient in a familiar setting or in a distant spot under an assumed name? Was detection certain, probable, possible, or unlikely? Did the patient try to attract attention or to avoid discovery? A self-induced laceration in front of a lover during a quarrel carries a far different prognosis than does an overdose taken alone in the depths of the Maine woods.

### Evaluation

**Evaluation of mental status.** Is the patient presently psychotic? Are there signs of a psychotic depression, schizophrenia, or organic brain syndrome? The type and extent of psychopathology become a guide to the type and intensity of precautions. They also signal what type of psychiatric treatment will be needed. The presence of any of the aforementioned diagnoses, in the face of a suicide attempt, no matter how trivial, should be an indication for psychiatric hospitalization.

**Evaluation of patient affect.** The consultant also needs to evaluate the emotional tenor of the suicidal person. We have found that some suicide-prone people are looking for escape—release and relief. Others are looking for payback—revenge. The most serious potential for a suicide, according to the experience of the Los Angeles Suicide Prevention Center,[7] is associated with feelings of helplessness, hopelessness, exhaustion, and failure, the feeling of "I just want out." The danger of lethal behavior is generally reduced when the predominant affect is anger, rage, or frustration. Acting out feelings or ventilating can be rapidly effective in decreasing the suicidal perturbation seen with acute anger. But the affect of acute depression in the suicidal patient often lasts longer, is less readily discharged in a benign manner, and can therefore be lethal.

**Evaluation of premeditation versus impulsivity.** Was the suicide attempt premeditated or impulsive? The risk of subsequent suicide attempts is somewhat less if the attempt was impulsive.

**Evaluation of extent of future plans.** Does the individual have a detailed plan for a subsequent attempt? Many people who are thinking of suicide will tell their examiner that they have a vague plan, but if the patient has a plan replete with meticulous attention to detail, the consultant must clearly consider the necessity for hospitalization. When a suicidal patient focuses mainly on the manipulative elements of the behavior, the risk of subsequent lethality is somewhat diminished, especially if nonlethal methods are threatened.

**Evaluation of psychosocial support systems.** Finally, the consultant must also assess the adequacy of potential psychosocial support systems available to the suicidal patient after discharge. Unfortunately for the consultant, there are no simple, hard-and-fast rules to be used in the assessment of the adequacy of psychosocial support. If the suicide attempt has not accomplished its explicit or implicit goal, whether that be, for example, reunion with a lover, revenge on a significant key person, or escape from despair, available community outpatient support systems may not suffice. There is no easy mathematical way of assessing this. Nor is there yet any good pencil-and-paper predictive test of subsequent suicidal behavior.[8]

## Disposition

In making the decision to transfer the suicidal patient to a psychiatric unit, the consultant can usually rely on certain absolute and relative criteria for hospitalization. Indications for mandatory hospitalization pertain if the patient is (1) psychotic (even if the suicide attempt was trivial), (2) over age 45 (unless there is a long history of manipulative suicide gestures), or (3) a survivor of a violent, near-lethal, premeditated attempt. Indications for possible hospitalization pertain if the patient (1) took precautions to avoid being rescued alive, (2) regrets having survived the attempt and demonstrates a rising level of perturbation, (3) refuses help, (4) shows signs and symptoms of the presuicidal syndrome, including constriction of affect, associations, behavior, human relationships, and values,[9] or (5) is living alone without a viable social support system.

Most suicidal patients who come to a general hospital emergency room go home the same day. An intensive study of one-hundred patients randomly selected from the 347 people who were alive when brought to Massachusetts General Hospital following a suicide attempt[10] reveals that 67% went home the same day, 11% signed out against medical advice or eloped, 5% died in the hospital of medical complications, and 17% were sent to a psychiatric unit. As determined by the risk-rescue ratio,[5] 8% of these patients had a high rating for lethality, 45% a moderate rating, and 47% a low rating.

Research into the subject of decision-making in the emergency room has proved particularly difficult because many cases of suicidal behavior are disguised by patient or family. Even the physician's notes in the chart may include euphemisms such as drug ingestion, drug intoxication, or toxic-metabolic coma. Self-induced laceration of the wrist is sometimes coded as laceration of the wrist; jumping under a subway train may be described on the chart as crush amputation, left leg; carbon monoxide poisoning may be coded as cerebral anoxia, secondary to carbon monoxide; and gunshot wounds witnessed by others as self-inflicted and intentional are not infrequently signed out as gunshot wound, left chest, accidental. Indeed, the "self" of self-inflicted wounds is not often the first interest or thought of surgeons trying to save a life in an emergency trauma situation.

The number of patients with medically serious suicide attempts who are subsequently referred to psychiatric units for further care varies considerably from institution to institution. The ready availability of beds on a psychiatric ward in a good general hospital or in a nearby well-regarded psychiatric hospital tends to increase referrals to inpatient psychiatric facilities. By contrast, such referrals to psychiatric facilities are made less frequently when the psychiatric inpatient facilities are not held in high regard, when there is a failure to detect the self-induced nature of the attempt by family or staff, and when the patient's family or local physician resists the idea of psychiatric care. Still another factor that may lower the referral rate to psychiatric units is the necessity of a lengthy medical or surgical hospitalization. In this situation the consultant is often able to provide adequate psychopharmacological or psychotherapeutic treatment while the patient remains on a nonpsychiatric service. Another factor tending to lower the rate of transfer of patients to psychiatric services is the extent of alcoholism in a given population. It is not uncommon for an alcoholic patient, for reasons that never become clear, to make an impulsive yet severe suicide attempt. When sober, the patient is stunned at what has happened. The alcoholic patient begins to function well again and leaves the hospital confidently disdaining the need for further help.

The decision to send a suicidal patient to a psychiatric unit is always a difficult one for consultants. They do not want their permissiveness to be an agent in a patient's destruction. On the other hand, they do not want to overburden often crowded facilities; to subject patients in a brief, benign, self-limited crisis to the indignities of unneeded hospitalization; or to reward crisis-seeking, histrionic behavior. Fortunately statistics can lighten the burden of this decision. More than 99% of patients discharged after a suicide attempt are alive at the end of 1 year.[11]

## THE SUICIDAL PATIENT ADMITTED TO THE MEDICAL OR SURGICAL WARD

What happens to the suicidal patient who lives long enough to be admitted to the medical or surgical ward? What are the chances of surviving if medical danger passes? Will the individual be a management problem for the staff? One unpublished but detailed survey of all emergency admissions to a university hospital indicated that 95% of all patients who had clearly inflicted injury to themselves in an acute suicide attempt survived.[10]

### Subsequent suicide attempts in the hospital

Subsequent overt suicidal acts of a suicide survivor while in the hospital seem to be rare. Moreover, systematic surveys reveal that those who do commit suicide in the general hospital are primarily patients admitted for nonpsychiatric conditions.[12-14,16] The involved, concerned, and usually vigilant staff presumably serves as an efficient deterrent. Many times the alerting staff member will be the psychiatric consultant, but often this role is filled by a nurse. Recent overt suicidal behavior sensitizes a network of observers to respond to any increment of anguish, rage, or despair.

There are a few patients admitted for medical care following suicide attempts who are extreme risks of subsequent hospital suicide attempts. Such patients are either young and schizophrenic, or middle-aged and melancholic. There may be auditory hallucinations of a persecutory nature or severe self-loathing. Schizophrenic patients may fear that they will be killed or dismembered unless they can successfully escape their persecutors. To relieve their perturbation they may attempt to leap out a window, slit their own throats with a safety razor, or hang themselves from a light cord or sheet in a desperate attempt to control their own destiny. They are readily perceived as "crazy" by the staff and may well be in four point restraint with a nurse in attendance. If lithe and terrified, they may be able to disengage the restraints during a change of shift, or during a nurse's trip to the bathroom. For such patients, continuous, uninterrupted surveillance is mandatory. If patients have a recent history of self-destructive behavior and continue to hear voices threatening them with execution or urging suicide, extreme precautions must be taken at all times until antipsychotic medication has not only completely calmed them, but also stopped the frightening hallucinations and delusions.

It is unclear why there is a moratorium on self-destructive behavior in the vast majority of suicidal patients after admission to medical and surgical wards. Possible explanations include (1) the cathartic effect of the recent suicide attempt, (2) the attention and close supervision from an anxious staff intent on avoiding subsequent attempts from the suicidal patient, (3) the painful (punishing) hospital treatments cathecting autoaggressive energy, and (4) the uniting of a shattered family or the emergence of the hospital as a caring and concerned pseudo-family.

Although suicidal patients rarely make further attempts on medical or surgical services, many continue to have suicidal ideation and longing for death. Suicidal patients also often think of effective methods to use in the general hospital. Subsequent to discharge, the first 30 to 90 days represent a period of vulnerability to suicide for medical, surgical, and psychiatric patients.[17,18]

## Management

Several emotionally charged issues face the consultant. Is the patient still suicidal? Is there still a risk of a suicide attempt on the ward? If the patient is suicidal, how suicidal and what level of observation is needed? Precautions range from basic, simple precautions, with removal of sharp objects in the room, brief room check to ensure that there are no hoards of medication, window locks on the patient's room as well as adjacent rooms, and room checks every 15 minutes to intensive, strict suicide precautions with one-to-one accompaniment at all times and restraints when necessary as determined by the patient's level of activity and impulsiveness. Because of the staff anxiety generated by such a patient, the consultant will initially need to visit the floor several times daily, being available both psychologically and physically.

The psychiatric consultant called to see a patient identified as suicidal on the medical-surgical ward is also faced with making the decision about postdischarge disposition. At times social manipulation, the use of psychoactive drugs, and individual or family psychotherapy while in the hospital makes transfer to a psychiatric unit unnecessary. In other instances, the institution of antidepressant therapy (generally with a rapidly acting tricyclic antidepressant such as nortriptyline or desipramine plus individual or family-centered psychotherapy) can obviate the otherwise necessary transfer to a psychiatric unit. Sometimes patients who become dangerously, impulsively suicidal following a mild social upset while drinking actually lose their inclination toward self-destruction and no longer pose an active suicide threat. However, cases in which there is severe threat to life caused by a premeditated attempt certainly deserve the offer of referral to a psychiatric unit. Commitment to a psychiatric unit is often reserved for those patients who are actively psychotic or who fit the state's legal definition for commitment.

If the patient has recently been suicidal, the consultant will need to reassure the staff that the consultant will still be available on an emergency basis if anything should happen, and that the consultant in the meantime will continue to actively follow the patient while on the medical-surgical ward. Patients who have made suicide attempts oftentimes are very frightening or threatening to the staff and this requires an extra amount of the consultant's attention.

Not all patients are overt about the self-destructive behavior that resulted in their hospitalization. Some patients are very covert about this, neither confessing nor admitting, for example, that the "accidental tumble" in front of the subway train was actually a swan dive.[19] The hospital course of these covert cases is usually placid and benign. Once discharged, though, the subsequent risk of acting out lethal impulses may be very serious.[19]

## THE PATIENT WHO BECOMES SUICIDAL ON THE MEDICAL-SURGICAL WARD

For the patient whose self-destructive tendencies emerge while in the hospital, it may be that the hospital environment itself has become nontherapeutic or antitherapeutic. The noxious element is not always the attitude of hospital staff or of the patient toward illness. At times suicidal ideation and even suicidal action can be impelled by fragmented, frightened thinking while in a toxic psychosis (as in delirium tremens[16], or steroid-induced depressive psychosis). Only rarely does the previously mentally stable individual respond to the severe pain and debility attendant to a terminal or chronic illness with suicidal ideation.[12,16]

Little systematic information is available about patients who profess or act our their self-destructive desires while on medical or surgical services. For the sake of this discussion these patients are arbitrarily divided into Threateners, Attempters, and Completers.

### Patients who threaten suicide

Threateners seem to be dramatizing people. Typically, a Threatener is a woman who has for many years moaned to her family in times of stress with such comments as, "Oh, my God, I wish I were dead!" or, "God, take my life!" Rarely is there a history of a bona fide suicide gesture or attempt. The patient may have a history of wishing to be dead (passive), but hardly ever wishing to die or to be killed.[20,21] When questioned on the ward about the so-called suicide threat, the patient adamantly denies intended suicide, but readily admits to a recent increase in feelings of loneliness and hopelessness.

The staff's increased attentiveness following such a threat is therapeutic in itself. Suicide precautions usually do not become necessary. Many times these patients are not referred for psychiatric consultation because their problems are handled rapidly and effectively at a staff level with added attention. For this reason prevalence studies for this type of behavior are lacking.

### Patients who attempt suicide on medical-surgical wards

Several studies have examined attempted suicide on general hospital wards. A recent study[12] surveyed overt suicidal activity in a teaching hospital. There were seventeen attempts and no fatalities over a 7 year span. All attempts were impulsive. None of the patients gave warning, left notes, expressed suicidal thoughts, or appeared to be seriously depressed. In none of the cases was immediate suicide risk suspected by the staff, but after each attempt close study revealed that the patient did give signs of rising tension with anger, agitation, acute psychosis, or sudden change of mood. And each episode was associated with a stress not directly related to illness, pain, or disability. Suicide attempts were precipitated by loss of emotional support. In fifteen of the seventeen cases, this loss involved disruption in relationships with medical personnel, and in two of these cases there was also overt conflict with key family members. The critical determinant of underlying suicidal behavior was the psychological susceptibility of the patient. The most frequent source of this vulnerability was the presence of antecedent mental disorder (fifteen out of seventeen cases). In those two cases without prior psychopathology, both patients made their attempts when they found that specific treatment programs were failing and when the staff attitude changed from optimism to discouragement.

## Patients who kill themselves in a general hospital

There are several studies of patients who have completed suicides. Farberow[13] reviewed the records of cardiorespiratory patients who committed suicide and compared them to a matched control population who did not attempt suicide. The suicide fatalities were more emotionally disturbed and had poor relationships with hospital staff and family. They were previously seen as problem patients with provoking, complaining, and demanding behavior. Additionally, they seemed to be dependent and dissatisfied people.

In a study of Veteran's Administration (V.A.) patients, Farberow[14] isolated as predictors of suicide potential (1) emotional stress over and above the physical and psychological aspects of the disease process itself, (2) low tolerance for pain and discomfort, (3) excessive demanding and complaining behavior with a strong need for attention and reassurance, (4) controlling and directing activity (insistent requests or refusals of treatment and medication), (5) relative alertness and orientation, (6) exhaustion of physical and emotional resources, including feeling of lack of support and attention from family or hospital, and (7) prior or present suicidal threats or attempts.

In another study from a V.A. facility, the important factors leading to suicide appeared to be acute toxic-metabolic disturbances and physical features in the hospital that failed to restrain confused, hallucinating patients from falling to their deaths. Pollack[16] reported on eleven patients who committed suicide in the hospital. Seven of these had an acute organic brain syndrome at the time they killed themselves. Three of these patients had severe diurnal variation in sensorium with nocturnal confusion. Associated diagnoses for these organic brain syndrome patients were alcoholism and convulsive disorder. Of all eleven patients, only one had been given a psychiatric diagnosis and that was the only one with a history of a suicide attempt. None of these patients had ever been given a diagnosis of a psychosis during previous hospitalizations. Curiously, just before the suicide, most of these patients were believed to be improving by the staff. Hence, there were few markers from the past to alert the staff to the possibility of suicide. All the patients needed to be in a general hospital for medical treatment, and only one was near death at the time of suicide.

Another aspect of suicide in the general hospital concerns patients with chronic renal failure (see Chapter 18). Nonsystematic studies reveal that although patients with carcinoma have low risks of suicide, patients on renal dialysis have a suicide rate 400 times that of the general population.[22] About 5% of all dialysis patients die by suicide according to a survey of 201 hemodialysis centers. Issues contributing to this self-destructive behavior included object loss outside of the health sphere, failure of patient-staff communications, and the miserable quality of life without hope for release from chronic illness and its disrupting treatment.[23]

Experiences at MGH with those who are prone to kill themselves in a medical setting are exemplified by the case of a middle-aged, semi-skilled machinist.

> He was a boxer in his youth. Married to an aggressive woman, he had become increasingly passive and dependent during the past 2 decades. At age 55 he developed rapidly advancing Hodgkin disease with only brief remissions from a variety of increasingly toxic chemotherapeutic agents. He was compliant and friendly, but his hospital insurance was about to stop, the final drug had failed, his private physician was about to transfer him to ward service, and his wife had become fed up. Under these circumstances he jumped out the window at 7:00 A.M. when the night nursing shift was giving report. He had given only the vaguest clues of suicidal thoughts before he chose an active way out of his dilemma.

> Another example of a high-risk patient was a middle-aged grandmother, active in civic affairs and president of several organizations. A charming, dramatic woman with a high need for control, she had once mentioned that she would drive her Rolls Royce over a cliff herself if she ever developed the same kind of agonizing carcinoma that afflicted her mother. On developing such similar symptoms from the same disease, she became increasingly despondent. Without any warning she made a major in-hospital attempt, ingesting hoarded chloral hydrate. Like the first patient, she had no psychiatric history. Later, after recovering from her attempt, and after having come to peace with herself and her family, she was given an option of having a morphine-chlorpromazine intravenous drip as her pain increased. She demurred, fearing she might miss something, vomit in her sleep, or lose control. She died in sepsis with her family beside her.

Treatment of the patient who becomes increasingly suicidal in the hospital is based on (1) keeping the patient safe, (2) giving the patient needed attention, and (3) giving the patient control insofar as is medically possible.

## SUMMARY

The consultant treating the suicidal patient in the general hospital must deal with the anger of the medical staff, the anxieties of the nursing staff, the ambivalence of the family, and the despair of the patient. The consultant often must be knot tier, lip reader, social mediator, psychotherapist, psychopharmacologist, and friend.

Those patients who refuse help may prove difficult to evaluate and even more difficult to give treatment on a long-term basis.[15] Another group that offers a particular challenge to detection and treatment are those patients whose desires for self-destruction emerge while in the hospital. Hospital environment, illness, and often even family and physician become toxic for these few patients.

## REFERENCES

1. Stengel, E.: Suicide and attempted suicide, Baltimore, 1964, Penguin Books.
2. Maltsberger, J. T., and Buie, D. H.: Counter-transference hate in the treatment of suicidal patients, Arch. Gen. Psychiatry **30:**625-633, 1974.
3. Granacher, R. P., and Baldessarini, R. J.: Physostigmine: its use in acute anti-cholinergic syndrome with anti-depressant and anti-parkinson drugs, Arch. Gen. Psychiatry **32:**375-380, 1975.
4. Dublin, L. I.: Suicide. A sociological and statistical study, New York, 1963, The Ronald Press Co.
5. Weisman, A. D., and Worden, J. W.: Risk-rescue rating in suicide assessment, Arch. Gen. Psychiatry **26:**553-560, 1972.
6. Littman, R. E., and Farberow, N. L.: Emergency evaluation of self-destructive potential. In Farberow, N. L., and Shneidman, E. S., editors: Cry for help, New York, 1961, McGraw-Hill Book Co.
7. Brown, T. R., and Sheren, T. J.: Suicide prediction: a review, Life Threat. Behav. **2:**67-98, 1972.
8. Rosen, D. H.: The serious suicide attempt: five-year follow-up study of 886 patients, J.A.M.A. **235:**2105-2110, 1976.
9. Ringel, E.: The pre-suicidal syndrome, Life Threat. Behav. **6:**131-149, 1976.
10. Stirling-Smith, R.: Personal communication, 1970.
11. Ettlinger, R. W.: Suicide in a group of patients who had previously attempted suicide, Acta Psychiatr. Scand. **40:**363-378, 1964.
12. Reich, P., and Kelly, M. J.: Suicide attempts by hospitalized medical and surgical patients, N. Engl. J. Med. **294:**298-301, 1976.
13. Farberow, N. L. McKelligott, J. W., Cohen, S., and Darbonne, A.: Suicide among patients with cardiorespiratory illness, J.A.M.A. **195:**422-428, 1966.
14. Farberow, N. L., Shneidman, E. S., and Leonard, C. V.: Suicide among

general medical and surgical hospital patients with malignant neoplasms, Med. Bull. V. Adm. **9:**1-11, 1963.

15. Guggenheim, F. G.: Strategies and tactics in the outpatient management of severely suicidal patients. In Lazare, A.: Diagnosis and treatment in outpatient psychiatry, Baltimore, The Williams & Wilkins Co. In press.

16. Pollack, S.: Suicide in a general hospital. In Shneidman, E., editor: Clues to suicide, pp. 152-163.

17. Robbins, E., and others: Some clinical considerations in the prevention of suicide based on a study of 134 successful suicides, Am. J. Public Health **49:**888-899, 1959.

18. Dorpat, T. L., Anderson, W. F., and Ripley, H. S.: The relationship of physical illness to suicide. In Renik, H. L. P., editor: Suicidal behaviors, Boston, 1968, Little Brown & Co., pp. 209-219.

19. Guggenheim, F. G., and Weisman, A. D.: Suicide in the subway: publicly witnessed attempts of 50 cases, J. Nerv. Ment. Dis. **155:**404-409, 1972.

20. Guggenheim, F. G., and Weisman, A. D.: Suicide in the subway: psychodynamic aspects, Life threat. behav. **4:**43-53, 1974.

21. Menninger, K.: Man against himself, New York, 1938, Harcourt Brace Jovanovich, Inc.

22. Abram, H. S., Moore, G. L., and Westervelt, F. B.: Suicidal behavior in chronic dialysis patients, Am. J. Psychiatry **127:**1199-1204, 1971.

23. McKegney, F. P., and Lange, P.: The decision to no longer live on chronic hemodialysis, Am. J. Psychiatry **128:**47-54, 1971.

# 14

# Coping with illness

**AVERY D. WEISMAN**

Coping is problem-solving behavior designed to bring about relief, reward, quiescence, and equilibrium. However, this definition is hardly adequate. After all, doing arithmetic is problem-solving behavior; driving an automobile through heavy traffic is problem-solving; raising children is, at the very least, problem-solving. The common denominator of coping is to have a problem. The common task of physicians, including liaison psychiatrists, and patients is to solve problems related to being sick, that is, the medical plight beyond mere physical changes and consequences. Coping, therefore, is an integral part of medical practice as well as illness. With the same disease at comparable stages, and with more or less equivalent treatment, patients may have different problems, and physicians may themselves respond with a wide variety of reactions, diagnoses, and management.

Coping strategies, that is, the processes by which the end result of coping is reached, are not the same as defense mechanisms, certain writers notwithstanding. In common parlance, coping means that one has overcome a threat or mastered a risky situation. To liaison psychiatrists this definition is unsatisfactory because they want to know more about the intermediary steps required to define and to master the incipient calamity. How patients cope is a complicated mixture of cognitive appraisal and reappraisal, initial responses and corrected responses, strung out along a time continuum. Some investigators such as Murphy and Moriarty distinguish between COPE I for external problems, and COPE II for intrapsychic conflicts, thereby doing away with the imagery of defense mechanisms. Regardless of how complicated coping processes are, the liaison psychiatrist is expected to perceive the key problems that distress a patient, to evaluate the degree of emotional turmoil, and to do something about it.

## THE MEDICAL PLIGHT

Being sick is a problem in itself. But the fact of being sick sends waves into the far reaches of a patient's life, undoing psychosocial balance, and even initiating illness in significant others (family, friends, and so forth). However, because a hospital-based liaison psychiatrist usually is asked to evaluate individual medical and surgical patients, I shall consider only the coping problems related to the medical plight, as seen through the eyes of the physician and patient. Much of what follows applies also to the nurse, social worker, chaplain, or other professional who is engaged in psychosocial interventions, whether as a primary responsibility or not.

The medical plight consists of problems related to (1) disease, (2) sickness, and (3) vulnerability. Being sick means that a patient not only feels sick but also fills a sick role within the hospital structure and its relationships. Patienthood imposes certain tacit obligations. There are rules and regulations that define proper comportment and medical expectations. In return for being a "good" patient, one is promised an average expectable outcome. Patients with a "good" doctor-patient relationship are usually less distressed and probably do better during hospitalization than those who are unable to abide by expectations. Many psychiatric consultations stem from the staff's intolerance of aberrant behavior. Those patients who insist on their own way, struggle for power, or manipulate the staff too obviously may be forced to sign out, or at least be labeled "uncooperative," "resistant," or "passive-aggressive." There are other patients who are quietly uncooperative, and simply surrender themselves. They are not often referred to the liaison psychiatrist unless a nurse or social worker is alert to what is happening.

These remarks should not be construed to mean that patients are hapless victims who must go along to get along. Too often physicians and other members of the professional staff see their work thwarted by patients and families. Their jobs are made difficult because of unnecessary outside problems that hinder progress.

It is futile to judge faults. But even the most cooperative patients find that they must communicate in the lingua franca of sickness and "hospitalese." To be fully accepted by their colleagues liaison psychiatrists must also codify their findings in medical format, trying to be objective in the most subjective of specialties. For example, patients who feel vaguely disconsolate, lonely, bored, irritated, and discouraged even when their medical progress is satisfactory may not be able to say exactly what is bothering them. While intellectuals might call their feelings "anomie," patients may fret or fume until, finally, they agree to the suggestion that they are "depressed." The difference between their private feelings and the self-derogatory delusions of a melancholic patient could hardly be greater. From the time of conceding "depression," however, the noun becomes the diagnosis, and no further attention is given to how these patients actually cope with their medical plight.

## Disease-related problems

Different diseases have their own special complications with which almost every victim must cope. A disfiguring scar, ataxia, a colostomy, a restrictive diet, and so forth require some form of primary rehabilitation and retraining that entails coping processes. Not every patient seen by a liaison psychiatrist suffers from mental or emotional troubles. As a rule, however, the liaison psychiatrist is not called on merely for disease-related problems. There are paramedical and professional specialists in a variety of fields who are much more expert than the primary physicians. Liaison psychiatry in a general hospital deals with psychosocial problems. Some of these are complications of rehabilitative procedures. For example, it is not uncommon for an elderly person to prefer a wheelchair to a prosthesis after a leg amputation. The patient may be able to walk well when assisted by a physiotherapist but be reluctant to venture beyond his room when he returns home. The liaison psychiatrist will talk about the amputation with the patient, then about the living arrangements, the emotional support received or not received from others, and fears about walking unaided or alone on a crowded street. The liaison psychiatrist will recognize that the patient suffers from an agoraphobia related to the recent amputation, prosthesis notwithstanding. This condition may yield to psychotherapeutic suggestions by the psychiatrist working in conjunction with the physiotherapist, visiting nurse, or members of the family who can be motivated for the task.

Liaison psychiatrists are now being asked more often to consult patients suffering "diseases of progress." Almost every advance in medicine is followed by an unexpected complication. Treatments that save patients from one disease may expose them to several others. The secondary problems of immunosuppression are prominent examples that require psychosocial intervention. While medicine can disregard or minimize the psychosocial fallout of sickness, there is no "impersonal" disease.

## Sickness-related problems

Illness has its interpersonal and intrapsychic qualities that may undo medical and surgical efforts. When the limits of medicine and surgery have been reached, psychosocial problems may just be gathering momentum. For example, a young father who develops carcinoma of the lung is not just physically sick. He worries about his job as well as about the other psychosocial complications of illness and its treatment. He may complain to and about the physicians, argue with his wife, and even blame his children for his plight. All these objectionable results may conceal deep pessimism about survival and fear of abandoning people closest to him.

The liaison psychiatrist should not forget that for the layman sickness is usually serious business, and serious sickness cannot help but evoke fears about death, regardless of the actual prognosis. Fear of being irreparably harmed or incapacitated reflects similar existential concerns. Perhaps the first question that a liaison psychiatrist should ask is, "How has this illness been a problem for you and for the people closest to you?" Fears about dying are more difficult to inquire about because patients with conscious fears resent the question as self-evident, while those with unadmitted fears may defend themselves by asserting that they have not been told everything.

For some people, patienthood is easier than functioning in the outside world. A person who submits courageously to a series of operations may not be able to work when recovered and thereby becomes an even greater liability than before the surgery began. Every illness should be presumed to carry a balance of gains and losses for the individual. An unexpected improvement or recovery in a patient who has become accustomed to invalidism and the sick role may induce relative ego impairment if too many psychosocial responsibilities are thrust on the patient too quickly. Psychiatrists are trained to identify hypochondriacal patients who suffer from heightened visceral sensations and morbid convictions of incurable disease, but there are other patients who derive benefits from being ill, just as there are losses and secondary illness-related solutions that permeate any aspect of life. Survival, support, and self-esteem are only three important problems faced by chronically ill patients, including those who are rescued from invalidism through newer medical and surgical treatments.

### Vulnerability

Vulnerability refers to the emotional distress that is the most personal aspect of illness. It reflects impairment of competence, control, and consciousness. Consequently, vulnerability not only signifies distress in the here-and-now, but a disposition to behave or conduct oneself at less than full efficiency.

Endless is the list of human frailties; unexpected are human strengths. The ways in which the human being is vulnerable are both endless and unexpected. While motivated by an understandable wish to simplify, it is yet sheer arrogance to pretend that even a well-trained liaison psychiatrist can unerringly pierce the defensive shell surrounding every distressed patient. However, the psychiatrist can approximate both generality and specificity by recognizing distress and disposition in vulnerable patients. For example, depressed patients are dejected and hopeless about the future. Time is closed, so they feel unable to take action on their own behalf. Their sense of doom leads to an apparent apathy and indifference. On the other hand, truculent patients feel angry, victimized, resentful, and misled. When approached by physicians or nurses, they may be curt or monosyllabic, feeling that it is useless to buck the system. The inner distress of these two types of patients is quite different, but their outward behavior, which is about all the outsider has to go on, may be identical. Both kinds of patients discourage others from coming to their aid or from entering their world. Depressed patients and the truculent patients may both feel, "What's the use?" Depression has a disheartening effect on the outsider; truculence has a distancing effect through hostile recalcitrance. Nevertheless, "Let me alone, but don't desert me," is perhaps as good a slogan of truculence as of depression.

The boxed material lists thirteen common types of vulnerability found among hospitalized medical and surgical patients. This is, in fact, a very short list that leaves out a variety of emotional states, but the liaison psychiatrist would do well to begin by differentiating these thirteen types, rating patients according to the extent as well as the kind of vulnerability each demonstrates.

In evaluating patients liaison psychiatrists must realize that the moment of consultation may not be typical, but rather a moment of crisis for the patient, for the staff, or for both. Anyone can have a good day or bad day. Liaison psychiatrists should always evaluate the significance of the timing of the referral. "Why now, at this time, not yesterday or last week, am I being called?"

## HOW DO PATIENTS COPE OR FAIL TO COPE WITH PROBLEMS?

The immediate work of a psychiatric consultation involves both an encounter and an evaluation. It is a wise policy not to differentiate the two very sharply. Not only is differentiation difficult, but the liaison psychiatrist must recognize that both the encounter and the evaluation depend on the evaluator as well as on the problems being evaluated.

# VULNERABILITY

**Hopelessness**

Patient believes that all is lost; effort is futile; there is no chance for recovery.

**Turmoil/perturbation**

Patient is tense, agitated, restless, indicating inner distress.

**Frustration**

Patient is angry about inability to resolve problems and get relief.

**Despondent/depressed**

Patient is dejected, withdrawn, tearful, often inaccessible to interaction.

**Helplessness/powerlessness**

Patient feels unable to initiate positive action; complains of being too weak to struggle; surrenders and defaults decisions.

**Anxiety/fears**

Patient has specific fears or dreads; feelings of panic or impending doom.

**Exhaustion/apathy**

Patient feels depleted and worn out; expresses indifference to outcome.

**Worthlessness/self-rebuke**

Patient feels no good, defective; blames self for weakness, shortcomings, and failures.

**Painful isolation/abandonment**

Patient feels lonely, ignored, alienated from others who allegedly don't care.

**Denial/avoidance**

Patient speaks or acts as if unwilling to recognize threatening aspects of illness; minimizes complaints or findings.

**Truculence/annoyance**

Patient is embittered, feeling victimized or mistreated by someone or something outside, beyond control.

**Repudiation of significant others**

Patient rejects, turns away from, or antagonizes sources of potential help and support, usually a family member or friend.

**Closed time perspective**

Patient foresees a very limited future; day to day existence.

The encounter is not just a matter of beholding the patient. Success depends on the readiness with which the psychiatrist facilitates communication and distinguishes the predominant problems and obstacles of the particular plight in which the patient is immersed.

Vulnerability and the variations of coping have a somewhat reciprocal relationship, at least from the clinical viewpoint. Few patients use only one or two strategies to cope with very important problems, because in coping with important problems patients recall past experiences and portend future obstacles. A very simple problem does not exist except possibly in the mind of the examiner. Nevertheless, given a suitable combination or sequence of strategies, the patient who copes effectively will experience reduction of distress, relief, and perhaps even resolution of problems.

Every patient for whom consultation is sought has a plight that may cause high or low concern. In any event, at least one or two problems can be found, the degree of distress can be estimated, and the prevailing coping strategies can be identified. The boxed material shows fifteen such strategies that serve as the starting point for more specific identification. Although this list is neither complete nor precise, it does show the variety of possible coping strategies that can be used in any sequence or combination.

While psychological inventories and tests are also available that purportedly measure how the individual copes, clinical expediency necessitates immediate empirical evaluation of the problem, the vulnerability level, and the coping strategies in use. Of the three principal parts of a patient's plight, coping is by far the most difficult to detect. The distress of vulnerability is usually far more obvious because high levels of vulnerability are what prompted the consultation in the first place.

Two groups of patients present the most difficult diagnostic problems for the liaison psychiatrist. These are patients who claim to have no problems and patients who inundate the psychiatrist with problems of every sort. Patients who disavow any problems and, despite overt symptoms, reject the notion of being distressed usually cope by suppression, withdrawal, and projection of blame. The liaison psychiatrist may assume that such patients also repress, but this so-called mechanism means only that their experiences are not available by ordinary means. The equilibrium between denial and awareness is always precarious. When denial predominates, the psychiatrist must approach the patient indirectly. Instead of directly asking about problem areas, which would be denied anyway, the psychiatrist poses

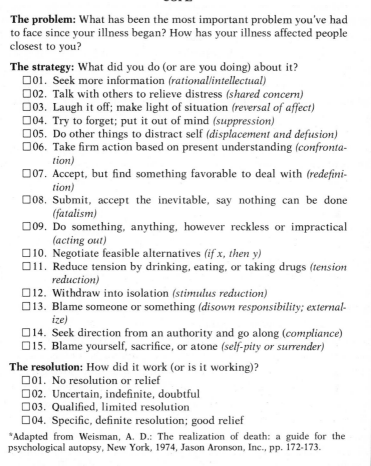

**COPE***

**The problem:** What has been the most important problem you've had to face since your illness began? How has your illness affected people closest to you?

**The strategy:** What did you do (or are you doing) about it?

□ 01. Seek more information *(rational/intellectual)*
□ 02. Talk with others to relieve distress *(shared concern)*
□ 03. Laugh it off; make light of situation *(reversal of affect)*
□ 04. Try to forget; put it out of mind *(suppression)*
□ 05. Do other things to distract self *(displacement and defusion)*
□ 06. Take firm action based on present understanding *(confrontation)*
□ 07. Accept, but find something favorable to deal with *(redefinition)*
□ 08. Submit, accept the inevitable, say nothing can be done *(fatalism)*
□ 09. Do something, anything, however reckless or impractical *(acting out)*
□ 10. Negotiate feasible alternatives *(if x, then y)*
□ 11. Reduce tension by drinking, eating, or taking drugs *(tension reduction)*
□ 12. Withdraw into isolation *(stimulus reduction)*
□ 13. Blame someone or something *(disown responsibility; externalize)*
□ 14. Seek direction from an authority and go along *(compliance)*
□ 15. Blame yourself, sacrifice, or atone *(self-pity or surrender)*

**The resolution:** How did it work (or is it working)?

□ 01. No resolution or relief
□ 02. Uncertain, indefinite, doubtful
□ 03. Qualified, limited resolution
□ 04. Specific, definite resolution; good relief

*Adapted from Weisman, A. D.: The realization of death: a guide for the psychological autopsy, New York, 1974, Jason Aronson, Inc., pp. 172-173.

hypothetical "what if" questions. This approach does not challenge the patient who rigidly represses problems, but merely asks consideration of general issues. An example of the approach is "What if you had a father who threatened you whenever a boyfriend came to the house so that you had to meet him outside or lie about seeing him?" "What if nothing you did ever pleased your boss?" "What if these pains kept you out of work so that you didn't have to face problems there? I do not necessarily mean you, but anyone in your situation." The idea is to go from the general to the particular without becoming too conjectural. The liaison psychiatrist generalizes the plight in such a way that nothing can be denied, dismissed, or rejected out of hand. In effect, the gambit is, "What if this were a problem? What would you advise someone with this problem to do?"

For the patient with many problems the psychiatrist needs another approach. Here the problem is how to sort out the most urgent and timely issues. The liaison psychiatrist must ignore many complaints before using the "if–then" strategy. For instance, the psychiatrist might ask, "If you feel as sad (angry, anxious, etc.) as you seem to, then what have you done or are you doing about it?" A profusion of complaints usually means lack of focus, so efforts are made to limit confrontation to only the most important problems. The "if–then" approach starts with the distress but quickly goes to the general coping strategy. Emotional distress is connected with a coping strategy, after the psychiatrist singles out a specific problem from the many reported. In contrast, with the "what if" approach the psychiatrist begins with general hypotheses and goes to the particular case of coping. "What if" and "If–then" are two ways of stating a problem.

It is imperative to preserve any patient's self-esteem. Consequently, distress may be difficult to report. The psychiatrist may have to prepare the ground by avoiding problem areas—a paradoxical maneuver that can create an alliance—and by concentrating instead on acceptable coping strategies. Sometimes paraphrasing what a patient says about feelings or about previous coping situations helps clarify current coping strategies. There is no interpretation so sagacious or correct that the patient cannot avoid or ignore it completely. Relevant interpretations do not require fancy verbiage. Insight is not of much value unless its clarity is followed by an appropriate action. In other words, good insight usually is a product of good coping, not the reverse. There are, unfortunately, many patients who have abundant insight, that is, "intellectual insight," but are practically paralyzed with indecision and conflict.

## WHO ARE THE BEST COPERS?

For the liaison psychiatrist, the medical plight is a three-legged stool, supported by the problem, vulnerability, and coping strategies. In a study of newly diagnosed cancer patients who were subsequently followed for at least 6 months after the initial impact, it was found that the most effective copers used cope strategies 1, 2, 5, 6, 7, and 14 (see p. 269), but not necessarily in that order. One individual's method may be another's madness. But if these findings can be generalized to other chronic illnesses, then we can add correlations with interview variables. For example, good copers also have good doctor-patient relationships. They are optimistic and resourceful, can directly confront problems, and then can revise them in "cope-able" terms. Suppression and denial are only temporarily effective and, thus, should be considered as only expediencies and not as strategies to be fostered. It is not appropriate to dwell on possible future misfortunes but rather to seek suitable distractions to drain off tensions that accumulate. The main idea is that good copers are flexible in using all available options, just as they faced difficult situations in the past. Moreover, the illness is the unique possession of the patient, not just another problem. When the patient then consents or yields decisions, agreement is given willingly, not by default or surrender.

In contrast, patients who are poor copers tend to have higher emotional distress (by definition) and do not clearly recognize pertinent psychosocial problems. The habits of avoiding, nullifying, and disguising problems as well as the failure to be clear and communicative are diagnostic signs of poor coping. Blaming others or themselves is also an indication of poor coping potential, because patients who use these methods discourage alliances and distort the past. It is usually important to ask about time perspective and anticipated recovery, since these give a clue to how pessimistic or realistic the patient's view of the illness is.

## HOW DO PSYCHIATRISTS COPE WITH ILLNESS?

Liaison psychiatry makes unusual demands on a physician who is also a psychiatrist. Knowledge of medication, psychodynamic theory, and descriptive psychiatry is necessary but insufficient to an understanding of the biosocial ecology of a hospital and the patients in it. Liaison psychiatry itself has an atypical, ambiguous role in the hospital setting because it is primarily concerned with how illness affects the human condition and which aberrations of the human condition complicate illness. It is not enough to have a warm heart and a brain filled with information. Successful liaison psychiatry depends on the ability of the psychiatrist to facilitate good communication. It is pragmatic but cannot be programmed. There is no consultation technique applicable to one and all. Every encounter is a separate challenge. Liaison psychiatrists must be aware of their own vulnerable points, and must not let their compassion get in the way of clinical separateness. They are always reevaluating and responding not only to what is said, but to how it is said or left unsaid.

Psychosocial interventions range from individual sessions with patients to group retraining and discussions with salient professionals (nurses, social workers, and so forth). First, however, the psychiatrist who works with patients needs experience in interview skills to deal with medical and surgical patients who are not primarily motivated to seek or use psychotherapeutic interventions. The following list suggests guidelines of a generally useful approach to the assessment of patients, whether the predominant problem is ward-centered, illness-related, or personality-related.

1. Do not use a set speech because each patient is different.
2. Introduce yourself, even to stuporous or confused patients. Touching is not only permissible, but may reinforce what you have to say.
3. Sit down and try to establish eye contact.
4. Avoid asking questions that can be answered yes or no. These are not real questions, but statements in disguise.
5. Learn how to listen and observe, but the wait-and-see technique of office psychotherapy should be shunned.
6. Respond as seems appropriate, but make sure that the patient has the opportunity to talk, too.
7. Monitor your own thoughts because they may mirror those of the patient, or help explain your difficulties in getting across.
8. Modulate and measure your answers according to the needs of the patient and prerogatives of the primary physician but without being deliberately evasive.
9. Always ask yourself what the patient was like before becoming ill.
10. Clarification, control, and cooling off are usually carried out simultaneously, just as perception, behavior, and emotion are a unit.
11. Use the most timely, informative, and evocative questions, such as:
    a. What has bothered you most about this illness?
    b. How has it been a problem for you?
    c. What have you done (or are you doing) about the problem?
    d. What has been the most difficult thing you've had to face until now?
    e. What did you do then?
    f. Whom do you rely on most, or expect will be most helpful to you?
    g. In general, how do things usually turn out for you?
    h. Tell me what you think about this whole situation.

Liaison psychiatry can be onerous and discouraging if the physician is overly pessimistic or too ambitious. A simple clarification—"least possible contribution"—may be more effective in reducing the impact of illness than a long-range psychotherapeutic program that can rarely be implemented. After all, the goal of liaison psychiatry is to do for patients with high emotional distress what other patients with lower emotional distress do for themselves. Good coping means good coping by the physician as well as by the patient. The aims are to modulate distress, to control behavior by keeping it within acceptable bounds, and to be clear about the immediate most difficult problems.

**SUGGESTED READINGS**

Bird, B.: Talking with patients, ed. 2, Philadelphia, 1973, J. B. Lippincott Co.

Coelho, G., Hamburg, D., and Adams, J., editors: Coping and adaptation, New York, 1974, Basic Books, Inc.

Feinstein, A. R.: Clinical judgment, Baltimore, 1967, The Williams & Wilkins Co.

Jackson, E.: Coping with the crises in your life, New York, 1974, Hawthorn Books, Inc.

Murphy, L., and Moriarty, A.: Vulnerability, coping and growth, New Haven, 1976. Yale University Press.

Weisman, A. D.: The doctor-patient relationship: its role in therapy, In Miles, H., Cobb, S., and Shands, H., editors: Case histories in psychosomatic medicine, New York, 1952, W. W. Norton & Co. Inc., pp. 22-40.

Weisman, A. D.: Confrontation, countertransference, and context. In Adler, G., and Myerson, P., editors: Confrontation in psychotherapy, New York, 1973, Science House, Inc., chap. 5, pp. 97-122.

# 15

# Brief psychotherapy

**JAMES E. GROVES and ANASTASIA KUCHARSKI**

"The tranquilizers can only do so much. I wish somebody
would *talk* to me about this cancer thing. . . ."
*Patient to consultant*, 1975.

---

Tranquilizers can only do so much for the medical or surgical
patient coping with psychological stresses imposed by illness and
hospitalization. The hospital staff can do only so much reassuring,
explaining, and talking to the patient. In fact, staff members had spent
hours talking with the patient quoted in the epigraph, yet the patient
felt no one "talked" about the "cancer thing." What patients in this
situation usually mean by "talking" is a specialized kind of listening
by the caregiver—listening and responding based on an understanding
of what the illness or surgery means to patients, to their self-image
and to their lives, careers, and families. This specialized kind of
listening, psychotherapy, is a complicated intellectual and empathic
relationship between the patient and the physician.

"Psychotherapy" can refer to transactions continuing for months or
years, but it can also refer to interactions of a few minutes in which
only a few sentences are exchanged—provided they are the right
sentences. Brief psychotherapy on the medical or surgical ward
deserves consideration in liaison psychiatry because psychiatrists
must combine a knowledge of medicine and surgery with an understanding of stress response syndromes. Psychiatrists should know
how to listen and to respond on three levels—medical, social, and
psychological—simultaneously. The role of the consultant who comes
to the stressed patient is mainly that of fostering optimal adaptation to
painful reality. How well the consultant succeeds in a small number of
interviews depends on the ability to understand how personality
interacts with illness to produce stress responses. Such work begins

with the consultant's understanding why psychiatric consultation is requested.

## WHY CONSULTATION IS REQUESTED

Cassem and Hackett[1] found that the three most common reasons for consultation requests to see myocardial infarction patients in a Coronary Care Unit (CCU) are patient anxiety (32%), depression (30%), and problem behavior (20%). Other reasons include the patient's hostility, delirium, depression, psychosis, delayed recovery, predilection to death, family problems, or sleep disturbance.[2,3] Also, the physician may seek medication advice. Behavior problems seem to stem from excessive denial of illness, euphoria, inappropriate sexual behavior, or hostile-dependent conflicts with the staff. Interventions by the consultant include medication, explanation and reassurance, changes in the patient's immediate environment, confrontation of disruptive behavior, and hypnosis.

Based on these and several other studies,[4-8] there are three broad categories of indications for psychotherapy in the general hospital:

1. Problems with *cognition*—delirium, psychosis, excessive denial, and other states in which the patient is not processing information the way caregivers think the patient should
2. Problems with *affect*—anxiety, depression, apathy, hostility, euphoria
3. Problems with *behavior*—dependency, expression of hostility, noncompliance, manipulativeness, withdrawal, flight

Clearly, these categories overlap; they are all found in responses to stress. In the following sections we will attempt to discuss stress responses under the category that is most relevant to the consultation.

### Therapy for disturbances of cognition

By "cognition" we mean the complicated mechanisms by which human beings process information: they attend (focus information-gathering apparatuses), they perceive (take in information), they register (encode new information), they recall (retrieve previously stored information that is relevant), they understand (integrate new information with previously stored and processed information), and they plan responses (anticipate consequences of the product of new with old information). Disorders of consciousness impair attention and perception; disorders of memory impair registry and recall; disorders of intellect impair understanding and planning. Medical and surgical illnesses typically engender more than one of these deficits. Delirium, for instance, especially affects the ability to attend and register; dementia affects the recall and integration of previously stored information. *Therapy for a disturbance of cognition consists mainly of recognizing the nature of the impairment and, as much as possible, helping the patient compensate for it.*

> The consultant was called to see an 80-year-old widow who had been hospitalized for treatment of viral pneumonia. Consultation was sought because the patient frequently awoke confused, dressed, packed, and tried to leave. When she was prevented from leaving, she invariably wept piteously. The consultee thought she might be depressed.
>
> When examined, the patient was fully oriented and seemed not to recall her nocturnal adventures. Her memory of recent events was impaired, but she was a storehouse of information about World War I when she was a nurse in France. She was optimistic about her improvement. She was dismayed by the quality of hospital food, especially since her appetite was returning. She especially missed the photographs of her husband and her children. These mementos had been left behind in confusion the day she was rushed by ambulance to the hospital.
>
> The consultant recommended that she be given 1 mg of haloperidol at bedtime as a sedative. Also, it was recommended that her mementos be brought from home, prominently displayed by her bedside, and brightly lit throughout the night.

Simple orienting objects such as clocks, calendars, and familiar possessions frequently suffice to correct cognitive disturbances such as those associated with senile dementia and "sundowning" in the aged. More severe disturbances, such as those accompanying toxic or metabolic encephalopathies, require environmental adjustment of a more restrictive sort (such as restraints) along with correction of the underlying cause of the organic dysfunction.

Another sort of disordered cognition arises when the patient is ignorant of certain aspects of the illness or medical procedure, or when there is misperception or miscommunication between physician and patient.

> A beefy, middle-aged longshoreman was convalescing unremarkably following a myocardial infarction until suddenly one afternoon he threw a glass across his room and roared out his intention to leave the hospital immediately. He refused to speak with his physician or with the psychiatric consultant who had been called soon after the incident started. When they pleaded with the patient to say what had upset him, he muttered that he knew "what fibrillation means," but would say no more. With the intern and the consultant half-blocking

the door to the patient's room, the consultant asked the physician to describe the clinical course of the patient during hospitalization. The patient had electrocardiographic and enzyme evidence of a recent myocardial infarction and tracings indicating a previous MI. He had also had episodes of atrial fibrillation that had responded to digitalization.

With the words "fibrillation that had responded" the patient sat heavily down and began to sob—as he later explained—with relief.

Late that afternoon when the patient was again settled in bed, he explained to the consultant the series of events that had led to his outburst. The previous day he had been told that he had had an earlier MI that left a scar on his heart. This scar he visualized as an ominously fragile, thin lesion in his heart wall similar to the "scars of tuberculosis that killed my dad." He had worried about the scar through the night and then on the morning of the incident heard the team talking at the foot of his bed about "fibrillation." Fibrillation, he said, filled him with dread because it " . . . is what the patient on the hospital shows on television always gets just before he dies."

The patient was an intelligent and keenly interested man who derived much satisfaction from following his own course and much comfort from learning some details of cardiology—such as the difference between atrial and ventricular fibrillation. He did well until his MI extended and he died suddenly the day before he was to go home.

In this example the patient required additional information in order to avoid flight. In the following, the patient appeared to flee from more information than he could tolerate.

A successful young businessman and father of three small children was hospitalized for treatment of fulminant acute myelogenous leukemia that had failed to respond to a succession of chemotherapeutic agents. He was dying and arrangements were being made to place him in a terminal care facility. Consultation was sought at the urgent request of his wife because the patient stoutly denied he was more than mildly ill. The wife knew the patient was dying. She explained to the consultant that although she hoped no one would think her mercenary, she was frantic because the patient had no life insurance. Also, he was a member in a limited partnership of a small electronics firm, and she believed the contract specified that if a partner died intestate, all interest reverted to the firm. The consultant understood her desire to provide for herself and the children, and suggested that she find an estate attorney while the consultant spoke with the patient.

The consultant found the patient to be an emaciated man who was slightly euphoric. Although he identified his illness as leukemia, he said firmly, "It's not going to kill me. I can assure you of that." The patient's history included extreme childhood poverty, an absent father, and a depressed, hypochondriacal mother who "was constantly dying."

The consultant briefly explained that leukemia is usually considered to be fatal, but that progress has been made in its treatment. The consultant also stated a belief that persons who were able to put the illness out of their mind or to fight it, as this patient was doing, were those who survived longest. After a period of silence, the consultant told the patient of his wife's concerns and asked why the patient had deferred making a will. The patient replied that his "one superstition" was that to make a will was to "invite trouble."

The consultant gently confronted this notion reminding the patient how hard he was "fighting it" and how that helped the prognosis. With these going for him, he had no need for such superstitions—especially when his wife was so distraught. For his wife's peace of mind, would the patient please make a will? The patient agreed to do so.

In this example, the patient's stalwart refusal to process information about his dying was responsible for maladaptive behavior. The consultant saw no harm in the patient's denial except that it prevented him from providing for his family. A direct assault on the denial of impending death would not have changed cognition but, rather, would only have alienated the patient and rigidified the behavior. The consultant supported the denial, strengthened it, and then confronted the behavior and unhooked it from the denial.

### Therapy for disturbances of affect

Affects—even negative affects such as anxiety, depression, anger—are not inimical to health and adaptation in the human organism. Perhaps they even facilitate growth by motivating change in cognition and behavior. Affects become a problem on the medical or surgical ward when they are (1) inappropriate, (2) too intense, or (3) autonomous—beyond the power of the individual or the environment to change them. They also tend to become a problem when they are based on inaccurate cognition or when they give rise to maladaptive behavior. *Therapy for disturbance of affect in a stressed patient consists mainly of recognizing the causes of disturbance and restoring appropriate affect and control over its intensity and expression.*

Anxiety, depression, and hostility that stem from a psychotic or depressive disorder presumably with a biochemical substrate seem to be autonomous, having "a life of their own" and existing apart from any ability of the individual or of the environment to change them. Psychological or environmental factors may obscure the evidence of biological illness.

A 50-year-old, single, female, classical languages professor whose mother had died a month before was brought to the hospital in a diabetic coma. After the correction of her metabolic imbalance, she refused further treatment saying, "Let me die. It's my right to die and I choose to do so." She also refused to be examined by a psychiatrist until the consultant haltingly interviewed her in Latin. Haughty and contemptuous of the consultant's grammar, she nonetheless consented to be interviewed in Latin and eventually agreed to use English.

The consultant found that the patient had suffered from early morning awakening and severe weight loss during the past year, starting some months before her mother became ill. Her mother had had two postpartum depressions and her father had died of alcoholic cirrhosis. The patient also displayed a paranoid delusion in which her academic rivals gave her diabetes by wireless devices in order to sabotage her work. She also had a plan to commit suicide at home.

Working with the hospital lawyer, the consultant obtained a court order that mandated treatment of both her depression and her diabetes. After eight unilateral electroconvulsive treatments her psychotic depression responded and she was given follow-up care by an internist and a psychiatrist after her discharge home.

In addition to being aware of the possibility of a functional psychosis, the consultant should be aware of the possibility that the illness or the medical regimen itself could be the cause of inappropriate, too intense, or autonomous affects.

Another middle-aged woman was hospitalized for regulation of her diabetic regimen. Because she was anxious and sleepless and had had an idiosyncratic reaction to sedative-hypnotics, she was given haloperidol in small doses as a sedative. After a few days in the hospital she became panicky, impulsive, uncooperative, and hostile. Her condition only worsened with an increased dose of her tranquilizing medication.

The psychiatric consultant believed that the patient had akathisia. Indeed, she improved within half an hour after being given intramuscular benztropine mesylate.

While disturbances of affect are occasionally caused by undiagnosed schizophrenia, manic-depressive illness, medication side effects, or metabolic disturbances related to the medical illness, more often, disturbances of affect encountered by the consultant are psychological or psychosocial reactions to the illness or surgery and require a psychodynamic formulation and psychotherapeutic intervention.

A 60-year-old truck farmer was hospitalized for radiation therapy for cancer of the larynx that was too extensive for surgery. The patient also had severe psoriasis, the history of which began in his childhood. Psychiatric consultation was sought because of the patient's severe depression, because of his extreme anxiety— extending as it did even to the most innocent and routine medical procedures, to which he attached the most dire significance—and because of a hostile dependent attitude. The patient had been given large doses of a tricyclic antidepressant for several weeks but this seemed to help little. The patient was very eager to consult the psychiatrist. He seemed anxious to go into great detail about his life-long struggle with psoriasis. When he spoke of his skin, his voice rose and he assumed a declamatory, vibrant posture. He was the youngest of seven children of a hard-working widowed seamstress.

He gave particular emphasis to an incident that had occurred when he was 6 years old. He was returning home from Sunday school with his entire family who boarded the trolley car. Because of crowds the patient had been sent to sit away from his mother at the other end of the car. He felt humiliated, he recalled, and sat feeling defective and ugly because his skin was "all broken out" that day. As he sat his rage grew until suddenly he jumped up and ran to his mother. "You treat me like a leper!" he accused her, pleased with the stares of the other passengers. "You treat me like a leper!" After a momentary pause, his mother picked him up, hugged him, and held him in her lap all the way home. Ever since then he had believed that he was his mother's favorite and, in fact, he had been her sole heir. With the inheritance money he bought his farm. "From that day on," he said, "I been a loudmouth and that's what I'll always be."

The consultant now understood that the patient valued most his ability to speak out and was depressed by the possibility that his most valued possession—his voice—would be taken away. The consultant recommended to the staff that they compliment the patient's loudness and forcefulness. Over a period of time the consultant reassured the patient that no one would take his voice away. He died several months later, after a discharge and subsequent readmission, shouting to the end.

For many patients, it is easier to be angry than to be sad. Sometimes culture, sometimes notions of gender-appropriate behavior, and sometimes simply aloneness prohibit the patient from being sad about losses and give rise to depression accompanied by hostility or uncooperativeness. "Nobody to cry with," one patient said.

A roisterous, elderly ex-convict delighted in shattering the surgical ward with the most vile, obscene, vituperative cussing that any staff member could ever recall. Patently psychopathic, he had "gotten by" until a dissecting aneurysm of the aorta had necessitated a Teflon graft. His postoperative course was punctuated by life-threatening crises. Hypotension, cardiac arrhythmias, septic emboli, a succession of febrile episodes, anemia, renal failure, stress ulcers, and more, all seemed destined, as he put it, "to do me in." Finally, the disruption of the ward became so intense one day when the patient had (1) stolen another patient's wallet, (2) kicked in a television set, and (3) grabbed three nurses that a psychiatric consultation was sought to find appropriate medication for the patient.

The consultant, tired at the end of a long day, sat down with the patient. A chain-smoker, the consultant managed somehow to get smoke in the eyes and tears began to stream out. "I know how you feel, Doc," the patient exclaimed. "It's not dying I mind—it's this rot, rot, rot all day long—and nobody to cry with that I mind." After that, the consultant made it a point to go at the end of a day to have a cigarette with the patient so they could be sad together. The patient's behavior improved—not a lot—but a little.

Losses stir up feelings of hopelessness and depression that—until there is time and opportunity for the patient to understand the possibility for repair—seem beyond the reach of any human help.

A young Vietnam combat veteran had lost a leg because of a shrapnel injury. In the hospital for revision of his below-the-knee amputation, he became increasingly despondent. The psychiatric consultant was called to evaluate his deteriorating psychological status. It was a bad war, a foolish war, the patient ruminated, a war that shouldn't have been fought. What possible sense did it make, and for what possible reason had the leg been lost? The consultant conceded the futility of the war and after a period of silence asked the patient what came to mind. "My son, my 3-year-old," the patient replied. "He's big into guns now. Bang! bang! bang! All the time. At times," he confided, "I hate him . . . hate his stupid playing." "Perhaps he only wants to be brave like you," the consultant offered. The veteran grimaced and said nothing. "Perhaps he sees you as a hero and wants to be a hero too."

The patient seemed to reject his idea but said he'd like to have the consultant come again. Through the many hours they sat together, the idea of the war came up again and again, often associated in the veteran's mind with his son. Eventually the consultant began to see that the son represented to the father a part of himself, albeit a stupid, immature, aggressive part. "You love that kid, I can tell. But he reminds you of yourself, going blindly off to the war—and you hate it, you just hate it. Maybe that's what you can use your lost leg for—to understand him and teach him about that part of all of us that has such a romantic fascination for violence." The veteran said nothing, but the staff later reported that the patient seemed gradually to have lost some of his despair and seemed to have some new motivation, some purpose.

While depression, sadness, and apathy are affective states, which the consultant has time and some leverage to deal with, there are emotions such as panic that require an emergency response not based on a leisurely examination and a stately approach to treatment.

A 36-year-old single man was hospitalized for revision of a colostomy for ulcerative colitis. Consultation was sought because the patient became anxious, hostile, paranoid, and completely noncompliant with staff during the evening shift.

The consultant found that the patient, a night watchman, was a self-described "loner" with no family or friends. He lived a simple, isolated existence most of his life in fantasy punctuated by occasional visits to pornographic films. The consultant believed that the patient had a stable schizoid or paranoid character structure that was threatened by the forced intimacies of the hospital situation. The consultant gingerly asked him why he became upset in the evening. "It's that faggot nurse Eddie!" the patient exclaimed and proceeded to aim a deluge of paranoid vituperation at the male licensed practical nurse on the ward, growing increasingly hostile by the second and developing loose associations.

The consultant was fearful and immediately told the patient that the hospital was aware of the "situation" with Eddie and that the consultant would "take steps" to ensure that the patient would be safe from Eddie. "Masculine men like yourself are often put off by people like Eddie, but I think you'll relax about it if you stop a second to realize that you're strong enough to protect yourself from anybody, including Eddie, and, besides, you don't go to sleep until 11:00 P.M. anyway, and by that time, Eddie's long gone." Immediately the patient calmed down. He showed no further panic during his hospitalization after the consultant recommended that only female nurses be assigned to work with the patient.

In each of the preceding examples, the consultant moved to restore appropriateness of affect and to give the patient control of its intensity and expression. Such interventions are based on an assessment of whether the affect is autonomous, that is, governed by metabolic or biochemical substrates, or whether it is amenable to psychodynamic formulation and explanation. When explanation is possible, its form depends on the personality and capacity of the patient to understand.

### Therapy for disturbances of behavior

Disturbances of behavior arise from some sort of disordered information-processing—cognition—or from some inappropriate, uncontrollable, or autonomous affect. *Therapy with a stressed patient having a disturbance of behavior consists mainly of understanding the behavior as it relates to the affects associated with it and cognition—the patient's picture of the self with an illness.* As shown by the examples already given, disruptive behavior results from affects of anger or depression based on cognitions that embody hopelessness or frustration of goals for successful adaptation. Noncompliance and therapeutic negativism are variations of these behaviors. Withdrawal and flight are maladaptive responses to the hospital environment mediated by incorrect cognitions and governed by fearful affects. Behaviors of hopelessness and their accompanying affects are related to incomplete perceptions of options for better adaptation.

Inappropriate sexual behavior by the medical or surgical patient usually represents an attempt to repair some real or imagined loss of masculine or feminine appeal rather than truly erotic aims. When the behavior is viewed in its proper perspective and "unlinked" by the consultant from guilt-inducing cognitions in the staff,[9] patients who display inappropriate sexual behavior respond dramatically to limits on inappropriate behavior coupled with reassurance that they are still attractive men or women.

> A middle-aged married male shop owner was hospitalized for treatment of a myocardial infarction. During his convalescence consultation was sought because the patient constantly fondled or pinched the female nurses who were caring for him. When examined the patient appeared quite anxious and concerned about his cardiac condition and asked many questions about how much it would impair his ability to "exercise." The consultant responded to these concerns and gradually brought up the subject of sexual functioning as an example of exercise. The patient was told how soon he could return to full sexual activity. "A lot of people are afraid that when they have a heart attack their sex life is over, but that's simply not true." After this interview the patient's anxiety was considerably lower and his inappropriate sexual overtures to the nurses ceased.

Such behavior is a good example of how disordered cognition ("I am sexually defective because of my heart attack") leads to intense and ungovernable affects (here, anxiety and despair), which, in turn, lead to a maladaptive attempt to repair the damage through undoing and acting-out.

Far more difficult are those consultations involving pathological dependency and its manifestations. Pathological dependency in the hospitalized medical or surgical patient presents as (1) intense, implacable, clinging behavior and constant requests for reassurance and attention, (2) constant requests for anxiolytic or pain medication, (3) manipulative and contradictory demands for emotional supplies, and (4) chaotic, destructive, hostile-dependent or passive-aggressive behavior that makes the staff furious or frustrated and that makes every encounter with the patient a ghastly chore. While mild or moderate forms of clinging and demanding behavior are often seen in emotionally healthy individuals who have regressed to an infantile dependence under the multiple stresses of hospitalization and illness, pathological dependency in its full-blown form typically occurs in persons with long-standing character pathology. Such persons usually feel empty and worthless even without a physical illness and have an intense desire for closeness but a simultaneous fear of intimacy. This pervasive fear of what they most long for leads them to thrash about emotionally, simultaneously demanding and rejecting help and then destroying whatever help is given. A conviction of interior emptiness and worthlessness, along with hurricanes of affect—rage, despair, terror, hate—are important in the genesis of pathologically dependent behaviors. Also important is the fact that while self-defeating and contradictory demands are obvious to the caregivers, such patients typically lack the ability to step aside and observe the nature and consequences of their own behavior. For this reason and because such individuals do not make good alliances with caregivers, interpretation of the self-defeating nature of the character pathology does not work; interpretations such as, "You are so hungry for care that you drive others away, fearful of your devouring needs," are either heard as sadistic or not heard at all. Such techniques simply do not succeed in the short-term treatment of such patients. They feel entitled to all they demand; but this feeling of entitlement is a fragile, primitive thing at best. Any interpretation that challenges the entitlement makes such a patient prey to intense despair and rage.

Psychotherapy with patients displaying pathologically dependent behaviors on the medical or surgical ward requires (1) clear communication among the staff and with the patient, (2) not challenging entitlement and needed defenses, (3) constant personnel and support but without too close a stance that threatens the patient's need for privacy and distance, (4) liberal use of major tranquilizers when indicated to help calm the hurricanes of affect, and (5) most importantly, firm, consistent, repeated limit-setting on demanding and self-destructive behaviors. This limit-setting reassures such patients that they cannot destroy the caregiving system, however much they may wish or fear it.

The behavior of such patients under stress stirs up sadistic feelings in caregivers, who, in turn, may flinch from necessary firm limits because such drastic control may somehow seem sadistic.

> An 18-year-old man, self-described as a "speed freak," terrorized the orthopedic floor where he was in traction following multiple long bone fractures received in a motorcycle accident. He demanded excessive doses of narcotics, ripped out intravenous lines, threatened extortion and litigation if he were not given his way, threw food, shouted, and was menacing toward the staff. The consultant recommended a treatment plan based on clear communication; constant

personnel; firm, consistent, noninterpretive limits; and 25 to 50 mg of chlorpromazine given intramuscularly or orally every 2 to 8 hours as needed. With the consultant present, the orthopedist informed the patient that his narcotics would be tapered very gradually but that any threatening or acting-out behavior would immediately result in the patient being restrained even more than he already was. Ten minutes later, the patient broke a drinking glass and inflicted superficial lacerations on his wrist. He was placed in four-point restraints and given chlorpromazine until heavily sedated.

Throughout his course, this regimen was followed. Any acting-out behavior immediately resulted in restraint and sedation. While this regimen did little to control verbal assaults and demanding behavior, it drastically reduced his physical destructiveness.

This is a behavioral response to stress occurring in a man with an obviously abnormal personality.

### STRESS RESPONSES, PERSONALITY, AND DEFENSES

With an understanding of cognition, affects, and behavior the consultant can proceed to the "four major features of the psychiatric consultation:

1. Rapid evaluation of the most pressing psychiatric problems
2. Explicit psychodynamic formulation of predominant conflicts
3. Proposal of a practical program of management
4. Active participation by the psychiatrist"[2]

But psychodynamic formulation presupposes an understanding of the personality and defenses as they relate to stress:

A 37-year-old married mother of two school-aged children was also a successful attorney. She had coped well with the multiple demands of home and career until she underwent a radical mastectomy for carcinoma of the breast. After the surgery she seemed to do well for a time but then developed anxiety, severe depression, insomnia, weeping spells, and angry outbursts that responded only partly to sedatives. Her surgeon had carefully explained the procedure and had discussed with her its impact on her self-image and sexual functioning, but she felt little better and eventually requested a psychiatric consultation.

"It's like a traffic accident!" the patient exclaimed. "I can't stand to look—but I can't look away either." On initial examination, the consultant found nothing that the surgeon had not already noted and it was not until the following day that an explanation became apparent. The patient reported a dream. "I am in court and trying the case of someone accused of larceny. My client is clearly guilty and the judge is overruling me time after time. It's an all-male jury and they go out to deliberate before I can even make my summation." Asked for her associations to the dream she promptly told the consultant that she felt that she had not really deserved to go to law school, even though she had graduated near the top of her class. She felt, she said, that her classmates had secretly suspected her of being a lesbian because she had been so orderly and logical. She became silent. After a long pause the consultant suggested that perhaps it was really she who was on trial for larceny. Perhaps her crime had been to succeed in a man's world and perhaps the punishment was to be made into a man.

"It's true, you know," she replied, "I guess I always expected that eventually I'd have to pay for becoming a lawyer. Did I tell you? My father is a lawyer."

The next day the patient told the consultant that she had had her first night of sound sleep in the hospital. She felt "at peace for some reason" and a few days later went home to convalesce uneventfully from both her surgery and her stress reaction.

There have been numerous descriptions of the personality and its cognitive, affective, and behavioral phases of response to a crisis. Cannon,[10] Lindemann,[11] Anna Freud,[12] Menninger,[13] and Caplan,[14] among others, have worked on various aspects of what Horowitz synthesizes as typical phases of response to a stressful event[15] (see Fig. 15-1). When confronted with a catastrophic event, the individual typically responds with outcry ("Oh God! Oh God! Oh God!"), denial ("It isn't true! You're joking! It's not true!"), or affective numbing and repetitive thoughts about the event. Not uncommonly the individual, like the patient with the mastectomy, will vacillate among these first three phases. As noted by Caplan[14] and Lindemann,[11] these initial reactions to catastrophe are reflexive and probably serve some adaptive function. Outcry is accompanied by an autonomic discharge like the flight-fight response described by Cannon,[10] and denial has a resemblance to dissociative mechanisms of ego defense.[12] Caplan traces the sequence of responses from the dazed impact or flight-fight response to affective flooding that, in turn, is followed by coping efforts.

The unwanted intrusion of thoughts and feelings about the stress event and the inability either to look or to look away probably represent an unstable equilibrium between the need to come to cognitive and affective completion in service of adaptation and the need to defend against affects that are painful. The need to process information about a crisis seems to be innate, and phenomena noted by Zeigarnik,[16] Festinger,[17] and Piaget[18] show that the human being remembers uncompleted tasks, experiences discomfort from doubt and dissonance, and generally moves in the direction of cognitive com-

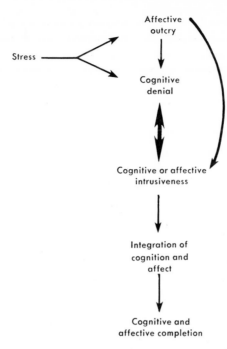

**Fig. 15-1.** Phases of response after a stressful event. (Adapted from Horowitz, M. J.: Stress response syndromes, New York, 1976, Jason Aronson, Inc. p. 56.)

pletion when possible in order to adapt to the environment. But the need to defend against painful feelings associated with a crisis is also adaptive. The consultant ought not to come to the consultation with a bias toward affective outpouring and a bias against cognitive denial. Hackett, Cassem, and Weisman[19-21] found that patients facing terminal illness who are able to defend well (major deniers) not only lower their anxiety and raise their hopes, but also survive significantly longer. The consultant should not confuse neurotic denial in nonemergency situations with "denial in service of the need to survive,"[22] nor apply concepts about long-term growth in the ability to master painful affects[23] to denial in the acute stress response.

The phase of cognitive and affective integration is best examined by referring to the model of the ego described by Hartmann[24] as that central, creative part of the personality that synthesizes, rationalizes, and makes do with whatever tools it has in order to bring to the individual the greatest possible peace and function during deviations from the "average expectable environment" that trauma violates. Integration is accomplished when the individual optimally balances mechanisms of defense[12] with the capacity for the tolerance of negative affects[23] and emerges with flexible yet realistic plans for dealing with trauma in the present and anticipating problems that may emerge in the future.[15]

Integration depends at least partially on the stressed individual's ability to shoulder what Lindemann aptly terms grief work.[11] Grief work is the process of experiencing the painful affects associated with mourning in order to gain emancipation from bondage to the lost object. For Lindemann, the major obstacle to doing grief work is the individual's unwillingness to suffer the pain of mourning. He noted that the psychotherapist's task in such work is evocative (vivifying the trauma), hortatory (encouraging grief), and supportive (being with the grieving individual).

While Lindemann focused on the affective response to trauma, Horowitz[15] explored the cognitive aspects of integration. A series of theoretically ideal steps emerge that can be applied, for example, to the cancer patient who had a mastectomy:

First, she should perceive the event correctly ("A total mastectomy has taken my breast, leaving me mutilated.")

Next, she should translate this preception into meaningful ideas about the world. ("By allowing myself to be mutilated, I have probably been cured of cancer.")

Next, she should relate these meanings to her attitudes about the world and her place in it. ("It is better to be mutilated than to die.")

Next, she should plan responses to the event appropriate to this idea of her place in the world. ("With a prosthesis and new wardrobe I will hide my mutilation. When I can't, as with my husband, I will work out new techniques to minimize the impact of this mutilation on him and me.")

Then, she should revise her habitual attitudes so that her plans are not sabotaged. ("It is not necessarily true of my body and relationships, as I had previously thought, that anything less than perfect is grotesque.")

And, finally, she should not ward off the full implications of the event, lest denial of some important aspect of reality impair her ability to work through the steps of information processing. ("I can't kid myself. This looks awful—awful enough to cause me to give up or to pull away in shame, which I must not do.")

In real life, the patient said that she could neither look nor look away. She needed to look because the trauma contained information essential for coping with reality. She needed to look away because it hurt. She was in the unstable equilibrium represented by the two-headed arrow in Fig. 15-1. Her paralysis was exacerbated by an unconscious, painful assumption or syllogism in addition to the terribly painful fact of the loss of her breast. The unconscious meaning of the loss was that it represented a punishment for something "bad" she had done—that is, she succeeded by "unfeminine" means. Her dream illustrated the unconscious idea that the "punishment" fits the "crime." Her associations to the dream revealed the basis of her guilt, an ambivalent identification with her father. By using the consultant's interpretation, she was able to unlink the loss of her breast from her neurotic syllogism and habitual information-processing about herself and subtract the unconscious painful affect of guilt from the total suffering she was experiencing. Thus, she could move the equilibrium forward into affective and cognitive integration.

It is when the patient is in this unstable equilibrium between intrusiveness and denial that the consultant is often called. Sometimes there is an unconscious conflict underlying the maladaptive paralysis; sometimes there is not. But in each consultation the psychiatrist must understand the patient's habitual ways of processing information and defending against negative affects.

Shapiro's[25] descriptions of neurotic styles of personality and Bibring and Kahana's[26] discussion of personalities encountered in the general hospital provide details of the leading traits and defenses of various personality types, their typical reactions to the stress of illness, and strategies of therapy for each. These styles are summarized in Table 15-1.

The patient who had the mastectomy had a mixture of styles:

> I guess the main thing my father taught me is to do one thing at a time, to make lists of priorities . . . hierarchies, you know. And then to work through them in a logical way—playing advocate to first one and then another idea before coming up with a judgement or decision. On the other hand . . . on the other hand I guess I also owe a lot to my mother because I inherited her "woman's intuition" as it's stupidly called. Sometimes I just *know* things. Sometimes I just get the big picture and make a snap decision and it's right! Call it a hunch or whatever, but I still do it and it pays off.

She processes information in at least two ways—one, orderly and sequential—the other, intuitive, holistic, gestalt-oriented.

**Table 15-1.** Personality types in the general hospital*

| "Name"/leading traits | Reaction to illness | Suggested management |
|---|---|---|
| *"Hysterical"* dramatic, vivid, likable, anxious, involved | As if illness were a punishment for or an attack on masculinity or femininity | Appreciation of attractiveness/courage; ventilation of fears; supportive but not detailed explanations |
| *"Obsessive"* orderly, dull, likable, anxious, involved | As if illness were a punishment for letting things get out of control | Detailed "scientific" explanations, intellectualizations, and making the patient a partner in therapeutic decisions |
| *"Narcissistic"* self-involved, strong, angry, independent, perfectionistic | As if illness were an attack on autonomy and perfection of the self; the leading fear (and wish) is of being taken care of | Supporting strength and integrity of the self by making patient equal, independent partner in own care |
| *"Oral"* clinging, demanding, attention-seeking | As if illness posed the threat of abandonment | Warm support but firm limits on undue neediness and manipulativeness |
| *"Masochistic"* long-suffering, depressed, help-rejecting | As if illness were a deserved, expected punishment for worthlessness | Appreciation of courage in suffering without undue reassurance or optimism; appeal to altruism |
| *"Schizoid"* remote, unsociable, uninvolved | As if illness threatened a dangerous invasion of privacy | Muted interest in patient but respect for need for privacy and distance |
| *"Paranoid"* wary, suspicious, aggrieved, querulous, blaming, hypersensitive | As if illness were an annihilating assault coming from everywhere outside the self | Honest, simple, full, repeated explanations; accusations neither disputed nor confirmed but explained as coming from illness rather than from someone trying to injure patient |

*Based on G. R. Bibring and R. F. Kahana[26], and adapted from an unpublished summary by T. F. Dwyer.

Horowitz[15] chooses three personality styles, their information-processing and problem-solving habits and their defenses to illustrate the interplay between stress and personality. The hysterical personality has as a perceptual mode a global, holistic intake of information without much attention to detail. Information-processing is impressionistic and affect-oriented rather than sequential, with a limited translation of images into words. Such a style is vulnerable to stereotyping and conclusion-jumping, and therefore problem-solving is rapid but prone to error and sometimes marred by avoidance or wishful thinking. The obsessive personality has as a typical perceptual mode a preoccupation with detail at the expense of gestalten. Information-processing is orderly but often neglects the importance of affects and fails to make meaningful connections between ideas and their emotional impact. Problem-solving may be active but it is slowed by prolonged reasoning back and forth, so that affective and cognitive integration is tediously late in coming. The narcissistic personality (resembling also depressive-masochistic, paranoid, and borderline personalities, some of which are included in Table 15-1) has as a perceptual mode a search from the environment for data that protect the self or blame others, as if the self were desperately fragile. Information-processing may be either too impressionistic or too detailed, but its aim is to hide damaging implications from the individual. Thus problem-solving behavior is poor and sometimes self-destructive since it is based on too few accurate cues from the environment and the emotions.

Therapy with the hysterical patient involves controlling affects and slowing down information-processing to include sequence and logic. Therapy with the obsessive personality involves eliciting overall views and blending in affects as tolerated. Therapy with the narcissistic patient involves shoring up primitive defenses, controlling affects, and lending reality-testing and logic—all within a firm, noninterpretive supportive relationship. The patient who had the mastectomy used very little narcissistic information-processing and her mixture of hysterical and obsessive styles actually helped each other once the neurotic assumption was interpreted away. Therapy with any patient involves helping the patient combine as many cognitive facts as are needed for adaptation with as much of their associated affects as the patient can stand—all without assaulting needed defenses.

To clarify the psychoanalytic concepts of ego defense mechanisms, Vaillant[27,28] proposes a theoretical hierarchy of defenses and ways of coping. Some defenses are associated with psychological health; some are less effective for adaptation than others. But *all* of them help the individual cope with painful affects. Table 15-2 presents this hierarchy.

Vaillant believes that narcissistic defenses are less effective and more costly than immature defenses, which are less adaptive, in turn, than neurotic defenses, and so on. In this schema defenses are not drawn up in a single line against a threat but rather form concentric

**Table 15-2.** Theoretical hierarchy of adaptive ego defenses*

---

**"Narcissistic"** defenses are common in "healthy" individuals before age 5 and in adult dreams and fantasy; such mechanisms alter reality for the user but to the beholder they appear "crazy"; they tend to be refractory to change by conventional psychotherapeutic interpretation but are altered by change in reality (for example, antipsychotic medication, removal of stressor); in therapy they can be given up temporarily by interpersonal support combined with direct confrontation with ignored reality.

1. *Delusional projection*—paranoid attribution of internal feelings as coming from outside "reality"
2. *Psychotic denial*—unshakably ignoring some aspect of external reality
3. *Distortion*—gross reshaping of external reality to suit inner needs

**"Immature"** defenses are common in "healthy" individuals between ages 3 and 16, in "character" and affective disorders, and in individuals in psychotherapy; such mechanisms mitigate the "dangers" of interpersonal intimacy for the user but to the beholder they appear socially undesirable and self-defeating; they may be altered by prolonged relationships with intuitive, mature individuals.

1. *Projection*—attribution of one's own undesirable, unaccepted, unacknowledged feelings to others
2. *Schizoid fantasy*—retreat into autistic daydreams for the purpose of conflict resolution and gratification
3. *Hypochondriasis*—transformation of reproach toward the self or others into somatic symptoms
4. *Passive-aggression*—overt compliance but covertly hostile behavior designed to punish others
5. *Acting-out*—direct behavioral expression of unconscious conflict in order to avoid consciousness of the affect that accompanies the conflict

**"Neurotic"** defenses are common in "healthy" adults with neurotic disorders and in mastering acute adult distress; such mechanisms alter private feelings or instinctual expression (sexual or aggressive) for the user but to the beholder appear as quirks or "hangups"; often they can be dramatically changed by conventional brief psychotherapeutic clarification of unconscious wishes or fears.

1. *Intellectualization*—subtraction of affective implication from reality with simultaneous overattention to detail
2. *Repression*—forgetting some aspect of reality often accompanied by highly symbolic behavior that suggests that the repressed idea is not really forgotten
3. *Displacement*—redirection of conflicted feelings toward a relatively less-cared-for object than the person or situation arousing the feelings (for example, jokes, phobias, hysterical conversion reactions)

---

*Adapted from Vaillant, G. E.: Theoretical hierarchy of adaptive ego mechanisms, Arch. Gen. Psychiatry **24**:107-118, 1971.

**Table 15-2.** Theoretical hierarchy of adaptive ego defenses—cont'd

4. *Reaction formation*—affect or behavior opposite to an unconscious, unwanted sexual or aggressive wish
5. *Dissociation*—temporary but drastic modification of character or of the sense of personal identity to avoid emotional distress (for example, amnesia)

**"Mature"** defenses are common in "healthy" adults during optimal functioning; they are often regarded as so adaptive and conscious as to be not defenses but rather "coping mechanisms"; for the user these mechanisms integrate conscience, reality, interpersonal relationships, and private feelings; to the beholder they appear as convenient virtues; under increasing stress they may change to less mature mechanisms.

1. *Altruism*—vicarious but constructive and gratifying service to others
2. *Humor*—overt expression of feelings without discomfort or immobilization and without unpleasant effects on others; it releases tension and is gratifying both for the user and for the beholder
3. *Suppression*—conscious decision to postpone paying attention to a feeling or fact and, indeed, later attending to and integrating the conflict
4. *Anticipation*—realistic planning for and experiencing future discomfort
5. *Sublimation*—indirect or partial expression of sexual and aggressive needs without either adverse consequences or loss of pleasure

**Regression and progression**—not defenses but, rather, reflected by shifts in levels of defenses.

walls about the vulnerable core person; the closer to the center, the more archaic the wall. Vaillant provides a pivotal clarification by subtracting from this hierarchy of defenses the mechanism of regression, which he chooses to see as reflecting shifts in levels of defenses toward the vulnerable center rather than to see regression as a mechanism of defense per se. This crucial point implies that all defenses at all levels are to be respected. Depending on their capacity, individuals may be able to use only primitive defenses in service of adaptation. Psychologically less healthy individuals such as paranoid and schizoid personalities typically use narcissistic defenses. Masochistic, oral, and narcissistic individuals (see Table 15-1) tend to use immature defenses. Hysterical, obsessive, and mixed personalities use neurotic and mature defenses. Stressors such as illness and surgery are associated with a regressive shift to lower levels of defenses. But environmental manipulation and therapeutic interpersonal intervention can facilitate shifts to higher levels (outer walls) of defenses—progression.

Both clinical and experimental evidence exists to support the concept of a hierarchy of defenses or responses to stress ranging from maladaptive to adaptive. The clinical work of Hackett, Cassem, and Weisman[19-21] concerning the responses of patients faced with life-threatening illness, such as myocardial infarction or cancer, parallels the experimental work of Funkenstein and colleagues[29] in which normal subjects were stressed in a laboratory situation. These experimental subjects appeared to respond in three ways to unexpected situations that required the mastery of stress in task-performance:

1. They did not notice the stress and remained "un-anxious" from start to finish, carrying out tasks smoothly throughout.
2. They mastered the stressful situation with some anxiety or were dysfunctional at first but went on to master the anxiety and successfully carry out tasks.
3. They were anxious from the outset and deteriorated in performance as the experiment progressed.

Those rarer individuals who either did not notice the stress or who noticed it too much represented extremes, whereas those numerous individuals who noticed stress but eventually overcame it represented the mean. Thus, to notice stress and be bothered by it but then eventually to master it seems normal.

Hackett, Cassem, and Weisman[19-21] find a similar set of phenomena in individuals who suffer life-threatening illness: "major deniers" tend not to notice the illness, to brush off its implications, to poo-poo the necessary medical regimen for its care. The average patient tends to be anxious and compliant with a medical regimen, but to go on to adjust to the illness. The "ontological denier" may resemble the major denier in avoiding compliance with the medical regimen, but this type of patient is angry, difficult to deal with, and displays to the observer—if not to the self—evidence of severe and dysfunctional anxiety. Hackett and Weisman[21] note that "bullies, braggarts and bigots are specialists in ontological denial: they attempt to destroy another person's autonomy simply because they feel challenged by his dissenting version of reality."

The consultant is called frequently for major deniers and ontological deniers because they stand out from the average patient who gets along. The major denier coolly refuses to process threatening information; the ontological denier hotly attacks the staff members as if they and not the illness were the threat. But although the noncompliance with a regimen may be similar, prognosis is not. Major deniers who can get to the hospital in time and who can be persuaded to follow enough of their regimen survive longer than normal persons.

Thus, although it is abnormal not to notice the threat of an illness, it does have adaptive value in major deniers; they illustrate the paradox that it can be healthier to be abnormal.

Ontological deniers are another story altogether: they resemble the less adaptive personality types, paranoid and schizoid, described in Table 15-1, and they utilize narcissistic and immature defenses. Unlike major deniers who settle comfortably into cognitive denial (see Fig. 15-1), the ontological deniers vacillate between denial and cognitive or affective intrusion (the two-headed arrow) and never seem able to arrive at a stage of cognitive and affective equilibrium.

The noncompliant night watchman in the homosexual panic and the "speed freak" who had the motorcycle accident provide examples of ontological denial. The man with leukemia who almost died without writing a will is a classic example of a major denier. The woman with the mastectomy falls into the large group of patients who at first experience dysfunctional anxiety but go on to master it—with or without the help of a psychiatrist. Under the stress of an illness and mutilation she had regressed from mature to neurotic defenses. By partially interpreting her sexual-agressive confusion, the consultant helped her move from behavior that seemed to reflect oral and masochistic personality traits to her customary hysterical and ob-sessive traits. This the consultant knew how to do by using the traditional clinical tools, the history and mental status examination, and by formulating her conflict in terms of (1) the stage of stress response—stuck between intrusiveness and denial, (2) personality style—mixed hysterical and obsessive, and (3) defenses—habitually mature or neurotic but now regressed. This patient occupies a central place in our discussion because she represents both a norm and an extreme—the norm, in that she is highly adaptive—the extreme, in that the consultant is rarely called to see such a healthy patient. In comparison to that of the major deniers, her denial is the flexible sort based on the defense of repression. Her affects, unlike those of the ontological denier, are tolerated over time, are governable, and eventually submit to cognition.

## CONCLUSION

The psychiatric consultant summoned to evaluate medical or surgical patients in the general hospital should be prepared to encounter a stress response in some phase of its evolution, manifesting problems in information-processing (cognition), feelings (affects), or behavior (the product of cognition and affect). The consultant should be prepared to encounter patients with distinctive personality styles, encompassing the capacity—or lack of it—to tolerate and master affects by utilizing a hierarchy of defenses. These patients will in all likelihood be in some state of regression from their customary levels of defenses. But whatever the state of the patients' defenses, the consultant's most intelligent and most appropriate strategy is to recognize that such defenses as they are *now* are the best available for the moment and not to be assaulted. Rather, they are to be strengthened and worked with in order to return the patients to their previous level of functioning. Meanwhile, the patients' cognitions of self and illness are assessed in order to help patients integrate, so far as personality and defenses permit, both painful affects and facts necessary for optimal adaptation.

## REFERENCES

1. Cassem, N. H., and Hackett, T. P.: Psychiatric consultations in a coronary care unit, Ann. Intern. Med. **75:**9-14, 1971.
2. Hackett, T. P., and Weisman,. A. D.: Psychiatric management of operative syndromes. I. The therapeutic consultation and the effect of noninterpretive intervention, Psychosom. Med. **22:**267-282, 1960.
3. Hackett, T. P., and Weisman, A. D.: Psychiatric management of operative syndromes. II. Psychodynamic factors in formulation and management, Psychosom. Med. **22:**356-372, 1960.
4. Meyer, E., and Mendelson, M.: Psychiatric consultations with patients on medical and surgical wards: patterns and processes, Psychiatry **24:**197-220, 1961.
5. Lipowski, Z. J.: Review of consultation psychiatry and psychosomatic medicine. I. General principles, Psychosom. Med. **29:**153-171, 1967.
6. Lipowski, Z. J.: Review of consultation psychiatry and psychosomatic medicine. II. Clinical aspects, Psychosom. Med. **29:**201-224, 1967.
7. Lipowski, Z. J.: Review of consultation psychiatry and psychosomatic medicine. III. Theoretical issues, Psychosom. Med. **30:**395-422, 1968.
8. Lipowski, Z. J.: Consultation-liaison psychiatry: an overview, Am. J. Psychiatry **131:**623-630, 1974.
9. Kucharski, A., and Groves, J. E.: The so-called "inappropriate" psychiatric consultation request on a medical or surgical ward, Int. J. Psychiatry Med. **7:**209-220, 1976-1977.
10. Cannon, W. B.: The wisdom of the body, New York, 1932, W. W. Norton & Co., Inc.
11. Lindemann, E.: Symptomatology and management of acute grief, Am. J. Psychiatry **101:**141-149, 1944.
12. Freud, A.: The ego and the mechanisms of defense, New York, 1946, International Universities Press.
13. Menninger, K. A.: The vital balance, New York, 1963, The Viking Press, Inc.

14. Caplan, G.: Principles of preventive psychiatry, New York, 1964, Basic Books, Inc.
15. Horowitz, M. J.: Stress response syndromes, New York, 1976, Jason Aronson, Inc.
16. Zeigarnik, B. W.: Über das Behalten von erledigter und unerledigter Handlungen, Psychol. Forsch. **9:**1-85, 1927.
17. Festinger, L.: A theory of cognitive dissonance, New York, 1957, Row, Peterson.
18. Piaget, J.: The construction of reality in the child, New York, 1954, Basic Books, Inc.
19. Hackett, T. P., and Weisman, A. D.: Denial as a factor in patients with heart disease and cancer, Ann. N. Y. Acad. Sci. **164:**802-817, 1969.
20. Hackett, T. P., and Cassem, N. H.: Psychological reactions to life-threatening illness. In Abram, H., editor: Psychological aspects of stress, Springfield, Ill. 1970, Charles C Thomas. Publisher.
21. Weisman, A. D., and Hackett, T. P.: Denial as a social act. In Levin, S., and Kahana, R., editors: Creativity, reminiscing and dying, New York, 1966, International Universities Press.
22. Geleerd, E. R.: Two kinds of denial: neurotic denial and denial in service of the need to survive. In Schur, M., editor: Drives, affects, behavior, vol. 2, New York, 1965, International Universities Press.
23. Zetzel, E. R.: The capacity for emotional growth, New York, 1970, International Universities Press.
24. Hartmann, H.: Ego psychology and the problem of adaptation, New York, 1958, International Universities Press.
25. Shapiro, D.: Neurotic styles, New York, 1965, Basic Books, Inc.
26. Bibring, G. L., and Kahana, R. J.: Lectures in medical psychology: an introduction to the care of patients, New York, 1968, International Universities Press.
27. Vaillant, G. E.: Theoretical hierarchy of adaptive ego mechanisms, Arch. Gen. Psychiatry **24:**107-118. 1971.
28. Vaillant, G. E.: Natural history of male psychological health, Arch. Gen. Psychiatry **33:**535-545, 1976.
29. Funkenstein, D. H., King, S. H., and Drolette, M. E.: Mastery of stress, Cambridge, 1957, Harvard University Press.

# 16

# The dying patient

**NED H. CASSEM**

Oncologists, cardiologists, and nephrologists, long accustomed to caring for the whole person, typify experienced physicians faced with the management of the dying person. These physicians have seen every variety of emotional reaction, so that the request for psychiatric consultation, at least in the beginning, may focus on special treatment modalities (such as TM, psychopharmacology, relaxation response, biofeedback, or hypnosis) or be reserved for the most difficult patient problems. Because the literature of the contemporary thanatology movement frequently accuses physicians of neglecting dying patients, the referring physician may fear that the consultation itself may be construed as failure to meet responsibilities as the primary-care physician. Sensitivity to these pressures on the referring physician will strengthen the relationship with the patient, a factor essential to the patient's well-being.

Problems prompting consultation requests are as varied as those for other general hospital patients. Most common are: anxiety—usually extreme, with panic and phobic concerns or extreme fear of dying; denial—refusal to accept diagnosis or treatment, unrealistic demands for miracles, or persistent failure to understand why there is no improvement; angry and hostile behavior—treatment rejection, hostility toward staff, or litigation threats; depression— including open expression of grief, hopelessness, the desire to die (but rarely involving suicidal threats), complete withdrawal, or giving up long before the illness seems terminal; pain—particularly if unresponsive to conventional analgesics or associated with marked anxiety; guilt—as experienced by mothers with daughters having vaginal cancer when they learned that the diethylstilbesterol taken during pregnancy was linked to the later development of cancer in their daughters; delirium or psychosis—with or without cerebral metastases or known metabolic or neurological disorder; unrelated bad news—for example, whether a dying person should be told of a relative's death when

300

ability to tolerate another trauma is seriously questioned. Finally, there is a more general consultation request that comes particularly from the physician comfortable with the consultant, expressed something like, "Very difficult situation for unfortunate 32-year-old man with two small children; any suggestions appreciated."

In about one-third of the consultations, the family of the dying person is included in or made the specific subject of the request. The family may be the first to alert the physician to one of the problems mentioned (as when the patient gives up) or may appear to be having more difficulty than the patient in facing the illness. Families who deny the illness—seem oblivious to it or express conviction about a cure, for example—and those who are hostile to staff and critical of care most commonly complicate treatment for the patient. Families are doubly vulnerable; they are faced not only with the dying person's emotional reactions but also their own.

The nursing staff is also helpful in bringing the physician's attention to problems of patient and family and, as the source indirectly initiating the consultation, can provide additional invaluable information to the consultant.

Confronted by this broad range of problems, the consultant can benefit from research findings derived from studies of the dying. These include what is known about dying as a psychophysiological process, goals of treatment, management recommendations, breaking bad news (the diagnosis), truth telling, function of religious faith and value systems, and emotional problems of physicians and nurses who care for the dying.

## PSYCHOPHYSIOLOGICAL PROCESS OF DYING

Dying is a process that keeps the body near the forefront of the mind. Having contracted a disease that may eventually cut him down (like heart disease) or devour him (like cancer), the patient interprets or even anticipates bodily changes as ominous. Symptoms are likely to produce fear when present, but fear is often present long before their arrival. The body, once regarded as a friend, may seem more like a dormant adversary, programmed for betrayal. Dying persons, even before disintegration begins, fear many things. Loss of autonomy, disfigurement, being a burden, becoming physically repulsive, letting the family down, facing the unknown, and many other concerns are commonly expressed. When all fears were compared for frequency in one sample of cancer patients,[1] the three that occurred most often were abandonment by others, pain, and shortness of breath. These fears were expressed before the patients were symptomatic. Patients thought that as their illness progressed family and hospital staff would gradually avoid them, their conditions would become increasingly more painful, or the illness would encroach on breathing capacity and suffocate them.

Because physicians and families also worry about what will happen to the dying person, it is helpful to know which difficulties are, in fact, the most distressing when the patient is terminally ill. Saunders[1] documented the exact incidence of practical problems in terminal cancer at St. Joseph's Hospital in London. She found that the three most common complaints were nausea and vomiting, shortness of breath, and dysphagia. Largely because of her efforts, avoidance of dying patients was not a problem at St. Joseph's Hospital, but one would expect to find it in most hospitals or nursing homes with chronically ill patients. It was striking that pain did not appear high on the problem list. Nausea and dyspnea are miserable psychophysiological states. Relief of these and other troublesome symptoms helps restore peace of mind.

Just as there are common reactions of the body (like nausea) to a fatal illness, so there are common reactions of the mind. To describe the psychological process that begins with getting the news about illness and ends in death, Kubler-Ross[2] presented a framework of five stages experienced by the dying person.

1. The stages begin with *shock and denial*. In this stage the patients say, "No, not me!" They may simply be numb and appear completely unaware of the bad news, disagree with the diagnosis, or remain oblivious to its implications. Denial may persist for moments or pervade the rest of their lives. More characteristically it fluctuates, waxing and waning over the course of the illness.

2. In the stage of *anger* patients say, "Why me?" Angry outbursts may be directed toward hospital menus, treatment regimens, physicians, families, life in general, or God. Past life may be reviewed, usually with inability to find self at fault for hygienic or moral reasons. A sense of unfairness, frustration, and helplessness generate a normal sense of outrage that may turn into periods of bitterness.

3. In the stage labeled *bargaining* patients say, "Yes, it is me, but . . .," and put a condition on acceptance, such that they hope or plan for something that can mitigate disappointment. A characteristic hope is that life be extended until some special event occurs, such as a wedding, birth, or graduation.

4. In the stage called *depression* patients confront the sadness of the reality: "Yes, it is me." They may do considerable weeping, be

intermittently withdrawn or uncommunicative, brood, and be weighed down by the full impact of their condition. Despair and suicide are common preoccupations during this period.

5. The final stage of *acceptance* is conceptualized as a state reached through emotional work, such that losses are mourned and the end is anticipated with a degree of quiet expectation. It is seen as a restful albeit weary time, almost devoid of feeling.

The concept of stages of adaptation is by no means new and is not restricted to dying. As a dynamic process, dying is a special case of loss and the stages represent a dynamic model of emotional adaptation to any physical or emotional loss. A common misdirection in caring for dying patients is the attempt to help an individual through the stages one after the other. It is more accurate and therapeutically more practical to regard the stages as normal reactions to any loss. They may be present simultaneously, disappear and reappear, or occur in any order. Responding to the emotional distress of the dying often reduces physical distress. Pain, in particular, diminishes when a patient is helped to feel understood, less anxious, and less alone.

In fact, some investigators have introduced experimental psychological measures to combat illness directly. Simonton[3] uses relaxation techniques patterned after Jacobsons's techniques[4] to induce remission or even cure in cancer patients. Once patients are relaxed or in a modified trance, suggestions are made that they picture their white cells and immune mechanisms mobilized in concentrated attack on their malignancy. These reports are anecdotal and await controlled replication. The rationale is much the same as that suggested by Surman and others[5] who demonstrated the effectiveness of hypnosis in the removal of warts; that is, a person may in some way be able to influence immune defense systems.

## CARE AND MANAGEMENT OF THE DYING

Questions far outnumber answers wherever people care for the dying. Many controversies remain unresolved. The investigators mentioned earlier have outlined objectives that the physician can consider from the time treatment of the terminally ill begins. Because the patient's bedside can be an uncomfortable place for the physician, several practical considerations for management are added in support of the goals.

### Goals of treatment

Deutsch[6] observed from his clinical sample of dying patients that the decline in vital processes is accompanied by a parallel decline in the intensity of instinctual aggressive and erotic drives. With the reduction of these drives, fear of dying is also reduced. The illness could be viewed by the patient as a hostile attack by an outside enemy such as God or fate, or as a punishment for being bad. Since patients could complicate their conditions by reacting with increasing hostility toward outside objects or with self-punitive actions to offset guilt, Deutsch's therapeutic objective is a "settlement of differences." The ideal stage is reached when all guilt and aggression are dissipated.

For Eissler,[7] therapeutic success depends on the psychiatrist's ability to share the patient's basic beliefs in immortality and indestructibility. The main forces in the psychiatrist's supportive relationship with the patient are the abilities to share the patients' defenses and to develop a strong admiration for their inner strength, beauty, intelligence, courage, and honesty. Kubler-Ross[2] has described the unfinished business of the dying—reconciliations, resolution of conflicts, and pursuit of specific remaining hopes. Saunders[18] has said that the aim is to keep patients feeling like themselves as long as possible. For her, dying is also a "coming together time" when patient, family, and staff help one another share the burden of saying appropriate goodbyes. LeShan[8,9] has deliberately chosen not to focus on dying (the minor problem), but searches aggressively with patients for what they wish to accomplish in living (the major problem). Weisman and Hackett[10] have coined the term "appropriate death." To achieve this patients should (1) be relatively pain-free, (2) operate on as effective a level as possible within the limits of their disabilities, (3) recognize and resolve residual conflicts, (4) satisfy those remaining wishes that are consistent with their conditions and ego ideals, and (5) be able to yield control to others in whom they have confidence.

Perhaps more important than any other principle is that the treatment be individualized. This can be accomplished only by getting to know the patients, responding to their needs and interests, proceeding at their pace, and allowing them to shape the manner in which those in attendance behave. There is no one "best" way to die.

### Treatment recommendations

Most of what we know about dying patients comes from them. All investigators have emphasized the reversal of expertise that is manifest in care of the dying. In this field patients are the teachers, while those who take care of them have more to learn. Over the years, observations made by patients on various aspects of their management have helped in the formulation of nine essential features in the care and management of the dying patient.[11]

**Competence.** In an era where some discussions of the dying patient seem to suggest that love covers a multitude of sins, it would be unfortunate to encourage the misconception that competence in physicians and nurses is of secondary importance to dying patients. Competence is reassuring, and when one's life or comfort depends on it, personality considerations become secondary. Being good at what one does brings emotional as well as scientific benefits to the patient. For example, no matter how charming physicians, nurses, or technicians may be, the person who is most skillful at venipuncture brings the greatest relief to a patient anxious about having blood drawn.

**Concern.** Of all attributes in physicians and nurses none is more highly valued by terminal patients than compassion. Although they may never convey it precisely by words, some physicians and nurses are able to tell the patient that they are genuinely touched by his or her predicament. A striking example came from a mother's description of her dying son's pediatrician: "You know, that doctor loves Michael."

Compassion cannot be feigned. Although universally praised as a quality for a health professional, compassion exacts a cost usually overlooked in professional training. This price of compassion is conveyed by the two Latin roots, *com-*, "with", and *passio*, from *pati*, "to suffer", which together mean "to suffer *with*" another person. One must be touched by the tragedy of the patient in a literal way, a process that occurs through experiential identification with the dying person. The process of empathy, when evoked by a person facing death or tragic disability, ordinarily produces uncomfortable, burdensome feelings to which internal resistance can arise defensively. Who can bear the thought of dying at 20? It is not perverse but natural for us to discourage discussion of such a topic by the individual facing it. Also, students are sometimes advised to guard against involvement with a patient. When a patient becomes upset, hasty exits or avoidance are likely.

Few things infuriate patients more than contrived involvement. For this reason, the patient may excuse even an inability to answer direct questions when the inability stems from genuine discomfort on the physician's part. One woman preferred to ask her physician as few questions as possible, even though she wanted more information about how much longer she could expect to survive with stage IV Hodgkin disease. "Whenever I try to ask him about this, he looks very pained and becomes very hesitant. I don't want to rub it in. After all, he really likes me."

What are the emotional traumas a compassionate nurse or physician must sustain? They can be summarized by the stages the terminally ill patient experiences. Since the stages describe emotional processes in the terminally ill patient, it is only logical that these processes evoke similar reactions in a sympathetic observer. As the physician and patient view the patient's predicament together, the physician, depending on his or her sensitivity, is likely to experience shock, denial, outrage, hope, and devastation.

Involvement—real involvement—is not only unavoidable, but necessary in the therapeutic encounter. Patients recognize it instantly. As a hematologist percussed the right side of his 29-year-old patient's chest, his discovery of pleural effusion brought the realization that a remission had abruptly ended. "Oh shit!" he muttered. Then, realizing what he had said, added hastily, "Oh, excuse me, Bill." "That's all right," the young man replied. "It's nice to know that you care."

**Comfort.** With the terminally ill patient, comfort has a technology all its own. "Comfort measures" should not indicate that less attention is paid to the patient's needs. In fact, comforting a terminally ill person requires meticulous devotion to myriad details. Certain things are basic, such as narcotic medication to relieve pain. The most common mistake is inadequate dosage or frequency of medication. For example, even though the average duration of action of meperidine (Demerol) is 3 hours, it is common to find orders written for administration every 4 hours. Pain medication orders for patients with continuous pain are too often written p.r.n., which can demean the patients by forcing them to beg for pain medication. The goal of narcotic administration is pain relief with a dosage and frequency adequate to dispel pain and prevent its return. The fear of addiction, often covert, is not justified by experience. Fewer than 1% of hospitalized medical patients given narcotics for pain develop a serious problem of addiction.[12] Allowing patients to share control of their medication can dramatically relieve their fear that none will be available if they suddenly need more. For a patient with painful bone metastases the order could read: "Morphine sulfate, 2 mg to 15 mg subcutaneously every hour as needed, patient to specify amount or refuse; if two consecutive 15 mg doses are required, call M.D." The last order ensures that the physician will be notified if pain suddenly worsens.

Some comfort measures, such as pressor infusions to ward off pulmonary edema, are dramatic; others, such as providing fresh air and sunlight in the room, are simple. Attention to detail demands systematic vigilance by physicians and nurses. An excellent example is mouth care for terminally ill patients. While most people appreciate the comfort of fresh taste and breath, few can imagine how an entire book could be written on this topic as it relates to the terminally ill patient.[13] Yet the mouth is the instrument by which one speaks, tastes, chews, drinks, sucks, bites, and grins. Its care involves the face, teeth, dentures, tongue, gums, lips, and larynx. Pain, dryness, infection, odor, secretions, drooling, hemorrhage, and nutrition are all complicated problems that cause much discomfort. There are myriad technical aspects of comfort, such as isotonic saline and Karo mouth washes for stomatitis or potassium chloride rinses for dry mouth. Dumping syndrome may result because the tip of the nasogastric tube slipped into the duodenum. Pain in the jaw may be due to vincristine. The ingenuity of skillful, thoughtful providers of care can be taxed in bringing comfort to the terminally ill patient.

The principles of drug use apply as much to patients living on borrowed time as they do to patients living under more fortunate circumstances. Alcohol can be of great advantage to those patients who want it and can profit from its effects. Orders are best written specifically (for example, two old-fashioneds before dinner, as needed, or six bottles of beer per day, as needed, etc.). Tranquilizers can be helpful in some anxiety states with the patient being the best judge of their effectiveness. When tachycardia and sweating appear related to anxiety, beta blockade (10 mg of propranolol given four times a day or as needed) has been helpful. Although difficult at times to establish, when five of the eight research diagnostic criteria for depression are present, antidepressants may bring additional relief to the patient. The flexibility mentioned for narcotics also applies to tranquilizers and antiemetics.

Psychedelic drugs were first used for dying patients by Kast[14] in 1964 and have been studied extensively at the Maryland State Psychiatric Research Center since 1955.[15] The investigators there used lysergic acid diethylamide (LSD) or dipropyltryptamine (DPT) as an adjunct to brief courses of intense psychotherapy. Cancer patients who were feeling pain, depression, anxiety, and psychological isolation and who also sensed staff feelings of frustration and inadequacy were selected. After an average of 10 hours of psychotherapy there was a single psychedelic session averaging 20.2 hours. Flowers and stereophonic classical music were provided on the day of treatment, and after patients returned to their usual state of consciousness persons important in their lives (spouse, children, parents, friends) were invited to be present at the final period of the psychedelic drug session. All but six of the forty-one ratings for depression, anxiety, pain, fear of death, isolation, and ease of management showed significant changes.

According to global index ratings, 36% were dramatically improved, 36% moderately improved, and 19% were unimproved. Only 8.3% were worse. There were no changes in amount of narcotics consumed before and after psychedelic drug therapy. Goldberg and his associates have edited a book[16] on the use of psychopharmacological agents for the terminally ill. A recent finding of great promise is Sallen and his associates' demonstration[17] of the antiemetic efficacy of oral cannabis for patients receiving cancer chemotherapy. The relief of nausea induced by chemotherapeutic agents remains extremely difficult.

**Communication.** Talking with the dying is a paradoxical skill. The wish to find the right thing to say is a well-meaning but misguided hope among persons who work with terminally ill patients. Practically every empirical study has emphasized the ability to listen over the ability to say something. Saunders summarizes it best when she says, "The real question is not, 'What do you tell your patients?' but rather, 'What do you let your patients tell you?' "[18] Most people have a strong inner resistance to letting dying patients say what's on their minds. If a patient presumed to be 3 months from death says, "My plan was to buy a new car in 6 months, but I guess I won't have to worry about that now," a poor listener would say nothing or, "Right. Don't worry about it." A better listener might say, "Why do you say that?" or, "What do you mean?"

Communication is, however, more than listening. Getting to know the patient as a person is essential. Learning about significant areas of the patient's life—such as family, work, or school—and chatting about common interests are the most natural if not the only way the patient has of coming to feel known. After a 79-year-old man of keen intellect and wit had been interviewed before a group of hospital staff members, one of the staff said, "Before the interview tonight I just thought of him on the ward as another old man in pain." It is not necessary to talk about esoteric things to a dying person. Like anybody else these individuals get self-respect from a sense that others value them for what they have done and for their personal qualities. Allowing dying persons to tell their own stories helps to build a balanced relationship. The effort spent getting to know them does them more psychological good than trying to guess how they will cope with death.

The physician can help dissolve communication barriers for staff members by showing them the uniqueness of each patient. Comments such as "She has thirty-four grandchildren" or "This woman was an Olympic sprinter" (both were actual patients) convey information that helps the staff find something to talk about with the patients.

Awkwardness subsides when a patient seems like a real person and not merely "a breast cancer." This rescue from anonymity is essential to prevent a sense of isolation.

Communication is more than verbal. A pat on the arm, a wave, a wink, or a grin communicates important reassurances, as do careful backrubs and physical examinations.

Patients occasionally complain about professionals and visitors who regard them as "the dying patients," not as unique individuals. A wise precaution is to take conversational cues from the patient whenever possible.

> A woman in her early fifties with breast cancer that had metastasized to bone, brain, lungs, and liver entered the hospital for a course of chemotherapy. During her entire 6-week stay she was irascible, argumentative, and even abusive to the staff members. To their surprise, she got a good response with a substantial remission and left the hospital. She later told her oncologist, apologizing for her behavior, "I know that I was impossible. But every single nurse who came into my room wanted to talk to me about death. I came there to get help, not to die, and it drove me up a wall."

Had staff members tuned in to this patient as an individual with a courageous attitude toward her illness, instead of treating her as "a dying patient," their efforts to comfort would not have backfired.

**Children.** All investigators have learned that the visits of children are as likely to bring consolation and relief to the terminally ill patient as any other intervention. A useful rule of thumb in determining whether a particular child should visit a dying patient is to ask the child whether he or she wants to visit. No better criterion has been found.

**Family cohesion and integration.** A burden shared is a burden made lighter. Family members must be helped to support one another, although this requires that the physician get to know each member of the family as well as the patient. Conversely, when patients are permitted to give support to their families, the feeling of being a burden is mitigated.

The often difficult work of bringing the family together for support, reconciliations, or improved relations can prevent disruption when death of the patient begins the work of bereavement. The opportunity to be present at death should be offered to family members, as well as the alternative of being informed about it while waiting for the news at home. Flexibility is the rule, and the wishes of the family and patient are paramount. After the patient has died, family members who wish to should be offered a chance to see the body before it is taken to the morgue. Parkes[19] documented the critical importance to grief work of seeing the body of the dead person.

**Cheerfulness.** Dying persons have no more relish for sour and somber faces than anybody else. Anyone with a gentle and appropriate sense of humor can bring much relief to all parties involved. "What do they think this is?" said one patient of his visitors. "They file past here with flowers and long faces like they were coming to my wake." Patients with a good sense of humor do not enjoy dead audiences either. It is their wit that softens many a difficult incident. After an embarrassing loss of sphincter control, one elderly man with a tremor said, "This is enough to give anybody Parkinson's disease!"

Wit is not an end in itself. As in all forms of conversation, the listener should take the cue from the patient. Forced or inappropriate mirth with a sick person can increase feelings of distance and isolation.

**Consistency and perseverance.** Progressive isolation is a realistic fear of the dying person. A physician or nurse who regularly visits the sick room provides tangible proof of continued support and concern. Saunders has emphasized that the quality of time is far more important than the quantity.[18] A brief visit is far better than no visit at all and patients may not be able to tolerate prolonged visiting anyway. Patients are quick to identify those who show interest at first but gradually disappear from the scene. Staying power requires hearing complaints.

> Praising one of her nurses, a 69-year-old woman with advanced cancer said, "She takes all my guff, and I give her plenty. Most people just pass my room, but if she has even a couple of minutes she'll stop and actually listen to what I have to say. Some days I couldn't get through without her."

**Equanimity.** The capacity to be comfortable with a dying person is another valued quality.

> A 68-year-old woman with two primary pulmonary malignancies fought, as did her physicians, a steadily losing battle against shortness of breath. She often complained that death would be preferable. Nevertheless, she also worried that her criticisms and unanswerable questions were an unfair burden to her physicians. After making such an observation to one of her physicians, she suddenly fixed her piercing blue eyes on him as she said, "You know, you're just like an old shoe—comfortable."

Equally prized by the physician, equanimity not only greatly contributes to but is produced by enriching encounters with terminally ill persons.

## Breaking bad news

Because so many reactions to the news of diagnosis are possible, it is helpful to have some plan of action in mind ahead of time that will permit the greatest variation and freedom of response. When the diagnosis is made and it is time to inform the patient, it is best to begin by sitting down with the patient in a private place. Standing while conveying bad news is regarded by patients as unkind and an expression of wanting to leave as quickly as possible. The patient should be informed that when all the tests are completed, the physician will sit down with him again. Spouse and family can be included in the discussion of findings and treatment. As that day approaches, the patient should be warned again. This permits those patients who wish no or minimal information to say so.

If the findings are unpleasant, for example, a biopsy positive for malignancy, how can it best be conveyed? A good opening statement is one that is (1) rehearsed so that it can be delivered calmly, (2) brief— three sentences or less, (3) designed to encourage further dialogue, and (4) reassuring of continued attention and care. A typical delivery might go as follows: "The tests confirmed that your tumor is malignant (the bad news). I have therefore asked the surgeon (radiotherapist, on-cologist) to come by to speak with you, examine you, and make his recommendations for treatment (we will do something about it). As things proceed, I will be by to discuss them with you and how we should proceed (I will stand by you)." Silence and quiet observation for a few moments will yield valuable information about the patient, his emotional reactions, how he deals with it from the start. While observing one can decide on how best to continue with the discussion, but sitting with the patient for a period of time is an essential part of this initial encounter with a grim reality that both patient and physician will continue to confront together, possibly for a very long time.

## Telling the truth

Without honesty, human relationships are destined for shipwreck. If truthfulness and trust are so obviously interdependent, how can there be so much conspiracy to avoid truth with the dying? The paradoxical fact is that for terminally ill patients the need for both honesty and the avoidance of the truth can be intense. Sir William Osler is reputed to have said, "A patient has no more right to all the facts in my head than he does to all the medications in my bag." A routine blood smear has just revealed that a 25-year-old man has acute myelogenous leukemia. If he were married and the father of two small children, should he be told the diagnosis? Is the answer obvious? What if he had had two prior psychotic breaks with less serious illnesses? What if his wife says he once said he never wanted to know if he had a malignancy?

Most empirical studies in which patients were asked whether or not they should be told the truth about malignancy overwhelmingly indicated desire for the truth. When 740 patients in a cancer detection clinic were asked prior to diagnosis if they should be told their diagnosis, 99% said they should be told.[20] Another group in this same clinic was asked after the diagnosis was established and 89% of them replied affirmatively, as did 82% of another group who had been examined and found free of malignancy. Gilbertsen and Wangensteen[21] asked the same questions of 298 survivors of surgery for gastric, colonic, and rectal cancers and found 82% wanted to be told the truth. The same investigators questioned ninety-two patients who had advanced cancer and were judged by their physicians to be pre-terminal and found that 79% of the patients thought they should be told their diagnosis.

How many don't want to know the truth or regard it as harmful? Effects of blunt truth telling have been empirically studied in both England and the United States. Aitken-Swan and Easson[22] were told by 7% of 231 patients explicitly informed of their diagnosis that the frankness of the consultant was resented. Gilbertsen and Wangensteen[21] observed that 4% of a sample of surgical patients became emotionally upset at the time they were told and appeared to remain so throughout the course of their illness. Gerlé, Lunden, and Sandblom[23] studied 101 patients who were divided into two groups. Members of one group were told, along with their families, the frank truth of their diagnoses. In the other group, an effort was made to maintain a conspiracy of silence with family and physician excluding the patient from discussion of the diagnosis. At first, greater emotional upset appeared in the group where patient and family were told together, but the investigators observed in follow-up that the emotional difficulties of the families of those patients shielded from the truth far outweighed those of patients and families who were told the diagnosis simultaneously. In general, empirical studies support the idea that truth is desired by terminally ill patients and does not harm those to whom it is given. Honesty sustains the relationship with a dying person rather than retarding it.

Dr. Hackett saw in consultation a 57-year-old housewife with metastatic breast cancer, now far advanced. She reported a persistent headache, which she attributed to nervous tension and asked why she should be nervous. Turning the question back to her, he was told, "I am nervous because I have lost 60 pounds in a year. The priest comes to see me twice a week, which he never did before, and my mother-in-law is nicer to me even though I am meaner to her. Wouldn't this make you nervous?" . . . [He] said to her, "You mean you think you're dying." "That's right, I do," she replied. He paused and said quietly "You are." She smiled and said, "Well, I've finally broken the sound barrier; someone's finally told me the truth."[24]

Not all patients can be dealt with so directly. A nuclear physicist operated on in Massachusetts General Hospital greeted his surgeon on the day following exploratory laparotomy with the words, "Lie to me, Steve." Individual variations in willingness to hear the initial diagnosis are extreme. And diagnosis is entirely different from prognosis. Many patients have said they were grateful to their physician for telling them they had a malignancy. Very few, however, reacted positively to being told they are dying. In my experience, "Do I have cancer?" is a common question, while, "Am I dying?" is a rare one. The question about dying is more common from patients who are dying rapidly, such as those in cardiogenic shock.

Honest communication of the diagnosis (or of any truth) by no means precludes later avoidance or even denial of the truth. In two studies patients who had been explicitly told their diagnosis (using the words "cancer" or "malignancy") were asked 3 weeks later what they had been told. Nineteen percent of one sample [22] and 20% of the other [21] denied that their condition was cancer or malignant. Likewise Croog, Shapiro, and Levine[25] interviewed 345 men 3 weeks after myocardial infarction and were told by 20% that they had not had a heart attack. All had been explicitly told their diagnosis. For a person to function effectively truth's piercing voice must occasionally be muted or even excluded from awareness. On 4 consecutive days I spoke with a man who had a widely spread bone cancer. On the first day he said he didn't know what he had and didn't like to ask questions. The second day he was "riddled with cancer." The third day he didn't really know what ailed him. The fourth day he said that even though nobody likes to die that was now his lot.

Truth telling is no panacea. Communicating a diagnosis honestly, though difficult, is easier than the labors that lie ahead. Telling the truth is merely a way to begin; but since it is an open and honest way, it provides a firm basis on which to build a relationship of trust.

### Role of religious faith and value systems

Investigation of the relationship between religious faith and attitudes toward death has been hampered by differences in methodology. Lester[26] and Feifel[27] have reviewed much of the conflicting literature on the relationship between religious faith and fear of death. Other research has tried to clarify the way belief systems function within the individual. Allport[28] contrasted an extrinsic religious orientation in which religion is mainly a means to social status, security, or relief from guilt, with an intrinsic religious orientation, in which the values appear to be internalized and subscribed to as ends in themselves. Feagin[29] provided a useful twenty one item questionnaire for distinguishing the two types of believers. Experimental work[30] and clinical experience indicate that an extrinsic value system, without internalization, seems to offer no assistance in coping with a fatal illness. A religious commitment that is intrinsic, on the other hand, appears to offer considerable stability and strength to those who possess it.

Many patients are grateful for the chance to express their own thoughts about their faith. For assessing religious faith a useful question that can be asked during discussion of the illness is "Where do you think God stands in all this?" This question leads to others. "Do you see your illness as imposed on you by God? Why? What sort of a being do you picture God to be?" Answers can be scrutinized for feelings of guilt and for the quality of relationship the individual describes with God. Belief in afterlife is another useful area for questioning and helps to assess tolerance of doubt, an important quality of mature belief. In general, those persons who possess a sense of the personal presence of God, of being cared for or watched over, are more likely to manifest tranquility in their struggle with terminal illness. The presence of firm religious convictions indicates that consultation of the chaplain (patient's own minister/rabbi) is important. He or she will usually provide many valuable facts and insights about the patient and family that can smooth the patient's overall course.

## DIFFICULTIES OF THOSE WHO CARE FOR THE DYING

Cultural taboos spare no one from their subtle pressures. The "American way of not dying" (Paul Ramsey's phrase) pervades the population. Even in the arenas where death most frequently occurs— general hospitals, nursing homes, and chronic care facilities—staff members may become uncomfortable at even the mention of death. It is not discussion of death and dying that is the focus here but rather the bedside discomfort of health professionals who attend the dying. In a careful study of the activities of nurses on a general hospital floor Glaser and Strauss[31] showed that the more ill the patients and the closer they were to death, the less time the staff spent with them, even though they were located closer to the nursing station. Despite a general consensus that dying persons fear abandonment, avoidance of them is the rule rather than the exception.

Why does the physician tend to avoid dying patients or, if not avoid, become quite uneasy in their presence? Encounters with dying persons tend to represent either personal threats to professionals or threats to their relationships. A personal threat can arise from exposure to serious disability or dying. The dictum that "there is to be no mention of the word death here" can represent a denial that death will ever claim the physician. The surgeon who does not allow such orders as "do not resuscitate" may be denying that failure is possible in the struggle against death. Avoidance of paralyzed or disfigured patients may protect the physician from the realization that the same fate could befall him or her. It is very difficult to absorb and respond to a dying person's plight. Compassion can impose a heavy burden on the sympathetic professional. The sentence, "I don't think I can take another story like the one I just heard," expresses a familiar and realistic worry.

A dying person poses a threat to the professional's own human attachments. First of all, the physician is reminded that death means loss of the relationship with the patient and all the investment and caring that has gone into it. Second, imminent loss of a patient reminds professionals of their own losses and of threatened losses. Caring for a dying woman, for example, can remind physicians of the past or feared death of their own mother, sister, or spouse. Wounds of an incompletely grieved loss are reopened. Losses in life are not discreet; they are cumulative. Those who care for the dying sustain repeated bereavement.

Because of the repeated stresses posed by these threats, professionals develop defenses. One course is to avoid involvement with patients in order to minimize personal loss or discomfort. This is the probable cause of fixed styles of relating to patients. Physicians who follow the initial communication of the diagnosis to the patient with a standardized, nonstop monologue detailing diagnosis, treatment, and course of the disease are not trying to baffle, overwhelm, or lose the patient altogether, but rather they are trying to minimize their own anxiety by handling every initial bad news session the same way. Intellectualizing or depersonalizing by referring to the dying person as an interesting "problem" or "case" is also a protective defense. Some professionals say the patients "can't take it," which is often a projection of their own fear onto patients. Other examples would illustrate other defense mechanisms. The point is that the physician's discomfort and avoidance of patients arise mainly from instincts of self-defense rather than any desire to alienate or harm patients.

Criticism of physicians tends to be widespread and can generate unfortunate hostilities. Common accusations are that physicians are more afraid of death than other persons and that this fear prompted them to enter the medical field in the first place. Sophisticated critics refer to Feifel's[32] study of physicians' attitudes toward death that showed that physicians spent significantly less time in conscious thought about death than did two control groups of professionals. Feifel and others[33] also found more fear of death in medical students than in two control samples. Dissatisfaction with physicians' communication patterns, avoidance of patients, and their manner in the sickroom compounds the alienation.

In response to such criticism some physicians have become defensive or even hostile. When forced to assume the adversary role, physicians are at a distinct disadvantage. It would be well for physicians and those who work with them to keep certain reflections in mind. Although everyone is fascinated with death, physicians grapple with it more frequently than others and are sought out by those who wish to prevent or postpone it. Conflict or discomfort in the presence of death is intensified by the combination of two factors: frequent exposure and high responsibility. The findings of Feifel and others[33] may also be accounted for by the increased exposure of medical students to death and to the widespread belief of the population that the physician is the last barrier against it. Natural disappointment that a terminally ill person cannot be saved can lead to resentment. As one who could not reverse the illness, the physician may become the object of some or all of the family's resentment and blame. Finally, those who accuse physicians of inability to communicate with the dying patient seem to forget that everyone has this difficulty, including members of the patient's family.

What can be done to decrease the defensiveness of the physician? Physicians pay for enjoying the exercise of greater responsibility in helping prevent or postpone death by having stronger feelings of failure and guilt when their hopes and the patient's hopes are disappointed. If one notes a surgeon or an oncologist who is particularly gruff, a sympathetic approach will accomplish much more than a hostile one. One could say, for example, "It must be difficult to work with patients whose illnesses always have such poor odds for cure or recovery." Or to the surgeon after an untimely failure one might say, "It's been a tough day, but you did everything you could." Such sympathetic comments have a greater likelihood of turning tense situations into mutually supportive times. Finally, more systematic efforts need be undertaken to help health personnel who work on the front lines deal with their own feelings about suffering, disappointment, failure, and death. Ideally this should begin early in training, so that the repeated exposure to these traumatic experiences can be accompanied by emotional growth in compassion and equanimity, its major features.

### REFERENCES

1. Saunders, C.: Care of the dying, 6 parts, Nursing Times, October 9 to November 13, 1959.
2. Kubler-Ross, E.: On death and dying, New York, 1969, Macmillan, Inc.
3. Simonton, O. C., and Simonton, S.: Management of the emotional aspects of malignancy, delivered at the symposium New Dimensions of Rehabilitation for the Handicapped, University of Florida, Gainesville, June, 1974.
4. Jacobson, E.: Progressive relaxation, Chicago, 1938, University of Chicago Press.
5. Surman, O. S., Gottlieb, J. K., Hackett, T. P., and Silverberg, E. L.: Hypnosis in the treatment of warts, Arch. Gen. Psychiatry **28:**439-441, 1973.
6. Deutsch, F.: Euthanasia, a clinical study, Psychoanal. Q. **5:**347-368, 1933.
7. Eissler, K.: The psychiatrist and the dying patient, New York, 1955, International Universities Press.
8. LeShan, L., and LeShan, E.: Psychotherapy and the patient with a limited life span, Psychiatry **24:**318-323, 1961.
9. LeShan, L.: Psychotherapy and the dying patient. In Pearson, L., editor: Death and dying, Cleveland, 1969, Case Western Reserve University Press, pp. 28-48.
10. Weisman, A. D., and Hackett, T. P.: Predilection to death: death and dying as a psychiatric problem, Psychosom. Med. **23:**232-256, 1961.
11. Cassem, N. H., and Stewart, R. S.: Management and care of the dying patient, Int. J. Psychiatry Med. **6:**293-304, 1975.
12. Marks, R. M., and Sachar, E. J.: Undertreatment of medical inpatients with narcotic analgesics, Ann. Intern. Med. **78:**173-181, 1973.
13. Kutscher, A. H., Schoenberg, B., and Carr, A. C.: The terminal patient: oral care, New York, 1973, Columbia University Press.
14. Kast, E. C.: The analgesic action of lysergic acid compared with dihydromorphinone, Anesth. Analg. **43:**285-291, 1964.
15. Kurland, A. A., Grof, S., Pahnke, W. N., and Goodman, L. E.: Psychedelic

drug–assisted psychotherapy in patients with terminal cancer. In Goldberg, I. K., Malitz, S., and Kutscher, A. H., editors: Psychopharmacologic agents for the terminally ill and bereaved, New York, 1973, Columbia University Press, pp. 86-133.

16. Goldberg, I. K., Malitz, S., and Kutscher, A. H., editors: Psychopharmacologic agents for the terminally ill and bereaved, New York, 1973, Columbia University Press.

17. Sallen, S., Zinberg, N., and Frei, E.: Antiemetic effect of Δ9 THC in patients receiving cancer chemotherapy, N. Engl. J. Med. **293:**795-797, 1975.

18. Saunders, C.: The moment of truth: care of the dying person. In Pearson, L., editor: Death and dying, Cleveland, 1969, Case Western Reserve University Press, pp. 49-78.

19. Parkes, C. M.: Bereavement: studies of grief in adult life, New York, 1972, International Universities Press.

20. Kelly, W. D., and Friesen, S. R.: Do cancer patients want to be told? Surgery **27:**822-826, 1950.

21. Gilbertsen, V. A., and Wangensteen, O. H.: Should the doctor tell the patient that the disease is cancer? Surgeon's recommendation. In American Cancer Society, The physician and the total care of the cancer patient, New York, 1962, American Cancer Society, pp. 80-85.

22. Aitken-Swan, J., and Easson, E. C.: Reactions of cancer patients on being told their diagnosis, Br. Med. J. **1:**779-783, 1959.

23. Gerlé, B., Lunden, G., and Sandblom, P.: The patient with inoperable cancer from the psychiatric and social standpoints, Cancer **13:**1206-1217, 1960.

24. Hackett, T. P., and Weisman, A. D.: The treatment of the dying, Curr. Psychiatr. Ther. **2:**121-126, 1962.

25. Croog, S. H., Shapiro, S. D., and Levine, S.: Denial among male heart patients, Psychosom. Med. **33:**385-397, 1971.

26. Lester, D.: Religious behaviors and attitudes toward death. In Godin, A., editor: Death and presence, Brussels, 1972, Lumen Vitae, pp. 107-124.

27. Feifel, H.: Religious conviction and fear of death among the healthy and the terminally ill, J. Sci. Study Religion **13:**353-360, 1974.

28. Allport, C.: The nature of prejudice, New York, 1958, Doubleday & Co., Inc.

29. Feagin, J. R.: Prejudice and religious types: focused study, Southern Fundamentalists, J. Sci. Study Religion **4:**3-13, 1964.

30. Magni, K. G.: The fear of death. In Godin, A., editor: Death and presence, Brussels, 1972, Lumen Vitae, pp. 125-138.

31. Glaser, B. G., and Strauss, A. L.: Awareness of dying, Chicago, 1965, Aldine Publishing Co.

32. Feifel, H.: The function of attitudes toward death. In Group for the Advancement of Psychiatry; Death and dying: attitudes of patient and doctor, Symposium 11, 1965, Vol. 5, pp. 633-641.

33. Feifel, H., and others: Physicians consider death, Proceedings of 75th Annual Convention of American Psychological Association, 1967, Vol. 2, pp. 201-202.

# 17

# The setting of intensive care

**NED H. CASSEM and THOMAS P. HACKETT**

"Intensive care" is a relatively new term for an ancient idea. Constant attendance of the critically ill or the dying began with the death watch. During the last 3 decades mechanical devices have slowly taken more space by the bedside pushing personal vigilance to the side. Intravenous and continuous suction apparatuses and oxygen tent have led the way for today's awesome array of life-support and monitoring systems. With this machinery and computerized environment has come a new cadre of medical caregivers, physicians and nurses especially trained to treat the complicated cardiac and respiratory problems, burns, and surgical recoveries of the critically ill patient. Despite their specialization, intensive care areas share some common features. Severity of illness and readiness of the staff to launch dramatic life-saving interventions combine to lend a unique air of danger, urgency, and heroism to these settings. A new phrase, "intensive care syndrome," has even been coined with reference to this new "disease of medical progress."[1]

In this chapter the practical issues and problems of the intensive care setting and some basic approaches to their solution are presented. The difficulties can be viewed from two vantage points—that of the patient and that of the staff. This chapter is divided into two parts: (1) problems for which the patient requires assistance and (2) difficulties that affect staff members working in the intensive care setting.

## DIFFICULTIES CONFRONTING THE PATIENT

Any illness serious enough to warrant admission to an intensive care unit (ICU) evokes in the patient predictable emotional reactions. These reactions share common features regardless of the illness. Whether admitted after myocardial infarction, motor vehicle accident, or valve replacement, patients may become sufficiently upset to complicate their own medical management.

**319**

## Some typical problems and their timing

Reactions to myocardial infarction can serve as a model for emotional reactions in an intensive care setting. They illustrate typical problems as well as their characteristic timing. Fig. 17-1 diagrams the timing of consultation requests for emotional difficulties in 149 coronary patients admitted over a 15 month period. Most problems of the first 2 days stem from fear and anxiety. Denial (here mainly illustrated by the desire to sign out) follows shortly thereafter, with depression, sometimes persistent, not far behind. A final group of management problems, related mostly to dependency issues, round out the sequence.

From this grouping of consultation requests, it is possible to describe a somewhat typical course for the patient who has had a myocardial infarction. During admission, fear and anxiety are commonly present. As symptoms stabilize or subside, patients are likely to decide that the symptoms were a false alarm. In some cases such

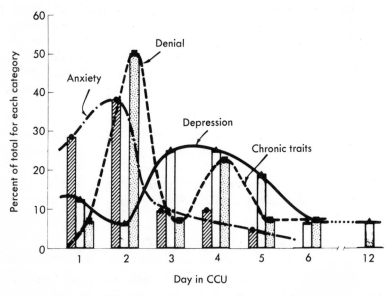

**Fig. 17-1.** Hypothetical sequence of emotional and behavioral reactions of a coronary care unit (CCU) patient, derived from the frequency of psychiatric consultation for each category of reaction. (From Cassem, N. H.: What is behind our masks? AORN J. **20:**79-92, 1974.)

patients may even insist on signing out of the hospital. However, after diagnostic tests confirm the presence of myocardial infarction, feelings of demoralization start. As the hospitalization progresses, personality problems, such as a passive-aggressive personality, may complicate interactions between the patient and hospital personnel and lead to psychiatric consultation.

This model can be of practical assistance in our care of patients in an ICU. For example, if they seem impossible to deal with on the day of admission to an ICU, the reason is very likely underlying fright. Nothing else distorts personality quite like panic. Staff members often comment 3 or 4 days later that the patient seems like a completely different person. On the other hand, when patients become impossible to deal with after 4 or 5 days and there has been no new and frightening event, their behavior most likely reflects a lifelong style of coping with stress. In contrast to patients who are frightened when admitted, those who demonstrate personality problems later are not likely to become favorites of the staff no matter how long they stay in the unit. If by nature they have typically handled threats to their self-esteem with hostility or with machismo, they can be expected to continue to do so in the ICU. The consultant here must be content with directing efforts at minimizing destructive behavior rather than encouraging the hope that it will go away.

**Characteristic problems of specific intensive care settings.**

Specific settings of intensive care have characteristic problems. The patient who has had a coronary bypass, for example, for whom anxiety was a preoperative difficulty, enters the surgical ICU unconscious. A

**Table 17-1.** Frequency of consultation requests according to intensive care setting*

| Coronary care unit* | Surgical ICU | Respiratory ICU |
|---|---|---|
| 1. Anxiety | 1. Delirium | l. Depression |
| 2. Depression | 2. Depression | 2. Anxiety weaning |
| 3. Management of be- | 3. Anxiety weaning | from respirator |
| havior (sign out, de- | from respirator | 3. Management (drug |
| pendency) | | dependency, depen- |
| 4. Hostility | | dency) |
| 5. Delirium psychosis | | |

*Modified from Cassem, N. H. and Hackett, T. P.: Psychiatric consultation in a coronary care unit, Ann. Intern. Med. **75:**9-14, 1971.

coronary care unit (CCU) can seem quite tame by comparison, at least until a cardiac arrest occurs. Table 17-1 lists the incidence of consultation requests in three different intensive care settings—a coronary care unit, surgical intensive care unit, and a respiratory intensive care unit. In this table the frequency of consultation requests in the CCU is based on 450 consecutive admissions,[2] whereas those listed for the surgical and respiratory units are based on unsystematic clinical impressions. Delirium or psychosis, for example, a rare problem in the CCU, is the most frequent reason for consultation requests received from the surgical ICU. (At Massachusetts General Hospital the surgical ICU is almost exclusively for postoperative cardiac patients.)

Despite the variation in incidence of these difficulties, any patient in an intensive care setting is normally susceptible to the mental distress caused by fear and anxiety, depression, delirium or psychosis, special anxiety of weaning from the respirator, cardiac arrest, interpersonal problems characteristic of each personality, and death. Since the treatment of these difficulties is basically the same no matter where they arise, they are discussed one at a time.

**Fear and anxiety.** In the intensive care unit anxiety and illness are symbiotic. Admission to an intensive care setting almost invariably means a threat to life. The bottom line in the content of fear or anxiety is death. Even when death does not haunt their awareness patients may fear that they will be maimed by the illness or by its treatment. As common as fear is, it may assume many guises. Verbosity and silent withdrawal are both behaviors typically produced by fear.

Fear is treated by medication and by the quiet dialogue of reassurance. Unless panic has begun to encroach on rationality, the drugs of choice are the benzodiazepines. These drugs, their common dosages, and their appropriate use are described in Chapter 26. If the patient's condition (for example, myocardial infarction) is one in which autonomic lability is a hazard, routine prescription of one of these agents is warranted whether the person looks anxious or not. About 8% of patients given this drug treatment will object to feeling sedated. The drug can then be reduced or discontinued. The most sensitive measure for dosage adequacy remains the perception of the ICU nurse. A general rule is to prescribe the simplest and shortest-acting effective drug. For example, 15 mg of oxazepam is given four times per day. With the physician's permission the nurse can hold this if it seems excessive or report if the patient seems undermedicated. For the longer-acting agents like diazepam, whose half-life varies between 20 and 50 hours, the physician can assume saturation after 2 or 3 days and administer only a bedtime or twice-daily dose thereafter. While parenteral forms of chlordiazepoxide and diazepam are available, intramuscular absorption is erratic and less complete than absorption when the drugs are taken orally. For this reason oral or cautious intravenous administration is recommended.[3] Chlordiazepoxide and diazepam can on rare occasions produce paradoxical rage or hostility; since oxazepam is not known to do this, the physician should start with oxazepam if the patient already seems hostile.

If fear is sufficiently intense to impair reason or if the patient appears to be in a state of panic, an antipsychotic agent is the drug of choice. When such fearful individuals are barely in control, the minor tranquilizers can sometimes serve only to further compromise an already diminished ability to cope. Panic can produce a transient psychotic state in these settings. The preferred drug is haloperidol, which can be administered in oral or parenteral form. (See under delirium.)

Explanation and reassurance can also have very soothing effects for anxious patients. When physicians sense fear, they can safely assume that the patient regards the illness as an overwhelming threat to well-being. This is often based on what the individuals already know or think they know about the disease. Questions such as, "Have you ever known anyone with these symptoms (gastric bleeding, a heart attack, or whatever pertains)?" or, "What is your idea of a heart attack (Hodgkin's disease, or whatever pertains)?" can be used to uncover threatening or erroneous concepts. When misconceptions emerge, they can be corrected. When a family member has died of the same condition, his or her age at death may figure heavily in the patient's fear, that is, the patient may expect that fate will take him at the same age. After false ideas have been corrected, it is important to mention positive aspects of the treatment plan, for example, that myocardial healing is complete in 5 to 6 weeks, that normal activities can be resumed, and that the patient can plan to be placed on an exercise program. Even when the prognosis is grave, as in lung cancer, a calm statement of the treatments planned to counteract and contain the malignancy is of value to the anxious patient. The more ominous the prognosis, the more important it is to encourage the patient to specify the fear, so that the specific valid reassurances (for example, that medication can control pain) can be given. False reassurances are not recommended because they rob the physician of credibility and, therefore, of the ability to reassure the patient later in the illness.

Equanimity of the physician has a soothing effect on the patient. Anxious patients have a way of making people who take care of them anxious as well and a vicious circle develops. A calm person can break that deleterious circle.

**Depression.** The subject of the depressed patient is considered in detail in Chapter 10 and is especially pertinent here.

**Delirium or psychosis.** A more complete discussion of these difficulties is given in Chapter 6 in which careful distinctions are made between delirium, psychosis, and dementia. The practical approach to the treatment of these states begins with a checklist of all possible contributing organic factors in order to eliminate all but the most pertinent. The treatment is always the same when specific causes cannot be found. Delirium is a rare problem in the CCU and it is so uncommon to discover a patient in a psychotic state in the CCU that the standard response to the onset of a delirium in a CCU patient is to think immediately of a lidocaine or atropine reaction or delirium tremens. Many patients experience some neurological symptoms when the flow rate of lidocaine has reached 2 mg per minute and almost all patients will experience some symptoms when the flow rate reaches 4 mg per minute. Fortunately, the half-life of this antiarrhythmic agent is short and other group I antiarrhythmic agents are routinely added if ventricular irritability persists. In persons over 60, atropine in doses of less than 1 mg can produce an organic brain syndrome. In fact, a liaison psychiatrist in a CCU would do well to advocate that all patients over 60 years of age with bradycardia be treated with parenteral propantheline bromine (Pro-Banthine), a quaternary ammonium compound that does not cross the blood-brain barrier and is equally effective in treating bradycardia.

In the treatment of delirium or psychosis in the ICU, the physician should consider the probability of an acute brain syndrome until proved otherwise. Because of this the differential diagnosis is mandatory. Of course this can become cumbersome and hard to remember when checking for metabolic (as sodium, potassium, calcium, magnesium, blood urea nitrogen, or others), traumatic (skull fracture), neoplastic (metastasis), vascular (thrombosis), hematologic (hemorrhage, vitamin $B_{12}$, folate), hypoxic, endocrine (thyroid), or toxic (alcohol, carbon monoxide, drugs) causes. In the CCU setting, recalling the common organic possibilities soon becomes second nature. The consultant does not always have the luxury of being a liaison psychiatrist present every day in a specific unit setting. Since it is actually easier to check laboratory tests than it is to run through a list of possible diagnoses, the consultant can facilitate the differential diagnosis by carrying a small card with appropriate laboratory tests listed on it. The boxed material shows what such a card might contain. This approach has been used in screening for dementia.[4,5] The first and most important step in making a differential diagnosis of acute brain syndrome is the identification and elimination of any possible exogenous or endogenous toxic agent. Using laboratory data and vital signs readily available in the ICU patient's chart is a simple, practical, "check-the-numbers" approach that is systematic and can identify potential problems. Every patient's chart should have a complete blood count, fasting blood sugar, blood urea nitrogen, and electrolyte

---

**LABORATORY AND ASSORTED CHECKPOINTS
IN SCREENING CAUSES OF DELIRIUM\***

Prior psychiatric history
Withdrawal: alcohol, barbiturates, benzodiazepines, meprobamate
Drugs: steroids, levodopa, amphetamines, psychotropics, digitalis,
  lidocaine, anticholinergics
Temperature
Blood pressure
Hematocrit, mean corpuscular volume greater than 96, vitamin $B_{12}$,
  folic acid
Erythrocyte sedimentation rate, lupus erythematosus preparation
Electrolytes, magnesium, calcium, phosphates, tetraiodothyronine
Blood urea nitrogen
Fasting blood sugar
Oxygen pressure (arterial)
Carbon dioxide pressure (arterial)
Ammonia, liver function tests
Venereal disease report
Electrocardiogram
Skull roentgenograms
Electroencephalogram
Brain scan
Cerebrospinal fluid proteins, cells
Computerized tomography scan

\*Adapted from Fox, J. H., Topel, J. L., and Huckman, M. S.: Dementia in the elderly—a search for treatable illnesses, J. Gerontol. **30:**557-564, 1975; and Jacobs, J. W., Bernhard, M. R., Delgado, A., and Strain, J. J.: Screening for organic mental syndromes in the medically ill, Ann. Intern. Med. **86:**40-46, 1977.

test results. It is our philosophy at MGH that all medically ill patients with mental abnormalities should also have serum tetraiodothyronine, calcium, and phosphorus checked as a matter of routine.

Once the implication of a distinct organic cause of the brain syndrome has been confirmed, treatment is imperative. In the intensive care setting agitation is that component of the brain syndrome that leads to the call for help in the first place and its decrease becomes the treatment goal against which drug effects are titrated. When an agitated person becomes susceptible to self-harm by pulling out pacemaker wires, sumps, sutures, and similar therapeutic lifelines, prompt sedation is mandatory. Haloperidol is the drug of choice and can be administered orally or parenterally. Its effects on blood pressure, pulmonary artery pressure, heart rate, and respiration are even milder than those of the benzodiazepines, making it an excellent agent for severely ill patients with impaired cardiorespiratory status. A loading regimen should be followed and unless the agitation is mild, the route should be parenteral. Two to ten milligrams of haloperidol should be administered every half hour until adequate sedation is achieved. The peak effect of each dose is reached in about 10 minutes; one should never expect to see immediate effects of haloperidol, even if it is administered intravenously. In healthy volunteers the mean half-life of haloperidol varies from 14 hours for an intravenous dose to 24 hours for an oral dose.

Once the patient has been sedated, the aim of therapy is maintenance of a blood level gradually declining to the minimum dose necessary to maintain calm. A very rough formula for the dosage needed to treat acute delirium is to add up the total initial quantity of drug required to quiet the patient. The subsequent dose given the patient should be about half this total dose. For example, if 2 mg, then 5 mg, and then 10 mg doses of haloperidol were administered one-half hour apart (increasing the dose each time until adequate sedation was reached), then about 8 mg would be prescribed for 12 hours later or at bedtime, whichever came later, provided agitation remained under control. If the 17 mg total provided sedation for less than 12 hours, then 8 mg would be given at the point where agitation recurred, on the assumption that an adequate dose of the drug had not been achieved. If agitation had not been controlled for more than 12 hours by an initial series of parenteral doses, the next dose (here 8 mg) would be given parenterally as well. If agitation remained absent, the next dose could be given orally, even though the total effective drug absorbed would be about half that of the parenteral dose. A common mistake in the prescription of antipsychotics is the use of a regular repetitive dose, such as 5 mg every 6 hours. With such a regimen excessive sedation is a hazard. Delirium in intensive care settings is ordinarily a transient phenomenon; therefore, the ideal treatment is that of a loading dose followed by diminishing maintenance doses. For two or three nights after complete disappearance of the acute state, a small nighttime dose, 1 to 3 mg, should be given to prevent recurrence, which is most likely at night.

On rare occasions a patient becomes more agitated after increasing sedative doses of haloperidol. If the haloperidol dose has been pushed to 60 mg and this happens, the physician should consider the possibility of brain syndrome resulting from anticholinergic drugs (especially if other anticholinergic drugs are being given simultaneously). Brain syndrome caused by anticholinergic agents is immediately responsive to and can therefore be immediately checked by a 1 ml intravenous dose of physostigmine. There are also occasional paradoxical responses to haloperidol; in such cases administration of the drug should be stopped. At this time it is not clear what an adequate loading dose of haloperidol is. The estimate of 60 mg is conservative; on occasion this has been exceeded by a factor of three with successful results. Paradoxical responses, although rare, are a reality. An excellent alternative to haloperidol for very ill, unstable medical patients would be thiothixene or a piperazine phenothiazine like trifluoperazine.

In addition to pharmacologic treatment, other efforts are important in neutralizing a confusional state. A familiar family member is almost always helpful in quieting a patient. Staff members can help patients maintain better contact with reality by habitually identifying themselves by name, supplying a clock and calendar, letting patients know that not all remarks overheard are about them, reducing lighting at night, and providing stereo, radio, or television. (See also Chapter 6.)

**Anxiety which inhibits weaning from the ventilator.** Persons who suffer acute and chronic respiratory failure and therefore require mechanical ventilation for a prolonged period of time may become so anxious when the weaning process begins that a psychiatric consultant is called for assistance. The anxiety generated by this attempt may so increase the metabolic demands and cardiac work of the patients that they are rendered physically incapable, at least transiently, of further weaning. No consultation problem presents more complicated psychophysiological difficulties.

Most physicians who are not respiratory specialists have become somewhat bewildered by the burgeoning technology of contemporary respiratory assistance devices. For this reason, the consultant must unconditionally accept the verdict of the referring physician who says that the patient is physiologically ready for weaning. A consulting psychiatrist who faces this problem fairly often will profit from reading Feeley's[6] very clear description of how a respiratory physician determines a patient's readiness for weaning. Basically, Feeley states that six criteria must be met before a patient is considered ready for weaning.

1. The patient must have a vital capacity of at least 10 ml to 15 ml per kilogram of body weight.
2. The maximum inspiratory force exerted by the patien† with a totally occluded tracheostomy tube should be greater th. $H_2O$. (This does not require the cooperation of the patient.)
3. The oxygen gradient, $AaDO_2^{1.0}$, should be less that 300 mm to 350 mm Hg.
4. The ratio of dead space to tidal volume ($V_D/V_T$) should be less than 0.6.
5. Cardiovascular stability is a must.
6. Metabolic balance must be present.

When these six criteria are met, the patient is hooked up to a T-piece or Brigg's attachment with a heated nebulizer, the inspired oxygen concentration is raised 10% higher than is required for controlled ventilation, and weaning begins. It is quite systematic and logical. Vital signs are taken every 5 minutes and after 20 minutes arterial blood gases are drawn. If the arterial oxygen pressure is less than 70 mm Hg or the pH is less than 7.25 the patient is put back on the ventilator. If not, weaning continues. In addition, many units will use positive end expiratory pressure (PEEP) or continuous positive airway pressure (CPAP). Another device available is intermittent mandatory ventilation (IMV). With the IMV system the number of controlled expirations per minute can be preset and all other breaths must be taken by the patient unassisted. Some physicians believe that the use of IMV by an anxious patient may promote smoother progress to independent breathing.

Another psychophysiological complexity in weaning the anxious patient from the ventilator stems from the fact that the lungs are the organ of relaxation. Most behavioral exercises aimed at relaxation encourage the subject to take slow, deep, easy breaths. This is one of the quickest and surest ways of inducing relaxation. This is precisely what patients with respiratory problems cannot do, however, and precisely what makes them so anxious. Whatever means for combating anxiety are used, this common one is unavailable.

Before proceeding with specific treatment, it is well for the consultant to think of a brief list of exclusions. Failure to wean may be due to hypoxemia or hypercapnia. Arterial blood gases can change and the consultant who fails to check them is doing both the patient and the consulting physician a disservice. If the arterial oxygen tension has not changed, the physician can quickly check the pH to make sure that it is not less than 7.25. Common causes for onset of hypercapnia might be an increase in the dead space, poor muscular function due to weakness or starvation, lack of coordination between the muscles of the diaphragm and the intercostal muscles, bronchospasm, tumor, tracheal stenosis, or a tracheostomy tube that is too narrow.[6]

Once the preliminaries have been checked, treatment can proceed. Treatment is best thought of as multimodal. Pharmacological agents can be quite helpful. A benzodiazepine can be administered prior to weaning periods or an antipsychotic such as haloperidol can be helpful if the patient is thought to be near actual panic. Patients can be very helpful in pointing out whether a drug is effective and which drugs are more helpful than others. In some cases it may be possible to use a mixture of nitrous oxide if the respiratory physician or anesthesiologist is present to begin administration. Hypnosis or relaxation techniques have often been helpful in distracting the patient from the weaning process itself. The instruction to breathe easily must be completely omitted from hypnotic suggestion, while concentration on either a tranquil scene such as a beach or a single concept (mantra) such as that proposed in Benson's method of the relaxation response can be encouraged.[7] The patient may be helped by the explanation that the weaning process can be expected to produce anxiety. Despondency as well as anxiety can become a problem impeding weaning. Specific mention is made in Chapter 10 of the depressed patient who experiences no progress in weaning.

**Cardiac arrest.** The ultimate complication, cardiac arrest, leaves distinctive marks on the minds of patients and staff. After cardiac arrest, the survivor almost invariably shows some natural increase in apprehension, even though it may not be verbalized. Most patients (two out of three in MGH studies) are amnesic for the arrest episode itself, but manifestations of emotional turmoil such as nightmares of violence and fires are common.[8,9] This turmoil is usually transient; the overall capacity of the survivor to adjust is high. Those who adjust poorly usually have prior histories of emotional disturbance.[9] The ability of patients to negotiate such extreme adversities successfully is considerable.[10] Cardiac arrest does not necessarily justify concomitant pessimism. Studies indicate that the occurrence of ventricular fibrillation in acute myocardial infarction bodes no worse for its survivor than for patients who have not had such a cardiac arrest.[11-13] Myerburg and others demonstrate that the frequency of recurrence of cardiac arrest can be successfully minimized.[14] Lemire and Johnson reviewed the course of 1,204 patients resuscitated in a general hospital, of whom 230 (19.1%) survived to discharge.[15] Regardless of the nature of the underlying disease, survival rates of those patients discharged were 74% surviving for 1 year, 59% for 2 years, and 51% for 3 years. A study of randomly chosen survivors showed that their functional capacity before and after resuscitation was unchanged. In general, the literature supports the emotional adaptability of survivors of cardiac arrest.[16-18] The consultant armed with these facts is likely to communicate more subjective, tranquil optimism in assisting the patient recovering from cardiac arrest. After arrest the patient's fear of recurrence often takes the form of anxiety at being left alone. Then emphasis on the watchdog value of the monitor is helpful along with the reminders from the staff that the nurses are never far from the patient.

In his book, *Life After Life*, Moody has stirred tremendous interest in the death experience with reports by survivors of near-death experiences like cardiac arrest and their reports of "out of body" pleasant experiences.[19] Based on the reports of these individuals, Moody has listed the following fifteen characteristic aspects described by such survivors: participating in an ineffable and indescribable experience; hearing bystanders pronounce them dead; feeling peaceful and quiet; hearing an unusual noise of some sort such as a buzzing, whistling, or windy sound; traveling through a dark space such as a tunnel; being out of the body; meeting with significant others such as family, God, or the saints, who are often viewed as spiritual rather than physical beings; encountering a very bright light; watching one's life pass in review before the mind's eye; approaching a border such as a fence, shore, or line; feeling a need to "come back" (often with regret); being reluctant to tell others despite their conviction of reality; feeling a dramatic change in their lives; having a new and fearless view of death; and being assured that elements of the story, such as words actually uttered by bystanders, can be corroborated. We have spoken with a number of MGH patients who have had experiences such as those described by Moody. The actual incidence of these experiences in all survivors of cardiac arrest is not known, but we estimate it at about 2%. It would also be inaccurate to give the impression that these "out of body" experiences are all pleasant. Moody describes survivors of attempted suicide who awaken with guilt and remorse after having been transported to a frightening place. We have not interviewed any of these individuals, but two patients who had altered mental states during cardiac arrest reported unpleasant experiences.

One woman described seeing all the dead members of her family awaiting her on the other side of a fence. She had no desire whatsoever to join them and resisted desperately their efforts to pull her through the fence. She "came back" with considerable relief.

A 32-year-old psychologist who had a cardiac arrest in the emergency ward experienced himself as a piece of meat in a supermarket being carried along a conveyor belt to the check-out counter. He found himself shouting that he would not be "checked out" and reentered consciousness in the emergency ward to the sight of several physicians and nurses dressed in white. "Jesus, there are a lot of people in this supermarket!" he exclaimed, a remark that mystified the medical team until he later explained it.

### Denial: the threat to sign out

Denial is often useful to the acutely ill person.[10] The ability to minimize or to exclude the threatening implications of one's disease is essential in order to avoid panic. If panic sets in, a person may get the urge to flee; this is the most common propellant leading acutely ill people toward the hospital exit. Although the threat to sign out can mean that the individual does not take the illness seriously (that is, is not frightened enough), the threat to sign out issued by an acutely ill patient should be assumed to be a reaction to panic unless proved otherwise. Because such persons are desperate, antagonism flares when efforts are made to detain them. This difficulty should be approached without threat and with heavy emphasis on the positive aspect of proposed treatment that will reverse the illness and restore health. A gentle approach is essential. For example, the psychiatrist might begin by saying, "I am not here to force you to do anything; what I ask is that you just hear me out." Such patients need to hear the truth—that they are seriously ill—expressed in direct but quiet, calm terms. The most important feature in the explanation, however, is the part that can quiet their panic—that is, that their illness is manageable. "Your heart is damaged and needs to be carefully monitored to avoid further damage and risk, but it's much like the process of cement setting. At first any kid can poke a finger through freshly poured cement, but as it firms up it can hold up a building. The same can be true of your heart muscle if you give it a chance to repair itself." As the patient calms down, other questions aimed at decreasing fear (as described in the section on fear and anxiety) can be asked: Does the person know anyone else with a similar illness? How does he picture the illness he has? Family members should be informed and mobilized. If calm is achieved, it should not be expected to last. The patient should be medicated promptly, according to the guidelines suggested in the section on fear and anxiety.

**Other common management problems presented by the acutely ill person**

**Refusal to obey the rules.** Rule violators harass physicians and nurses by their refusal to comply with limitations—eating while under restrictions of no eating, getting out of bed when confined to it, smoking, and the like. Such individuals often have long-standing conflicts about dependency. For example, many dependent people when placed in a dependent position react by hyperindependent behavior. Therapeutically, the physician tries to restore their sense of control wherever possible and to avoid fights over limits. For example, "Look, no one here really has any intention of playing policeman. We can only explain the nature of your illness and how to make it better and after that we depend on you to let us know how we can get the job done." On some issues the staff can bend and on others compromise is medically contraindicated. At best it is usually helpful to let patients know that no one can make them do anything they do not want to do anyway. For more specific limits, a sample statement might include: "Your Pronestyl and Garamycin should be taken on schedule for your own safety, but your Valium and Colace can be postponed or refused." Any statement is meant to reassure patients that they are respected and that the treatment regimen is not intended as a put-down. At times gentle humor, exaggerated in the direction of acknowledging what the patient can do, can diffuse some of the anger and soften conflict when used naturally. For example, "If finally you have to stand up to void, fine; let us know. But you're forbidden to do a handstand from your intravenous pole until we can sell tickets to watch it."

**Hostility.** Hostile patients are difficult and complicated to manage. Angry persons are threatened persons; they fight because they feel endangered or because they feel demeaned. If they have just entered the hospital or if they have suffered a setback, patients may be frightened. In this case all the methods for dealing with fear come into play. On the other hand, a general anger and resentment about being sick are common. The patient who is not irritable at some point during the illness is unusual. If a person launches a tirade against the hospital food, the nurses (especially the night staff), and the house staff and then searches for other targets, the physician should patiently hear out the gripes and take them seriously. It can also be helpful, after listening, to insert a little sympathy into the conversation. For example, "I'm sorry to hear that you've been having such a tough time; even if everything were perfect, it's a rotten break to be sick at all." Some patients may take this opportunity to verbalize the feelings of "why me?" that occur naturally in response to the damage done by illness. Sometimes past experiences can be elicited with a question like "Have you had bad experiences with other hospitals and physicians?" In more complicated instances, some persons relive the turbulent circumstances of a sick parent. Maintaining a hostile stance can also serve to protect a person from lapsing into profound despondency. Under such circumstances hostility can be prolonged and the psychotherapeutic intervention more time-consuming.

**Dependence.** Dependent patients, who, under the threat of hospitalization, regress to a helpless state and plead by word or action to be fed, comforted, reassured, and pampered, are among the most irritating to physicians and nurses. Call lights are on constantly and family visits are an occasion for displays of almost abject helplessness. Many of these individuals, resenting their own dependency needs and the caregivers they feel so dependent on, are hostile; pleading insatiable requests can be replaced by angry insatiable demands. This behavior is another manifestation of how threatened these patients are by the illness, especially if they fear being driven into inescapable dependency. The fear of illness itself promotes regressive tendencies in such individuals. The principles of dealing with fear and anxiety can be used successfully here. It is important to learn what the illness means to such persons and why their conception of it is frightening. Like the rule violators, these individuals often do not perform activities expected of them. Staff members, often angrier than they realize at such patients, hesitate to be firm or to make demands because when they do it seems more like an expresson of anger than an expression of concern. The demands are therefore not made and the regression becomes worse. The consultant can emphasize that reinforcement of limits and steady mobilization are essential to the patient's health and reassuring words can be aimed at fear of illness without encouraging further despondency. For example, "It is necessary at this point that you begin getting out of bed. I know how frightening it must be to try to take a few steps, but this is essential for you to get better. You'll be all right. Don't be afraid."

### Rites of passage: transfer out of the ICU setting

Klein and others[20] have documented the dramatic rise in catecholamine excretion in coronary patients on the day of transfer out of the CCU. Passage from intensive care is generally both bad and good news—bad, because it means reduced coverage and observation; good, because it means that the patient's condition is sufficiently improved to warrant graduation from the ICU setting. Both aspects must be addressed. Preparation for transfer is best done soon, the earlier the better, so that the patient clearly learns the association between improvement and release from the ICU. If the date can be predicted, so much the better—hopefully it can be made definite at least 24 hours before the fact. Warnings about less frequent checks and fewer nurses should be explicit, as well as the assurance that these security supports will no longer be necessary. Patients interviewed about their transfer experiences gratefully remember being reassured by the congratulations of the staff on their graduation from the ICU.

### STRESS ON THE STAFF OF THE INTENSIVE CARE UNIT

The emotional stress that comes in the wake of critical illness holds more than the patient in its grip. Delivery of intensive care in modern units proceeds at a hectic pace, under high tension, and usually in the midst of pain, delirium, and death. What happens to the personnel working in such settings? Recently several studies have been devoted to this question.[21-28]

**Specific stresses.** At MGH the direct study of CCU nurses began in 1968. Like most intensive care personnel these nurses were especially perceptive and astute in detecting the emotional problems of their patients. With practice they also became skillful in indentifying their own stresses and emotional responses. These nurses were asked to rate by questionnaire the most difficult stresses associated with their work.[25] A partial list of individual ratings is included in Table 17-2. Each stress was given a score of 1, 2, or 3 according to each nurse's judgement of its frequency and of the magnitude of the item. The sum of scores for both measures gives the "conflict score" of each item.

**Atmosphere assessment scale.** In 1972 an effort was made to study the relationship between unit morale and specific CCU events such as

**Table 17-2.** Combined frequency and severity scores of conflicts rated by CCU nurses (n = 16)*

| Conflict score | Item |
|---|---|
| 57 | Heavy lifting. |
| 46 | Balloon research. |
| 44 | The scheduling is unpredictable. |
|  | Feeling the weight of personal responsibility. |
| 42 | The family is overwrought, anxious. |
| 40 | The pace is too hectic. |
| 38 | The families annoy the staff. |
| 36 | The severity of the patient's illness or prognosis. |
|  | Not enough time off, poor distribution of time in scheduling. |
| 35 | Personal feeling of insecurity. |
| 34 | Patient's behavior or personality is troublesome. |
| 31 | Personality conflicts with other nurses. |
| 30 | Elderly patients are depressing. |
|  | Physicians not available when wanted. |
|  | Poor communication with physicians. |

*From Cassem, N. H. and Hackett, T. P.: Sources of tension for the CCU nurse. Copyright © 1972, American Journal of Nursing Company. Reproduced with permission from American Journal of Nursing, August, Vol. 78 No. 8.

---

**FOUR SUBSCALES OF THE ATMOSPHERE ASSESSMENT SCALE**

| Anxiety | Discouragement |
|---|---|
| tense | discouraging |
| frightening | sad |
| overwhelming | blue |
| uptight | heavy |

| Conflict | Harmony |
|---|---|
| frustrating | smooth |
| in conflict | coordinated |
| hostile | together |
| irritating | harmonious |
| complaining | close . |
| catty | |

From Cassem, N.H.: What is behind our masks? AORN J. **20**:79-92, 1974.

ATMOSPHERE ASSESSMENT SCALE
(Rapid first impressions are best. Place an X on the line at the
number which seems to best convey your impression.)

Admissions _____        Census:                      Date _____

Discharges _____            Start of shift _____    Initials _____

Transfers _____             End of shift _____      (circle) _____ shift = D-E-N

                                                          _____ perm-float

Today the unit seems or feels:

|  | None 1 | Some 2 | Moderate 3 | 4 | Much 5 | 6 | Extreme 7 |
|---|---|---|---|---|---|---|---|
| 1. Tense |  |  |  |  |  |  |  |
| 2. Smooth |  |  |  |  |  |  |  |
| 3. Frightening |  |  |  |  |  |  |  |
| 4. A fast pace |  |  |  |  |  |  |  |
| 5. Discouraging |  |  |  |  |  |  |  |
| 6. Pleasant |  |  |  |  |  |  |  |
| 7. Relaxed |  |  |  |  |  |  |  |
| 8. Coordinated |  |  |  |  |  |  |  |
| 9. Frustrating |  |  |  |  |  |  |  |
| 10. Friendly |  |  |  |  |  |  |  |

**Fig. 17-2.** The Atmosphere Assessment Scale used in a study done in 1972 to assess the effect that death and other events have on CCU staff members. The adjective checklist was filled out by nurses on each shift studied. Additional characteristics, numbers 11 to 30, are: lively, in conflict, apathetic, overwhelming, hostile, cheerful, irritating, a disaster, together, sad, complaining, up tight, secure, blue, harmonious, heavy, catty, boring, close, and the way I like it. Space is also available for comments (arrests, emergencies, DNRs). (From Cassem, N. H.: What is behind our masks? AORN J. **20:**79-92, 1974.)

cardiac arrest. In order to do this the Atmosphere Assessment Scale (AAS) was devised.[29] The AAS is an adjective checklist filled out by nurses on each shift studied. Figure 17-2 gives an example of this scale. The scale contains four subscales: anxiety, discouragement, conflict, and harmony (see box).

Figure 17-3 displays AAS scores as the expected death of a young coronary patient approached. This man was a 34-year-old man whose grandparents had died in their fifties, his parents in their forties, a brother at 41, and two sisters at 38 and 41. They all died of coronary heart disease. He had had angina since age 14, but with this hospital admission he had experienced his first myocardial infarction, a large

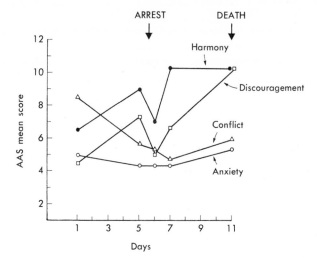

**Fig. 17-3.** AAS mean scores of CCU nurses' reactions to an expected death.

anterior lesion, that left him with a large aneurysm and in cardiogenic shock. The intraaortic balloon pump rescued him from shock, but only temporarily, for angiography revealed that he had severe inoperable triple vessel disease. Figure 17-2 shows that after the first episode of ventricular tachycardia arrest, from which he was resuscitated, staff discouragement scores rose steadily. The staff experienced feelings of despondency because they knew he was dying and felt helpless to do anything about it. Despite the significant elevation in feelings of discouragement, the feeling of harmonious group action was unaffected, or possibly even enhanced. Nevertheless, the fatal implications of heart disease affect staff as well as patient. This fact cannot be disregarded in intensive care settings.

**Nature of the ICU nurse.** Are ICU nurses different from nurses who work in other settings? Gentry and others[26] compared ICU nurses with personnel in non-ICU settings and found that although they did not show any distinctive personality patterns on psychological tests, ICU nurses reported significantly more depression, hostility, and anxiety than non-ICU nurses. We regard this as a factor of the setting rather than as an innate difference in the personalities of the individuals involved.

Some difficult conflicts are also generated by the ICU, intensified more by the setting than by the personalities of the individuals involved. ICU nurses are often viewed as elite prima donnas and sometimes resented by non-ICU personnel, who may well be envious of the special status of the intensive care person. These feelings are critical whenever patients are transferred out of the ICU to the regular floor. Criticisms about the way orders are written or not written are usually due to such feelings of competitive envy. These emotions can be mitigated if there is open discussion between the two units. When there is little or no opportunity for communication, bad feelings usually intensify.

### Group meetings for ICU personnel

Group meetings are an excellent method for dealing with poor morale and for helping individuals on the staff to support one another in their very difficult work. Simon and Whitely[28] describe stages in the development of such a group. In the early phase the group meeting tends to be programmed with scheduled formal content and emphasis on didactic information coming from the leader. In the middle phase

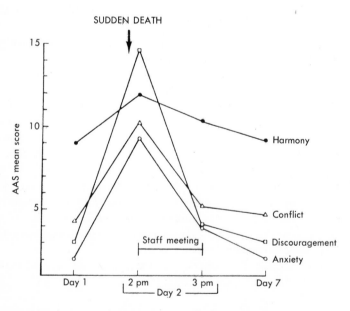

**Fig. 17-4.** Morale scores of CCU nursing staff after a sudden death on morning rounds, with assessments before and after a staff meeting.

tensions and anxieties tend to emerge as the feelings of participants are stirred into awareness. At this stage the staff is satisfied to let the meeting content develop spontaneously, although fluctuation in the group between resistance and intense feelings is characteristic. In the late stage, informality, spontaneity, openness, and high-level participation are characteristic in an atmosphere of trust.

The value of such meetings receives some suggestive validation from an MGH experience with a sudden, unexpected death in the CCU. Figure 17-4 presents the AAS scores on the afternoon following a sudden cardiac arrest of a 51-year-old man admitted on the preceding night with a routine inferior myocardial infarction. His cardiac arrest occurred during morning rounds. Instant efforts at resuscitation progressed smoothly, but failed. Postmortem examination confirmed ventricular rupture. All subscale scores taken approximately 5 hours later were the highest recorded for a 15 month period. The value of a 1 hour staff meeting in reducing anxiety, depression, despondency, and conflict scores among the staff is shown in Fig. 17-4. Scores indicated ICU staff tension returned to the levels they were at before the cardiac arrest.

Other explicit difficulties that arise in dealing with the approaching death of an irreversibly ill patient are treated in Chapter 32. Working with intensive care unit staff is an extremely rewarding experience for the liaison psychiatrist.

### Recommendations for maintaining ICU morale

The following practical recommendations for the maintenance of unit morale may further this worthy cause.

1. Group reactions to ICU crisis are best handled in group meetings. Even 15 minutes taken at the time of report can be helpful for this.
2. The steps required for successful group resolution of conflict could be summarized as: (a) identification and acknowledgment of feelings, (b) sharing of and reaction to these feelings by the group, (c) review of the experience with criticism, support, and praise, (d) integration of what is learned with application to future experience.
3. The closer the meetings are to the site of action, the better. Personnel must be free to come and go at any moment.
4. Units function better where a strong medical director is present who can work in close conjunction with the head nurse. It is impossible to overemphasize the truth of Safer's insight that

intensive care unit personnel are happier under a benevolent dictator than they are under a disorganized or passive democracy.[30] This physician-leader must have special competence in critical care and the strength to keep the ICU staff from being caught between physicians of various disciplines who may be feuding over who is in charge of the patient.

5. A quiet, reasonably secluded place with a coffee pot is very helpful to unit morale.

6. Families should be made into allies wherever possible. This can reduce their function as distractions or obstacles to care. They should be allowed to share in the realities of the intensive care setting, whether these be optimistic or tragic.

## SUMMARY

Intensive care settings reveal humanity at its best and at its worst. This is as true for the staff as it is for the patients. Those who serve in intensive care settings in a true sense risk their own lives, their own feelings, their own self-esteem, and their own self-respect. Those who face these risks receive opportunities to mature, while those who avoid them must face the dehumanization of themselves or of their patients. The unit that faces these responsibilities together does best.

## REFERENCES

1. McKegney, F. P.: Intensive care syndrome: definition, treatment and prevention of new "disease of medical progress," Conn. Med. **30**:633-636, 1966.
2. Cassem, N. H., and Hackett, T. P.: Psychiatric consultation in a coronary care unit, Ann. Intern. Med. **75**:9-14, 1971.
3. Greenblatt, D. J., and Shader, R. I.: *Benzodiazepines in clinical practice*, New York, 1974, Raven Press.
4. Fox, J. H., Topel, J. L., and Huckman, M. S.: Dementia in the elderly—a search for treatable illnesses, J. Gerontol. **30**:557-564, 1975.
5. Jacobs, J. W., Bernhard, M. R., Delgado, A., and Strain, J. J.: Screening for organic mental syndromes in the medically ill, Ann. Intern. Med. **86**:40-46, 1977.
6. Feeley, T. W.: Problems in weaning patients from ventilators, Resident and Staff Physician, **22**:51-55, August, 1976.
7. Benson, H. A.: The relaxation response, New York, 1975, William Morrow & Co., Inc.
8. Druss, R. G., and Kornfeld, D. S.: The survivors of cardiac arrest, J.A.M.A. **201**:291-296, 1967.
9. Dlin, B. M., Stern, A., and Poliakoff, S. J.: Survivors of cardiac arrest, Psychosomatics **15**:61-67, 1974.
10. Hackett, T. P., Cassem, N. H., and Wishnie, H. A.: The coronary care unit: an

appraisal of its psychological hazards, N. Engl. J. Med. **279**:1365-1370, 1968.

11. Dobson, M., Tattersfield, A. E., Adler, M. W., and McNicol, M. W.: Attitudes in long-term adjustment of patients surviving cardiac arrest, Br. Med. J. **3**:207-212, 1971.

12. Lawrie, B. M.: Long-term survival after ventricular fibrillation complicating acute myocardial infarction, Lancet **2**:1085-1087, 1969.

13. McNamee, B. T., and others: Long-term prognosis following ventricular fibrillation in acute ischemic heart disease, Br. Med. J. **4**:204-206, 1970.

14. Myerburg, R. J., and others: Long-term antiarrhythmic therapy in survivors of prehospital cardiac arrest, J.A.M.A. **238**:2621-2624, 1977.

15. Lemire, J. G., and Johnson, A. L.: Is cardiac resuscitation worthwhile? N. Engl. J. Med. **286**:970-972, 1972.

16. Minuck, M., and Perkins, R.: Long-term study of patients successfully resuscitated following cardiac arrest, Anesth. Analg. **49**:115-118, 1970.

17. White, R. L., and Liddon, S. C.: Ten survivors of cardiac arrest, Psychiatr. Med. **3**:219-225, 1972.

18. Hackett, T. P.: The Lazarus complex revisited, Ann. Intern. Med. **76**:135-136, 1972.

19. Moody, R. A., Jr.: Life after life, Atlanta, 1975, Mockingbird Books.

20. Klein, R. F., and others: Transfer from a coronary care unit: some adverse responses, Arch. Intern. Med. **122**:104-108, 1968.

21. Koumans, A.J.R.: Psychiatric consultation in an intensive care unit, J.A.M.A. **194**:633, 1965.

22. Vreeland, R., and Ellis, G. L.: Stresses on the nurse in an intensive care unit, J.A.M.A. **208**:332, 1969.

23. Gardam, J.E.D.: Nursing stresses in the intensive care unit, J.A.M.A. **208**:2336, 1969.

24. Hay, D., and Oken, D.: The psychological stresses of intensive care unit nursing, Psychosom. Med. **34**:109, 1972.

25. Cassem, N. H., and Hackett, T. P.: Sources of tension for the CCU nurse, Am. J. Nurs. **72**:1426, 1972.

26. Gentry, W. D., Foster, S. B., and Froehling, S.: Psychologic response to situational stress in intensive and nonintensive nursing, Heart Lung **31**:793, 1972.

27. Cassem, N. H., and Hackett, T. P.: Stress on the nurse and therapist in the intensive care unit and the coronary care unit, Heart Lung **4**:252-259, 1975.

28. Simon, N. M., and Whiteley, S.: Psychiatric consultation with MICU nurses: the consultation conference as a working group, Heart Lung **6**:497-504, 1977.

29. Cassem, N. H.: What is behind our masks? AORN J. **20**:79-92, 1974.

30. Safer, P.: Quoted in Hosp. Trib., vol. 9, March 17, 1975, p. 20.

# 18

# Repetitive dialysis

**HARRY S. ABRAM**

Since the early 1960s when I began to work with patients suffering terminal renal failure, I have been repeatedly asked by nephrologists in one form or another, "What is so special psychologically about the reactions of these patients to hemodialysis? They respond no differently to their disease than patients with other chronic illnesses (for example, those with diabetes, heart failure, and so forth)." The question in itself is a revealing one and can be answered at various levels. It shows that the nephrologist has insight into the process of chronic illness but denies the unique stresses associated with dialysis. Indeed, understanding the psychological aspects of this illness and its treatment does throw light on how patients with other chronic diseases feel and react because it highlights their plight so vividly. In addition, there is no doubt that the treatment of terminal renal failure with repetitive hemodialysis has brought to the forefront an entirely new perspective on the role of modern medical advances as they relate to life-extending technologies, particularly to the maintenance of life through artificial means. Thus, to regard this form of treatment as similar to the use of insulin for diabetes or digitalis for heart failure (in spite of the many similarities) is to deny the impact of the prolongation of life by a mechanical process that raises psychosocial and ethical issues of major proportions.

## CONFLICTS OF BEING MACHINE-DEPENDENT

Central to understanding patient response to chronic dialysis is the consideration of the patient's adaptation to a life dependent on a machine, the artificial kidney or hemodialyzer, and the conflicts this dependence imposes. In this discussion I use various terms interchangably and in various combinations: dialysis, chronic dialysis, repetitive dialysis, and hemodialysis. All refer to the same mode of treatment— the long-term treatment (life-long unless the patient acquires a renal transplant) for terminal kidney failure by mechanical means to remove human byproducts normally excreted by the healthy kidney. The

342

dialysis patient is occasionally called the "dialysand" in a manner similar to the "analysand" or the patient undergoing psychoanalysis. (The adage "urinalysis before psychoanalysis," speaking of the necessity to consider uremic symptoms in the differential diagnosis of the psychotic patient, was coined long before the advent of dialysis.) From a psychological viewpoint some have commented, perhaps in too farfetched a fashion, that "dialysis" is an unfortunate word choice in that it uses the syllable *dy-* ("die"), which conjures up the concept of death in a group of patients already concerned enough with dying.

The central conflict of the dialysand is the dilemma between independence and dependence. The dialysand receives two simultaneous but disparate messages. He is a sick person who must remain dependent on a rigorous treatment program requiring that he be "hooked" to a machine (the "artificial kidney" or dialyzer), that he restrict his dietary and fluid intake, and that he accept the side effects of his illness and its treatment (for example, weakness, lethargy, and malaise). For the other hours of each day he must react in an independent, responsible fashion as if he were totally healthy. Although I have obviously overdrawn and simplified the situation, the dialysand is torn between sickness and health, living and dying, and autonomy versus submission. How patients resolve these conflicts dramatically influences their overall adaptation to dialysis. Some respond favorably by accepting both horns of the dilemma. Others react with excessive dependence, begin to cherish the "sick role," and remove themselves from responsibilities and the mainstream of life. Still others to whom dependence is too frightening (perhaps because of its allure) rebel against the disease and its treatment. By looking at adaptation or maladaptation in the light of this conflict between dependence and independence, the consultant sees the noncompliant or rebellious patient as one threatened by dependence and responding with excessive independence. Patients who seem to give up and to be unable to return to their positions as functioning citizens involved in everyday life, on the other hand, have surrendered to dependence. Well-adjusted patients accept their illness and treatment (and the dependence associated with it) and remain independent when they are not on dialysis.

**Prolonging life versus prolonging dying**

When I first began working in this area I found it difficult to tease out and assess the potential psychosocial aspects of dialysis. Indeed if I had been aware of its multiple ramifications at that time I probably would have been overwhelmed and given up in discouragement. There were few psychiatrists with whom I could communicate and commiserate and little background information existed in the medical or psychiatric literature. Although the subject of dialysis seemed a logical extension of my clinical research with patients who had heart surgery (representing other forms of treatment with mechanical devices derived from modern technology such as the heart valve itself, extracorporeal circulation, the intensive care unit, and so forth), I gradually discovered that the stresses and experiences of dialysis took me in a direction all their own. The dialysand is preoccupied with the problems inherent in prolonged life rather than preoccupied with fears of death. Although the threat of death remains omnipresent, as it does with any patient who is physically ill or, indeed, with every human being, the dialysand's problem is that of returning to a life of normalcy when confronted with the restrictions of the condition. Put into more dramatic terms, the question becomes "When does the prolongation of living turn into the prolongation of dying?" Generally the life forces in the patient outweigh those of death and the patient learns to live with the complications of the illness and dialysis, adjusting both psychologically and physiologically to a lowered hematocrit, to the risks of intercurrent infections, to progressive arteriosclerosis, and to other associated pathological states. When the scale tilts in the other direction and suffering outbalances the gains of life, self-destructive behavior may become evident.

**Early observations of emotional complications**

Although there were no psychiatric reports in the early 1960s when dialysis first became clinically feasible, there was some brief discussion of emotional complications of dialysis published in medical literature. Brown and his coworkers[1] first described such disturbances in three patients on chronic dialysis. One patient developed "an acute paranoid psychosis" after 1 month on dialysis and another "a severe mental depression" after 2 months. The third patient became "apprehensive . . . very withdrawn and irritable" during the seventh month. He subsequently experienced "intense fear of night . . . insomnia," restlessness, anorexia, and "a general decline in well-being." Brown concluded that "any evidence of emotional instability, overt or latent, should be considered a contraindication for chronic dialysis" and recommended that "psychological and psychiatric testing . . . become an integral part of the preacceptance evaluation."

Gombos and associates[2] in a medical presentation in 1964 were probably the first to point out the psychological stresses associated with dialysis:

> Psychological factors were clearly recognized as important considerations in the treatment program. Not withstanding its life-prolonging promise, hemodialysis was felt to be an obviously stressful affair. Immediately apparent were potential stresses of disrupted work patterns, diminished income, and generally altered life activities. It was agreed that anxiety was a more subtle, but important, factor surrounding treatment by dialysis. The possibility arose that an individual might not be able to tolerate the degree of dependency necessitated by the program.

It is noteworthy that Gombos, a nephrologist working when dialysis first became clinically feasible, made the important observation that dependency played a major role in the patient's overall adaptation to the treatment regimen. Gombos also originally drew attention to dietary indiscretions and self-destructive behavior that have continued to be of clinical importance.

The first psychological study appeared a year later and also touched on many points that remain of interest to psychiatrists. Shea and her associates[3] observed that "the emotional reactions to the need for dialysis may represent the greatest obstacle to successful rehabilitation." All of the nine patients in their report "manifested significant psychological reactions while on the dialysis program." Two of these patients experienced schizophrenic-like episodes, another became psychotically depressed, and five of the remaining six had "severe neurotic depressive reactions." Shea additionally raised the crucial issues of suicide and dependence, as well as drawing attention for the first time to both denial and body image distortions in these patients.

> . . . they [the dialysands] try but never quite accept the shunt as part of themselves. The cannulae are constant reminders of their condition and their dependence on the dialyser. A few patients, either as an attempt to deny their illness or as an expression or a gesture of suicide, frequently subjected their cannulated arm to unnecessary trauma. . . .

> To one adolescent patient, the dialyser more clearly represented a threat to his identity. Being attached regularly precipitated a variety of hysterical outbursts. His ultimate loss of personal identity was graphically represented in figure drawings that were obtained shortly before his death. The mechanical appearing drawings consisted of a head and a torso with a cylindrical contour, quite similar in appearance to the dialyser.

As happened with the pioneering psychological articles in cardiac surgery, many of the main themes of the psychology of chronic dialysis were outlined in the above presentations and forgotten or unmentioned by later investigators. The conflict between depending on the regimen and striving toward independence in life emerged as the central issue.

**Body image and the machine**

Body image distortions must be recognized and studied if we are to understand the patient's adaptation to dialysis. They offer an avenue for gaining insight about the relationship between man and his survival by machine.[4] Much like the cardiac surgical patients in intensive care units following surgery, dialysands project and introject the external environment (in this instance the dialyzer) into their body schemata. Dialysands may unconsciously begin to think of themselves as machine-like and as an extension of the dialyzer. Or they may endow the dialyzer with human qualities and make it an extension of themselves. Although psychosis is rare in this group of patients, there is an interesting case report by Cooper[5] of a woman who developed hypomanic psychosis while on dialysis. In her psychotic state she personalized the dialyzer, expressing:

> . . . considerable hatred of the machine, endowing it with human motives. She expressed the view that the machine somehow knew of her dependence for her life on it and enjoyed, patronizingly and sometimes contemptuously because of her weakness, a feeling of total power.*

Cooper observed:

> The patient's attitude to the machine was exteriorized during the psychosis. She clearly resented her dependency upon it but also feared the pain it could bring her. She referred to it vehemently, almost as if it had human attributes, as "that hateful thing," "I despise it," and "I sometimes feel like destroying it." In fact, the patient threw a bottle of saline, intended for infusion, through a window; this can be seen as a symbolic act of destruction directed at the machine.*

Much of the material related to body image distortion is evident with dialysands only at an unconscious level and emerges in the rare patient on dialysis who becomes psychotic as in the case just described or in the rare patient who is also involved in intensive psychotherapy or psychoanalysis. Another source, however, is found in the fantasies or dreams of personnel who take care of the dialysand.

---

*Cooper, A. J.: Hypomanic psychosis precipitated by hemodialysis, Comp. Psychiatr. 8:168-174, 1967. By permission.

I can well remember my own reactions when first entering a dialysis unit. It was in the evening. The lights were turned down and there was an eerie glow from the television set that each patient was watching. The patients were connected to their dialyzers via plastic cannulae filled with blood running into and then out of the dialyser. Additionally I could hear the faint humming and swishing of these artificial kidneys. My overall impression was that these patients were being rejuvenated or brought back to life. At that time (the early 1960s) a television series entitled "The Invaders" depicted aliens from another planet. They resembled humans but each night had to be connected to electronic devices to restore their energy. The dialysis unit scene did not seem dissimilar and the thought that dialysands were also not entirely human entered my mind. Litin[6] also observed that some dialysands had fantasies of themselves as Frankenstein-like monsters with tubes in their necks similar to their external cannulae or shunts.

There is also interesting symbolism related to the dialyzer-as-placenta with the arterial and venous cannulae representing the umbilical vessels. Indeed some patients curl into the fetal position while on dialysis.

Another common theme is that of the dialysand as zombie or not totally alive. This motif has a quality of Lazarus arising from the dead, not unlike the heart and kidney transplant patients who believe that they are reborn. It is evident that a blend of realism and symbolism exists, for in truth the dialysands would be dead if it were not for a machine, and in this sense they have risen from the dead. The sallow color of the dialysand adds to the fantasy of being the "walking dead."

> A minister shortly after starting dialysis gave a sermon on "the rather singular story of Jesus raising someone from the dead" and described himself as a present-day Lazarus saved by "the miracle . . . of advanced medical science."

Another patient[7] spoke of his complexion as a "half-olive color" and spoke of himself as looking "like a candidate for a downtown morgue." He also humanized the dialyzer and fantasized conversations with it.

> I used to think if it [the machine] could talk, it would say emphatically, "Do you love me?" and I would say, emphatically, "No!" Then it would say, "but do you respect me?" and I would shout, "Yes! Yes I do!"

Another dialysand once stated,

"We're sort of zombies. . . . sort of close to death . . . I guess we're like the living dead. . . . someone who should be dead but who isn't. . . . We're sort of just marking time. In essence we're dead anyway. I'll never have the feeling of being a whole human being. Even if I have a [kidney] transplant one of these days, I'll never get over the feeling I'm already dead."

At one point he wondered if he could be held responsible for murder if he killed someone, since in essence he was "already dead" and really only kept alive by artificial means. He described dialysis as similar to being given a death warrant that was signed and dated. At one point he remarked, "What a piece of junk I've become!" as if his body were becoming the dialyser.

Again in a science fiction manner patients may think of themselves as a robot or an android (a robot who appears human). One dialysand, for example, described himself as "half-robot, half-machine"—an interesting slip instead of "half-man, half-machine" or "half-robot, half-man" as Borgenicht,[8] who discusses the patient, noted. He also described a patient whose physician told her, "If you learn to run the machine, you'll get closer to it." To this suggestion she replied bitterly, "I don't want to be buddy-buddy with the machine . . . It's a machine . . . if it does its job, I'll do mine."

Concerning distorted body imagery Kemph[9] described a patient who "depicted himself quite graphically as a broken man, a disjointed man, jerked about and completely controlled by the straps to his arms. At this time he had a blood pressure apparatus on one arm and the dialyzer on the other."

## LOSSES DUE TO RENAL FAILURE
### Loss of physical function and bodily integrity

At this point I shall shift from problems of conflict and adaptation to the multiple losses experienced by the dialysand. Obviously these subjects interrelate and blend. In discussing the loss of bodily integrity the previously described body image distortion comes into play. As in any chronic illness, patients with end-stage renal failure face the loss of a functioning healthy body. I stress the concept of loss in these patients because depression is so prevalent and, indeed, may be universal. In my experience depression is most easily understood from the viewpoint of loss—whether it be the loss of a loved one, the loss of self-esteem, the loss of approval, or another loss. For the dialysand, loss of bodily function relates to a loss of autonomy and the loss of ability to perform in an independent manner. Weakness, malaise, lethargy, debilitation, and the threat of other physical complications, with the ever-present ultimate possibility of death, all represent losses to the dialysand.

**Loss of family stability and economic security**

There are also other losses associated with dialysis, such as those brought about by diminished sexual functioning. Shambaugh,[10] in his group work with spouses of patients receiving dialysis, was the first to emphasize the inherent problems involved in such situations, especially the problem of hostility toward the dialyzed partner.

> They [the spouses of the dialysands] had to cope with many stresses including their marital partners' severe medical complications, possible death, and regressive behavior. In response to these unhappy changes they reacted with intense feelings of deprivation and primitive urges toward psychological closeness to their partners and with enormous hostility, often giving rise to intense guilt. Those who operated the artificial kidney machine had their infantile fantasies confirmed in reality, for their partners were likened to their machines and could be destroyed.

As an example, "a husband fantasied taking an axe to the kidney machine."

The ultimate fate of Shambaugh's group therapy was disastrous in that he found it necessary to disband the group. Apparently the hostility could not be handled effectively and the group's use of denial was threatened to the point where the meetings had to cease. The finding that the healthy spouse not infrequently had extramarital affairs may well have added to the group's anxiety and undermined its denial. Until recently group therapy with dialysands and their families has not been common, perhaps because of Shambaugh's results. In general I have found that dialysands do not seek each other out as do patients who have had colostomies or cardiac operations. This is not to say that dialysis "consumer" organizations have not been effective in legislative changes to make dialysis available through governmental funding. Indeed they have; but this is a separate issue.

Borgenicht also describes marital discord and the development of murderous impulses toward the dialyzed spouse.[8]

> In one case example a dialysand died after her husband "used the wrong dialysate in the dialysis machine." Following this event the husband disappeared with the wife of another dialysand for whom she had responsibility. The two healthy spouses met when they started driving together to Cleveland several times weekly to the dialysis clinics with their ill mates.

In another example a repartee between husband and wife demonstrates vividly the underlying hostility:

*Wife:* Roll over, please, I have to take your blood pressure.
*Patient:* (joking and addressing remarks to observer) She's always pestering me.
*Wife:* Come on, dear, it will just take a second.
*Patient:* (joking to wife) Can't you let a guy sleep. I'm going to have to get a new nurse.
*Wife:* (joking to husband) Turn over or I'm going to pull the plug out of the machine and then I'll get a new husband.

Role reversal occurs within the family structure of the dialysand when the husband must take time from his work to dialyze his wife or when he is the patient, and the wife must assume financial responsibility and be away from the home during the day to support the family. Under such circumstances, economic as well as emotional strain is placed on the family and the standard of living may drop. Even though governmental funding has now made dialysis available for most patients with end-stage renal failure, the illness and its treatment remain catastrophic in nature and take their toll on patient and family. Sullivan[11] has also shown that dialysis in itself is full-time work and that to expect patients or their families to maintain occupations outside the home may be unrealistic.

**Loss of sexual function**

Ever since dialysis became clinically feasible, there has been anecdotal evidence of sexual dysfunction, especially of reduced potency in men. Even before dialysis there were endocrinoligical studies of the effects of azotemia on spermatogenesis and gonadal functioning. In the early 1970s two reports appeared that specifically addressed the subject of sexual dysfunction in the dialysis population. With several co-workers I conducted one study[12] on reduced potency in thirty-two male married patients either on chronic dialysis or after receiving renal hemografts. We conducted our study at a local Veteran's Administration Hospital. In addition to interviewing our sample population with a structured interview directed at obtaining a detailed sexual history, we talked with eleven wives. Our definition of reduced potency was a decrease in frequency of sexual intercourse to at least 50% when compared to the patient's premorbid (before end-stage renal failure) state. We found that 20% of the patients experienced no reduction in potency after the onset of chronic renal disease, dialysis, or kidney transplantation; 45% had reduced sexual potency after the onset of renal disease; and 35% suffered reduced potency after the institution of dialysis. Forty percent showed an improvement in sexual functioning after beginning dialysis treatment. Most patients were interested in and cooperative with the study. They looked on reduced potency as if it were a function of physical factors. They made such statements as, "When you're sick, sex is the farthest thing from your mind." They noted that sexual functioning was at its lowest ebb after a dialysis run. As one patient remarked, he felt figuratively and literally washed out under such circumstances. On the other hand, the wives were more defensive and generally estimated that sexual intercourse occurred less frequently than reported by their husbands. They typically replied with such questions as, "I'm really interested in whether my husband lives or dies. Why are you asking about our sex life?" As noted, 40% with reduced potency improved after transplantation, but at least one such patient expressed anxiety about damaging his transplanted kidney during intercourse. The other report by Levy[13] was a questionnaire study based on mailing to a national organization of several thousand dialysis patients. His findings with both males and females were similar to ours, that is, a general deterioration in sexual functioning. Obviously this problem is a complex one in need of further study. Physical factors cannot be separated from psychological factors in the etiology of these sexual difficulties.

**Loss, depression, and suicide**

Taking into account all of these losses naturally leads to a consideration of depression and the occurrence of suicide in this group of patients. Depression is practically a universal phenomenon among dialysands—depression related to multiple losses, all of which ultimately boil down to loss of autonomy and eventually to loss of life itself. The existential question is: When does the prolongation of life become the prolongation of death? Under such circumstances and in such a predicament the question of suicide becomes understandable and even legitimate. The subject of suicide in dialysis patients warrants far more attention in medical literature than it has had. Our study[14] on the subject is the only one to appear, although anecdotal evidence can be found beginning with the clinical reports of Gombos[2] mentioned previously. I suspect that this lack of attention is related to confusion in defining suicide in this particular patient population. For example, is it considered suicidal when patients will not adhere to their dietary restrictions and die because of this behavior? In discussing an experience with a patient requiring dialysis Rubini[15] noted,

> We have had one suicide. He was a chap who, as a child, didn't like his teacher or his parents. As an adult he didn't like his bosses; they all told him what to do. After he was dialysed two years, he didn't like dialysis either, as we tried to tell him what to do also. He picked the Easter weekend. He went on a tremendous feed, almost a Roman orgy. He started off at the San Francisco docks, where he purchased a number of kinds of shellfish and a jug of chianti. He went home, put a suckling pig on the spit; he partook of all these goodies and more. When admonished by his visiting mother, he retorted he knew better than his doctors how to take care of himself. He returned to the hospital with severe hyperkalemia, suffered a cardiac arrest and he died.

Clearly such behavior contains a self-destructive element. Whether termed suicidal or not, it fits into a spectrum from active to passive suicide. At one end of this spectrum are those patients who actively seek self-destruction through hanging, gunshot, cutting, and so forth. In the spectrum's midrange are those patients who, like the man just described, bring about their own death through a behavior inconsistent with maintaining life. This includes those patients who refuse to be dialyzed. At the passive suicide end of the spectrum are those patients who passively fail to comply with their regimen—patients who do not adhere to their diets or take care of their shunts. I look on all such behavior as somewhat suicidal. Yet there are others who do not agree with this formulation. Many prefer to view noncompliance with the regimen as a desire not to conform totally that is unrelated to self-destructive tendencies. There are undoubtedly multiple levels of understanding such behavior (for example, denial of illness, rebellion against the regimen and the attendant enforced dependency), but to state that patients do not stay with a treatment program essential to their life just because they get "tired of it" or "don't like it" seems psychologically naive. Even before our suicide study, newspaper articles appeared describing patients who withdrew from dialysis programs. One such item,[16] entitled "It's Time to Die, Ailing Man Decides" from the Associated Press, described a dialysand with a "wasting body and . . . demoralized mind" who decided, "I'm taking myself off the machine . . I'm ready to die." It noted that "a day later, he signed a waiver removing himself from treatment." Later he remarked "When I signed the waiver I knew what kind of symbol that was, like signing your own [death] certificate. . . ." In this example and in other clinical instances, there are obvious indications that the patients want control over their lives and deaths rather than to surrender to the ravages of disease, despair, and suffering.

In our study we sent questionnaires to dialysis centers throughout the United States requestioning information concerning suicidal behavior among their patients. At that time I was struggling with the suicides of two patients in the dialysis program at the University of Virginia. One exsanguinated after severing her external shunt. Another gorged himself and imbibed to the point where he literally drowned in his own fluids. I subsequently became aware of two similar situations at another institution and, with the help of Gordon Moore from the psychiatric division of the Mayo Clinic, we conducted our questionnaire study. Receiving replies from 127 of 201 dialysis centers we discovered that of 3,478 dialysands, twenty patients died following active suicidal attempts (overdoses, severing shunts, and so forth), seventeen similar attempts were unsuccessful, twenty-two patients withdrew from dialysis programs and subsequently died, 117 died as a result of not following the regimen, nine died from "accidental" causes that may have been suicidal in nature, and there were 107 such accidents that did not result in death. The number of deaths from active suicide and from withdrawal from programs indicates that the incidence of suicide is significantly higher in this group of patients than in the normal population. The suicide rate of forty-two (twenty active suicides and twenty-two withdrawals) patients out of 3,478 dialysands (1.21%) is significantly higher than the normal population's suicide rate of approximately 1 per every 10,000 people (.01%). If suicide is interpreted more broadly to include the 117 who died from not adhering to the regimen, the death rate is approximately 4.6% (161 patients out of 3,478).

The failure of medical professionals to recognize self-destructive behavior in this group of patients is of interest to me. From the beginning of our study, we received comments on the questionnaires such as, "You're barking up the wrong tree looking for suicide in dialysis patients. They kill themselves no more often than anybody else." Others have asked if the suicide rate is higher than in patients with other chronic or terminal physical illness. It is revealing that there is so little available data. Farberow[17] studied suicide among patients with cardiorespiratory illnesses and with malignant neoplasms. With the former group he noted that patients with emotional disturbances and with poor relationships with hospital staff and family were more likely to commit suicide. They also were more likely to be considered problem patients because of their dependent behavior. Dorpat[18] observed that there was a high incidence of suicide among patients with peptic ulcer, cardiovascular disease, and malignancies. Other studies are needed to verify or disagree with our figures on the suicide rate among dialysis patients.

No matter what the figures, the psychiatric consultant is confronted with the clinical and ethical problem of dealing with patients suffering a fatal illness who contemplate and carry through with suicidal acts. I have come to the conclusion, that dialysands who kill themselves may well be doing it for justifiable reasons and that, indeed, physicians may be helpless from a clinical viewpoint to do anything about it. Seneca's[19] argument in 1 B.C. for suicide seems to hold remarkably true today for this group of patients and for other patients with chronic fatal illness:

> I will not raise my hand against myself on account of pain, for so to die is to be conquered. But if I know I must suffer without hope of relief, I will depart, not through fear of pain itself, but because it prevents all for which I would live.

### Problem of denial

As in all phases of adaptation to illness, denial plays a prominent and pervasive role not only for the patient but for family and hospital personnel. Psychiatrists must learn to work with or around this defense or they find themselves at times unwittingly representing a threat to the successful use of denial by the staff as well as by the patient. They are told, "There's nothing unusual or stressful about dialysis. Why should it be of interest to a psychiatrist?" As dialysis has become more of an accepted procedure, this form of denial has become less necessary and those involved with it have been able to look at it more objectively.

The description of denial by patients in dialysis by Short and Wilson[20] remains, in my opinion, a classic one:

> The capacity for denial in these patients is phenomenal, but what are they denying? Previously, it was pointed out that these patients accept their conditions and the inevitability of their outcome. What is denied is that it is happening now. When their bones become bowed from osteomalacia, and they go from a cane to a walker, and then to a wheelchair, they continue to expect and to hope that this process will be reversed. When clotting, bleeding, or infections occur at the cannula site, they accept this as a singular occurrence, only to have it happen again. . . .
> In view of the foregoing, it would appear that denial would be an inevitable consequence of chronic hemodialysis. However, in ac-

tuality, it may be necessary that these patients be allowed to maintain their capacity to repress in order to cope with their life situation.

It is important to consider the positive aspects of denial and to question whether the psychiatrist should attempt to alter or tamper with it. In my experience this defense mechanism is usually so well entrenched that it cannot be changed even if one wants to do so. As such it appears similar to a delusion and reminiscent of the futility of trying to convince someone that a tenaciously held false belief is not true. There are also positive, protective components to denial in everyday life and in physical illness. If people did not deny many of the mishaps that could happen to them hourly or daily, they could not function. Hackett and Cassem[21] have pointed out the protective qualities of denial in patients with myocardial infarction in coronary care units. Those patients using denial had lower morbidity and mortality rates; those patients overwhelmed with anxiety were more likely to develop cardiac irregularities and to die. My experience with denial by the dialysand is that when it works, it does so quite effectively; but when it begins to crack, it falls apart precipitously, resulting in psychosis or total despair, culminating at times in suicide. Denial also becomes destructive to dialysands when it takes the form of obliterating their view of their illness and the concomitant need for treatment. Thus, some patients develop a psychotic denial in which they exclaim they are miraculously cured and do not need dialysis.

**Crisis intervention**

Over the years I have noted a gradual acceptance of the importance of considering and, when necessary, treating the psychosocial problems of dialysis. Now there is a plea for psychiatrists to become more involved in the field. In my opinion, the most effective mode of action for the psychiatrist is to offer crisis-oriented, short-term psychotherapy and to work with the personnel caring for the dialysand.[22] Intensive long-term psychotherapy is rarely indicated and is limited to patients with neurotic problems that may or may not be related to dialysis. There are just not enough therapists to provide such treatment, nor, in my experience, are there many dialysands who want psychotherapy enough to seek it out.

**Role of psychiatrist vis-à-vis hospital personnel**

In addition to crisis intervention, psychiatrists may well find their time effectively spent with the dialysis unit personnel, especially the nurses who really (as in most instances of medical care) spend more time with the patient than anyone else, including the physician.

Transference and countertransference problems can arise between dialysand and nurse with such long-term and intimate care. It is not uncommon for dialysis nurses and others closely associated with dialysands to dream of being dialyzed themselves or of having shunts. For example, a nurse reported the following dream:

> I had a dream just today about cannulae and the kidney. I didn't ever think I would this soon after starting to work with them. Anyway, I barged in unexpectedly on a class at a college and started talking about the artificial kidney. I told the teacher that I "just had to tell these people all about the kidney." So I did. I had a cannula in my leg, by the way. I woke up just after leaving the classroom, but the teacher was running after me and yelling, "You forgot to show them your cannula!"

Sexual fantasies may also develop; the sight of male patients openly masturbating while on dialysis may give rise to anxiety in nursing personnel. The masturbating behavior may reflect the dialysand's anxiety, boredom, and need to prove masculine prowess due to reduced sexual potency. (The subject of patient behavior during dialysis has received no attention whatsoever. Most patients watch television or hibernate with the sheets pulled up over their face. Little time is spent on creative activities such as reading or writing. Similarly there is little socializing among dialysands either on the unit or away from it.) Explaining possible reasons for the patient's need to masturbate and suggesting that the nurse accept but not necessarily condone such behavior in a nonthreatening manner is effective in quelling anxiety for both nurse and patient.

Other problems in the dialysand-personnel relationship center around the arousal of hostile feelings, particularly when dialysands will not cooperate with the program.[23] In essence, cooperation may mean meeting the needs and expectations of the hospital personnel. The role of "good" patients who makes personnel feel wanted and appreciated and who return to a productive life-style may be more necessary for the morale of the dialysis staff than it is for patient morale. As noted earlier, Sullivan[11] cogently points out that "work" for dialysands may indeed be the full-time job of maintaining themselves on dialysis and that to require more from some patients is unrealistic.

### Psychopharmacology

I have not found psychopharmacological medication especially helpful for the dialysis patient except under specific circumstances. Transient anxiety states usually respond to diazepam and psychotic episodes of a schizophrenic nature usually respond to a phenothiazine derivative or haloperidol. Because in my experience dialysis patients react poorly to the antidepressants, I am hesitant to use them except in cases of severe depression or chronic insomnia. In such situations I usually administer a small dose of amitriptyline or doxepin first, and gradually increase the dose to an effective therapeutic level.*

When dialysis was a new procedure, when it was carried out in research or intensive care units, schizophrenic-like episodes were frequently reported; however, with the establishment of units for long-term dialysis the incidence dropped dramatically and now, schizophrenic episodes are rarely reported. I suspect that these early reports of psychoses were not unlike those reported in intensive care units following open heart operations and that as dialysis became more of an accepted procedure and the atmosphere of dialysis units became less frightening, this type of psychosis occurred less frequently.

**Psychological phases in adaptation to dialysis**

There have been various phases reported in adaptation to dialysis in which one may see specific psychiatric syndromes. In the early phases of dialysis, anxiety[24] is likely, whereas in the later stages depression is more common. When patients begin dialysis they may feel anxious, but they usually accept its mechanics and come to rely on the process. On the whole they are generally euphoric following dialysis and look on themselves symbolically and realistically as having arisen from the dead—a recurrent theme in the psychology of patients with artificial and transplanted organs. They may be euphoric during this early phase with depression manifesting itself only after they return to normalcy and the responsibilities of everyday living. As opposed to open heart operations, where anxiety stems from an acute threat of death, in chronic hemodialysis the distress is related to a life that in Unamuno's terms[25] may become "too long."

Alfrey and coworkers have recently described a syndrome that they call "dialytica dementia."[26] Psychosis can appear as a manifestation of this rare entity, which is also characterized by speech impairment progressing from slow articulation and stuttering to partial aphasia, intellectual deterioration, seizures, myoclonus, fascicular twitching especially around the lips, and paroxysmal slowing in the electroencephalogram. The course of this state is progressively downhill, worsening with dialysis and ending in death.

---

*Table 18-1 and the section on its use are included as a guide for those who do use psychopharmaceuticals.

**Table 18-1.** Sedatives, hypnotics, and tranquilizers

See explanation of abbreviations at bottom of table. Asterisks and daggers within table

| Drug | Major excretion routes | Half-life | | Normal dose interval | Plasma protein binding | Method |
|---|---|---|---|---|---|---|
| | | **Normal** | **ESRD** | | | |
| | Pharmacokinetic Variables | | | | | |

| Drug | Major excretion routes | Normal | ESRD | Normal dose interval | Plasma protein binding | Method |
|---|---|---|---|---|---|---|
| | | *hours* | | | % | |
| **Barbiturates** | | | | | | |
| Pentobarbital* (Nembutal*) | Hepatic | 17 to 50 | 17 to 50† | 8 | 61‡ | D |
| Phenobarbital | Hepatic (Renal) | 37 to 96 | 117 | 8 | 20 to 40 | I |
| Secobarbital (Seconal) | Hepatic | 30 | ? | 24 | 44 | D |
| **Benzodiazepines** | | | | | | |
| Chlordiazepoxide (Librium) | Hepatic* | 6 to 30† | ? | 6 to 8 | 86 to 93 | D |
| Diazepam (Valium) | Hepatic (Renal*) (GI†) | 20 to 90‡ | ? | 8 | 97 to 98 | D |

Abbreviations used in table: T¹/₂ =biological half-life: ESRD =end stage renal disease. I =interval extension method of dosage adjustment, data units are percent of usual maintenance dose; H =hemodialysis; *Use of the table:* Because dosage adjustments for renal failure depend on knowledge of drug handling under major route of drug disposal (excretion or metabolism), the usual interval between maintenance doses, the

If the major pathway of drug excretion is renal, or if a removal exists, the designation "renal" is used by parentheses.

To adjust dosage in patients with renal insufficiency, the intervals between individual doses can be Alternatively, the size of individual doses can be reduced keeping the interval between doses normal. This is desired. In the tables, following identification of the method used (D for dose reduction or I for interval filtration rate (GFR). In the dose reduction method the percent of the usual dose that should be given at the doses of normal size is given.

The qualitative effect of standard clinical dialysis on drug removal is shown for hemodialysis (H) and insure adequate therapeutic blood levels, whereas "No" refers to the lack of need for dosage adjustment should be given after dialysis. The designation "No" in the tables does not preclude the use of dialysis or

Nephrotoxicity and systemic adverse effects and information specifically related to patients with denoted by asterisks.

| Adjustment for renal failure | | | | Toxic effects and remarks |
|---|---|---|---|---|
| GFR (ml/min) | | | | |
| >50 | 10 to 50 | <10 | Dialysis | |
| | | | | *May increase osteomalacia in hemodialysis patients; $T^{1/2}$ decreases with chronic therapy due to hepatic microsomal enzyme induction; hemodialysis more effective than peritoneal dialysis in overdoses; all agents in this group may cause excessive sedation |
| Unch. | Unch. | Unch. | No (H,P) | Group toxicity and remarks *Pharmacokinetics of amobarbital are similar †$T^{1/2}$ may decrease in ESRD but metabolic clearance rate is normal ‡Decreased in ESRD |
| 8 | 8 | 8 to 16 | Yes (H,P) | Group toxicity and remarks |
| Unch. | Unch. | Unch. | No (H,P) | Group toxicity and remarks |
| Unch. | Unch. | Unch. | No (H) | All agents in this group may cause excessive sedation Group toxicity *Active metabolite excreted by kidneys †Chronic therapy prolongs $T^{1/2}$ |
| Unch. | Unch. | Unch. | No (H) | Group toxicity *Active metabolites excreted by kidneys †Enterohepatic circulation exists ‡Increased metabolism with prolonged therapy |

*Continued.*

method of dosage adjustment, data units are hours between maintenance doses; D =dose reduction
P =peritoneal dialysis; Unch =unchanged; GI =gastrointestinal; GFR =glomerular filtration rate
normal circumstances, various pharmocokinetic variables in normal subjects are given. These include the
plasma or biological half-life, and the extent of drug binding to plasma proteins.
in the column headed "Major Excretion Route." Other important avenues of drug disposition are enclosed

lengthened keeping the dosage size normal. This method is known as the "interval extension" method.
"dosage reduction" method is recommended especially for drugs in which a relatively constant blood level
extension), recommendations are given for various levels of renal function as estimated by glomerular
normal dose interval is shown, whereas for the interval extension method the number of hours between

peritoneal dialysis (P). "Yes" refers to the removal of enough drug to require a dosage supplement to
with dialysis. To insure efficacy when information about dialysis loss is not available, maintenance doses
hemoperfusion for drug overdoses.
renal disease are shown in the column "Adverse Effects and Remarks." The latter relate to specific points

From Extracorporeal Medical Specialties, Inc., King of Prussia, Pa., November, 1977.

**Table 18-1.** Sedatives, hypnotics, and tranquilizers—cont'd

| Drug | Major excretion routes | Half-life Normal | Half-life ESRD | Normal dose interval | Plasma protein binding | Method |
|---|---|---|---|---|---|---|
| Flurazepam (Dalmane) | GI* (Renal) | 47 to 100 | ? | 24 | ? | D |
| Ethchlorvynol (Placidyl) | Hepatic* (Renal) | 21 to 105 | ? | 24 | 35 to 50 | D |
| Glutethimide (Doriden) | Hepatic* | 10 to 45** | 10 to 45 | 24 | 45 | D |
| Halopendol | Hepatic (Renal GI) | 13 to 35 | ? | 8 | ? | D |
| Lithium carbonate | Renal | 5 to 40* | ? | 8 | 0 | D |
| Meprobamate | Hepatic (Renal 10%)* | 9 to 11 | ? | 6 | 30 | I |
| Methaqualone | Hepatic | 0.9 (Part)* 16 to 42 | ? | 8 | 80 | D |
| Phenothiazines | | | | | | |
| Chlorpromazine | Hepatic | 2 to 31 | ? | 6 to 12 | 90 | D |

| Adjustment for renal failure | | | | |
|---|---|---|---|---|
| GFR (ml/min) | | | | |
| >50 | 10 to 50 | <10 | Dialysis | Toxic effects and remarks |
| Unch. | Unch. | Unch. | ? | Group toxicity<br>*First pass hepatic metabolism; excretion routes pertain to active metabolites |
| Unch. | Unch. | Unch. | Yes (H, D) | May cause excessive sedation; ? nephrotoxic<br>*Proportion of hepatic and renal excretion uncertain |
| Unch. | Unch. | Avoid | No (H,P) | May cause excessive sedation<br>*Enterohepatic circulation exists<br>†$T^{1/2}$ increases with dose and hypotention |
| Unch. | Unch. | Unch. | ? | May cause hypotension, excessive sedation |
| Unch. | Avoid | Avoid | Yes (H,P)** | Nephrogenic diabetes insipidus; renal tubular acidosis; toxic effects increased by sodium depletion; blood levels best guide to dose<br>*Plasma $T^{1/2}$ does not reflect extensive tissue accumulation<br>†Plasma levels rise after dialysis as reequilibration with tissue stores occurs |
| 6 | 9 to 12 | 12 to 18 | Yes (H,P) | May cause excessive sedation<br>*Renal excretion may be increased by saline and furosemide<br>†Hemodialysis twice as efficient as peritoneal dialysis |
| Unch. | Unch. | Unch. | Yes (H) | May cause excessive sedation; contaminant (orthotoluidine) may cause hemorrhagic cystitis<br>*Biexponential pharmacokinetics; longer $T^{1/2}$ more clinically important |
| | | | | *All agents in this group are anticholinergic and may cause urinary retention, prototype chlorpromazine |
| Unch. | Unch. | Unch.* | No (H,P) | Group toxicity<br>*May need to decrease dose and increase interval if excessive sedation occurs |

*Continued.*

**Table 18-1.** Sedatives, hypnotics, and tranquilizers—cont'd

| Drug | Major excretion routes | Half-life Normal | Half-life ESRD | Normal dose interval | Plasma protein binding | Method |
|------|------------------------|------------------|----------------|----------------------|------------------------|--------|
| Tricyclic antide-pressants | | | | | | |
| Amitriptyline (Elavil) | Hepatic* (Renal <5%) | 117 to 73.5 | ? | 8 | 96 | D |
| Desmethylimipra-mine (Norpramin) | Hepatic (Renal <5%) | 4 to 53 | ? | 8 | 90 to 92 | D |
| Imipramine (Tofranil) | Hepatic* (Renal <5%) | 3.5 to 16 | ? | 8 | 96 | D |
| Nortriptyline (Aventyl) | Hepatic (Renal <5%) | 14 to 93 | ? | 8 | 94 | D |

### Selection of patients—an issue of the past

Fortunately, a discussion of selection of patients is no longer necessary except from a historical viewpoint. Because of federal legislation and funding, dialysis is now available to most patients who require it. Indeed it has become the first catastrophic illness to receive such financial backing. Selection committees making "life or death" decisions are no longer in existence. From an ethical as well as from a psychological perspective, this change seems highly advantageous because it bypasses the necessity for making judgments of "social worth" (deciding that one person's life is worth more than another).[27] It also is a relief because in fact it never was possible to predict which patients would adapt emotionally to the procedure and which would not. Because of this new federal legislation and funding, however, hospitals and physicians are faced with more patients accepted for dialysis who must learn to live or die with the multidimensional problems discussed in this chapter.

| Adjustment for renal failure | | | | |
| --- | --- | --- | --- | --- |
| GFR (ml/min) | | | | |
| >50 | 10 to 50 | <10 | Dialysis | Toxic effects and remarks |
| | | | | All agents in this group anticholinergic and may cause urinary retention; may decrease hypotensive effects of guanidium drugs; enterohepatic circulation and genetic variation in metabolism exist; increased excretion in acid urine (total remains small) |
| Unch. | Unch. | Unch.* | No (H,P) | Group remarks<br>*Metabolized to nortriptyline |
| Unch. | Unch. | Unch. | No (H,P) | Group remarks |
| Unch. | Unch. | Unch. | No (H,P) | Group remarks<br>*Metabolized to desmethylimipramine |
| Unch. | Unch. | Unch. | No (H,P) | Group remarks |

## REFERENCES

1. Brown, H. W., and others: Clinical problems related to the prolonged artificial maintenance of life by hemodialysis in chronic renal failure, Trans. Am. Soc. Artif. Intern. Organs **8**:281-291, 1962.
2. Gombos, E. A., Lee, T. H., Harton, R., and Cummings, J. W.: One year's experience with an intermittent dialysis program, Ann. Intern. Med. **61**(3):462-469, 1964.
3. Shea, E. J., Bogdan, D. F., Freeman, R. B., and Schreiner, G. E.: Hemodialysis for chronic renal failure. IV Psychologic considerations, Ann. Intern. Med. **62**(3):558-563, 1965.
4. Abram, H. S.: Survival by machine: psychological aspects of chronic dialysis, Psychiatr. Med. **1**:37-50, 1970.
5. Cooper, A. J.: Hypomanic psychosis precipitated by hemodialysis, Comp. Psychiatr. **8**:168-174, 1967.
6. Litin, E. M.: Discussion of three papers on man and the artificial organ, read at the 123rd Meeting of the American Psychiatric Association, Detroit, May, 1967.
7. Chadd, K., and Estlack, M.: Transplant . . . a layman's account of a kidney transplant, unpublished.
8. Borgenicht, L., Younger, S., and Zinn, S.: Psychological aspects of home dialysis, unpublished.

9. Kemph, J. P.: Renal failure, artificial kidney and kidney transplant, Am. J. Psychiatr. **122:**1270-1274, 1966.

10. Shambaugh, P. W., and others: Hemodialysis in the home—emotional impact on the spouse, Trans. Am. Soc. Artif. Intern. Organs **13:**41-45, 1967.

11. Sullivan, M. F.: The dialysis patient and attitudes towards work, Psychiatr. Med. **4:**213-219, 1973.

12. Abram, H. S., and others: Sexual functioning in patients with chronic renal failure, J. Nerv. Ment. Dis. **160:**220-226, 1975.

13. Levy, N. B.: Sexual adjustment to maintenance hemodialysis and renal transplantation. National survey by questionnaire: preliminary report, Trans. Am. Soc. Artif. Int. Organs **19:**138-143, 1973.

14. Abram, H. S., Moore, G. L., and Westervelt, F. B., Jr.: Suicidal behavior in chronic dialysis patients, Am. J. Psychiatry **127:**1199-1204, 1971.

15. Rubini, M. I.: Proceedings, the Conference on Dialysis as a Practical Workshop, New York, 1966, National Dialysis Committee.

16. Klobuchar, J.: It's time to die: ailing man decides, Associated Press, 1969.

17. Farberow, N. L., and others: Suicide among patients with cardiorespiratory illnesses, J.A.M.A. **195:**422-428, 1966.

18. Dorpat, T. L., and Ripley, H. S.: A study of suicide in the Seattle area, Compr. Psychiatry **1:**349-359, 1960.

19. Fedden, H. R.: Suicide, a social and historical study, London, 1938, Peter Davies, Ltd.

20. Short, M. J., and Wilson, W. P.: Roles of denial in chronic hemodialysis, Arch. Gen. Psychiatry **20:**433-437, 1969. Copyright 1969, American Medical Association.

21. Hackett, T. P., Cassem, N. H., and Wishnie, H. A.: The coronary-care unit: an appraisal of the psychological hazards, N. Engl. J. Med. **279:**1365-1370, 1968.

22. Abram, H. S.: Psychotherapy in renal failure, Curr. Psychiatr. Ther. **10:**86-92, 1969.

23. Abram, H. S.: The "uncooperative" dialysis patient: a psychiatrist's viewpoint and a patient's commentary. In Levy, N. B., editor: Living and dying: adaptation to hemodialysis, Springfield, Illinois, 1974, Charles C Thomas, Publisher.

24. Abram, H. S.: The psychiatrist, the treatment of chronic renal failure and the prolongation of life: II. Am. J. Psychiatry **126:**157-167, 1969.

25. Unamuno, M.: The tragic sense of life, New York, 1921, MacMillan, Inc.

26. Alfrey, A. C., and others: Syndrome of dyspraxia and multifocal seizures associated with chronic hemodialysis, Trans. Am. Soc. Artif. Intern. Organs **18:**257-260, 1972.

27. Abram, H. S., and Wadlington, W. W.: On the selection of patients for artificial and transplanted organs, Ann. Intern. Med. **69:**615-620, 1968.

# 19

# Renal transplantation

## HARRY S. ABRAM

Although presented here as a separate chapter, the psychology of renal transplantation occurs within the context of repetitive dialysis and cannot be separated from it in the final analysis. In essence end-stage renal failure patients who receive kidney transplants have been dialysands and will become so again if they reject their homograft. Thus the two forms of treatment are inextricably intertwined.

### PSYCHOSOCIAL BACKGROUND

Just as chronic dialysis offers a unique opportunity to investigate the human being's relationship with a machine on which survival depends, renal transplantation provides a similar avenue to understanding the acceptance of another's internal organ into the body and the individual's attitudes toward such a vital donation. Also, renal transplantation allows insight into the motivation of the donor and the family dynamics involved in such a decision. I know of no similar situation in the psychological study of surgical procedures that gives us these opportunities, even though future technological advances will undoubtedly lead to the clinical feasibility of the use of other transplanted organs. Once again there will be a science fiction motif, in this instance the effect of transplantation on personality such as in Curt Siodomak's *Donovan's Brain* and Robert Heinlein's *I Will Fear No Evil*. The themes of death and rebirth will again dominate the subject matter as they do in the following commentary by a renal transplant recipient.[1]

> Perhaps the healthiest attitude can develop only when one has experienced what I now term my "post mortem life." Then one feels that everything is an end in itself. One is reconciled with death and no longer fears it. Everything becomes piercingly important, and one actually becomes stabbed by things, flowers, babies, and beautiful objects: the very act of living and walking, of breathing and eating, of

having friends and chatting. One then feels a debt of loyalty and duty to the entire human species.*

It also becomes evident that most patients with end-stage renal failure look on receiving a transplant as a release from the rigors of dialysis and as a return to a life of freedom and independence. There is a panacean quality to such thinking that more often than not is more fantasy than reality. Even though the constraints of dialysis are lifted (making concerns with shunts, dietary restrictions, dependence on a machine, and other problems of dialysis no longer necessary) and the patient's sense of well-being is enhanced, the patient must learn to contend with the side effects of immunosuppressive and steroid medications and the ever-present possibility of organ rejection. Body image changes (acne, moon-like facies, and other somatic effects of corticosteroids) may occur and physical complications (diabetes mellitus and hypertension) may severely hamper the patient's return to health. The overall mortality rate of patients undergoing dialysis is approximately the same (around 10% per year) as that of transplant recipients and is usually related (as with dialysis) to arteriosclerotic vascular disease. With a living, related kidney donor the 5 year survival rate for the kidney is 85%, while it is 45% to 50% from a cadaveric donor. Because a return to dialysis is necessary following organ rejection, suicidal potential may be more likely at this time. The cost of a transplant in 1977 was approximately $30,000 with an additional $3,000 yearly for medication as compared to $25,000 yearly for center dialysis. Home dialysis was considerably cheaper at $7,000 yearly. Financial funding for transplantation as well as for dialysis is sponsored mainly through federal, state, and third-party insurance coverage. Nevertheless, there are many psychosocial hazards associated with transplantation and it seldom meets the utopian fantasies of the patient.

## RELATION TO HEMODIALYSIS

The relationship of dialysis to transplantation is an intricate one. At one level the two are obviously interdependent. Yet a dichotomy between the two has developed with nephrologists and transplant surgeons seldom being in total agreement, leaving the patient caught in the middle. Although at one time dialysis was regarded as a

---

*Beleil, O. M.: Landmarks in organ transplantation: a historical review by a kidney transplant recipient, Transplant. Proc. **5**:1031-1033, 1973. By permission.

treatment unto itself, transplantation is now generally considered an extension of it (or, more specifically, dialysis is viewed primarily as a necessary and cumbersome stepping-stone to transplantation). For some patients with severe adaptational problems to dialysis, transplantation may represent a way out of what appears to be an impossible situation. I suspect that difficulties arise mainly when physicians are too narrow or too chauvinistic in their attitudes toward treatment or when the patient's expectations are unrealistic. Probably the most vivid example of a patient caught in the Scylla and Charybdis dilemma of dialysis and transplantation[2] is that of Chad Calland, a cardiologist who received five renal transplants and who ultimately died a tragic, bitter death. He ends his autobiographical account on "Iatrogenic Problems in End-Stage Renal Failure"[3] with the plea:

> The physician is more often a voyeur than a partaker in human suffering. I am a cardiologist who has undergone chronic renal failure, dialysis and multiple transplants. As a physician-partaker, I am distressed by the controversial dialogue that separates the nephrologist from the transplant surgeon, so that, in the end, it is the patient who is given short shrift. I have observed that both nephrologist and transplant surgeon work alone in their own separate fields, and that the patient becomes lost in a morass of professional role playing and physician self-justification. As legitimate as their altruistic but differing opinions may be, the nephrologist and the transplant surgeon must work together for the patient, his circumstances, his needs and the quality of his life.

Calland also vividly portrays some of the psychosocial consequences of receiving a transplant and the interrelationship with dialysis:

> Patients on dialysis are accustomed to being told by the doctor, "You are doing fine"—usually after the electrolytes and treatment. The patient then thinks to himself, "If I'm doing fine, why do I feel so rotten. . . ?"
>
> On the other hand, after successful transplants, patients have even greater difficulties to cope with because almost without exception, they have undergone the problems of hemodialysis. They can now view life from a different perspective, free from machines, tubes, dialysates, supplies, dietary, fluid and travel restrictions, anemia, the mess of cleaning up after a run, and all the shunt or fistula problems that plague the patient on hemodialysis. Nonetheless, patients with transplants continue to share the anxieties of their friends who remain on hemodialysis, and, in addition, they carry the constant burdens of fear of rejection and the primary complications of immunosuppressive therapy. . . .
>
> They may also face worse mental depression. Despite a successful graft, their employment, marital, insurance, mortgage and financial

situations have not improved because not enough data have yet been gathered about life expectancy after successful transplantation. The longest known survival is 15 years, and this fact does not satisfy anyone, let alone insurance writers.

After giving short examples of some of these complications Calland asks, "Is transplantation 'the true answer' for all patients?" The answer to his rhetorical question seems to be in the misery he describes.

## DONORS

Aside from blood donation, the renal donor provides an unusual opportunity for the psychiatrist to investigate the concept of altruism and the giving of a vital organ to another person. Kemph's[4] pioneering work with end-stage renal failure patients gives us early insights into the psychology of the donor just as it made us aware of the problems of chronic hemodialysis. He observed:

> Although all donors were consciously altruistic, there was considerable unconscious resentment toward the recipient and toward those hospital personnel who requested or encouraged the transplant. There was consistent hostility on the part of the donor for the greater amount of attention shown the recipient. This led to a moderate degree of post surgical depressive reactions in all the adult donors.

As the limelight shifts from donor to recipient, depression in the donor is likely. In an elaboration on the matter Kemph[5] noted:

> In contrast to the [recipient], the donor tended to withdraw emotionally and appear harassed as the operative date approached. The loss of a part of his body was rapidly becoming a reality. Previously he felt compensated for the altruistic sacrifice he was making, but when surgery was imminent he realized more fully the significance of losing an organ through major surgery in terms of narcissistic threat, fear of damage to sexual organs, and the vital dangers of major surgery.

In this passage Kemph touches on important psychological and ethical issues related to renal donations that are still unsettled and controversial. Is the donation an altruistic act, a true "gift of life" or is it a masochistic, neurotic act? Does it harm or does it benefit the donor? How does one make the decision to donate? Undoubtedly there are multiple factors involved in such a decision. After an extensive study of the matter Fellner and Marshall[6] came to the conclusion that the decision whether or not to donate was based on unconscious forces and occurred in an impulsive manner rather than being well thought out and rational. They aptly used the phrase "the myth of informed consent" to emphasize that the would-be donor really decides at an emotional level without taking into account objective reasons for doing or not doing so. In general Fellner and Marshall regarded donation as a positive act and found that donors have few or no regrets over their decision.

## Living unrelated donors

Sadler, Davidson, and Carroll[7] studied living donors who were unrelated to recipients and reached similar conclusions. Although this type of renal donation is no longer in clinical use and, indeed, was never popular, the findings are interesting and relevant to the subject. They studied a group of people who gave or wanted to give one of their vital organs, a kidney, to a total stranger. Like Fellner and associates, Sadler and coworkers believed that these patients were truly altruistically motivated, that the donation represented to them a type of peak experience, and that such an act was not neurotically based. To them the donor was not harmed but reaped benefits from the experience that represented "growth" and reaching toward a "Christian ideal." Sadler responds to his own question, "Have any donors been harmed, especially if they had obvious psychological problems?" with the emphatic answer, "No, none of the 18 [living unrelated] donors have been harmed." Bieber,[8] in a discussion of Sadler's original article, nevertheless remained skeptical of this statement. Whereas Sadler's donors described their postoperative feelings with such exclamations as, "A wonderful renewal! I can reach people now," "I've grown so much," and "A privilege to do something worthwhile," Bieber found evidence of significant psychopathology in each of Sadler's patients. In contradistinction to Sadler, Bieber regarded these same donors as "acting out of highly subjective neurotic motives" and warned that "avowed altruism as motivation for irreversible acts of self-sacrifice or denial is almost always suspect. . . . Altruism may be a motive if, after careful psychiatric survey, neurotic gains cannot be demonstrated." Bieber strongly recommended that "donors should be examined by at least three psychiatrists preferably from different institutions," and that a "minimum of six months should elapse before accepting a willing donor, during which time the necessary social study, psychiatric examinations and evaluations may be completed." Bieber's position was that "many practical and moral questions have evolved as a result of spectacular advances in the surgical techniques of organ transplantation. I trust that the American Psychiatric Association and the American Medical Association will deem it important enough to issue guidelines and policy statements regarding donor-recipient managements, a problem that has immediate relevance in our lives today." To my knowledge neither of these organizations has officially looked into the matter.

Perhaps an analogous situation to that of the living, unrelated kidney donor and one that gives insight into the psychodynamics and motivation involved is that of the would-be heart donor—an even smaller population than those wishing to donate a kidney to a stranger! In the only study on the subject (of a person wanting to trade his heart for the sick heart of an awaiting recipient) Christopherson and Lunde[9] observed, "In most instances they [the living would-be donor] appeared to be profoundly depressed and suicidal and viewed heart donation as a process which would make their suicide a meaningful event and perhaps relieve some of their guilt." Blachly,[10] probably tongue-in-cheek, has suggested that potentially suicidal people be allowed to donate a kidney, for example, as a form of expiation to prevent suicidal behavior, "a partial sacrifice for a total sacrifice. . . . Such a sacrifice could enhance the person's sense of dignity and self-determination, while permitting him to rejoin the human race on his own terms."

I do not believe it wise to spend an excessive amount of time on the living, unrelated donor except to point out how it highlights the problem of what motivates donation of a vital organ. The situation is a singular one in that there is no blood relation between donor and recipient. Obviously it is not feasible with heart transplantation! And with renal donation the use and success of cadaver kidneys and those from living relatives make the living, unrelated donor unnecessary to the point of extinction.

### Living related donor

With the living related donor the problem becomes more complex in that one must consider the donation of an organ to extend the life of a relative who may be emotionally close to the donor. The ambivalence and interdependency between donor and recipient may be intense prior to the need for a transplant and enhanced when it does become necessary. Again the question must be raised about the effects of donation and how a donor is selected out of a family, several of whom are potential matches. These are not only academic concerns; conflict can develop between recipient and donor or elsewhere within the family structure if a certain member is selected or not selected. Legal precedents have also been based on psychiatric opinions of the potential harm or benefit from donation and ethical questions have been raised about the acceptance or rejection of donors on psychological grounds. For example, a judge's decision to allow a twin who was a minor to donate a kidney to his brother centered around a psychiatrist's testimony that to deprive the twin of the chance to donate would give rise for excessive guilt in the future. In one of the landmark decisions in the early history of transplantation Judge Counihan[11] declared, "I am satisfied from the testimony of the psychiatrist that grave emotional impact may be visited upon Leonard [the potential twin donor] if the defendents refuse to perform this operation and Leon [the potential twin recipient] should die, as apparently he will. . . . Such emotional disturbance could well affect the health and physical well-being of Leonard for the remainder of his life."

## Donor selection

There are also interesting psychological and ethical issues centering around donor selection. Some psychiatrists believe that donor screening should be mandatory to prevent emotional disturbances; others consider it necessary under unusual circumstances or when the surgeon is in doubt. If a potential donor is rejected because of psychiatric reservations or questionable motivation, a tradition has built up that he not be told the real reason for rejection but instead be told that there is tissue incompatibility or a physical contraindication. Fox and Swazey[12] comment, "In an unplanned, consensual way, these protective mechanisms [not telling the potential donor that his rejection is for emotional reasons] have been independently instituted by several of the kidney transplant groups with which we are acquainted. That physicians are willing to violate at least two important norms of medical ethics by telling a deliberate untruth and by withholding a chart entry indicates how grave they consider the consequence of revealing 'psychological incompatibility.' " This practice may well have been perpetuated by some psychiatrists such as Cramond,[13] a strong advocate of "careful psychological screening" with "strict psychological standards" for donor selection. These standards seem exceptionally vague: "those which current clinical experience and theoretical understanding suggest are sound, reliable and valid"! Cramond suggests that if a potential donor rejected on "psychiatric grounds" that he not be told this fact "in order to spare the feelings of the person" and that the rejection be "ascribed to some minor physical variation." Eisendrath,[14] on the other hand, takes an opposite approach and states that such psychiatric screening is rarely necessary. He notes, "We do not agree with Cramond and his associates that a psychological assessment is essential per se because the donor is healthy and thus deserves special protection, since no evidence exists that such a routine will provide it." As I understand Eisendrath's position, it is similar to my stand on the selection of hemodialysis patients; that is, just as the psychiatrist cannot predict which patients will adjust to dialysis, the psychiatrist cannot predict donor reaction. Although I do not agree with his statement that "the decision to donate a kidney need not be a matter for psychiatric study" or that the transplant surgeon can necessarily select or reject potential donors based on intuitive assessment, I suspect that he is correct in his underscoring that psychiatrists often emphasize the importance of psychological screening in this area when our ability and the evidence that we can effectively do so are lacking. Certainly it is a subject worthy of study, if for no other reason than that psychiatrists know so little about it. Some psychiatrists are now hypothesizing that a conflict between renal donor and recipient can lead to organ rejection.

Before turning to the reactions of the recipient per se I shall briefly discuss the potential conflicts of the donor with the recipient and the role of family dynamics in donor selection. Concerning the conflicts of the donor with the recipient Cramond[3] noted the "ambivalent dependency that may develop between recipient and donor." He also noted that the "donor experiences emotional and physical investment in the patient, and seeks to overprotect." In a manner similar to Kemph, Cramond is describing the ambivalence of the donor and the recipient with the donor being invested in the loss of the kidney and its fate and the recipient feeling beholden to the family member who donates.

The manner in which the family can select the donor is of interest. Most investigators who have studied the phenomenon of donor selection believe that family dynamics play a major role. Indeed, a network is set up by which potential family members are selected or rejected. Simmons[15] notes that transplant surgeons, because of a conflict of interest, must remove themselves as much as possible from the process. "While attempting to influence a potential donor, the doctor is placed in an ethical or role conflict between his obligation to the donor and his commitment to save the life of his patient." Fellner[16] observes that "the family system of donor selection is clearly at its most efficient level very early in the selection process and works primarily in the direction of excluding some family members from participation. Once the potential donors are known and made available to the renal team, the power of the family system to influence the medical selection process diminishes greatly." The motives for the family decisions vary greatly. For example, the most expendable member or the black sheep may be chosen to expiate past misdeeds. The spouses of recipients may find themselves in the position of recruiting or bargaining for kidneys from their in-laws, obviously a difficult and touchy position. On the other side of the balance, spouses of potential donors may well be protective and stand in the way of the donation.

In sum, the problem of donation is complex and multidetermined. Motives seem to range from true altruism through unresolved guilt to outright masochism. The decision whether or not to donate clearly appears to take place at an unconscious level and is heavily weighted by family structure and dynamics. There are some psychiatrists who demand total psychiatric screening while others want to abolish it. There are even some who apparently wish to eliminate the use of organs from living donors because of the inherent conflicts. As cadaver kidneys are not that plentiful and at times not that successful, I believe (at least for the time being) the use of kidneys from living, related donors will remain with us and, indeed, donors themselves may benefit from the act of giving. There is still much to learn about the matter.

**RECIPIENTS**

In the giving-receiving relationship, the responses of the recipient involve the inherent consequences of the acceptance. In my experience these reactions are more subtle and less dramatic than those to the other transplant procedures. Postoperative psychoses after receiving a kidney are relatively rare. When they do occur, they are usually transient and more likely related to steroid medication than to surgery. Kemph[4] was the first to report on the psychological complications of renal transplantation as well as of chronic dialysis. He observed a postoperative lifting of depression in the recipient and a "rapid recovery of mental capacity and personality within the first few days after surgery in those cases where the new kidney began to function immediately." Kemph postulated that a functioning kidney filters substances that account for depression from the blood previously not filtered by the "artificial" kidney. Be that as it may, the patient is often euphoric postoperatively, especially if the transplanted kidney is functioning well. As a patient ecstatically told me, "It's great to be able to pee again!" This succinct exclamation symbolically and realistically states the plight of the transplant patient. Kemph made two observations, the second of which became particularly important in studies made some years later.[5] First, after hospital discharge and on long-term interviews bouts of severe depression were frequently reported by recipients. Second, "the recipients were all concerned with body damage and some of them with a fear that they might be rendered sexually impotent or sexually damaged by the operation." Thus, the theme of body image distortions so common in the psychology of artificial and transplanted organs again becomes evident. In this instance, as we shall see later, the theme takes on special importance in the potential for acceptance or rejection of the renal transplant. Before discussing this somewhat speculative issue, I shall briefly touch on some of the general psychological themes expressed by renal recipients as well as some of the psychiatric complications.

Two prominent themes are those of rebirth and the effects of the transplant on personality structure. In my introduction to this chapter I used a quotation from the recipient with the "postmortem life," a typical expression of a transplant patient or indeed any patient given a reprieve from a fatal illness by advances in modern medical or surgical technology. As mentioned in Chapter 18, dialysands also speak of returning from the dead. After heart surgery patients allude to "birthdays" on the anniversary of their operations, and Hackett[17] writes about the "Lazarus complex" in patients who survive a cardiac arrest. It is not uncommon for the renal recipient to make such remarks as "You appreciate the fact that you're alive and can experience life going on about you, even the trees and grass," "You try not to waste a day," or "It's just something to be living. It's like coming back from the living dead." In the recipients of kidneys from both cadavers and living, related donors, one encounters fantasies that personality changes may result from the donation (that the recipient takes on the characteristics of the donor). For example, patients who receive kidneys from the same cadaver may think of themselves as "twins" or "kidney cousins." They also describe a type of bonding that develops between them and become excessively concerned with what happens to the other. The source of the cadaver kidney can potentially develop into an obsession for the recipient and attempts are made to discover facts about the previous life of the donor. In some ways acquiring a kidney from a cadaver is similar to adopting a baby. The mother of the adopted infant must remain anonymous to the adopting parents. The name and origins of the cadaver kidney donor remains unknown to the recipient. There are also anecdotal reports of male patients wondering if they would have to sit down to urinate after receiving a kidney from a female donor, patients feeling that they became smarter if the donor was of high intelligence, or more docile or belligerent depending on the donor's personality. In one instance a patient who had been "a Grand Dragon in the Klu Klux Klan became an active member of the National Association for the Advancement of Colored People after receiving a kidney from a black patient."[18] Ferris reports a similar incident.[19]

The problem of defining the postoperative complications following renal transplantation is a complicated one. A review of the available literature on the subject leads to a confusing and incomplete array of data in that psychiatric complications are defined variously by different investigators. In addition, some studies are of recipients of kidneys from living, related donors while others are of recipients of kidneys from cadavers. Kemph[4] in his initial 1966 study of twelve recipients of kidneys from living, related donors noted that "hysteria, phobia, confusion, anxiety, and psychosis occasionally developed." Colomb and Hamburger[20] in a 1967 report of forty-four similar recipients found evidence of depression in one patient and "overt or partly concealed anxiety" in eight. In a mixed small series (also in 1967) of five recipients of kidneys from both living relatives and cadavers Cramond[13] described the previously discussed ambivalence and also hostility and dependence. Two years later Short and Harris[21] observed severe depression of psychotic proportions in nineteen recipients of kidneys from living, related donors. In 1969, Ferris[19] noted that of fifty-four recipients of kidney transplants psychiatric complications (mainly psychosis and depression) developed in 31% of those receiving cadaver kidneys and 57% of those receiving kidneys from living relatives. In 1971 Penn,[22] reporting on 292 recipients of kidneys from living, related and cadaver donors, noted that ninety-four patients (34%) had adverse postoperative reactions, mainly of a depressive nature, with seven recipients eventually committing suicide. Penn also observed that "at some stage, practically all patients experienced episodes of anxiety and/or depression secondary to a complication, a painful treatment, drug therapy, fear of death, or an unresolved grief reaction to the loss of organs. . . . Often depression was transient and cleared once the complication was satisfactorily treated." The following year I observed in a study of renal recipients of cadaver organs that seven or 23% had moderate psychiatric complications or evidence of psychosocial upheaval postoperatively.[18]

I find it extremely difficult to weigh these psychiatric complications or to compare them with repetitive hemodialysis. I suspect it is safe to conclude that it is less difficult to receive a cadaver kidney than one from a living relative. This conclusion is in agreement with Ferris' belief that potential harm can come only to recipients of cadaver organs as opposed to two people when the donors are living. Nevertheless, there is guilt and ambivalence over accepting a cadaver organ if recipients think that their continuing lives are based on the deaths of others.

## PSYCHOLOGICAL INCORPORATION

The relationship of organ rejection to psychological conflict is, not surprisingly, of interest to psychiatrists since it centers around problems of body image and the somatic acceptance of a foreign internal organ. From a psychological viewpoint, such words as "rejection," "incorporation," and "internalization" are integral parts of our psychiatric and psychoanalytic terminology. The influence of placing another's internal organ inside one's body is a common theme in science fiction literature, and such authors as Thomas Mann ( in *The Transposed Heads)* have considered the subject, usually in the form of placing a brain in another's body. The symbolic relationship of the effect of the mind on the body seems evident in these writings. Psychiatrists such as Kemph and Cramond noted early that the transplanted kidney could well have sexual meaning (for example, if a kidney from a donor of the opposite sex was given to a recipient) and that disruptive relationships between a recipient and the related donor were distinct possibilities. The next step then occurred when some psychiatrists began asking if such disruption and conflict could lead to actual kidney rejections. My biased position is that I remain skeptical in spite of the attractiveness of such hypotheses. They may, nevertheless, be of heuristic value and, indeed, of clinical importance when we have a better understanding of autoimmune responses. That conflict between donor and recipient can occur is self-evident; there are anecdotal accounts of recipients who have committed suicide when they discovered their transplant came from a relative they hated. Yet, I still have doubts that such conflict can bring about physiological rejection. That "leap" is still too great for me. I am not denying that psychological factors play a strong role in the overall adaptation of the renal recipient. This is well supported by Kemph and others. Undoubtedly, the acquiring of a kidney (either from a living, related donor or from a cadaver) has special psychological meaning for the recipient. The ambivalence, hostile dependency, and premorbid relationship between recipient and donor is of obvious importance, as are the recipient's attitudes and fantasies toward the unknown cadaver donor. Muslin[23] was the first to emphasize this form of "psychological internalization." He says "the assimilation of the new tissues has as a counterpart the ego's integration of a new object in its care (at first periphery)—or psychological transplant"—and describes three "stages of internalization" or "psychological passage" of the transplanted kidney; (1) the "foreign body stage," (2) the "stage of partial incorporation," and (3) the "stage of complete incorporation." Although Muslin declares that "the process of internalization . . . of the new kidney is a universal phenomenon," his proof is scanty and anecdotal. Following up on Muslin's ideas, Basch's work[24] on the "intrapsychic integration" of the renal homograft is "based upon clinical observations without a preconceived research design." Even though he states in his introduction that his "findings must be viewed as suggestive rather than conclusive," he asserts that "psychic conflict about the new kidney and donor appeared to contribute to physiological changes, possible transplant rejection and, in at least two cases, death." Viederman[25] believes that "the degree of comfort and safety which a person will experience in accepting a transplanted organ will depend on the quality of his relationship with the donor, both real and fantasied." He also theorizes that whether the transplant is "hostile introject" or a "benevolent introject," relates to whether the graft is rejected or accepted. In my opinion, Eisendrath[26] presents the only convincing study along these lines. He found that "eight out of 11 patients who died following renal transplantation were noted to have suffered a sense of abandonment by their families or to have experienced panic and a sense of pessimism about the outcome of the operation, to a degree not observed among patients who survived."

## SUMMARY

In these two chapters I have described the psychology of renal failure. I have taken the reader through the meaning of survival by machine and the experience of hemodialysis that symbolically and realistically brings life out of death—but at the price of weighing autonomy against submission. With renal transplantation, one has the unique chance to examine the psychology of giving a gift of life[27] and the hazards involved in such an acceptance.

In closing I must remind the reader that prior to these treatments patients died the slow and, at times, agonizing death of progressive terminal uremia. Thanks to such courageous pioneers as Wilhelm Kolff and John Murray, who, as Fox and Swazey[12] aptly observed, had the "courage to fail," these deaths are now avoided and, indeed, the lives of many are preserved, prolonged, and allowed to continue in a productive manner, contributing much to our society. It is ironic that the most vivid account (the only autobiographical one to my knowledge) of a patient dying of terminal renal failure was written at the time that Kolff in German-occupied Holland was secretly just beginning to apply the principles of dialysis to saving the lives of patients dying of renal failure. A 31-year-old ex-Royal Canadian Air Force pilot, Martin Roher,[28] describes in his diary (while a patient at Duke University under the care of Dr. Walter Kempher) tragically but beautifully his courageous but losing battle against uremia. At one point he writes:

> The cheeks and lips feel sodden and heavy as a thick velvet curtain hanging from a string. Inside the head is a dullness unequalled by the sense of anesthesia, fogging over thoughts until they are reduced to impotent washes of indiscriminate hue and wavering outline which indicate nothing . . . All semblance of hope for the morrow is gone. When the swelling comes rolling in like some dreamy kind of wave and spreads over the mind rendering it impossible to think beyond the second.

Even though Lewis Thomas[29] cites both dialysis and transplantation as prime examples of "halfway technology," I believe they will both be with us for a while. Moreover, since dialysis and transplantation represent the forerunners of other artificial and transplanted organs yet to come, it behooves us to understand the way they affect the lives of those who use them.

**REFERENCES**

1. Beleil, O. M.: Landmarks in organ transplantation: a historical review by a kidney transplant recipient, Transplant. Proc. **5**:1031-1033, 1973.
2. Abram, H. S.: Renal dialysis and transplantation: Scylla and Charybdis of medical progress. In Fuente, R., and Weisman, N. editors: Proceedings of the Fifth World Congress of Psychiatry, Mexico, D. F. New York, 1973, American Elsevier Publishing Co., Inc.
3. Calland, C. H.: Iatrogenic problems in end-stage renal failure. Reprinted by permission. From the New England Journal of Medicine (287; 334-336, 1977).
4. Kemph, J. P.: Renal failure, artificial kidney and kidney transplant, Am. J. Psychiatry **122**:1270-1274, 1966. Copyright 1966, the American Psychiatric Association. Reprinted by permission.
5. Kemph, J. P.: Psychotherapy with patients receiving kidney transplant, Am. J. Psychiatry **124**:623-629, 1967. Copyright 1967, the American Psychiatric Association. Reprinted by permission.
6. Fellner, C. H., and Marshall, J. R.: Twelve kidney donors, J.A.M.A. **206**:2703-2707, 1968.
7. Sadler, H. H., Davidson, L., and Carroll, C.: In Castelnuovo-Tedesco, P. editor: Psychiatric aspects of organ donation, New York, 1971, Grune & Stratton, Inc.

8. Bieber, I.: Discussion of paper by Sadler, H. H. and others: The human phenomenon of the unrelated kidney donor, American Psychiatric Association meeting, Miami Beach, 1969.

9. Christopherson, L. K., and Lunde, D. T.: Heart transplant donors and their families, Semin. Psychiatry **3:**26-35, 1971.

10. Blachly, P. H.: Can organ transplantation provide an altruistic-expiatory alternative to suicide? Life Threat. Behav. **1:**1-9, 1971.

11. Curran, W. J.: A problem of consent: kidney transplantation in minors, N. Y. U. Law Rev. **34:**891-898, 1959.

12. Fox, R. C., and Swazey, J. P.: The courage to fail: a social view of organ transplant and dialysis, Chicago, 1974, University of Chicago Press.

13. Cramond, W. A.: Renal hemotransplantation; some observations on recipients and donors, Br. J. Psychiatry **113:**1223-1230, 1967.

14. Eisendrath, R. M., Guttmann, R. D., and Murray, J. E.: Psychological considerations in the selection of kidney transplant donors, Surg. Gynecol. Obstet. **129:**243-248, 1969.

15. Simmons, R. G., and others: Donors and non-donors: the role of the family and the physician in kidney transplantation. In Castelnuovo-Tedesco, P., editor: Psychiatric aspects of organ transplantation, New York, 1971, Grune & Stratton, Inc.

16. Fellner, C. H.: Selection of living kidney donors and the problem of informed consent. In Castelnuovo-Tedesco, P., editor: Psychiatric aspects of organ transplantation, New York, 1971, Grune & Stratton, Inc.

17. Hackett, T. P.: The Lazarus complex revisited, Ann. Intern. Med. **76:**135-136, 1972.

18. Abram, H. S.: The psychiatrist, the treatment of chronic renal failure, and the prolongation of life III, Am. J. Psychiatry, **128:**1534-1539, 1972.

19. Ferris, G. N.: Psychiatric considerations in patients receiving cadaveric renal transplants, So. Med. J. **62:**1482-1488, 1969.

20. Colomb, G., and Hamburger, J.: Psychological and moral problems of renal transplantation. In Abram, H. S., editor: Psychological aspects of surgery, Boston, 1967, Little, Brown and Co.

21. Short, M. J., and Harris, N. L.: Psychiatric observations of renal homotransplantation, So. Med. J. **62:**1479-1482, 1969.

22. Penn, I., and others: Psychiatric experiences with patients receiving renal and hepatic transplants, Semin. Psychiatry **3:**133-145, 1971.

23. Muslin, H. L.: On acquiring a kidney, Am. J. Psychiatry **127:**1185, 1971.

24. Basch, S. H.: The intrapsychic integration of a new organ: a clinical study of kidney transplantation, Psychiatr. Q. **42:**364-384, 1973.

25. Viederman, M.: The search of meaning in renal transplantation, Psychiatry **37:**283-290, 1974.

26. Eisendrath, R. M.: The role of grief and fear in the death of kidney transplant, Am. J. Psychiatry **126:**381-387, 1969.

27. Abram, H. S., and Buchanan, D.: The gift of life: a review of the psychological aspects of kidney transplantation, Int. J. Psychiatry Med. **7**(2):153-164, 1976-1977.

28. Roher, M.: Days of living, Toronto, 1959, Ryerson Press. Reprinted with permission of McGraw-Hill Ryerson Ltd.

29. Thomas, L. T.: The lives of a cell, New York, 1974, The Viking Press, Inc.

# 20

# The accident victim

## JERROLD F. ROSENBAUM

In this section, the psychiatric liaison experience with accident victims is briefly considered. Despite apparent randomness, accidents often appear clinically to have been partly determined by the victim's recent emotional state and life events. At times after diligent investigation and at other times serendipitously, psychological explanations of these seemingly chance occurrences frequently and convincingly become accessible to the psychiatric consultant. Case examples of accident victims who illustrate common psychological issues in accident pathogenesis are presented, and the implications for psychiatric intervention are discussed.

## ACCIDENTS

The general hospital patient population can be thought of as comprising two categories of individuals—the ill and the injured. While the injured patients may be distinguished from the ill patients by a number of characteristics such as age (younger) and prior physical condition (healthier), a primary distinction is that injured persons or accident victims—formerly whole and healthy—suddenly and unexpectedly alter the course of their lives in a traumatizing encounter with the physical environment. In a single moment, unanticipated and unprepared for, accident victims begin a frequently complicated process of injury, coping, and rehabilitation.

Accident victims can be found on orthopedic, general, and plastic surgery services, in burn units and intensive care units, and on rehabilitation and physical medicine wards. Accidents are the leading cause of death for individuals under the age of 37[1] and are responsible for disabilities accounting for several billions of dollars of annual payments through insurance companies and workmen's compensation funds.[2] The sum total of pain, suffering, disability, and shattered dreams is not measurable. For all these reasons, that crucial moment of "the accident" clearly deserves close scrutiny. Psychological understanding can perhaps contribute to the prevention of serious accidents and to the treatment of their consequences.

In *The Psychopathology of Everyday Life*[3] Freud discusses how unconscious motivation, discerned from psychoanalytic observation, appears to play a primary role in ordinary, daily accidents. An accident could be useful in a number of ways: as a self-punishment to alleviate guilt, as an excuse to avoid an unpleasant situation, as a symbolic castration, and so forth. In considering serious or fatal accidents, Freud invoked the concept of a death instinct.

> Anyone who believes in the occurrence of half-intentional self-injuries will be prepared also to understand that in addition to consciously intentional suicide, there is such a thing as half-intentional, self-destruction—self-destruction with an unconscious intention, capable of making skillful use of the stress of life and disguising it as chance mishap.

Other analytical writers, including Menninger[4] expanded the notion of man's innate self-destructive forces.

Whether life-threatening behavior and subintentional suicide are manifestations of Thanatos, a basic death instinct, or, on the other hand, are even adequate explanations for most accidents is controversial. While psychodynamic theory offers self-destructiveness as a plausible component of the moment of self-injury, the data examining its primacy as a cause of most accidents are mixed. Sobel and Margolis[5] underscore how repeated accidental poisoning in children reflects family pathology. One study of people who attempted suicide[6] revealed an 81% higher accident rate than the rate for control individuals and another report on patients with self-destructive tendencies[7] described an accident frequency twice that of the control population. Tabachnick,[8] however, found that self-destructiveness is not a significant cause of accidents. Selzer, Rogers, and Kern[9] noted a 21% incidence of suicidal proclivity (compared to 8% in the matched control group) in ninety-six drivers involved in fatal accidents.

While suicidal and self-destructive drives are not clearly shown to be specifically and consistently linked with self-injury, the data for more general psychological factors are much more impressive. A number of reports demonstrate the importance of a variety of life changes, vocational and interpersonal stresses, and recent emotional upset in the causation of traffic accidents.[10-12] Using a modified Holmes-Rahe Scale, Selzer and Vinokur[13] emphasize the role of life events and subjective stress as precipitants of accidents. In one study, ten of fifteen drivers killed in traffic accidents either had recently been given positions of increased responsibility or were considering such a change.[14] In another study, 20% of ninety-seven drivers involved in fatal accidents[9] were noted to have been acutely upset in the 6 hour period prior to accident, usually as the result of violent quarrels with wives or girlfriends. Alcoholism has been repeatedly indicted as a crucial contributing factor to traffic accidents.[8,15,16] Acute or chronic alcoholism is presumed to be a reflection of acute or chronic emotional stresses and the inability to cope with them.

The observation that a small percentage of individuals is responsible for a relatively high percentage of industrial and traffic accidents[17,18] led Dunbar, Alexander,[19,20] and others to posit accident-prone individuals who have certain personality traits, such as impulsiveness and resentment against authority, that make them vulnerable to accidents when under certain stresses that threaten their sense of independence. The recent literature suggests, however, that proneness to accidents as a life-long and enduring condition is not a concept consistent with the data. While a few accident victims may be chronically accident-prone, the group of accident repeaters appears to change from one time period to the next; most accidents seem to reflect a transient accident syndrome, involving a variety of personality traits and recent life stresses, rather than a chronic process.[21,22] In studies of the psychopathology in groups of individuals who have a high incidence of accidents, impulsivity, aggressiveness, paranoid traits, unmet dependency needs, and depressive tendencies have been prevalent.[9,14,23,24]

While the foregoing material is of interest and highlights the importance of psychosocial factors in accident causation, its relevance to the individual, hospitalized, accident victim is less clearly evident. These studies do alert clinicians to the role of emotional issues in accident victims, and, therefore, lend credibility to the pursuit of psychological explanations in individual cases. However, the clinical psychiatric approach to the patient in hospital is more problematic. At first sight, most accidents do, indeed, appear to have been chance events. Even when historical data are readily available indicating recent emotional upset or major life changes, the issue of unconscious causation is often still rather vague; that is, information suggesting psychological stress prior to accident is rarely sufficient evidence to conclude that a direct causal link to the accidental trauma exists.

Unconscious dynamics that may be implicated as accident precipitants are often only accessible after extended investigation in interview. This investigative interviewing, while often dramatically revealing, is too rarely accomplished. To the liaison psychiatrist, the reasons for doing it are often not clear and to the physician, surgeon, patient, and much of the rest of the world, the rationale for it is obscure; after all, most people do tend to accept "it was just an accident" as a reasonable accounting of causality. However, as Rome[25] has stated:

> Very little in nature is truly capricious, deserving of the designation "accident." For the most part, our use of the term actually means that the antecedents of the event have not been analyzed in sufficient detail to establish the logical, scientific basis required for a suitably parsiminious explanation of its pathogenesis.

The weight of evidence implicating psychodynamic causes for accidents will often become available through psychological detective work. Alexander [26] emphasized that traditional psychological testing failed to provide the evidence necessary to define the psychological aspects of accident causation. He believed that detailed psychiatric interview provided the most reliable method. Our work in the Liaison Service at Massachusetts General Hospital has time and again revealed striking examples of psychological causalities for accidents leading to fracture, burn, and multiple trauma. For the moment, clinical cases remain the best proof of the existence of psychological determinants in the accident process.

## ACCIDENT "VICTIMS"

If the foregoing comments appear to overstate the degree of importance of psychosocial and psychodynamic issues in accident causation, the primary reason is that the error is all too often made in the opposite direction, overlooking the unconscious motivations. While there are indeed "true" or "pure" accidents, such as a flowerpot or a brick falling off a ledge and striking an unaware pedestrian (assuming the pedestrian had not ignored potential warnings), most often the victim is in some way an agent or prime mover for the sequence of events.

The accident victims seen on the MGH Liaison Service show a broad spectrum of ages and injuries. There is some consistency in the affects most keenly experienced prior to the time of the accident, especially anger, guilt, grief, or loneliness. Most accident victims possess personality characteristics that are manifested in one or more of the following three ways:

1. Chronic masochistic character traits or transient masochistic defenses with anger leading to guilt and self-punishment

2. Grief, sadness, loneliness, or depression
3. Counterdependent defenses acutely threatened by increased dependent feelings, with predominant themes of overindependence, bravado, impulsiveness, or rebelliousness, coexisting with neediness

The use of the term "masochism" in the first of these three accident victim categories refers to the process whereby angry feelings toward important others are intolerable and generate severe guilt feelings that are relieved only by self-punishment, by being hurt. Punishment expiates the guilt these individuals feel at their anger, especially when their anger is directed toward people on whom they are dependent for nurturance:

> A 32-year-old housewife was admitted to the surgical service after accidentally shooting off her right foot with a rifle. She stated she was routinely putting away the weapon, which her husband used for hunting. Interview revealed a history suggestive of masochistic personality traits including physical abuse by her husband. At the end of one interview, the psychiatrist did not have adequate evidence to implicate an acute psychological motivation. On return visit, the interviewer heard that the patient had just recalled that hours before the accident, the husband had pointed the rifle at her and had threatened to kill her.

The masochistic person often follows a pattern of introjecting other people's anger, taking it in, feeling it is deserved, feeling guilty and worthless. This woman quite concretely directed her husband's rage at herself.

Even when the patient does not have masochistic personality features, a history of rage toward spouse, lover, or parent is often followed by self-injury. A rather frequent scenario is the following:

> A 23-year-old woman was admitted for fractures and lacerations from an automobile accident. She had been having an on-going conflict with her boyfriend. After a particularly violent argument that appeared to threaten the relationship, she stormed furiously out of his apartment and drove off. Within minutes she had lost control of her car and struck a tree. Noting her anger at her boyfriend she said, "Hurting myself was the last thing I wanted to do."

Again, rage toward an emotionally significant person eventuated in self-injury. In the words of another patient, acknowledging that he was angrier than he had admitted, "Of course I'm angry!. . . . at myself."

The second category of psychological predisposition to accidental trauma includes depressive affects, sadness, loneliness, and grief:

A 78-year-old man was admitted for treatment of severe chemical esophageal burns. He was living at home alone and had gotten up at night to take a dose of a liquid antacid. Instead, from the medicine chest shelf he opened a bottle of a drain cleaner and took a swallow before realizing his error. He came to the emergency ward immediately. The psychiatrist was suspicious of suicidal intent from the history but, after interview, was satisfied that the patient had no history of suicidal ideation, intent, or plan but, rather, in the darkness had made a tragic error. During routine information gathering, however, the interviewer learned that the date of the ingestion was 5 years to the day since the death of his wife. It was the anniversary of her death.

In addition to sadness and loneliness, guilt feelings are common concomitants of the grief process. The following case emphasizes this point and also serves as a reminder of how psychological determinants can go undiscovered.

One day on Liaison Service rounds, the residents presented a case of "an accident that was just an accident"; the psychiatric resident had been originally called to see the patient for a transient delirium.

The patient was an 18-year-old man who had been visiting friends in an apartment building and was just leaving when the building caught on fire. He was trapped by smoke in a stairway leading to the outside. No one else had been injured, but the patient was badly burned and had suffered smoke inhalation. To the surprise of the hospital residents, the interview by the staff psychiatrist revealed that at the first sign of fire the patient had gone back up the stairs, not out of the building. The patient stated that he wanted to rescue others, all of whom had already reached safety.

*Psychiatrist:* That was a generous act.

*Patient:* My father would have done the same thing.

*Psychiatrist:* Your father?

*Patient:* He was killed in an accident at the shipyard 2 months ago, caught by a rope and crushed between a ship and the dock. No one was there to help *him*.

Acute grief and associated guilt feelings played a part in determining this individual's seemingly chance injuries.

The third category of psychological predisposition to accidental injury includes individuals, similar to the description of accident-prone personality, who are impulsive and aggressive, or who act very independent but have much difficulty with dependent feelings. As noted before, some people manifest these traits for years and have difficulty during periods of stress, such as times of separation. Other individuals appear to fit this description only transiently.

A 16-year-old boy was admitted to the Burn Unit after sustaining multiple burns from a flash fire that he touched off while climbing a utility pole. He dropped to the ground unconscious. That night he had been out drinking with friends and, in a spirit of carousal and daring, had climbed the pole. This was unusual behavior for him, and he later could not answer why he had placed himself at such risk. The request for consultation came as a result of his behavior on the unit. He was alternating between periods of anger at the staff for leaving him alone and for causing pain when changing the dressing and periods of contrition and remorse when he begged forgiveness for his anger.

When interviewed he related that he had been living at home alone for the past 3 weeks while his parents were traveling out of the country. This was the first time in his life that he had been left alone, since his older brother had left for college that year. He spontaneously offered, "I wasn't angry that my parents were away." Unit staff reported that his first question on regaining consciousness was, "Are my parents on their way back?"

He had sustained one prior serious accident in his life. At age 4 he tripped and fell and lost part of a digit in his lawn mower while he was running across his yard to greet his parents who arrived home from a trip abroad.

This young accident victim had been engaged in an unaccustomed act of bravado and fearlessness at a time when he was feeling most lonely and needy. His behavior on the ward also suggested problems with guilt resulting from angry feelings toward caregivers. Other victims who fit in this category of pseudo independent behavior have often had an acute falling-out with someone whom they need for support, despite their feelings of angry self-sufficiency. Traffic accident victims in particular seem to fit in this category.

These three categories are not exhaustive, but represent the most familiar themes elicited on interview with accident patients. Other issues, conflicts, needs, fears, and stresses may be involved as precipitants of accidents. In general, there are a variety of stresses that can render many different individuals accident-prone or vulnerable to having an accident at certain periods in their lives.

A 33-year-old man suffered a posterior dislocation of his knee that severed his posterior tibial artery when he walked into a pothole. The patient, formerly in good health, had now been hospitalized three times in the past 6 months. The first admission was for a circumcision; the second was for a concussion suffered in an automobile accident. In an interview the psychiatrist learned that the patient was a chronic loner with a schizoid personality. Six months before, the patient had become married for the first time.

At times an accident appears to be an attempt to resolve a conflict acceptably. In this case a wish to escape from a conflictual situation—closeness with another person—seems to have led the patient to his frequent hospitalizations.

At times there appears to be, in addition to psychological motivation for self-injury, particular significance attached to the nature or site of the injury, much in the same manner attributed to certain conversion symptoms.[27] These may have symbolic meaning, resolve a particular conflict, indicate identification with another injured person, and so forth:

> A 21-year-old woman was admitted after she severed the distal third of the ring finger of her left hand in an industrial accident. She recalled being angry at her employer that day for having been switched to an unsafe machine that her mother, employed by the same company, used to operate. Later in the interview she mentioned that the day prior to her accident, she had broken off her engagement to her fiancé.

While the injury to her ring finger seemed quite psychologically overdetermined to the psychiatrist, ward staff members were previously quite certain that this was a chance accident.

Hirschfeld and Behan[21,28,29] have reviewed 300 cases of industrial accidents and injuries and have emphasized the concept of the accident process. They note that accidents do not just occur but "rather, they are events which are captured by the personality for the purpose of solving the individual's life problem." The process begins with the build-up of conflict and anxiety that are resolved by the accident. Since the accident and resulting injury succeed in resolving the antecedent conflict, the patient becomes a high risk for ongoing disability and for failure to respond to rehabilitation measures or pain relief:

> A 47-year-old married father of five was admitted for evaluation of intractable pain. Four years earlier he had fallen off a loading dock and broken his left ulna and radius. After surgery he had complained of constant pain despite apparently normal neurological findings. He had been on disability payments since that time and had a suit pending against the employer.
>
> When interviewed, he described his childhood as "never had one." His father, who was abusive and alcoholic, abandoned his mother and three sisters when the patient was 11. At age 12 the patient began taking part-time jobs to help support the family and at age 16 he left school to work full-time.
>
> He had never had a respite. At times he had held two jobs to support his own family. Shortly before the accident, he had been passed over for promotion to foreman, a position he felt he deserved.

In this case the patient had never had relief from the burden of work and financial pressures. In addition, he was furious with his employer. The accident and subsequent disability provided short-and long-term resolutions to his conflicts about his anger. They also offered him relief from the pressures of providing for others, a relief to which he felt entitled.

## THE PSYCHIATRIST'S THERAPEUTIC ROLE

The preceding discussion emphasizes the detective and diagnostic aspects of the evaluation of the accident victim to determine the nature and extent of psychological motivation. While instructive about unconscious processes, the foregoing begs the question of the therapeutic utility of these endeavors. There are indeed, however, clinical reasons for the rigorous psychological evaluation of the accident victim.

The search for the unconscious antecedents of accidents has repeatedly uncovered preexisting psychopathology that often had been compromising the patient's general functioning—psychopathology such as unresolved grief, depression, or acute situational disturbances. Generally these three conditions offer the psychiatrist opportunities to make dramatic clinical interventions with a variety of short-term therapeutic modalities. Since these states once predisposed the patient to accidental injury, failure to diagnose and treat these states could lead to a missed prophylactic opportunity, leaving the patient vulnerable to future injury in the same way. Since accident repeaters are a changing group, a person injured for the first time may be one of these transiently accident-prone individuals.

More chronic psychopathology, such as masochistic personality traits, success neurosis, or unresolved dependent feelings, is, of course, more resistant to treatment. However, some of the people with these conditions will improve their patterns of interpersonal relationships and their response to life change in long-term dynamic or supportive psychotherapy. When, for various reasons, these patients are not candidates for treatment, a very direct explanation of their vulnerability to specific stresses should be offered. Masochistic persons might well be spared repeated trauma if instructed about the role of unacceptable anger in their self-injury and if cautioned to be wary of certain situations that bring increased danger. For those who have a success neurosis, who injure themselves at times of moving ahead in life, a warning about times of critical risk can easily be communicated. Such a warning would be humane and ethical, if not certainly therapeutic.

Another important therapeutic role for the psychiatrist evolves from the understanding of the accident-process concept. Many individuals have a high risk of permanent disability after they have captured the accident moment. As time passes these patients will become increasingly resistant to physical and psychological interventions. Early discovery of the anxieties, stresses, and conflicts involved in the accident process will increase the likelihood that psychiatric treatment can be directed to these underlying factors, possibly avoiding enduring disability. Psychological consultation with those involved in the physical rehabilitation and treatment of these patients can at least increase the effectiveness of their work and minimize the possibility of increasing disability for the patients.

A number of emotional sequelae of accidents may be discovered by the therapist in interviews. Feelings of guilt and responsibility are at times evident, especially if others were injured or killed. Whether or not other people were involved, the patient may have a semiawareness of the role of recent upsets or angry feelings in accident causation and be troubled by this. A chance to talk openly with the psychiatrist is then likely to relieve some of this vague uneasiness and to facilitate coping with hospitalization. A dramatic example of such emotional sequelae is the following:

A surgical ward requested consultation for a 19-year-old man who was acting very nervous and agitated. He was in the hospital for multiple fractures and lacerations sustained in a motorcycle accident. The nursing staff was frustrated and angry because the patient was "always on the light" (the signal for assistance). When they responded, he would make such apparently trivial requests as a Kleenex, sip of water, fluffing of the pillow, and so forth. His behavior was generating anger in nursing and house staff members although they knew the patient was anxious. They asked the consultant to suggest an antianxiety agent.

The psychiatrist learned that the patient had had a young girl passenger on the motorcycle; she was killed in the accident, a fact which family and staff knew but had not told the patient. They believed he had lost his memory of the events of the accident day. The staff and family had agreed to keep the secret until he was "strong enough to know." He told the psychiatrist that he feared he was going crazy.

The psychiatrist was convinced that the patient knew more than others suspected, that the secret was the toxin in the environment, and that the patient accepted the conspiracy of silence fearing there was some terrible reason why he was being held ignorant. Meetings with staff and family were held and the parents agreed to tell the secret. The following morning the patient told the psychiatrist, "My memory came back." He proceeded to tell of the young girl and he cried. Then he said, "At least I know that people still love me." The aggravating behavior on the ward subsided dramatically.

The time and effort involved in eliciting detailed history from accident victims are more than justified by the pain and cost of their injuries to themselves, to their families, and to society. Accidents are a major public health issue. The more that is learned about the causes of accidents, both at the individual and at the population level, the closer we will be to more effective prevention.

## SUMMARY

A variety of emotional factors and life stresses can be implicated as important causes of many apparently fortuitous accidents. Usually the accident results from the momentary convergence of psychological vulnerability, transient life stresses, and the physical opportunity for the accident at one point in time. A detailed, investigative psychological interview will often elicit evidence indicting the psychological determinants and will thus permit the consideration of various therapeutic options.

## REFERENCES

1. National Academy of Sciences, Division of Medical Sciences, Committee on Trauma, Committee on Shock: Accidental death and disability: the neglected disease of modern society, Washington, D.C., 1966, U.S. Department of Health, Education, and Welfare.
2. Dickerson, O. D.: Health insurance, Homewood, Illinois, 1963, Richard D. Irwin, Inc.
3. Freud, S.: Complete psychological works, London, 1960, The Hogarth Press Ltd.
4. Menninger, K.: Purposive accidents as an expression of self-destructive tendencies, Int. J. Psychoanal. **17**:6-16, 1936.
5. Sobel, R., and Margolis, J.: Repetitive poisoning in children, a psychological study, Pediatrics **35**:641-651, 1965.
6. Crancer, A., Jr., and Quiring, D. L., Jr.: Driving records of persons hospitalized for suicidal gestures, Behav. Res. Highway Safety **1**:33-43, 1970.
7. Selzer, M. L., and Payne, C. E.: Automobile accidents, suicide, and unconscious motivation, Am. J. Psychiatry **119**:237-240, 1962.
8. Tabachnick, N. D., editor: Accident or suicide? Destruction by automobile, Springfield, Illinois, 1973, Charles C Thomas, Publisher.
9. Selzer, M. L., Rogers, J. E., and Kern, S.: Fatal accidents: the role of psychopathology, social stress, and acute disturbance, Am. J. Psychiatry **124**:1028-1035, 1968.
10. McMurray, L.: Emotional stress and driving performance: the effect of divorce, Behav. Res. Highway Safety **1**:100-114, 1970.

11. McFarland, R. A., and Moseley, A. L.: Human factors in highway transport safety, Cambridge, Massachusetts, 1954, Harvard School of Public Health.

12. Selzer, M. L., and others: Automobile accidents as an expression of psychopathology in an alcoholic population, Q. J. Stud. Alcohol. **28:**505-516, 1967.

13. Selzer, M. L., and Vinokur, A.: Life events, subjective stress, and traffic accidents, Am. J. Psychiatry **131:**903-906, 1974.

14. Tabachnick, N. D., and others: Comparative psychiatric study of accidental and suicidal death, Arch. Gen. Psychiatry **14:**60-68, 1966.

15. Selzer, M. L.: Alcoholism, mental illness, and stress in 96 drivers causing fatal accidents, Behav. Sci. **14:**1-10, 1969.

16. Waller, J. A., and Turkel, H. W.: Alcoholism and traffic deaths, N. Engl. J. Med. **275:**532-536, 1966.

17. Greenwood, M., and Woods, H. M.: Preliminary report on special tests, Sacramento, 1919, California Department of Motor Vehicles.

18. Motor vehicle traffic conditions in the U.S., House Document 462, Part 6, Washington, D.C., 1938, 75th Congress, 3rd Session.

19. Dunbar, F.: Psychosomatic diagnosis, New York, 1943, Paul B. Hoeber, Inc.

20. Alexander, F.: The accident prone individual, Public Health Rep. **64:**357-362, 1949.

21. Hirschfeld, A. H., and Behan, R. C.: The accident process: I. Etiological considerations of industrial injuries, J.A.M.A. **186:**193-199, 1963.

22. Schulzinger, M. S.: Accident syndrome, Arch. Indust. Hyg. Occup. Med.**10:**426-433, 1954.

23. Conger, J. J., and others: Psychological and psychophysiological factors in motor vehicle accidents, J.A.M.A. **169:**1581-1587, 1959.

24. Tillman, W. A., and Hobbs, G. E.: The accident-prone automobile driver: a study of psychiatric and social background, Am. J. Psychiatry**106:**321-331, 1949.

25. Rome, H. P.: Emotional problems leading to cardiovascular accidents, Psychiat. Ann., July, 1975, pp. 6-14.

26. Alexander, F.: Psychosomatic medicine, New York, 1950, W. W. Norton & Co., Inc.

27. Engel, G. L.: Conversion symptoms. In MacBryde, C. M., and Blacklow, R. S., editors: Signs and symptoms, Philadelphia, 1970, J. B. Lippincott Co. pp. 650-668.

28. Behan, R. C., and Hirschfeld, A. H.: The accident process: II. Toward more rational treatment of industrial injuries, J.A.M.A. **186:**300-306, 1963.

29. Hirschfeld, A. H., and Behan, R. C.: The accident process: III. Disability: acceptable and unacceptable, J.A.M.A. **197:**125-128, 1966.

# 21

# The emergency department

**WILLIAM H. ANDERSON**

Psychiatric consultation in an emergency department is a task that differs from other consultation services in several important ways. The physical and psychological environment of the emergency ward is unique in the hospital setting. The time frame, the nature of decision, and the expectations of staff and patients all combine to present the psychiatrist with unusual challenges. In contrast to other patient care areas, the physical and psychosocial environment is highly unpredictable. There is no way to know from minute to minute whether the number of patients will be increased suddenly or whether another arrival will require diversion of therapeutic resources. It is a place where unusual and even unreasonable demands are made frequently. The clinical problems are full of ambiguity and often without an obvious method of approach. Often the physicians who work in the emergency service are not based there primarily and thus are not familiar with the routines of ancillary services. These factors combine to distract the physician from the critical decision-making tasks.

**Emergency decisions.** Decision-making in an emergency department is quite different from that which is usually practiced on other services and at other locations. The physician is usually most comfortable and familiar when approaching questions of diagnosis and treatment in an systematic way. The emergency department has concerns that come even before diagnosis. The first branch of the decision tree concerns a judgment as to the seriousness of the condition. Those patients perceived to have life-threatening emergencies are, of course, examined first. This judgment is often based on nonclinical considerations such as the fanfare with which the patient enters. Next comes the decision to admit the patient or to attempt final diagnosis and treatment in the outpatient service. This decision is also heavily influenced by nonclinical factors such as the availability of beds. Then a decision must be made concerning the service to which the patient should be admitted. When behavioral abnormalities are the presenting symptoms, this decision is not always obvious. Psychiatry, neurology, general medicine, or neurosurgery may be the most appropriate service for definitive management, depending on the circumstances.

**Time frame.** Among the uppermost considerations in patient evaluation is the passage of time. In contrast to other patient-care environments, the emergency department most frequently has a rigid requirement that patients may not stay beyond a designated small number of hours. Problems of psychiatric assessment are not always easy to fit into such time restrictions. The psychiatric consultant may not be notified of the patient's needs until much of the available time has expired. Furthermore, the patient may not be able to give a coherent history and may not be cooperative to examination. Nevertheless, the time frame is constrained for generally sound reasons and it is important for the psychiatric consultant to be comfortable in working within it. This requires that the consultant be familiar with methods of rapid diagnosis, treatment, and disposition that are not normally required on other clinical services. The consultant should see that the patient leaves the emergency area as soon as possible.

**Patients.** Patients who appear for psychiatric consultation in emergency services are not always similar to psychiatric patients in outpatient clinics or inpatient services. They may not define their problem as psychiatric, and they may be correct in this. They may be disruptive or violent, or they may be physically restrained prior to or during the consultation examination. If they are self-referred, they see their problem as extremely urgent and expect its early resolution.

**Staff.** Every consultation is defined by the desires and expectations of the physician or nurse who requests it. With inpatient consultation it is clear that the patient remains the responsibility of the original service and may be transferred only after the primary medical or surgical condition is resolved. In an emergency department this convention is less clear. Consultations are centered more on staff and institutional needs than on patient requests. Thus the consultant may be asked for advice on diagnosis or treatment, or, even more often, may be asked explicitly or implicitly to take over all responsibility for the case.

**Consultant.** The mission of the consultant is then to control the violent and disorderly and to treat those who have such chronic or poorly defined illnesses as alcoholism, drug addiction, depression, psychosis, or hypochondriasis. This type of consultation request, although blunt, represents a legitimate need of a busy general emergency service. It is equally important that the psychiatric consultant be satisfied that no concomitant acute medical or surgical illness exists. Frequently a patient will enter the emergency service with psychosis or other bizarre behavior that is brought about by acute organic brain disease. Because the behavioral manifestations are often much more prominent than other signs of illness and because these behavioral manifestations often compromise such routine measures as checking vital signs, taking a history, and making a physical examination, the psychiatric consultant must remain alert to the possibility of subtle organic disease. The consultant should never routinely trust another physician's judgment that organic disease has been ruled out.

## GENERAL PRINCIPLES OF EFFECTIVE EMERGENCY ROOM CONSULTATION

1. Respect the constraints of time. It is seldom possible to develop a thoroughly satisfactory psychiatric diagnosis of a patient's difficulty in the time and circumstances available in an emergency department. It is therefore necessary to assess the patient's condition quickly for any acute occult medical illness, for psychosis or other serious psychiatric illness, and for suicide potential. On the basis of these assessments make a decision clear whether the patient needs inpatient or outpatient care. In either case, expedite the decision.

2. Have confidence in a method of identifying major organic illnesses that may resemble psychiatric conditions. This requires that the psychiatrist be familiar with the relevant methods of history taking, physical examination, and laboratory work.

3. Clarify any ambiguity of responsibility at once. Be sure to determine whether the patient is yours to diagnose and treat as you see fit, or whether your role is the more traditional one of an advising consultant.

4. Give clear orders that will assure the necessary degree of safety and security for patient and staff. Write notes that are short and avoid jargon. Specify how medication is to be given and whether restraints or constant supervision is needed.

## PSYCHIATRIC EMERGENCIES
### Acute organic psychosis as distinguished from functional psychosis

Psychosis is one of the more frequent of the emergencies for which psychiatric consultation is requested. Psychosis is a disorder of information processing during which the patient has diminished capacity to receive, retain, process, recall, and act on information in a plausible or culturally acceptable manner. Numerous causes, both organic and functional, may be implicated. Physicians unfamiliar with psychosis are apt to make the assumption that any hallucinatory or delusional activity necessarily implies a diagnosis of schizophrenia or other functional psychosis. There are, of course, cases in which the distinction between organic brain disease and schizophrenia or mania can be extremely difficult and can require expert consultation and exhaustive laboratory tests. Such investigations are not practical in the emergency department setting. The emergency room consultant therefore requires a simple method of identifying first those medical and surgical conditions that cause death or irreparable damage in a short time and that may resemble functional psychosis. Fortunately, there are a few general principles that facilitate the recognition of acute organic brain disease.

1. In emergency department consultations it is important to retain a high index of suspicion for organic psychosis—to assume that the disordered information processing is a result of organic brain disease until serious medical and surgical conditions are excluded.
2. A psychosis is not functional simply because of a so-called precipitating psychological event. Most illness with rapid onset can be traced to an outside event if the psychiatrist is determined to find one. The "precipitating" event has little value in differential diagnosis.
3. It is dangerous to assume that an illness is functional because of specific mental content. Even the most classical schizophrenic delsuions are often seen in organic brain disease.
4. The more acute the onset of psychotic illness, the more the psychiatrist must suspect organic causes. Neither schozophrenia nor manic-depressive illness develops in hours or days as a general rule.
5. A first episode of acute psychotic illness in a person over 40 years of age most frequently implies organic cause.
6. A psychosis in a patient who has a previously diagnosed, serious, medical illness is usually a complication of the illness or of its treatment. A major malfunction of the heart, lung, liver, kidney, or endocrine system often announces itself by psychotic decompensation of the mental status. Numerous medications can produce similar changes.
7. Organic psychosis is not necessarily excluded by the absence of

localized signs. Many organic psychoses produce such signs late in their course or not at all.

**History.** As in all fields of medicine, the history often yields the most diagnostically helpful information. Psychotic patients will often give critical information if examining physicians are patient and tactful in their inquiries. Often the more rewarding inquiries are those about the use of drugs, medications, and alcohol and about any previous metabolic illness. The questioning of relatives and the perusal of medical records are often revealing. Examination of the contents of wallets and pockets is similarly helpful.

**Mental status examination.** The mental status examination is also a helpful tool. Most valuable are the evaluation of orientation, memory, and hallucinosis. Failure to identify time or place correctly is evidence for organic brain disease. Difficulty recalling five objects immediately and after 5 minutes is also an indication of organic disease. Visual or tactile hallucinosis generally suggests organic brain disease of the toxic or metabolic type.

**Physical examination.** A complete physical examination is always desirable, but not all aspects of it are equally productive of useful information. Checking vital signs however, including a reliable temperature, is absolutely indispensable. Most of the other important findings are available to careful inspection with a minimum of invasive action. Signs of autonomic dysfunction and abnormal motor activity are especially useful. Examination for head injuries, nystagmus, and pathological reflexes are often useful.

**Laboratory investigation.** Laboratory investigation has limited but definite value in otherwise uncertain cases. Among the most useful procedures are electroencephalography and blood tests for such chemical constituents as electrolytes, glucose, blood urea nitrogen, and toxic agents.

**Priorities in diagnosis.** It is important to recognize that there are clear priorities in diagnosis. In the milieu of the emergency department it is critical to first investigate and confirm or exclude those conditions that are life-threatening.

1. *Meningitis* and *encephalitis.* Fever, headache, elevated pulse or white blood cell count, or presence of meningeal signs should suggest this diagnosis.
2. *Hypoglycemia.* History of diabetes mellitus, weakness, and signs of sympathetic hyperactivity (sweating, dilated reactive pupils) make it necessary to check the blood glucose.
3. *Hypertensive encephalopathy.* Blood pressure measurement is sufficient to exclude this entity.

4. *Diminished cerebral oxygenation.* Cardiovascular and pulmonary conditions and severe anemia from any cause (including major unrecognized bleeding) may bring about an acute psychotic state. A change in mental status may be the first sign of decompensation of these systems.

5. *Poisonings.* In the absence of a patient history, the diagnosis of poisoning may be difficult to make. Tricyclic antidepressants are among the most commonly abused agents. These drugs are very toxic in acute overdoses. The presenting signs are consistent with delirium of the atropine type with peripheral signs of cholinergic blockade.

6. *Intracranial hemorrhage.* This condition is recognized by the presence of headache and meningeal signs.

7. *Wernicke encephalopathy.* Although Wernicke encephalopathy is not a life-threatening condition, the consequences of untreated Wernicke disease are so profound that they must be considered here. Acute confusional states in alcoholic individuals or others who are nutritionally deprived ought to be treated expectantly with parenteral thiamine. (50 mg given intravenously immediately and 50 mg given intramuscularly daily until normal diet is resumed.)

These conditions are medical and surgical emergencies that must be recognized and dealt with at once in order to avoid serious sequelae or death. There are other conditions less critical than those listed that may also appear at first to be acute functional psychosis and that require decisive early action. Among these are: (1) chronic subdural hematoma, (2) subacute bacterial endocarditis, (3) hepatic failure, (4) uremia, (5) thyrotoxicosis or myxedema, (6) delirium tremens, and (7) atropine delirium.

Many other conditions may resemble functional psychosis. These are listed in the box. The recognition of acute organic brain disease as an entity distinct from functional psychosis continues to be an important function of the consultation psychiatrist. In the setting of an emergency service, this function is especially critical. When the pattern of psychosis is consistent with organic brain disease, the first order of business is to make a diagnosis. This usually means admission to the general medical service, where diagnostic expertise and nursing care are apt to be optimum.

### Acute functional psychosis—schizophrenia and mania

**Diagnosis.** After having considered organic brain disease as a cause of psychosis and having rejected it as an hypothesis, the emergency

## METABOLIC AND STRUCTURAL DISORDERS WITH PRESENTING PSYCHOTIC FEATURES

**Space-occupying lesions**

Primary tumors
Metastatic carcinoma (lung, breast)
Subdural hematoma
Brain abscess (bacterial, fungal, gumma, cysticerosis)

**Cerebral hypoxia**

Pulmonary insufficiency
Severe anemia
Diminished cardiac output
Toxic agents such as carbon monoxide

**Metabolic and endocrine disorders**

Electrolyte imbalance
Calcium
Thyroid disease (thyrotoxicosis and myxedema)
Pituitary insufficiency
Adrenal disease (Addison and Cushing disease)
Hypoglycemia
Diabetes
Uremia
Hepatic failure
Porphyria

**Exogenous substances**

Alcohol (intoxication and withdrawal)
Barbiturates and other sedatives (intoxication and withdrawal)
Amphetamines
Lysergic acid diethylamide and similar compounds
Anticholinergic agents
Heavy metals
Digitalis
Corticosteroids
Levodopa
Reserpine
Cocaine
Bromides
Marihuana
Carbon disulfide
Isoniazid
Cycloserine

---

### METABOLIC AND STRUCTURAL DISORDERS WITH PRESENTING PSYCHOTIC FEATURES—cont'd

**Nutritional deficiencies**

Thiamine (Wernicke-Korsakoff syndrome)
Niacin (pellagra)
Vitamin $B_{12}$

**Vascular abnormalities**

Intracranial hemorrhage
Lacunar state (hypertension)
Collagen diseases
Aneurysms

**Infections**

Meningitis (bacterial, fungal, tuberculous)
Encephalitis (viral, for example, herpes)
Lues
Subacute bacterial endocarditis
Typhoid
Malaria

**Miscellaneous conditions**

Normal pressure hydrocephalus
Temporal lobe epilepsy
Huntington chorea
Alzheimer disease
Remote effects of carcinoma
Wilson disease
Pancreatitis

---

service psychiatric consultant is faced with the diagnosis of acute schizophrenia or mania. The task now is to determine whether the circumstances demand that the patient be admitted to inpatient psychiatric care or whether it is a plausible alternative to consider outpatient treatment as an option.

**Disposition.** There are three important questions to answer before determining appropriate disposition for these functionally psychotic patients.

1. Is there suicidal or homicidal danger?
2. Is there viable family or social support?
3. What is the initial response to medication?

The psychotic patient who has attempted suicide or who has thoughts of self-destruction must be considered to be in extreme danger and in general requires immediate hospital admission, rapid treatment of the psychosis, and close direct observation. For the psychotic patient, suicide is a highly unpredictable consequence. Any hint of impulsive behavior or active bad judgment as to safety should mandate hospitalization. A psychotic patient need not be intentionally suicidal in order to accomplish death. For example, a manic patient may have no intention of harming himself, but his judgment may be so impaired that he will attempt a 30 mile walk in subzero weather.

The next important consideration is the extent and quality of the patient's social support. A psychotic patient who has no available family or friends should be hospitalized. If the patient has a family that is alert, competent, and concerned, and that will provide the patient with environmental protection and will ensure the taking of medication and his continuous outpatient visits, hospitalization may be avoided.

Finally, the response to initial treatment must be considered. Many patients will respond to parenteral antipsychotic medication with a considerable remission of symptoms for several hours. When such a degree of remission occurs, oral medication may be continued in outpatient treatment.

**Method of initial treatment.** When the diagnosis of acute functional psychosis (mania or schizophrenia) has been made, antipsychotic medicine may be started in the emergency service. Parenteral high-potency drugs are generally preferred. High-potency antipsychotics such as haloperidol or trifluoperazine have relatively little sedative, hypotensive, or anticholinergic effect. The parenteral route is preferred because of more rapid response. Sedation, per se, is often an undesirable side effect for the patient who has acute psychosis. Lower potency drugs that have greater sedative properties, such as chlorpromazine, are less useful in rapid treatment because side effects limit the amount that can be used within a few hours in the emergency setting. A typical regimen might include an initial 5 mg dose of haloperidol that might be repeated hourly with 5 mg or 10 mg doses. Frequent observation is required to determine whether satisfactory improvement occurs or whether side effects will limit further treatment. First day remission will occur in about half of the cases with doses of intramuscular haloperidol ranging between 15 mg and 45 mg. There is no evidence that stronger doses promote further improvement on the first day. The physician should be alert for the development of acute dystonia, which occurs in about a third of the cases so treated. Benztropine mesylate is an effective treatment for this condition.

**Follow-up.** Unless a highly satisfactory remission of symptoms occurs, the patient should be transferred to an inpatient unit. If such a remission is present and all other factors are favorable, outpatient treatment may be continued. Oral medication may be substituted for the parenteral. For the first few days many patients require the same dose given orally as the total remission-inducing parenteral dose. Some patients will require more or less. The keystone of successful initial outpatient management is to adjust the dose on an individual basis for the first few days to allow for adequate continued remission with minimum side effects.

### Suicide

Suicide is the topic of Chapter 13 and is discussed in more detail there. Remarks will be restricted here to the special problems of consultation of a suicidal patient in an emergency department.

Patients who have made suicide attempts or who have suicidal ideation or even depression seem to elicit very little sympathetic understanding in the emergency milieu. Physicians and nurses often assume a punitive or derisory attitude that is, to say the least, countertherapeutic. Since the typical emergency department is not always suitable for on-the-spot staff education, often the most prudent choice is to remove the patient to more peaceful and less abrasive surroundings while evaluation takes place. At all times it must be kept in mind that the emergency room is a very fertile field for obtaining means of self-harm. Ideally the patient should be kept under constant observation with adequate security measures to abort further attempts.

Psychiatric consultants must remember that their basic task is to decide whether suicidal or depressed patients require inpatient or outpatient care. All other concerns are secondary, since time is not on the side of adaptive response in most cases. Several risk factors affect the decision for hospitalization.

**Risk factors.** Patients who attempt or contemplate suicide by violent means are among the gravest risks in the emergency room situation. Shooting, hanging, and mutilation suggest the more profound disturbances and argue for immediate hospitalization in a secure facility and expeditious treatment of the underlying disorder. A combination of a highly lethal method and survival only by good fortune should call for constant vigilance and security.

*Psychosis* with attempted or contemplated suicide is also an indication for the most zealous and watchful care. It is important to remember that manic patients often have the combination of impaired judgment and increased energy that makes a completed suicide or accidental death possible.

*Intoxication* presents some of the most difficult problems in emergency service psychiatry. Ideally, intoxicated patients should be kept under close observation until they are thoroughly detoxified from the alcohol or other sedative drug. A meaningful evaluation is hardly possible until this has been accomplished. Unfortunately it is not always possible to keep the patient in the emergency department for the length of time required. In such a case the best solution is to admit the patient to a psychiatric facility where adequate medical attention as well as suicide prevention is possible.

*Severe depression* is another risk factor that makes rapid decision necessary. This is especially true if the depression is mixed with agitation such that ample energy is available for self-harm.

### Violent and assaultive behavior

Violent and assaultive patients are among the most difficult patients the emergency service psychiatrist must face. An emergency service frequently becomes paralyzed when confronted by unrestricted violence. Consultants can find themselves without the accustomed help from colleagues. Three tasks are defined; the situation must be controlled, the presumptive etiology identified, and the patient treated.

It is best to marshal more than sufficient force before the initial confrontation to keep the situation under control so that evaluation can be made. It is worse than useless to attempt to interrupt violence with inadequate or marginal countermeasures. Fewer injuries and less damage will result if the counterforce is overwhelming and rapid. It is best if there is a trained security force to accomplish the task of applying physical restraint.

Once the patient is under control, the task is to identify possible underlying causes of the violence. Violent behavior of organic etiology includes sedative intoxication and withdrawal, amphetamine intoxication, thyroid dysfunction, hypoglycemia, and temporal lobe epilepsy. Functional etiologies include the psychoses with paranoid features, catatonic excitement, impulse character disorder, and antisocial personality.

Adjunctive chemotherapy is often valuable even before a diagnosis is made. High potency antipsychotic drugs in adequate parenteral dosage are the most useful agents. Nonspecific sedatives such as barbiturates or benzodiazepines are likely to make the situation worse by promoting further disinhibition unless the cause of the violence is sedative withdrawal.

### Alcoholism

Chronic abusers of alcohol are vulnerable in an emergency room milieu. Often in spite of the best intentions, the staff of the service tends to give less than complete evaluation to the alcoholic patient's somatic complaints.

The psychiatric interventions for the alcoholic patient are nonspecific and in general not amenable to the routine of the emergency department. The psychiatric consultant's task, in addition to attempting to organize ongoing care, is to try to make certain that no related somatic condition coexists. Common complications of alcoholism include delirium tremens, hypoglycemia, subdural hematoma, hepatic decompensation, epilepsy, and Wernicke-Korsakoff syndrome.

### Acute anxiety

Acute anxiety with hyperventilation is one of the most frequently seen psychiatric difficulties in the emergency department. The psychiatric consultant's first task is to make certain that the anxiety is in fact psychogenic and not merely the most visible sign of an underlying acute medical condition. The classical picture is one of very rapid and deep breathing, paresthesia of extremities and face, and possible tetany. The physical symptoms arise from respiratory alkalosis. Among the medical illnesses that resemble this condition are:

1. Toxic conditions; aspirin ingestion, amphetamines, caffeine, and steroids
2. Alcohol or sedative withdrawal
3. Metabolic disturbances; hypoglycemia, hypocalcemia, hyperthyroidism, Cushing disease
4. Temporal lobe epilepsy
5. Acute blood loss
6. Incipient anaphylaxis

Most of these entities can be excluded by taking a careful history. Typically the patient is a young person with acutely emergent neurotic conflict. Such other psychiatric disorders as agitated depression or phobic-anxiety state may also be present. The investigation for the psychiatric differential diagnosis is best pursued in the outpatient department. A rebreathing bag is usually sufficient to control the acute symptoms of anxiety and to demonstrate the underlying physiological substrate.

## The overnight ward

The Massachusetts General Hospital emergency area has a small ward, known as the Overnight Ward, distinct from the general Emergency Room. Patients may be admitted from any service and may stay for a maximum of 72 hours. This allows for rapid multiple consultations from several services and for laboratory investigation for those cases in which diagnosis is uncertain or for which a short period of intensive observation is ideal. Such a ward is very convenient for solving some of the problems descibed in this chapter. Many emergency patients who appear to have psychiatric problems can be admitted to such a ward to determine quickly whether medical or surgical intervention is indicated. In addition to the benefits to the patient, the house staff from every service has an opportunity to observe closely a number of patients and diagnoses that would be unlikely to be seen otherwise. It represents a very useful adjunct to the emergency service and promotes efficient hospital utilization.

### SUGGESTED READINGS

Anderson, W. H., and Kuehnle, J. C.: Strategies for the treatment of acute psychosis, J.A.M.A. **229:**1884-1889, 1974.

Anderson, W. H., and Kuehnle, J. C.: Rapid treatment of acute psychosis, Am. J. Psychiatry **133:**1076-1078, 1976.

Benson, D. F.,and Blumer, D.: Psychiatric aspects of neurologic disease, New York, 1975, Grune & Stratton, Inc.

Detre, T. P., and Jarecki, H. G.: Modern psychiatric treatment, Philadelphia, 1971, J. B. Lippincott Co.

Plum, F., and Posner, J. B.: The diagnosis of stupor and coma, Philadelphia, 1966, F. A. Davis Co.

Shader, R. I., editor: Manual of psychiatric therapeutics, Boston, 1975, Little, Brown and Co.

# 22

# The burn unit

**GORDON HARPER**

Burn units exist in general hospitals and in self-contained burn hospitals. They offer the burned patient specialized treatment, including extraordinary protection against infection, by specially trained surgical and nursing staff. Such units bring together patients whose overwhelming injuries involve nearly every kind of medical, surgical, and psychological problem; whose care is protracted and painful; and whose survival is uncertain. A distinct set of psychological problems comes to be expected among both patients and staff of burn units.[1-4] Accordingly, many units[4,5] have made the psychiatric consultant a formal member of the treatment team responsible for the care of all burn patients rather than a consultant to be called on when a particular problem arises. Being severely burned is considered sufficient indication for examination by a psychiatrist.

The psychiatric consultant in the burn unit deals with disorders of the sensorium due to toxic states, infections, and disordered metabolism; with problems associated with the psychological reactions of patients and families to trauma and life-threatening illness; with the problems experienced by staff working in specialized intensive care units; and with the long-term psychological and social consequences of disfigurement, especially of the face.

## MODALITIES OF INTERVENTION

The burn unit consultant's role will vary according to the phase of a patient's illness, as indicated below. The consultant may provide consultation to nurses or physicians; recommendations to staff concerning both psychological and psychopharmacological management; diagnostic or therapeutic interviews with patients, including hypnosis for relief of pain; and diagnostic and therapeutic interviews with

□This section was written while the author was supported by a grant from the Commonwealth Fund.

family members. Discussions of these modalities are presented in other sections of this book.

The small size of most burn units and the regularity with which psychological problems emerge there have led to the use of psychiatric measures less common on other units offering intensive care. A routine introductory interview shortly after the patient's admission gives the consultant a chance to assess the patient and to discuss with staff the ways in which this kind of person may be helped to cope with his illness (see Chapter 14). This interview facilitates any subsequent consultation and expresses concretely to the patient the staff's awareness that sustaining and recovering from a severe burn is an extraordinarily stressful experience during which the patient may use resources, including the psychiatrist's help, he might not otherwise need. A weekly nurses' group meeting with the consultant is believed by many to be a necessary support to the staff members who deal firsthand with the patients and their pain. Such meetings give an opportunity for catharsis, for mutual support, and for sharing of information concerning the ways different individuals cope with stress, loss, and grief. Weekly patients' group and family group meetings conducted by the psychiatrist serve similar purposes for patients and relatives.

Nurses need both specialized skills and emotional equanimity to care for burn patients. The developmental stage of the staff as a whole is important to consider in assessing many problems arising on the unit. A cohesive and seasoned staff with experienced leadership will use the skills of the consultant in a way quite different from the staff that is in an earlier stage of development. For example, after a change in leadership on a unit or after the replacement of several experienced nurses by recent graduates, the consultant may receive fewer consultation requests or be requested to help suppress behavior, with special emphasis on medication, at the expense of understanding the distress behind the behavior. Bernstein[5] has described the prominence of requests for and use of hypnosis at an early stage in the development of a pediatric burn unit. At such times consultants may also find an increase in conflicts within the staff, between nursing and surgical staff, or between the staff and themselves as consultant. The same personnel a few months later may be working together smoothly and effectively and seeking consultation more out of a wish to understand and help than out of frustration.

Operating schedules and the limited time physicians spend with patients may make it difficult to arrange regular contacts between the psychiatric consultant and surgical staff. Nevertheless, the development of that relationship will greatly enhance the consultant's understanding of the unit and its patients and his effectiveness on behalf of both. It would behoove the psychiatrist to go out of his way to meet regularly with his surgical colleagues until he becomes known and trusted by them.

## Acute phase

The patient's first days on the burn unit are dominated by the physiological shock of the burn, with fluid loss and electrolyte imbalance, and by medical and surgical efforts to stabilize the patient. Such emergency surgical procedures as removal of dead tissue, amputation, or tracheotomy may be performed.

Immediately after the burn, the patient may show a dissociated calm, in which he is lucid, not anxious, emotionally unconnected to the catastrophe that has occurred. His calm may be upsetting to relatives or staff to whom this state can be clarified as a short-term way of coping with overwhelming injury. Soon an acute traumatic reaction supervenes, reflecting physiological compromise of cerebral function as well as emotional instability and marked by an exaggerated startle response and day and nightmares in which the injury is relived. This reaction may clear or it may blend into delirium (see Chapter 6), characterized by disorientation, insomnia, variable levels of consciousness and awareness, and often agitation. Delirium can continue off and on until most of the burned areas are covered by successful grafts or new skin.

Management includes careful:
1. Fluid and electrolyte regulation
2. Review of possible deliriogenic side effects of medications, especially sedatives, atropine derivatives, and opiate analgesics
3. Use of reorienting statements by all personnel
4. Constant bedside presence of trusted relatives and friends
5. Symptomatic use of sedatives and antianxiety drugs. Chlorpromazine is especially useful; its potential hypothermic effect is outweighed by its sedative, antisingultic, antipruritic, antiemetic, and narcotic-analgesic–potentiating effects. The benzodiazepines (chlordiazepoxide and diazepam) may also have a role.
6. Avoidance of barbiturates because they further impair cerebral function
7. Education and reassurance to family that these mental symp-

toms are transient and do not mean that insanity will be added to the patient's problems. Those treating delirium may have to contend with the feeling that the patient should be left delirious, "better off not knowing about all this." This attitude, which may reflect failure to distinguish one's own from the patient's perspective, can be countered by pointing out the terror that the delirium itself causes in the patient.

In this phase, family members experience acute shock and the beginnings of grief. Support for them includes opportunity for catharsis, explanation of the normality of the patient's reactions and of their own feelings as well, and help with the practical aspects of life during a crisis.

A role has been proposed for hypnosis in the acute phase as a means to attenuate burn depth by reducing the inflammatory reaction to the thermal insult.[6] The clinical reports behind this proposal await replication.

For the unit as a whole, the appeal of some patients and their injuries in this phase may elicit extraordinary mobilization of personnel, effort, and hope. When patients fail to respond dramatically, or when they die, staff let-down and discouragement affect morale and care of other patients and become issues for staff discussion. We at Massachusetts General Hospital have found it valuable to hold a meeting with nurses and physicians (if the latter will attend) immediately after a death where heroic efforts were made to sustain life. A communal ventilation of feeling often averts a dangerous drop in morale.

### Intermediate phase

After initial stabilization, the patient must undergo weeks to months of repeated attempts to cover his burned areas with skin grafts. Each procedure may result in a successful graft or sloughing. Because of this, patients' moods range from hope to dispair. Infection is inevitable in severely burned individuals. Vigorous treatment of infection may include tracheotomy and use of assisted ventilation. Debridement of dead tissue and changes of dressings are frequent, painful experiences. Limb and even trunk immobilization may be necessary during grafting. If patients' backs are burned, they may be prone for a month or more. Patients with extensive burns have huge caloric needs. They must consume 5,000 to 6,000 calories per day despite anorexia and nausea. Parenteral hyperalimentation may have to be used.

Psychologically , although delirium may continue to be a problem at times, the patient is now aware of the extent of his injuries. The psychological work now consists of coping with these extraordinary stresses and maintaining hope while beginning to grieve for what has been lost. Losses may include appearance, limbs or the use of limbs, genital tissue or genital function, and the ability to do accustomed work or to work at all. The patient must undertake the task of surviving deprived of most of his usual ways of coping. He lies in bed, often immobilized, infected, exhausted, and in frequent or constant pain—pain that becomes agonizing when dressings are changed.

The discussions in Chapter 5 and Chapter 14 are relevant to this phase. The particular coping patterns of burn patients have been described in some detail by Hamburg[7] and Andreason[4]. In the adaptive phase, the spectrum includes delusion (verbal equivalent: "I am not in this situation at all, but in a better one"); denial ("I may be in the hospital, but I am not hurt or hurt only slightly"); repression ("I have no feelings about my injury"); constriction ("I know I am severely hurt, but have no feelings about anything"); and suppression ("I know how serious my situation is, but I will not let myself think about it"). Many patients experience psychological regression marked by low frustration tolerance, demanding infantile behavior, exaggerated dependency needs, and unaccustomed hostile outbursts. On the other hand, overstrenuous efforts not to be dependent but to be in charge of all aspects of their own care, may also be observed. In the recovery phase, such coping mechanisms as mobilization of hope, reinvolvement with others, restoration of relationships, use of humor, active participation in their own care, and participation in group activities appear.

While premorbid personality is relevant to all behavior in the hospital, one aspect of burn patients' premorbid situations is especially relevant to their course—their possible unconscious contribution to their own injury. While a few patients are severely burned in acknowledged suicide attempts, many more do not acknowledge or are not aware of such self-destructive motivation. The exploration of this possibility clearly calls for circumspection, if only because of the forensic aspects of accidental fires. Nonetheless, the role of so-called victims in their own injury should be considered because many problems of apathy, anorexia, antagonistic behavior, or extreme regression in the unit will otherwise not be understandable. Psychiatrists are so often accustomed to thinking of depression in the burn patient as reactive in nature that they may overlook an important preburn depression.

The management problems associated with patients' own contributions to their injuries are of three kinds:

1. In some cases when depression preceded the injury and the burn may be seen as a suicide equivalent, depression manifest on the burn unit must be assessed in the context of the patients' lives before the injuries and not simply as reactions to the burns themselves.

2. With patients who before the accident consistently neglected their safety, the burn accident may be seen as a continuation of that pattern. Problems of overdependency, regression, or lack of cooperation manifested on the burn unit must be related to these longer-standing patterns as well.

3. Tension between burned patients who were pure victims of fate and those who seem to have contributed to their injury may be an issue on the unit, especially when those burned in the same fire are present. Strain and conflict between these two groups may extend to patients and families. Staff may feel and act quite differently toward patients according to the circumstances of their injuries, seeing the so-called victims as undeserving of care or sympathy.

Assessment of these issues requires exceptional tact and discretion. Patients, family, and staff may have great investment in unconscious denial of the patient's depression, characterological self-destructiveness, or sense of entitlement. Denial of such problems may be adaptive for them during this phase. Accordingly, consultants may keep their appreciation of these issues to themselves, or share it only with appropriate staff. Once appreciated, depressive or characterological problems should be managed according to the principles in Chapter 10.

Young men are overrepresented in burn units, primarily because of their occupational and recreational exposure to accidental fires. They find inactivity and dependency particularly stressful. While lying in bed all day and requiring help in many intimate acts of self-care are stressful for all patients, they represent the greatest change for young men who are accustomed to activity as a way of life and for young men whose physical movement is a major part of their identity. Usually these are individuals who prefer to cope with stress through bodily activity. They may become uncooperative, disruptive, or they may regress to an exaggerated degree of helplessness and dependence. Such adaptations can alienate staff and prevent the patient himself from mobilizing his own hope and determination behind the will to survive.

For all burn patients and for active young men in particular, management includes presenting the patients' role as a job to be done ("lying there and taking the pain is hard work") and offering full information and active choices in determining as many aspects of their own care as possible. They can be encouraged to participate in daily events like choosing the order in which nursing procedures are done, or their time of day; arranging their own rooms; indicating a preferred site for venipuncture; or, when possible, making major choices such as the order or timing of surgical procedures.

For men whose injury includes genital damage or loss, both the emotional meaning and the endocrine consequences of that loss may exacerbate problems in coping. A syndrome of tearful emotional collapse and feelings of helplessness that is responsive to testosterone replacement has been described in men with testicular loss.[8]

For others, inability to talk due to facial burn or tracheotomy can be extremely stressful; all efforts should be made to give the patient alternate means of communication, such as materials for writing, a communication board, or for those unable to use their hands, the assistance of those skilled in lip-reading.

Pain and depression are issues for all burn patients in this phase. Then the principles discussed in Chapters 4 and 10 are relevant. In the burn unit, the issue of patients' pain is complicated by the inevitable exacerbation of pain with dressing changes. The nurses are acutely aware of the role they themselves have in the patient's worst pain. "Leave me alone. Stop hurting me and let me die," most patients will say or imply at some point. Such an experience puts a strain on the nurses and makes patients' pain not just a psychophysiological event, but an interpersonal and social ordeal as well. The consultant's role in dealing with such pain must include the ward team and take account of the developmental phase of the unit. Teaching nurses the use of relaxation techniques or hypnosis that can be incorporated into the procedure of changing dressings is sometimes extraordinarily helpful to patients in terms of reducing their discomfort. It is equally useful in assuaging the nurse's sense of guilt about inflicting pain.[9]

Patients for whom antidepressant medication is indicated will be relatively few considering the universality among burn patients of depressive symptoms. Medication will be useful for those patients whose depression is severe and likely to be prolonged, for those who have accompanying vegetative signs of depression, and for those whose depression preceded their injury. While antidepressants of the tricyclic group are likely to be more useful than monoamine oxidase inhibitors for the same reasons that account for their greater general use, drug choice will depend on the individual physician's experience and preference.

In assessing the depression inevitably associated with the intermediate phase, it is especially important to consider (1) the possibility that depression preceded the injury, (2) the location and extent of the burn and the likelihood of permanent disability or disfigurement, and (3) the meaning to the individual of his current and future losses. Patients at this point begin to anticipate their lives after recovery and to integrate whatever deformity, disfigurement, or altered life possibilities are to be expected. At the same time they must be helped to focus their resources on the immediate problem of getting their uncovered bodies covered. They must be encouraged to defer detailed consideration of long-term issues until the time when these issues are real and not just potential concerns.

Especially helpful to patient, staff, and family here will be the consultant's ability to provide information about the inevitable components of grief, mourning, and depression; to accept the associated anger, sadness, and guilt; and to put into perspective the emotional reactions that can be troubling and appear to get in the way of critical medical and surgical procedures. The consultant can also serve as a much needed conduit of information between surgeon and family.

During the discouragements of the intermediate phase, staff may tend to prejudge patients' decision of what they will do with their lives and losses. "With losses like that," staff members may say, "no one would want to live. What are we doing?" Such reactions may reflect inappropriate identification with patients or the exhaustion and frustration that come with caring intensively for patients who don't get better, who don't get better fast enough, or who have already in some way died. Weisman has used the term "hypermature life" with regard to patients who live on after one or more occasions when their death seemed imminent.[10] Clinical staff and families alike are caught in a confusing mixture of anticipated and postponed grief. They feel angry with patients whose tenacious hold on life so alters the expected psychological work of mourning. They also, of course, feel guilty for having such feelings. Prejudging the patient's wish to live is also related to the high mortality in burn units (up to 50% or higher, depending on the severity of the burns of patients referred) and to the staff's conflicting needs to grieve the last patient who died while caring for the living patient. The value of team meetings becomes evident when these issues can be raised by the consultant and discussed by all.

Without such intervention, it is unlikely that caregivers would be aware of how their covert decisions about patients' future chances may influence the quality of care they provide. The goal for all should be to help patients recover to the point where they can decide for themselves what they want to do with their altered lives.

**Rehabilitative phase**

Once most of the body surface is covered with grafts and the danger from infection subsides, concern shifts from life-saving grafting to surgery intended to improve function and appearance, to rehabilitative physical therapy, and to social recovery. Patients may return to their previous lives, or, if their handicaps are great, to a radically altered life. Disfigured patients, especially the facially disfigured, are high risks for "social death."[11] Bernstein has described the high proportion of untraceable burn patients lost to follow-up and untraceable, without known addresses or telephone numbers, apparently living, if surviving, with extremely restricted social contacts.[5]

The shift from the intermediate to the rehabilitative phase can represent a great loss for patients, despite the obvious gains in physical well-being. They lose contact with personnel who have been intimately involved with them for months; they relinquish the special investment that the hospital staff makes in the critically ill; and also they leave behind a period when their biggest problems were susceptible to medical and surgical intervention. Because there are so many factors operating against the social recovery of patients in this phase, particular attention to psychosocial supports is indicated. On the burn unit itself visits from former patients with good adjustments, group discussion, and staged reentry into social situations are examples of such supports. Those burned in war, at least in England and France, have been known spontaneously to form clubs that provide mutual support and reduce social isolation. No such groups have been reported among civilians who recover from serious burns, probably because of their different situation. No patriotic or idealistic pride is associated with the circumstances of the civilian's injuries and considerable conscious or unconscious shame may be associated with injuries, especially those to which the individual may have contributed. The burn unit community itself, where patients engage in their personal struggle and where considerable pride is attached to their progress, can therefore have great continuing importance for the social recovery of physically recovered patients.

## REFERENCES

1. Cobb, S., and Lindemann, E.: Neuropsychiatric observations, Ann. Surg. **117**:814-824, 1943.
2. Lewis, S. R., and others: Psychological studies in burn patients, Plast. Reconstr. Surg. **31**:323-332, 1963.
3. Jorgensen, J. A., and Brophy, J. J.: Psychiatric treatment of severely burned adults, Psychosomatics **14**:331-335, 1973.
4. Andreason, N. J. C., and others: Management of emotional reactions of seriously burned adults, N. Eng. J. Med. **286**:59-65, 1972.
5. Bernstein, N. R.: Emotional care of the facially burned and disfigured, Boston, 1976, Little, Brown and Co.
6. Ewin, D. M.: Clinical use of hypnosis for attenuation of burn depth. Paper presented at the Seventh International Congress of Hypnosis and Psychosomatic Medicine, Philadelphia, July, 1976.
7. Hamburg, D. A., Hamburg, B., and DeGonza, S.: Adaptive problems and mechanisms in severely burned patients, Psychiatry **16**:1-20, 1953.
8. Money, J.: Personal communication.
9. Schafer, D. W.: Hypnosis use on a burn unit, Clin. Exp. Hypn. **23**:1-14, 1975.
10. Weisman, A. D.: Personal communication.
11. MacGregor, F. C., and others: Facial deformities and plastic surgery: a psychosocial study, Springfield, Illinois, 1953, Charles C Thomas, Publisher.

# 23

# The spinal cord–injured patient

**THOMAS D. STEWART**

Is there a role for psychiatry with the spinal cord–injured patient? Certainly the depression, denial, anger, and insecurity permeating such patients (and their caregivers) have a reality anchored in actual tragic loss. What could a psychiatrist trained to treat the pathological distortions of reality associated with neurosis and psychosis possibly offer?

Psychologists such as Wright and McDaniel have made far greater contributions to the understanding of the adjustment to spinal cord injury than have psychiatrists.[1,2] The views of spinal cord specialists about the role for psychiatry have covered the spectrum of possibilities. Munro, an early neurosurgical pioneer in this field, wrote that "it was therefore neither practical nor useful to call in psychiatric consultation in any case."[3] On the other hand, Kent believed "assistance from the psychiatrist was essential."[4] Sir Ludwig Guttmann, a leading authority in the management of spinal cord injury, has written that "formal psychiatric interviews and specialized psychology tests were necessary only in very selected cases and specialized psychiatric treatment was vary rarely indicated. . . ."[5]

My thinking has evolved through 5 years of intensive involvement in the care of spinal cord–injured patients. Two of these years were on the rehabilitation ward at Massachusetts General Hospital during my psychiatry residency. The ensuing 3 years have been at the West Roxbury Veteran's Administration Hospital. This experience has included direct medical management of spinal cord–injured patients, psychotherapy with patients individually and in groups, as well as leadership of family and staff groups. From this experience there has emerged an image of the possibilities and limitations for psychiatry in this setting. A fellow psychiatrist, while visiting West Roxbury with a group of first-year medical students, commented, "We can't make

---

**415**

it possible for them to walk or give them erections, but we can talk with them." This statement captures the theme of this chapter. Relating to spinal cord–injured patients is sometimes not easy, since paralyzed persons are an embodiment of one of man's most dreaded fears—helplessness. To avoid relating is to avoid confronting this fear.

In this chapter I describe a role for the psychiatrist in the initial evaluation and ongoing assessment of the spinal cord–injured patient with particular emphasis on the use of coping behavior. The treatment modalities available are reviewed, especially those involving staff groups and the use of psychotropic agents for physically disabled persons. Although the observations and conclusions in this chapter are based on spinal cord injuries, much of the content can also be applied to the understanding of a role for the psychiatrist in the broader areas of rehabilitation medicine and acute traumatology.

## INITIAL EVALUATION

The initial psychiatric evaluation lays the foundation for subsequent psychiatric involvement should any be necessary. It is done soon after the patient is admitted and involves interviewing someone who is still acutely injured. The focus is on assessing coping strategies that the patient has used to deal with past stresses and the need, if any, for further psychiatric involvement. In addition, this interview establishes the psychiatrist as a member of the medical team and, thus, as less of a stranger should subsequent psychiatric involvement be required.

Because of the physical and emotional impact of the recent trauma, the patient is approached with caution. Initial questioning centers on his physical state. "Are you in pain?" and "How is your sleep?" are asked. Pain is, of course, common, as is marked sleep disturbance. The latter is due to frequent turning and to the proprioceptive disruption in quadriplegia.[6] Further questioning is about postinjury body sensation. In the acute phase patients may have phantom sensations in which they feel as though their extremities are in positions that are patently impossible. For example, patients may feel as though they are astride a motorcycle.[7,8] Patients may experience this perception and be afraid to mention it for fear of being viewed as crazy. Responding to a question about strange feelings, along with the reassurance that such distortions are normal, can provide much relief. The responses to these questions enable the psychiatrist to assess the appropriateness of further questioning. If patients are too distraught, the interview should be postponed. If not, the second stage of the interview should be initiated.

This stage of the interview begins with questions about work history and social relationships. A stable work history is an important indication of an effective adjustment to the injury. Relationships are explored through traditional questioning about the quality of involvement in marriage or dating and other social interactions. Clues gained from this part of the interview can serve as guides for predicting the ease or difficulty with which patients will work with the hospital staff.

One question stands out in its ability to provide helpful data. It involves finding out whether the patient knows anyone else with a spinal cord injury. It is incredible to see how often the answer is yes when one considers that the injury is rare (30 per million people per year). If he does know someone else with this injury, his expectations about his prognosis will be profoundly influenced by this other individual's course. Since the acquaintance's injury and personality might be very different from the patient's, his outcome may be different as well. The psychiatrist needs to help the patient recognize the dissimilarities. This need is especially pressing when the other person was eventually able to walk and the patient lacks such good fortune.

## COPING STRATEGIES

The assessment of coping strategies is vital. Coping strategies can be viewed as behavior patterns designed to solve problems and/or reduce stress. A thorough discussion of the distinction between coping behavior and defense mechanisms is beyond the scope of this chapter but is well presented by White in *Coping and Adaptation*[9] (also see Chapter 13). For the purposes of this chapter, the difference centers on the fact that defense mechanisms attempt to avoid anxiety and pain often related to long-standing instinctual conflicts, whereas coping behavior attempts to maintain a sense of comfort and continuity in the face of drastic changes that defy familiar patterns of behavior. In an article on the coping behavior of the spinal cord–injured patient I reviewed the stages of coping with particular emphasis on depression and grieving.[10] Weisman has described a series of coping strategies that patients with cancer use.[11] These strategies are also applicable to the adjustment to the sudden stresses of spinal cord injury. A list of these strategies can be found in Chapter 14.

The determination of the predominate strategies of a particular patient provides the staff with clues for working with that patient. The answers to a few questions can provide a guide to the strategies favored by the patient. The question, "What is the most upsetting thing that ever happened to you before this injury?" is frequently quite productive. Once the patient answers, he is then asked, "What did you do to ease the frustrations it caused?" This answer will usually spell out one or several favored strategies. Sample answers are, "I kept myself busy" (displacement), "I started reading about it" (rational/ intellectual), or "I just got away by myself for a while" (avoidance).

This knowledge of the strategies employed by the patient in adjusting to past stresses allows the staff to work in concert with the patient's efforts to cope with the current situation. For example, displacement calls for active, early engagement of occupational and recreational therapy. The patient using rational/intellectual coping should be given especially thorough explanations of the condition and the required procedures along with available written information about the particular injury. The patient who needs to back off from stress may benefit from a corner bed that can be easily closed off with curtains if the patient uses such "getting away" as a springboard for aggressive rehabilitative efforts. Otherwise, such isolation could promote further withdrawal.

The assessment of coping behavior involves more than a few questions. Further observation during the course of hospitalization along with questions about how the patient managed vocational stresses will fill the picture. The protective denial frequently seen in the acute spinal cord–injured person sometimes makes this extended evaluation especially necessary because of the patient's initial refusal to acknowledge the existence of any problems creating stress.

### SYNTHESIS

The data from this interview along with information from the psychologist and social worker provide a working set of hypotheses concerning the psychosocial adjustment and potential problems of the patient. This synthesis of data should take into account several issues relating to disability. First, the impact of the injury on the effectiveness of the patient's coping strategies must be considered. For example, the patient who physically "acts out" to relieve tension is especially vulnerable to the restrictions of life in a wheelchair, particularly if that patient has a cervical injury. The patient's place in the life cycle can also provide clues to his particular vulnerability. Spinal cord injuries to a patient with an established social and vocational identity is a very different matter than a comparable blow to an adolescent for whom the uncertainty created by the injury adds to the turbulence associated with evolving activity/passivity and sexual identity conflicts. This disability in the young alters the life cycle by bringing the patient into contact with the feelings of loss and deterioration normally associated with aging. This patient must struggle with the sense of integrity versus despair—the issues of Erikson's eighth and final stage.[12] On the other hand, when this injury occurs to an older person the sense of decline present before the injury may be intensified.

The effect of this injury on the patient's ability to maintain self-esteem is a vital clue to its impact on the patient's life. Bibring's concept of self-esteem, which he saw as consisting of the sense of being strong, loving, and lovable, is a useful frame of reference.[13] The mechanism of depression, according to Bibring, consists of the ego's awareness of its helplessness in regard to what it must do to maintain self-esteem. From this model, two questions evolve. In what ways did this patient maintain his self-esteem? How will the sensory-motor losses he has suffered disrupt those efforts? Concerns about sexual and vocational functioning become especially relevant in this regard. This injury strikes an especially cruel blow to the patient whose coping efforts centered on physical activity to reduce tension and to increase self-esteem.

## INDICATIONS FOR PSYCHIATRIC INVOLVEMENT

There are several specific indications for psychiatric involvement during the initial posttrauma admission. Foremost among these is the history of a suicide attempt, even if the injury itself may not appear to reflect suicidal intent. Early regular involvement is important not only for ongoing assessment, but also for the development of rapport that may have future importance should suicidal behavior reassert itself. This psychotherapeutic investment for the future cannot be overemphasized. The injury may serve as temporary expiation for the driving force behind self-destructive forces in the patient. As a result, suicidal preoccupation may not be apparent initially. The relationship developed with the psychiatrist can increase the likelihood that the patient will reestablish contact after discharge from the hospital when feelings of despair and suicidal thinking recur. For this recontact to occur, however, it is critical that the psychiatrist clearly confront the patient with the fact that he is seen as a suicide risk. It should never be assumed that patients cannot kill themselves because they are too disabled. Vigilance and appropriate precautions are required regardless of the patients' level of injury. Suicide attempts during the hospitalization immediately after the trauma are always a possibility.[14]

Frequently, recently injured patients, particularly those with cervical injury, will be disoriented, delusional, and incoherent. It is vital for the psychiatrist to assess such patients and reassure the families and staff that this delirious state does not mean that they have lost their minds along with the use of their arms and legs. The reversibility of this state needs to be emphasized before such patients are irreversibly labeled as "mental."

A history of psychotic behavior, alcoholism, or drug abuse remains a traditional indication for psychiatric involvement. Special considerations with regard to medications useful in the management of these patients is presented in this chapter.

### RESISTANCE

There are many sources of resistance to psychiatric involvement and history taking. For the individual with acute and severe injury, the mind is the last bastion of intactness in an otherwise disrupted body. The intrusive questions of a psychiatrist can be viewed as efforts that may trouble the waters in the one otherwise intact area of the patient's life. As one patient said, "With quadriplegia I already feel helpless. Talking to a psychiatrist makes me feel even more so." By holding back with the psychiatrist, the patient can thus protect his remaining sense of intactness. The massive denial frequently found in response to acute stress further restricts the availability of affectively charged data. Weiss believes that this denial continues past the acute phase and becomes a feature of the patient's long-term adjustment.[15] He refers to this as "pseudohysteria." The personality style of the patient is often not suitable for verbal psychotherapeutic methods since spinal cord injuries frequently occur to physically active and impulsive young men whose tensions are acted out rather than talked out. Diller has confirmed the limited appeal of psychotherapy in a survey of 100 patients who had acute spinal cord injuries of whom only 10% showed any interest in psychotherapy.[16]

### STAFF GROUPS

Since individual psychotherapy is not acceptable for most patients, what can the psychiatrist do? Group involvement with the staff is an area where the psychiatrist's skills can be brought to bear. Familiarity with group dynamics, coupled with an understanding of the adjustment to traumatic disability, are especially useful. As a rule those with the most impact on the patient's adjustment are those with the most contact with the patient. Thus, groups are especially important for those in nursing and rehabilitation medicine (physical and occupational therapy). The "inversion effect" often applies to personal knowledge of the patient; that is, those with the least formal education often have the greatest exposure to the patient. Thus, it is important to include nursing assistants in group planning.

Several realities make staff group work in a rehabilitation setting necessary. Prolonged contact with shattered people is a depleting experience. The constant exposure to physical disability can challenge and drain the staff member's sense of intactness. The sharing and mutual support in a group can help offset this. Hospitals are hierarchical, quasi-military organizations in which resentments are passed down the chain of command. Patients often bear the brunt of these resentments since they are sometimes at the bottom of the power structure. Thus, patients may pay both the emotional and financial price of hospital administration. During group sessions these staff resentments are often vented. This ventilation may possibly reduce the pressure that might influence the patient-staff interaction. The prolonged patient contact that occurs in a rehabilitation hospital often activates gratifications and conflicts that staff members would experience in any long-term relationship. During group meetings the staff member is exposed to peer feedback and psychiatric input, both of which can give perspective to the staff member's distortions, which so easily arise in this work.

Recurrent themes have become evident from the group meetings. The most prominent involves the regressed and demanding behavior characteristic of some spinal cord–injured patients. Such patients will badger the staff with repeated requests for medication, food, and television channel changes. Often the staff is asked to do things that patients are able to do for themselves. Anger, often not expressed verbally, rapidly develops toward this type of patient.

> During one group session (not at West Roxbury) the nurses were discussing a man who insisted that they stay at his bedside regardless of other patients' needs. I pointed out that death wishes for such patients are not uncommon. Some nurses quickly denied this and others were silent. One nurse then shared her fantasy of pushing Lubefax into his tracheostomy site after he had been relentless with her. Other nurses then more openly shared their angry thoughts. The net effect seemed to be a reduction in the tension generated by this man.

Another common reaction is the feeling of "helplessness in the helpers," to use a phrase from Adler.[17] There is a deep wish to do more for the severely disabled than is actually possible. Guilt is a frequent sequel to this frustrated wish. Anger at other professionals for not doing more is also common. Some of the tension on a rehabilitation ward, however, may be unsolvable because such conflict serves the defensive purpose of distracting the staff members from the frightening human tragedies that surround them.

## PATIENT GROUP

Group sessions for patients were conducted for an eighteen month period by a social worker and myself. Meetings were held once per week for 1 hour. Such topics as sex, jobs, life in the hospital, and feelings about the injury were discussed. When attendance was adequate, the group provided several of the therapeutic functions described by Yalom.[18] One of these was the imparting of information. As a physician, I was able to provide information about both the medical and the sexual aspects of the injury. The social worker provided information about community resources. Altruism was apparent as the patients sought to help each other. Paraplegics would offer to help quadriplegics with tasks they could not manage. Older patients would share their experiences with the younger patients. Catharsis was another therapeutic function provided by the group with food and the staff being frequent targets. The feeling of universality, as the patients discovered that others shared some of their anxieties, helped to reduce their sense of aloneness in their struggle with the injury.

Consistent attendance, however, was a constant problem. Attendance varied from two to eight. Sudden medical problems, inadequate staffing, and time conflicts with other therapies interfered. Certainly the previously described resistance to individual therapy would apply to group efforts as well. Vigorous efforts on the part of the cotherapists did little to change the situation. A similarly frustrating experience with group therapy and patients who have spinal cord injuries was reported by Cimperman and Dunn.[19] Lipp, however, reported some success with a group involving acute amputees in a Veteran's Administration hospital.[20] His success is encouraging and may have been aided by the fact that the group meeting was essentially a social event and by the fact that he avoided anxiety-provoking techniques such as open-ended questions about the future. Lipp's efforts indicate that group work with spinal cord–injured patients may be plausible if mutual support is encouraged and defenses are not challenged.

## THE FAMILY

Severe disability is a blow to the family as well as to the individual. Prolonged absence of a member from the home, role changes, and grief over what has happened contribute to the stress. In my experience anger with the disabled person is one of the most painful and disguised problems faced by the family. Exclamations like, "How can I be so angry with him!" and "Look at all he's lost!" are common. By pointing out that anger over the personal upheaval caused by the injury is a natural reaction, the psychiatrist can help the family members who feel guilty see their feelings in a more compassionate light. The majority of individual and group family work at our hospital has been carried out by social workers with the psychiatrist serving in a supervisory role.

## SEX

Questions about postinjury sexual behavior can be handled by the psychiatrist if he or she is properly versed in the neurophysiology of the injury and is a person with whom the patient is comfortable. The psychiatrist's responses can be helpful on several levels. The first of these involves the interwoven themes of affirmation and grieving. The discussion of sexual possibilities with the patients serves to affirm the reality of sexual behavior and feelings after the injury, a reality the patient often doubts. This talking also presents the opportunity to share with the patient his sadness over what he has lost in both the sexual and nonsexual spheres of his life.

The next level involves the provision of specific information about sexual capabilities. While the patient must experiment to discover what he can do, there are generalizations that can help guide his efforts. After injury there are two types of erections—reflexogenic and psychogenic. The reflexogenic erections are mediated by sacral nerves and are initiated by physical contact with or without erotic meaning. Insertion of a catheter would be just as likely to cause an erection as the touch of a loving hand. Psychogenic erections, on the other hand, are a result of erotic thought and fantasy and are mediated by sympathetic nerves. Physical contact of which the patient is not aware can cause a reflexogenic, but not psychogenic, erection. Reflex erections occur in spastic patients and psychogenic erections in those who are flaccid. The probabilities that such erections will occur are given below.[21] The term "incomplete" is used here to mean that the neurological impairment below the level of injury is not total.

|  | Reflexogenic erections | Psychogenic erections |
|---|---|---|
| Spastic, complete | 93% | 0% |
| Spastic, incomplete | 98% | 0% |
| Flaccid, complete | 0% | 26% |
| Flaccid, incomplete | 0% | 83% |

The spinal cord–injured female retains the capacity to have intercourse. Like the male, she suffers a sensory loss and thus may not be able to climax, depending on the extent of her injury. Unlike most spinal cord–injured males, she retains fertility. Furthermore, she can have a vaginal delivery.[22]

The third level of response to sex-related questions involves individual and couple counseling. There are several articles in the literature dealing with this topic.[23-25] Such counseling is similar in some aspects to comparable efforts with the nondisabled. For example, issues relating to intimacy, mutuality, and self-esteem require attention. The first of these is the sense of vulnerability to rejection. During sex the disabled person must expose a damaged body over which he has limited control and must express tenderness with it. The potential for embarrassment, such as a bladder accident, serves to exaggerate whatever insecurity the patient has concerning rejection. Discussion of this feeling along with practical suggestions, like advising the patient to void before sex, help. Other issues requiring attention include feelings about oral or manual sexual contact and role conflicts should the sexual partner also be involved in intimate nursing care.

Affirmation, grieving, advice, and counseling offer a wide range of possibilities for psychiatric involvement. In many institutions, however, most of the sex counseling is done by social workers or psychologists.

## PSYCHOPHARMACOLOGY

Knowledge of the effects of psychotropic medication in the neurologically injured patient is a specific contribution that the psychiatrist can make for the spinal cord–injured person. The disabled individual, like anyone else, can suffer from conditions requiring such medications. This fact can easily be lost sight of, since the physical defects seem to serve as such obvious cause for depression or alcohol abuse. Autonomic side effects of psychotropic medications present a special threat to the spinal cord–injured patient since the paralysis includes the autonomic nervous system. These side effects in the nondisabled patient have been reviewed by Shader.[26] The anticholinergic effects of the major tranquilizers and antidepressants can serve to unbalance the already compromised function of the neurogenic bladder in the spinal cord–injured patient. The alpha adrenergic blocking properties of these medications can disrupt the tenuous control the quadriplegic has over his blood pressure since his thoracolumbar sympathetic outflow is disrupted. The result could be serious hypotension.

Proper questioning and medication selection can help avoid these pitfalls. Asking about the type of bladder drainage is crucial. The patient with an indwelling catheter, of course, will present no problem with regard to bladder function. It is quite a different matter for patients with condom drainage because his bladder empties by reflex contractions that are easily disrupted by parasympatholytic agents.

If antipsychotic or antidepressant medication is required for patients with condom drainage, it is important to select agents with fewer anticholinergic effects. Haloperidol or piperazine phenothiazines become reasonable choices.[27] This advantage is lost, however, if antiparkinsonian agents must be used in light of their anticholinergic properties. Care in the selection of antidepressants is equally important. Snyder and Yamamura have recently shown that the monomethylated tricyclic, desipramine, has fewer anticholinergic properties than the dimethylated forms.[28] Of the latter imipramine has less such effects than amitriptyline.

With respect to cardiovascular effects haloperidol and piperazine phenothiazines are again the choice due to the fact that they are less apt to cause a hypotensive episode. With respect to antidepressants there is no difference in alpha adrenergic blocking properties. They should be given exclusively at night when the patient, especially the quadriplegic, is supine.

If injection is required, the potent antipsychotic agents should be used because they appear to be less irritating than injectable chlorpromazine.[29] The irritated injection site on a spinal cord–injured person could become the focus for a bedsore.

Alcohol abuse and its management are frequent problems on a spinal cord unit. Disulfiram has a role in the treatment of this problem in spinal cord–injured patients as it does in the normal population. Special attention, however, must be given to the physiology of an adverse disulfiram reaction due to the autonomic paralysis in some spinal cord–injured patients. The patient with an injury at the T-4 level or above has a severely impaired capacity to regulate blood pressure. In fact, the pressure in such a patient is frequently around 90/60. It follows that such a patient would be especially vulnerable to the hypotension that occurs in a disulfiram reaction. As a rule I do not use this medication in patients with a T-4 level or higher. For paraplegics with injury levels of T-4 to T-12 I do not use dosages of more than 250 mg per day due to reduced sympathetic tone in the lower extremities. For the patient with an injury level of T-12 and below the full dosage can be used since sympathetic vascular control is intact.

Benzodiazepines are commonly used in the spinal cord–injured patients due to their spasmolytic properties. They can be employed for the management of anxiety in spinal cord–injured patients with little risk.

## CONCLUSION

Spinal cord injury shatters the crystal of human experience in every facet. Social relationships, intrapersonal dynamics, and neurological control of functions seen and unseen are involved. Nothing is spared. A role for psychiatry is obscured by the traditional emphasis on the treatment of emotional illness per se. Clearly, the anxiety and depression secondary to the injury are not an illness. A creative role for the psychiatrist can be carved, however, from the growing understanding of coping behavior. The psychiatrist's grasp of individual and group process can help the staff with their efforts to work in this setting.

Treatable psychiatric illness occurs in the disabled person as well as the able-bodied persons. This fact seems obvious and yet is not. The bias revealed in the phrase "mens sana in corpore sano" (a sound mind in a sound body) is all too widespread. The assumption is that a damaged body is to be equated with an unsound mind. Therefore, why should the psychiatrist treat this "unsound mind?" Such treatment is necessary and possible and requires a grasp of the side effects of psychotropic medications in the unsound body.

**REFERENCES**

1. Wright, B. A.: Physical disability—a psychological approach, New York, 1960, Harper & Row, Publishers.
2. McDaniel, J.: Physical disability and human behavior, New York, 1969, Pergamon Press, Inc.
3. Munro, D.: Rehabilitation of patients totally paralyzed below the waist with special reference to making them ambulatory and capable of earning

their own living: an end result study of 445 cases, N. Engl. J. Med. **250:**4-14, 1954.

4. Kent, H.: Potential for rehabilitation in quadriplegic teenagers, J.A.M.A. **169:**817-824, 1959.

5. Guttman, L.: Spinal cord injuries—comprehension management and research, Oxford, 1973, Blackwell Scientific Publications Ltd., pp. 478.

6. Adey, W., Bors, E. and Porter, R.: EEG sleep patterns after high cervical lesions, Arch. Neurol. **19:**377-383, 1968.

7. Conomy, J. P.: Disorders of body image after spinal cord injury, Neurology, **23:**842-850, 1973.

8. Wachs, H., and Zaks, M: Studies of body image in men with spinal cord injury, J. Nerv. Ment. Dis. **131:**121-127, 1960.

9. White, R. W.: Strategies of adaptation: an attempt at systematic description. In Coehlo, G., Hamburg, D., and Adams, J., editors: Coping and adaption, New York, 1974, Basic Books, Inc., Publishers.

10. Stewart, T. D.: Coping behavior and the moratorium following spinal cord injury, Paraplegia **15:**338-342, 1978.

11. Weisman, A. D.: The realization of Death, New York, 1974, Jason Aronson, Inc.

12. Erikson, E. H.: Childhood and society, New York, 1963, W. W. Norton & Co., Inc.

13. Bibring, E.: The mechanism of depression. In Greenacre, P., editor: Affective disorders, New York, 1953, International Universities Press.

14. Reich, P., and Kelly, M.: Suicide attempts by hospitalized medical and surgical patients, N. Engl. J. Med. **294:**298-301, 1976.

15. Weiss, A. J.: Reluctant patient—special problems in psychologic treatment of patients with myelopathy, N.Y. J. Med. **68:**2049-2053, 1968.

16. Diller, L.: Psychological theory in rehabilitation counseling, J. Counsel. Psychol. **6:**189-193, 1959.

17. Adler, G.: Helplessness in the helpers, Br. J. Med. Psychol. **45:**315-326, 1972.

18. Yalom, I.: The theory and practice of group psychotherapy, New York, 1970, Basic Books, Inc., Publishers.

19. Cimperman, A. and Dunn, M.: Group therapy with spinal cord injured patients, Rehab. Psychol. **21:**44-48, 1974.

20. Lipp, M. and Malone S.: Group rehabilitation of vascular surgery patients, Arch. Phys. Med. **57:**180-183, 1976.

21. Comarr, A. E.: Sexual function among patients with spinal cord injury, Urol. Int. **25:**134-168 (Karger, Basel 1970).

22. Comarr, A.: Observations on menstruation and pregnancy among female spinal cord injury patients, Paraplegia **3:**263-272, 1966.

23. Eisenberg, M., and Rustard, L.: Sex education and counseling on a spinal cord injury sercice, Arch. Phys. Med. **57:**135-140, 1976.

24. Griffith, F., and Trieschmann, R.: Sexual functioning in women with spinal cord injury: a review, Arch. Phys. Med. Rehabil. **56:**18-21, 1975.

25. Romano, M., and Lassiter, R.: Sexual counseling with the spinal cord injured, Arch. Phys. Med. **53:**568-572, 1972.

26. Shader, R. and Mascio, D.: Psychotropic drug side effects—clinical and theoretical perspective, Baltimore, 1970, The Williams & Wilkins Co.

27. Snyder, S., Greenburg, D., and Yamamura, H.: Antischizophrenic drugs and brain cholinergic receptors, Arch. Gen. Psychiatry **31**:58:-61, 1974.
28. Snyder, S. and Yamamura, H.: Antidepressants and the muscarinic acetylcholine receptor, Arch. Gen. Psychiatry **34**:236-239, 1977.
29. Hollister, L.: Clinical use of psychotherapeutic agents, Springfield, Illinois, 1973, Charles C Thomas, Publisher.

# 24

# The hospitalized child: general considerations

MICHAEL JELLINEK

The rapid evaluation of the developing child who is physically ill and in emotional distress in an unfamiliar environment is the complicated task requested of the child psychiatry consultant. The age and developmental level of the child serve as the basic framework for the consultation.[1,2] The consultant generates hypotheses based on his or her experience and expectations for age-appropriate behavior and intrapsychic functioning. For example, the consultant brings to a consultation with an 8-year-old boy definite developmental expectations of ego functioning, maturity of defenses, the ability to cope with certain levels of stress and anxiety, and cognitive functioning marked by concrete operations. The consultant also anticipates the presence of a range of probable fantasies, forms of play, social skills, and a hard-to-define, subjective quality of relatedness. The broad set of developmental expectations form the basis for a subset of hypotheses designed to begin to answer the referring pediatrician's question.

Initial hypotheses are modified and refined as more data are gathered and analyzed. The hypotheses generated on the basis of the patient's age, the specific problem that prompted the consultation request, and the patient's history then undergo careful assessment during clinical interviews with parents and child. The consultant balances his or her in-hospital "snapshot" evaluation with a longer-term, behavioral view. For example, a child seen in the hospital in a regressed state marked by depression or unusual anxiety and/or some bizarre ideational content may seem in better psychological health when the consultant reviews recent functioning and behavior. For the 8-year-old such a "behavioral review of systems"[3] would include previous recovery from stressful circumstances, school performance, peer relationships, style of play, mood in more familiar surroundings,

□I wish to thank Dr. Larry Selter for his helpful review of this manuscript.

and functioning within the family. The recommendations at the end of the consultation process are based on the consultant's subjective balancing of many current, historical, and interview variables viewed within a developmental context.

## AGE-SPECIFIC EFFECTS OF HOSPITALIZATION

The age-specific effects of hospitalization[4-7] parallel the concept of age-appropriate expectations or norms. For the infant, probably soon after birth, but certainly by age 6 to 8 months, the impact of hospitalization is almost entirely the stress of separation from the mother. Despite the best efforts at continuity of care, the infant is handled by numerous different medical and nursing personnel and, therefore, never achieves a stable relationship. Bowlby's work[8] is especially relevant here; his observations of separation anxiety are clearly seen in infants and elements of his model are seen in the regressed behavior of all preadolescent children. After careful observation of hospitalized infants, Bowlby described the following three phases of separation.

1. *Protest.* The infant acutely, vigorously, loudly, and thrashingly attempts to prevent departure of the mother or rapidly attempts to recapture her. In the older child this phase may appear as clinging, nagging, or bargaining as a parent is about to leave.

2. *Despair.* The infant is less active, may cry in a monotone with less vigor, begins to withdraw and appear hopeless. Sometimes the withdrawal phase is misleading since caregivers welcome the quiet and project their own hopes that the child is "settling in."

3. *Detachment.* The infant seems more alert and accepting of nursing care. However, these new attachments are superficial and the infant concomitantly shows a loss of affect or positive feeling when the mother appears. In chronic disease requiring numerous prolonged hospitalizations, the infant and child make many episodic inconsistent attachments and suffer numerous losses.

Bowlby[8] and Anna Freud[6] suggest that if this pattern of losses occurs repeatedly, the child may not reestablish the ability to attach and all future relationships will have a hollow, superficial quality. Tronick, Brazelton, and others have found antecedents of Bowlby's three phases of separation at very early ages and has demonstrated on film that the separation process occurs in microcosm over minutes if the mother is unresponsive to the infant's attempts at relating (entrainment).[9]

The school-aged child may share some aspects of the infantile separation phases, but in general develops multiple, often magical, fears about the nature of the illness. The child's artwork (drawings of a person, family, fantasy, or abstraction) during a clinical interview may demonstrate fears of mutilation, castration, or poisoning and may depict machines or rays from outer space. Sometimes the child feels that his illness is an appropriate punishment for angry thoughts. Often the illness creates family conflicts and the child responds by accepting responsibility for keeping the family together. The child's fear of abandonment may well be rooted in reality since severe or chronic illness often leads to a breakdown of the family unit. The stress of the child's illness may well either increase family cohesiveness or exacerbate areas of conflict.[5]

The adolescent is also sensitive to hospitalization and is especially concerned about maintaining a recently won sense of autonomy. Because of the adolescent's tentative identity formation and investment in peer acceptance, physical stigmata or limitations in daily activity arouse significant anxiety. Invariably the illness awakens dependency needs that may be defended against by aggressive assertiveness, denial, or refusal to follow medical regimens.

Anna Freud's classic work[6] emphasizes regression, especially in the younger child. The normal child between the ages of 2 and 4 will lose autonomous functioning (bladder and bowel control, body movement, ego autonomy) under the stress of physical illness and under the regressive, passive pull of nursing care. Prugh[4] found that a wide variety of reactions is common in hospitalized children. Virtually all children are anxious; some, seriously so. Older children tend to be irritable, restless, and withdrawn.

In general the maturity of a child's defensive style may help in coping with anxiety; however, defensive patterns are complex. The defense of denial, especially with some isolation and intellectualization, may be very successful in modulating anxiety.[10] Denial, particularly in a withdrawn child, can sometimes obscure psychopathology and prevent psychiatric referral.[11] The consultant must use a developmental perspective in understanding the normal range of responses to hospitalization and then use this understanding in the evaluation of a child's behavior, emotional state, and defensive style.

## SOME REASONS FOR CONSULTATION REQUEST

Why do children get referred for psychiatric consultation?[11-16] Some consultations are based on the child's difficulty in meeting developmental goals. In the infant, the consultant is asked to evaluate the role of emotional deprivation in "failure to thrive"—the failure to maintain physical growth, to form affective relationships, or to achieve early cognitive landmarks. If emotional deprivation is the final diagnosis in such a case, most of the consultant's efforts will be directed at the family.

School-age children may present with symptoms of unknown etiology and the consultant will be called on to help differentiate functional from organic complaints. A classic example is the child who presents with recurrent abdominal pain as a somatic defense against separating from home (school phobia). Other common referrals for children of this age are functional neurological presentations (seizures, paresis), urinary retention, and hyperactivity.[17,18]

The early adolescent comes with a variety of symptoms such as severe headache, chest pain, or dysmenorrhea in response to developmental pressures from peers (dating, rejection by group), or parents (inhibiting autonomy), or on the basis of intrapsychic conflicts (identity). The adolescent may also be referred if the pediatrician suspects anorexia nervosa, malingering, or early signs of sociopathy.

Referrals can also be based on detrimental parental interactions with a child or parental responses to the child's behavior or illness. The stressful demands of the toddler and the special dynamics of some parents (commonly young parents who are socially isolated or victims of child abuse themselves) can lead to abuse and, when recognized by the pediatrician, to psychiatric consultation.[19,20] The diagnosis of severe congenital abnormality or life-threatening illness often requires evaluation in an effort to help parents tolerate the ongoing stress of the child's illness.[21] The asthmatic child or adolescent is a classical referral, especially when attacks are frequent and manipulative. The consultant may find a pattern of asthmatic attacks with unconscious and even conscious precipitants rooted in and reflecting severely distorted family relationships. Some other reasons for consultation are obvious. The consultant is called quickly for the child who attempts suicide, refuses to cooperate with essential medical regimens, or drives the ward "crazy" with his behavior. Sometimes the reason is more obscure; referral can result from the pediatrician's subtle sense that a child is developing poorly, is not relating well, or seems to be in emotional distress.

## INITIAL STEPS IN THE CONSULTATION PROCESS

After the referral is received, the consultant should contact the pediatrician and, if necessary, clarify or explore the question being asked. Some pediatricians are especially sensitive to psychological concerns and have known the patient and family for several years. In university-affiliated hospitals, the consultant often deals with less experienced house staff on monthly rotating schedules and contact with the referring physician will be shifted toward teaching. A crucial function of ongoing consultation is the trust relationship that should develop between pediatrician, ward personnel, and consultant.[22] This trust creates an atmosphere in which the psychological needs of children are recognized and the consultant's recommendations are carried through even when this takes considerable time.

The next step in the consultation process is a thorough review of the hospital record. This often describes the course of chronic or acute illnesses (past and present), the utilization of medical facilities, the ability of the child and parents to comply with medical regimens, and a report of previous psychological observations in cases where there have been past problems of a similar nature.

For the current admission the registration sheet often contains relevant social and cultural data. The child's address will determine the availability of community resources. The family's socioeconomic status (SES) can be determined from address, parental level of education, and occupation.[23] The SES is one of the most reliable single indicators of general social stress; a low social class rating increases the probability of poor housing conditions, inadequate schools, unstable families, unemployment, and a high rate of mental illness.[24-26] The type of third-party coverage will place limits on available resources. This kind of information is necessary if the consultant's recommendations are to be realistic. Knowledge of race, religion, and cultural heritage can further refine the consultant's hypotheses.

In the current hospital record, the chief complaint and history of present illness require special attention; they describe the type of illness and, by implication, its probable course. Before considering psychological implications and formulations, the consultant should be keenly aware of the possible organic etiologies of psychological presentations. Some organic etiologies are clear. Head trauma may result acutely in a postconcussive confusional state with altered behavior and with chronic changes secondary to a subdural hematoma. An altered state of consciousness or unusual behavior may be the first sign of a viral encephalitis. Preinduction anesthesia medication or the anesthetic itself (especially ketamine) may produce an acute delirium. A psychotic-like state can be seen several days after some forms of major surgery[27] when the child is metabolically stable. Certain drugs, for example phenobarbital, can produce a paradoxical

reaction resulting in hyperactivity or, when used for seizure prophylaxis, may present as a child in a state of withdrawal if serum
levels become toxic. A frequently overlooked organic etiology is the
acute or chronic ingestion of lead that may present as irritability, poor
school performance, or aggressiveness. Drug abuse is an important
consideration for the adolescent. The consultant must also consider the
child's metabolic status. Frequently electrolytes, blood urea nitrogen
(BUN), and blood glucose are reviewed in the chart; however, less
attention is paid to calcium balance, thyroid status, and blood gases.
When a child presents acutely distraught, the consultant's focus on
action can block a careful review of organic possibilities.

> A 14-year-old diabetic patient had a history and initial assessment
> of moderate ketoacidosis. The patient had a history of difficult,
> uncooperative behavior that at this time was much worse and
> virtually prevented intravenous treatment. One hour after admission
> the patient was given 10 mg of diazepam intravenously for relief of
> anxiety with little effect. Soon thereafter the patient's pH was
> obtained with a value of 6.9. On recovery the patient had no memory
> of her admission to the hospital or of her subsequent behavior.

Some organic etiologies are much more subtle or rare. Frequently
the most important cue is the mother's vague sense that the child
"doesn't look or act right."

> A 7-year-old boy with a history of hydrocephalus treated suc-
> cessfully 5 years earlier by shunt presented first with altered behavior
> (stubbornness) and then a minimal increase in a long stable ataxia.
> The shunt was patent and there were no signs of infection. Despite
> good communication, the pediatrician, neurologist, and psychiatrist
> were perplexed. Finally the child developed a mildly edematous arm.
> Careful examination and radiological confirmation proved a venous
> embolus inhibiting drainage from both the arm and head. His
> behavior, arm, and gait returned to baseline with resolution of the
> embolus.

Physical illness can have a major impact on a child's development
and emotional life. Most children with acute illness, reasonably
sensitive treatment and parental support recover quickly from the
stress of hospitalization. Chronic illness is especially devastating[28-30]
and can serve as a prototype for illnesses leading to severe impairment
of self-image. A child may have physical signs of abnormality such as
cleft lip or loss of hair secondary to cancer chemotherapy that are a
ready basis for a poor body image and scapegoating. Heart disease[21] or
renal transplant[5,31] may limit physical activity and therefore radically
change peer relationships. Chronic bowel disease or diabetes may

require careful attention to diet. Such long-term regimens as medications after a renal transplant or pulmonary toilet for cystic fibrosis force the child into daily confrontation with his illness and decrease his sense of autonomy. Chronic disease changes the quality of play, of family and peer relationships, of daily activities, and potentially of every meal.

The family and social history will yield valuable information concerning patterns of family behavior. In addition to a history of the marriage and of parental employment, the chart may contain information that other family members have had illnesses similar to that of the child. Psychiatric histories of other family members may be noted here or in a social worker's note. The family's current capacity to deal with crisis may be predictable on the basis of past responses to stress.

Families respond to the illness of their child in a variety of ways.[21,32] There is an initial very anxious period of uncertainty; then there is shock when the diagnosis is confirmed. Families may begin to gather data and become heavily invested in the medical center staff's ability to manage the illness. At this point some parents do well and work with the child and pediatrician to maximize development. If the child has a more chronic, disabling, or life-threatening disease, less stable families may lose their respect for medical competency, become angry with the hospital staff, and feel guilty either for bringing about or not adequately protecting their child from the illness. As the disease continues or progresses the family may pull together, especially if they were previously cohesive, or, on the other hand long-standing tension may grow worse and result in open conflict and divorce. Such conflict will, of course, make the child anxious, guilty for having the illness, and depressed about the potential loss of parental support. Parents have many questions about the setting of limits on behavior. They may respond to matters of discipline and activity level by becoming either overprotective or indulgent. If the child's illness is life-threatening, parents will wonder what to tell the child. They may withdraw from the child as a result of anticipatory grieving for the child's unrealizable potential or eventual death.[32]

The other children in the family are frequently affected by their brother's or sister's illness. They may respond in a number of ways including attention-seeking behavior such as regressive nagging, withdrawal, poor school performance, or delinquency. Siblings may also harbor angry thought about the patient based on the reality of an altered family life-style forced to meet the needs of the ill child.

This anger may subsequently arouse feelings of guilt and depression.

In the review of the medical record, the consultant must pay special attention to the notes made in the chart by ward personnel. The pediatric nurse's observations may be the most helpful in a number of areas. The nurse is a surrogate mother on the pediatric ward and has considerable objective experience with children of similar ages and similar illnesses. When a child is admitted, the nurse takes a self-care and daily habit history emphasizing the child's healthy routine functioning. The nurse may also make the most careful observations of the child's level of anxiety, state of regression, and temperamental characteristics.[34,35] Because of the nurse's multiple contacts over days with the child, her impression of the child's quality of relating may be an important adjunct to the consultant's impression based on one or two interviews. The nurse's notes may be supplemented by other observations from additional personnel such as a child life worker.[36,37] The role of a child life worker, trained in child development, is to help children cope with the stress of hospitalization. By organizing group activities in the playroom or by celebrating a birthday on the ward, the child life worker may make significant observations about the child's ability to interact with peers. Child life workers may also have impressions of the child's intrapsychic life based on preoperative play sessions designed to decrease the child's anxiety about impending surgery. Also, some inpatient services have a social worker who reviews all admissions; this expanded social history may be very helpful before the consultant meets the family and child.

## BROADER CLINICAL AND ETHICAL ISSUES FACING THE CONSULTANT

I have discussed the approach to consultation before the consultant actually has clinical contact with the family or individual child. I have also reviewed what the consultant needs to know from past experience, from the referring pediatrician, from the chart, and from hospital personnel. Before proceding to the next chapter, it is important to discuss some issues that bear on the broader context of the consultation process.

Psychiatric consultation faces major barriers because of inadequate funding. The consultation itself may take several hours and require repeated visits with the child, the family, and ward staff. However, reimbursement guidelines do not recognize multiple evaluation visits or the time spent gathering data from other sources. The consultant's recommendations may include long-term psychotherapy or special school classes, both of which are expensive items. One of the major frustrations in consultation is the lack of financial support for the hours of consultant time or for implementing the consultant's recommendations. The future of inpatient psychiatric consultation to children depends on recognition by third-party payers that this is a necessary service and that it must be supported financially in all its facets.

The consultant faces some difficult clinical and ethical issues. The clinical interview of the family and child may yield very sensitive information. It is not uncommon to hear family secrets that are kept either from the child or from a spouse. In adolescent patients, the consultant frequently hears very private information about such matters as the first sexual contact, the use of birth control, or pregnancy. It is especially important clinically to build a confidential one-to-one therapeutic alliance; however, it may be therapeutically indicated, but quite complex, to negotiate release of information within a family. An additional problem is how much of all information and inference should be shared with the pediatrician, with the ward nurses, or written in the widely read medical record.

Another frustrating issue for the consultant is the lack of empirical bases for the psychiatric consultation process with children. The current state of the art in child psychiatry research has not developed a methodology to define diagnostic entities adequately or to evaluate interventions. There are too many variables, in both history and illness, to allow for accurate measurement or ready application to other consultations. It is apparent clinically that child psychiatric consultation is essential and useful; however, each consultant develops a personal system of evaluation with only limited systematic data or guidelines.

## SUMMARY

The psychiatric consultant meets the family and the patient after a thorough process of data-gathering and analysis. This process recognizes many sources of both historical and observational data and places special emphasis on developmental expectations for assessing the impact of physical illness. Considering each bit of data within a developmental framework allows the consultant to generate and refine hypotheses to answer the referring physician's questions. In Chapter 25 the next step in the consultation process—the direct contact between consultant, patient, and family—is discussed, several diagnostic categories are defined, and specific management interventions are discussed.

## REFERENCES

1. Eisenberg, L.: Normal child development. In Freedman, A. M., Kaplan, H. I., and Sadock, B. J., editors: The comprehensive textbook of psychiatry, ed. 2, Baltimore, 1975. The Williams & Wilkins Co., pp. 2036-2058.

2. Harper, G., and Richmond, J.: Normal and abnormal development. In Rudolph, A. M., editor: Pediatrics, ed. 16, New York, 1977, Appleton-Century-Crofts, pp. 61-95.

3. Jellinek, M., Evans, N., and Knight, R. B.: Evaluating the need for psychiatric referral: use of a behavior checklist on a pediatric inpatient unit, J. Pediatr., in press.

4. Prugh, D. G., and others: A study of the emotional reactions of children and families to hospitalization and illness, Am. J. Orthopsychiatry **23**:70-106, 1953.

5. Sampson, T. F.: The child in renal failure, J. Am. Acad. Child Psychiatry **14**:462-476, 1975.

6. Freud, A.: The role of bodily illness in the child. Psychoanal. Study Child. **7**:69-81, 1969.

7. Spitz, R.A.: Hospitalism, Psychoanal. Study Child. **1**:53-74, 1945.

8. Bowlby, J.: Separation anxiety, Int. J. Psychoanal. **41**:89-113, 1960.

9. Tronick, E., Als, H., Adamson, L., Wise, S., and Brazelton, T. B.: The infant's response to entrapment between contradictory messages in face to face interaction, J. Am. Acad. Child. Psychiatry **17**:1-13, 1978.

10. Knight, R. B.: Coping mechanisms used by children hospitalized for elective surgery, Dissertation, June, 1977, Yeshiva University.

11. Awad, G. A., and Pozanski, E. O.: Psychiatric consultation to a pediatric hospital, Am. J. Psychiatry **132**:915-918, 1975.

12. Monnelly, E. P., Ianzito, B. M., and Stewart, M. A.: Psychiatric consultations in a children's hospital, Am.J. Psychiatry **139**(7):789-790, 1973.

13. Looff, D. H.: Psychophysiologic and conversation reactions in children, J. Am. Acad. Child Psychiatry **9**(2):318-331, 1970.

14. Bolian G. C.: Psychiatric consultation within a community of sick children, J. Am. Acad. Child Psychiatry **10**(2):293-307, 1971.

15. Stocking, M., Rothney, W., Grosser, G., and Goodwin, R.: Psychopathology in a pediatric hospital: implications for the pediatrician, Psychiatr. Med. **1**:329-338, 1970.

16. Schowalter, J. E.: The utilization of child psychiatry on a pediatric adolescent ward, J. Am. Acad. Child Psychiatry **10**:689-699, 1971.

17. Millen, J. S.: Hyperactive children, Pediatrics **61**(2):217-222, 1978.

18. Eisenberg, L.: Hyperkinesis revisited, Pediatrics **61**(2):319-321, 1978.

19. Helfer, R., and Kempe, C.: The battered child, ed. 2, Chicago, 1974, University of Chicago Press.

20. Lystad, M. H: Violence at home: a review of the literature, Am. J. Orthopsychiatry **45**(3):328-345, 1975.

21. Glasser, H. H., Harrison, G. S., and Lynn, D. B.: Emotional implications of congenital heart disease in children, Pediatrics **33**:367-379, 1964.

22. Geist, R. A.: Consultation to a pediatric surgical ward: creating an empathic climate, Am. J. Orthopsychiatry **47**(3):432-444, 1977.

23. Redlich, F. C., and Hollingshead, A. B.: Social class and mental illness: a community study, New York, 1958, John Wiley & Sons, Inc.

24. Eisenberg, L.: Racism, the family, and society: a crisis in values. In Chess, S., and Thomas, A., editors: Annual progress in child psychiatry and child development, New York, 1969, Brunner/Mazel, Inc., pp. 252-264.
25. Birch, H. G.: Health and the education of the socially disadvantaged child. In Chess, S., and Thomas, A., editors: Annual progress in child psychiatry and child development, New York, 1969, Brunner/Mazel, Inc., pp. 265-291.
26. Rodman, H.: Family and social pathology in the ghetto. In Chess, S., and Thomas A., editors: Annual progress in child psychiatry and child development, New York, 1969, Brunner/Mazel, Inc., pp. 291-308.
27. Oanilowica, D. A., and Gabriel, H. P.: Postoperative reactions in hospitalized children: normal and abnormal responses after surgery, Am. J. Psychiatry **128**:185-188, 1971.
28. Bergman, T.: Children in the hospital, New York, 1965, International Universities Press.
29. Minuchin, S., and others: A conceptual model of psychosomatic illness in children, Arch. Gen. Psychiatry **32**:1031-1038, 1975.
30. Pless, I. B., and Roghman, K. J.: Chronic illness and its consequences, J. Pediatr. **79**(3):351-359, 1971.
31. Bernstein, D. M.: After transplantation—the child's emotional reactions, Am. J. Psychiatry **127**:1189-1193, 1971.
32. Friedman, S. B., Chodoff, P., Mason, J. S., and Hamburg, D. A.: Behavioral observations on parents anticipating the death of a child, Pediatrics **32**:610-625, 1963.
33. Gladston, R.: On borrowed time: observations on children with implanted cardiac pacemakers and their families. In Chess, S., and Thomas, A., editors: Annual progress in child psychiatry and child development, New York, 1970, Brunner/Mazel, Inc., pp. 517-523.
34. Graham, P., Rutter, M., and George, S.: Temperamental characteristics as predictors of behavior disorders in children, Am. J. Orthopsychiatry **43**(3):328-339, 1973.
35. Thomas, A., and Chess, S.: Temperament and development, New York, 1976, Brunner/Mazel, Inc.
36. Plank, E. N.: Working with children in hospitals, Cleveland, 1962, Western Reserve Press.
37. Vaughan, G. F.: Children in hospital, Lancet **272**:1117-1120, 1957.

# 25

# The hospitalized child: diagnosis and management

## JOHN E. O'MALLEY and GERALD P. KOOCHER

Working with hospitalized children in a psychiatric liaison capacity is substantially different from working with adults. While most adult patients can be realistically assessed as independent functioning people, it is virtually impossible to do a competent evaluation or intervention with a child unless the family is actively involved. In addition to general developmental and maturational factors, family issues are a most critical determinant of a child's ability to adjust to emotional and physical stress. Taking this into account, the consultant should not appear at the child's beside without advance parental contact. Aside from the legal right of parents to consent to such a procedure, there is often a special sensitivity about having one's child seen by a psychiatrist. Parental guilt often accompanies childhood infirmities. When this guilt is compounded by parental anxiety and by the behavior problems of the child, parents may be understandably sensitive about having psychiatric intervention for the child. Advance contact with the parents to outline the purposes of the consultation and to solicit their assistance as allies in helping the child to overcome specific difficulties will often help to reduce parental distress.

It is also difficult to assess the nature of a child's current problems accurately without some baseline data about usual family functioning, the nature of child-parent relations, special family problems, or other emotionally significant issues in the child's life that (not being strictly medical concerns) may not appear in the available records. There may well be instances where family issues are so central to the problem behavior that the significance of the child's physical complaints pales by comparison.

☐During the preparation of this chapter the authors were supported in part by National Cancer Institute Grant CA 18429-03 CCG.

While the usual medical consultation results in a report to the primary-care physician, the psychological or psychiatric consultation often leads to direct parent-consultant discussion. This happens because the emotional issues of concern to the child often do not evaporate at the end of the hospitalization and because subsequent intervention by mental health personnel is often required. Even when this is not the case, parents often ask the psychiatric consultant for guidance or management suggestions in dealing with their child's behavior, school, or emotional problems.

Developmental and maturational issues must always be kept in mind as the psychiatrist prepares to do a consultation. Mental status, ability to establish rapport, emotional reactivity, and other key variables are clearly a function of the child's stage of devlopement as well as of any psychopathology that may be present. It is important, therefore, that the consultant review basic child psychology and development prior to beginning service to a pediatric unit, especially if he or she has not recently worked with children. Just as the clinician who treats adults carries around a set of mental norms against which patients may be compared, the pediatric consultant recognizes the special developmental stages through which children pass and uses these as comparable guideposts (see Chapter 24).

## SYMPTOMS OF UNKOWN ETIOLOGY

Children are not infrequently admitted to a hospital for a further diagnostic evaluation of symptoms without apparent organic basis. Symptoms such as headache, abdominal pain, and other nonspecific pains are often refractory to outpatient medical evaluation and supportive treatment. Both a medical and a psychiatric evaluation should be carried out simultaneously while the child is hospitalized. In such situations the consultant has several responsibilities to the patient.

1. The medical history should be reviewed with the patient and with the referring physician.
2. Differential diagnostic possibilities of organic versus functional illness should be shared with the referring physician.
3. The consultant should arrange whatever other diagnostic tests or psychological investigations seem indicated (for example, psychological testing, neurological evaluation, and speech and language assessment).

Psychological testing can be a useful tool in assessing certain organic problems as well as in identifying critical emotional dynamics or themes that may not be developed in a less structured interview with the child.

The consultant must pay close attention to the correlation of deviant behavior and/or symptoms with the child's age and maturational level. Discrepancies in this correlation may suggest other avenues for inquiry in either the organic or the psychological spheres. Symptoms or behavior lie along a continuum from acceptable to extreme. In the latter case, intense emotional reactivity, uncontrollable behavior and anxiety, excessive withdrawal or anti-social reactions are the rule. In the middleground are the mild or transitory sorts of psychopathology including any and all of the above symptoms in less intense degree.

### Conversion (hysterical) symptoms

When considering the diagnosis of conversion reaction, both the absence of organic illness and the presence of sufficient emotional conflict to explain the symptom(s) are necessary. Neither is sufficient alone, and a full history and mental-status assessment of the child and parents are clearly indicated.

In our culture it is much more acceptable to seek relief from stress by being ill than by enduring the stress directly. Psychophysiological complaints are much more common than the "anesthesias" or "paralyses" of years gone by. The most common conflicts encountered in our experience with children showing hysterical symptoms include:

1. *Separation conflict:* Refusal to attend school is often masked by gastrointestinal problems. The psychiatrist should check the child's school attendance record and absences during the work-up.
2. *Dependency conflict:* Disinclination to act on one's own behalf, overcontrolling parents, and social immaturity may all be clues to dependency as a key issue.
3. *Chronic family turmoil:* In such situations the child may become an "identified patient" and show symptoms that are actually reflective of whole family distress.
4. *Avoidance of unpleasant experience:* In many cases, the hysterical symptoms have the additional gain of relief from pressures to perform academically or to otherwise live up to high levels of expectation.

### Diagnostic criteria for conversion hysteria

1. Original conflict centered around the use of repression.
2. Somatic dysfunction in bodily structure or function supplied by voluntary portion of the central nervous system.

3. Involvement of striated musculature and somatosensory apparatus (for example, paralysis, tics, blindness, deafness, seizures, weakness, vomiting, encopresis, and hyperventilation).
4. Presence of secondary gain (for example, absence from school).
5. Occasional overlap with other diagnostic categories (psychophysiological disorders; for example, abdominal pain).

**Management suggestions for conversion hysteria**

1. Appropriate tests must be given by the primary-care physician(s) to allay parental fears. What the parents fear most (for example, a brain tumor or other cancer) will generally be unfounded.

2. At the first hint of possible emotional conflict adding to the distress, an appropriate consultant should be called in. The consultant is then in a much better position to provide intervention or to suggest additional studies than if he or she were called in later.

3. With sensitive understanding the primary physician should indicate that there is no organic basis for the symptoms (supported by adequate medical studies), but that the symptoms are indeed real. For example, psychogenic headaches and nausea are just as painful and aggravating as those induced by physical disease. An explanation of how stress can lead to symptoms is also important.

4. The consultant should document for both the family and the child what the nature of the stress is.

5. Adequate follow-up for the psychotherapeutic intervention should be planned prior to discharge in conjuntion with the family's pediatrician. This should be carefully reviewed by all concerned including the parents and the child.

Jimmy, age 10, was referred by his family pediatrician following an extensive work-up for abdominal pain at a community hospital. This work-up failed to establish any organic etiology. Jimmy was admitted to Children's Hospital. The history taken there revealed that the abdominal pain occurred each morning before school, rarely on weekends, and was of such severity that his mother felt he could not be sent off to school. In fact, Jimmy missed 35 school days that term. His mother was sure something was missed by the doctors.

The family was in turmoil when Jimmy was admitted. The parents had been separated twice before and were thinking about separating again. Because of Jimmy's symptoms, his mother felt she had to quit her job and stay home to take care of him. He was always an excellent student and continued to complete his work at home. He had few friends and tended to enjoy adult company more.

Jimmy appeared to be a pleasant, quiet, bright, 10-year-old boy who related in a pseudomature manner. He showed little concern about his abdominal pain or hospitalizations. He remained quite guarded about his feelings concerning his parents' troubles, indicating only that he hoped it worked out. He said that he liked school, but would rather do his work at home where it was quiet. There was no evidence of a thought disorder.

What became clearer as the hospitalization continued was Jimmy's anxiety created by being out of sight of his mother. His need to be a guardian of the family was to ensure that his parents did not separate again. It was necessary to firmly indicate to the parents that all studies were negative, addressing their worst fear that Jimmy might have cancer. In addition, the physician showed that Jimmy was very anxious and that the abdominal pain was a manifestation of that anxiety.

Arrangements were made with the local pediatrician to be available each morning to see Jimmy before going to school if the pain continued. It was impressed on the parents that he must attend school. Also, the family was referred to a nearby mental health clinic in order to deal with the troubled marriage and provide support for Jimmy.

## DIAGNOSIS AND TREATMENT OF DEPRESSION

Very few people of any age are happy to be in the hospital, so it is not surprising that depression is a common psychological presenting problem. Once again, the history and other background data are of critical importance. The psychiatrist must be clear as to the relative chronicity or acuteness of the problem, the presence or absence of specific precipitants at home or in the hospital, and the appropriateness of the depression in light of recent life events. The manifestations of depression also shift in emphasis as a function of the child's developmental level.

### Universal issues

Children of all ages, as well as adults, can be expected to show signs of reactive depression in a number of hospital contexts. Precipitating factors can be:

1. Painful, invasive, or stressful medical/surgical treatments or physical illnesses
2. Uncertainty of outcome in cases of critical procedures
3. Loneliness, boredom, or lack of family supports while hospitalized
4. Concern about events at home (or work or school) while one is hospitalized

### Issues for younger children

In general, preteenagers are more likely than adults and teenagers to experience fantasies literally and to engage in magical thinking.

Special concerns in this group might include:

1. Fears arising from magical thinking or fantasies about the course in the hospital or physical illness
2. Concern about separation from parents, including withdrawal and isolation reactions
3. Fears of mutilation and abandonment
4. Concern about school or home issues related to care of a beloved pet, fears of falling behind scholastically, or concern about parental conflict

### Adolescent issues

While adolescents are not immune to any of the issues noted above, they often have a number of other specialized concerns including:

1. Loss of privacy and/or charge of their own activties as necessitated by hospital routine
2. Loss of contact with peers from the community and possible discomfort associated with having younger or less mature roommates

### Diagnostic criteria

1. General: Depression in childhood remains a controversial area. The symptomatology particularly in younger children (up to age 11 or 12) differs from that in older children.

2. Symptoms may include loss of appetite, sleep disturbances (nightmares, difficulty falling asleep, restless sleep), hypoactivity or hyperactivity, acting out behavior, wide mood swings, reemergence of phobias, and hypochondriasis.

3. The adolescent symptomatology of depression is similar to the adult's, including suicidal behavior. Children under the age of 10 do commit suicide, but it is rare.

### Management suggestions

1. Once the source of the depression has been determined, an intervention may be directed to the specific concern of the child.

2. In cases where fantasy or magical thinking is a source of depressive feelings, some explicit factual information or discussions, play demonstrations, or the opportunity to explore (for example, treatment rooms) in advance may reduce anxiety and depression.

3. In instances where the depression is realistically related to a serious medical problem or uncertain prognosis, sensitive, supportive listening often grants permission for the child to release sad feelings

while finding warm acceptance. Often parents or staff members may urge a child who is appropriately sad to cheer up, thus signaling that the child should not express sad feelings. The result is even more significant depression.

4. If loneliness or boredom is a causative factor, it may be possible to offer relief with some direct environmental manipulation. For example, placing a call button by the child's bed, providing the child with a roommate of or near the same age, encouraging parents to visit more often, or simply providing a television set (or recreational supplies) may be effective in specific cases.

5. If some home issue or event is identified as a key factor, some intervention with the parents and ultimately a family meeting with the child in the hospital may be a reassuring strategy with quite positive benefits.

6. The use of antidepressant agents may be considered for adolescent patients. The criteria for their use are the same as for adults, namely, somatic sequelae of depression (for example, decreased appetite, weight loss, insomnia, early morning awakening, and anxiety), and absence of contraindications (for example, allergy to the agents). There is little experience shared in the literature concerning the use of antidepressants for adolescents with a primary endogenous depression. Our experience suggests that the use of such medication can occasionally be helpful and well tolerated. Dosage schedules must, of course, be individualized but they approximate adult schedules.

> Alice, a 12-year-old seventh grader, was admitted to the hospital with the diagnosis of rheumatic heart disease.
>
> When first admitted, she was pleasant, cheerful, and outgoing. The nursing staff began to notice, however, after several days that she was not eating as well and was spending more time in her room away from other children. The night staff commented that she would try to spend as much time as possible watching television. When asked directly if something was bothering her, she denied any problems. The staff became increasingly concerned since the parents, who visited infrequently, would argue openly with her and between themselves.
>
> The consultant's role was to help evaluate her current status, offer support, and provide the beginnings of resolution. Alice was obviously depressed and with the consultant spoke of suicidal ideation, although she denied any intent to act on her thoughts. She could finally express the anger concerning her parents and their infrequent visits as well as how they embarrassed her when they argued. At the same time, she was deeply concerned about the possibility of their separating while she was in the hospital. Her role at home had been as mediator and buffer between them and now she could not do that.

After she was able to articulate some of her feelings her spirits improved, particularly when the consultant could relieve her of the responsibility of keeping the parents at peace with each other. In fact, the consultant quickly arranged joint meetings with the parents and Alice to define the problems and course of action. This was sufficient to provide substantial improvement in Alice's spirits and abatement of her depressive symptomatology. The rest of Alice's hospital course was uneventful and family counseling continued after her discharge.

## DIAGNOSIS AND TREATMENT OF BEHAVIOR PROBLEMS ON THE UNIT

The list of presenting complaints in such cases is limited only by the imagination of the children involved. Some recent examples we have encountered include the common refusal to take medication or to cooperate in treatment procedures and the rather unusual erotic advances of a 13-year-old boy toward his young female nurses. The problem behaviors may be merely humorous or annoying at the least, or actually life-threatening at their worst.

In such cases, the consultant is asked to assist in modifying or manipulating surface behavior. This is very much in contrast to the traditional psychiatric approach of dealing with deep-seated or unconscious issues that only incidently interrupt the symptom behavior. Because of the lack of time and the nature of the consultation process, only surface behavior is dealt with. By "surface behavior" we mean the actual observable behavior (for example, hitting a nurse or refusing to eat). This often means that the consultant may not fully probe the child's psyche to determine the why (for example, what is the origin of the sadistic impulse? What is the meaning of the refusal to eat?) Redl and Wineman have carefully outlined the use of such techniques, and we have modified a number of their concepts for presentation here. The adaptation (and possible corruption) of Redl's model for use by the consultant in the pediatric hospital is our work.

### Management suggestions*

**Selective ignoring.** Inappropriate behavior can sometimes be dealt with by simply not paying attention to it. Many times children need to relieve frustration and anger or want adult attention, but go about it in negative ways. If the behavior is ignored, it will run its course and

---

*These catagories were adapted from Redl, F., and Wineman, D.: Controls from within: techniques for the treatment of aggressive children, New York, 1952, The Free Press.

stop. The consultant has not added fuel to the fire by scolding, commenting, or drawing attention to it.

> Billy, age 10, was angry that his parents did not come to visit. He began to tear up the books given to him by his parents and throw the pieces around the room. The nurse elected not to scold Billy about the destruction, but instead waited until Billy stopped. She then helped him talk about how angry he was about his parents' absence. If the nurse had scolded him, fuel would have been added. Billy's anger would then have been directed toward the nurse.

**Distancing.** Separating two arguing children is often enough to interrupt inappropriate behavior. Likewise, the presence of an adult when a child is under stress (preoperatively, etc.) can calm and reassure an anxious child.

**Touch control.** Sometimes the presence of an adult is not sufficient to calm an anxious or unruly child. Touching the child by putting an arm around the shoulder or patting the child on the back can bring the additional control and reassurance.

> Sally and Jenny, both 10, were roommates who generally played well together. Sally was scheduled for surgery the next day and was quite anxious. She was irritable, hyperactive, and sullen. An argument about which television program both were going to watch resulted in screaming, name-calling, and tears. When a staff member arrived, he separated the two girls. Jenny settled easily with the separating and presence of an adult. Not so for Sally, who did not respond until a gentle arm was placed around her shoulder and reassuring words were given about the impending surgery.

**Taking an interest in the child's activity.** Hospitalization can be not only stressful for a child but also boring and lonely. Children occasionally react to boredom with difficult behavior. Interest in previously enjoyed activities can be revitalized if an adult shows enthusiasm in the activity.

> Billy, age 11, enjoyed putting model cars together to help pass time while his fractured femur healed. His interest waned and his behavior became difficult. The attending physician simply expressed great interest in the models, that is, how he did them, how long it took, how nice they looked, etc., which helped Billy regain his pleasure in assembling the models. The result was an improvement in behavior.

### Distraction

*Humor.* Humor used by an adult can provide a face-saving way for the child to stop the problem behavior.

*Activities.* For example, turning on a television set, giving a lump of clay, or having a child read a story or draw pictures can distract the child from pain or anxiety. Many children's units have a professional staff to help find pleasurable activities for children. Such services can be invaluable and should be utilized whenever possible.

*Shift of control.* Distraction can be enhanced by giving a child a different focus when an anxiety-provoking procedure or event is to take place. Giving the child control over part of the task to be done can distract the child from the discomfort of the task. For example, if an intravenous tube has to be placed, letting the child pick the site, cut the tape, and count the drips can take the focus away from the needle being placed as well as give the child more sense of control over what happens to his or her body.

**Stress help.** By being aware of and sensitive to areas of particular difficulty for a given child, an adult can give support by words or action for this brief period until the stress passes. The time just before a painful procedure may provoke great stress. The adult can offer most support at that time to get the child past this anticipatory stage until the actual procedure begins when such support may not be necessary.

Support can be given by several methods.

*Understanding and sympathy.*

*Firmness.* It is sometimes helpful for a child to have firm boundaries concerning expectations. ("I know it will hurt, but it must be done.")

*Restructuring activities.* Changing the schedule of daily events for an individual child may provide support. For example, if a child prefers the daily injection of an antimetabolite in the evening rather than in the morning, such flexibility should be allowed if at all possible. Having a rest hour in the morning rather than after lunch, giving treatments at different times, and so on can demonstrate to the child that a sensitive adult is aware of individual needs and can be responsive to them.

**Direct reasoning.** Appeals to a child's sense of judgment, consequences, or understanding of behavior may be quite effective and most direct. This assumes, of course, that the child has the age-appropriate conceptual and intellectual development as well as sufficient social maturity.

> Jimmy, age 8, was admitted for control of diabetes mellitus. Although initially quite compliant about injections and urine testing, his behavior rapidly deteriorated until the nursing staff believed he was unmanageable. He would scream, kick and knock needles out of the nurse's hand. Finally he kicked a nurse. The consultant was called, since short of physical restraint Jimmy would be without insulin. It was suggested that touch control might be helpful by one staff

member while another did the injection. With a supportive arm around his shoulder and soothing words, the injections could occur without incident. The touch control provided the additional support Jimmy needed against fear of loss of body integrity and dissolution.

## CONCLUSION

Psychological consultation to hospitalized children is a specialized, demanding, but rewarding task. It requires knowledge of child development, appropriate and inappropriate behaviors in childhood, and manifestations of psychopathology. In addition, the consultant must be aware of the ward milieu and establish meaningful work relationships with key staff members. Effectiveness of the consultation will also depend on the willingness to alter stereotypical procedures— working alone, low profile, not sharing with staff, etc. The consultant must also be willing to be on public display, to be tested as to helpfulness, availability, and common sense. To show respect for the staff's knowledge and insights, to be sensitive to their emotional needs, to be available at their request, will foster a working alliance in service of meeting the patients' needs.

Although techniques have been outlined, ultimately the success of the consultation effort will depend on the consultant's sensitivity, compassion, and understanding.

**SUGGESTED READINGS**

Geist, R. A.: Consultation on a pediatric surgical ward: creating an empathic climate Am. J. Orthopsychiatry **47:**432-444, 1977.

Langford, W. S.: The child in the pediatric hospital: adaptation to illness and hospitalization, Am. J. Orthopsychiatry **31:**667-684, 1961.

Miller, W. B.: Psychiatric consultation: a general systems approach, Psychiatry Med. **4:**135-142, 1973.

Monnelly, E. P., Ianzito, B. M., and Stewart, M. A.: Psychiatric consultations in a children's hospital, Am. J. Psychiatry **130:**789-790, 1973.

Oremland, E. K., and Oremland, J. D.: The effects of hospitalization on children, Springfield, Illinois, 1973, Charles C Thomas, Publisher.

Prugh, D. G. and others: A study of the emotional reactions of children and families to hospitalization and illness, Am. J. Orthopsychiatry **23:**70-106, 1953.

Redl, F., and Wineman, D.: Controls from within: techniques for the treatment of aggressive children, New York, 1952, The Free Press.

Rothenberg, M. B.: Child psychiatry-pediatrics liaison: a history and commentary, J. Am. Acad. Child Psychiatry **7:**492-509, 1968.

Rotmann, M.: A model of an integrated psychosomatic consultation service, Psychother. Psychosom. **22:**189-191, 1973.

Schowalter, J. E.: The utilization of child psychiatry in a pediatric adolescent ward, J. Am. Acad. Child Psychiatry **10:**684-699, 1971.

# 26

# Chemotherapy in psychiatry

JERROLD G. BERNSTEIN

In the past quarter-century the treatment of psychiatric patients has been revolutionized by the introduction of a variety of effective medications. Modern psychopharmacology began with the demonstration of the antipsychotic effects of chlorpromazine in 1952 by Delay and Deniker.[1] In recent years much has been learned about the mechanisms of action of a variety of chemical agents on the brain. The development and study of drugs effective in the treatment of psychiatric patients have helped also to elucidate some of the potential chemical and physiological mechanisms of psychiatric illness.

In some respects the introduction of chlorpromazine and other effective chemotherapeutic agents in psychiatry parallels the development of arsphenamine by Ehrlich in 1910. Ehrlich's compound "606" was seen as the "magic bullet" in the treatment of syphilis. Although we have no "magic bullet" in psychiatry there are a number of chemical agents that exert specific effects on brain function and, thereby, can be expected to bring about specific, clinically beneficial responses in psychiatric patients.

An understanding of pharmacological mechanisms of action of psychotropic drugs is essential to their appropriate clinical application. Although it is as difficult to distill the important knowledge of psychopharmacology into a single chapter as it is to reduce the *Talmud* into a single volume, in this chapter I will present a framework for the understanding and use of chemotherapeutic agents in psychiatric practice.

In order to prescribe psychotropic drugs rationally the psychiatrist needs to understand their mechanism of action. Furthermore, it is generally more desirable to learn the proper use of a few drugs and use them well than to prescribe any and all psychotropic drugs that exist. Table 26-1 presents functional and chemical classifications of the four important groups of drugs used in psychiatric treatment. In this chapter I will discuss mechanisms of action and practical aspects of

**Table 26-1.** Classification of psychotropic drugs

| Antianxiety drugs | Antipsychotic drugs | Antidepressant drugs | Mood-stabilizing drug |
|---|---|---|---|
| Benzodiazepine | Phenothiazine | Tricyclic | Lithium carbonate |
| Chlordiazepoxide (Librium) | *Aliphatic* | Amitriptyline (Elavil) | |
| Diazepam (Valium) | Chlorpromazine (Thorazine) | Imipramine (Tofranil) | |
| Chlorazepate (Tranxene) | *Piperidine* | Doxepin (Sinequan) | |
| Oxazepam (Serax) | Thioridazine (Mellaril) | Monoamine oxidase inhibitor | |
| Propanediol Carbamate | *Piperazine* | Phenelzine (Nardil) | |
| Meprobamate (Equanil) | Trifluoperazine (Stelazine) | Tranylcypromine (Parnate) | |
| Barbiturate | Fluphenazine (Prolixin) | Pargyline (Eutonyl) | |
| Phenobarbital (Luminal) | Perphenazine (Trilafon) | CNS stimulant | |
| Ethyl Alcohol | Thioxanthene | Dextroamphetamine (Dexedrine) | |
| Antihistamine | *Aliphatic* | Methylphenidate (Ritalin) | |
| Hydroxyzine (Atarax) | Chlorprothixene (Taractan) | | |
| Beta-adrenergic antagonist | *Piperazine* | | |
| Propranolol (Inderal) | Thiothixene (Navane) | | |
| | Butyrophenone | | |
| | Haloperidol (Haldol) | | |
| | Dihydroindolone | | |
| | Molindone (Moban) | | |
| | Dibenzoxazepine | | |
| | Loxapine (Loxitane) | | |

the clinical use of psychotropic drugs according to the system of classification presented in Table 26-1.

## ANTIANXIETY DRUGS

Drug treatment of anxiety is the oldest and the least pharmacologically specific area of psychiatric chemotherapy. For the most part, agents commonly employed for the treatment of anxiety may be viewed as central nervous system depressant drugs that, by virtue of this generalized effect on the brain, produce a diminution of the dysphoric feelings associated with nervousness and anxiety. Indeed, the use of alcohol as a sedative and tranquilizer extends back many millennia. Indeed, the central nervous system effects of alcohol were appreciated in Biblical times. Ethyl alcohol in a variety of forms continues to be used widely as a readily available drug by patients who self-medicate their dysphoria. Indeed, some individuals who abuse alcohol may do so in an attempt to medicate an undiagnosed psychiatric disturbance. Alcohol exerts a central nervous system depressant effect that is dose dependent and that may vary from mild tranquilization, through sedation, sleep, or in the case of excessive doses, death.

Having recognized the abuse and addiction potential of alcohol, medical science was pleased with the availability of barbiturate drugs in the early part of the twentieth century. Barbiturates, especially the longer acting compounds such as phenobarbital, were widely used to alleviate anxiety. Short-acting and intermediate-acting barbiturates such as pentobarbital (Nembutal) and amobarbital (Amytal), respectively, have also been used as sedatives and sleep-inducing medications. Because of increasing awareness of the addicting potential of barbiturates they have generally fallen into disfavor in modern clinical practice. However, phenobarbital in a dose of 30 mg once or twice daily may be a useful antianxiety agent. Unlike short-acting and intermediate-acting barbiturates, phenobarbital, which has a half-life of 24 to 48 hours, has little potential for inducing barbiturate addiction. Indeed, vast numbers of patients have been treated for decades with phenobarbital as an anticonvulsant without developing significant evidence of tolerance or physical dependence. Intermittent use of low doses of the very inexpensive drug, phenobarbital, may be highly beneficial for many patients. The major disadvantage to the use of phenobarbital to treat anxiety relates to its interaction with other drugs. Phenobarbital is capable of inducing hepatic microsomal enzyme systems and thus facilitating the metabolism of a variety of drugs including tricyclic antidepressants and warfarin-type anticoagulants. Barbiturates produce additive central nervous system depressant effects when used in combination with alcohol, meprobamate, benzodiazepines, and other sedatives.

Meprobamate was introduced into clinical use as an antianxiety agent in the mid-1950s. One of the prime virtues ascribed to meprobamate at the time it was introduced was that, unlike the barbiturates, it was non–habit forming and nonaddicting. Its clinical popularity grew rapidly, and it was widely prescribed. Within a short time following its extensive clinical use the development of meprobamate addiction was recognized.[1] Patients consuming moderately large doses of this drug over prolonged periods developed seizures following abrupt discontinuance of their medication. The mechanism of action of meprobamate is not significantly different from the generalized central nervous system depressant effect produced by barbiturates; therefore, addiction to meprobamate is not at all surprising. The ususal therapeutic dose of meprobamate is 200 to 400 mg for anxiety or 400 to 800 mg for sleep.[1] Meprobamate has no real specific antianxiety effect, and because of its significant potential for addiction should play little role in the chemotherapy of anxious patients. It is important to be alert to the possibility that patients using meprobamate may have a true barbiturate-sedative type of addiction. Patients addicted to meprobamate should be withdrawn using the same procedure that is employed in the treatment of barbiturate addiction.[1]

After the recognition of the addiction potential of meprobamate a new group of antianxiety drugs, the benzodiazepines, was introduced for the treatment of anxious patients. Benzodiazepine drugs currently available for the treatment of anxiety include chlordiazepoxide, chlorazepate, diazepam, and oxazepam. At the time that these drugs were introduced for clinical use, they were believed to be safer than the barbiturates and meprobamate by virtue of being nonaddicting. After considerable clinical experience, addiction to benzodiazepine drugs has been recognized. Prolonged use of high doses of these drugs produces tolerance and physical dependence. Patients may experience seizures following withdrawal of benzodiazepine-type antianxiety drugs.[1,2] Addiction to these drugs should be managed by detoxification following the same procedure employed with barbiturate addiction. Since benzodiazepines exert a generalized central nervous system depressant effect, it is not surprising that they may produce unwanted effects similar to those seen with other central nervous system depressants such as meprobamate and the barbiturates. One unique aspect of the pharmacology of the benzodiazpines is their apparent ability to produce a somewhat selective sedative effect on the limbic system. It is possible that this effect on the limbic system explains the clinical antianxiety action attributed to these drugs.[2] Nevertheless, the more generalized central nervous system (CNS) depressant effect of the benzodiazepines undoubtedly contributes significantly to their ability to reduce anxiety. These drugs, especially diazepam, are potent muscle relaxants. It is conceivable that relaxation of skeletal muscle by benzodiazepines may contribute to the sense of reduced anxiety associated with their use. Benzodiazepines inhibit the spread of generalized seizure activity and have found an important place in the clinical treatment of seizure disorders.[2]

In animal studies benzodiazepines have a disinhibiting effect and produce an attenuation of the behavioral consequences of fear, conflict, and frustration. The disinhibiting effect of this group of drugs is also observable clinically in that these drugs in modest doses may produce a state resembling mild alcohol intoxification that may be associated with paradoxical agitation and loss of behavioral control. For this reason these drugs should generally be avoided for patients with poor impulse control and a history of violent acting-out behavior. This disinhibiting effect may also be observed in elderly patients or those with organic brain syndromes.

The major guideline for appropriate therapeutic use of benzodiazepine drugs is that the dosage, frequency, and duration of administration should be minimized. Patients with long-standing anxiety are likely to remain anxious for a long time in the future and therefore are likely to consume, or to desire to consume, antianxiety medication for years. Such patients are perfectly set up to become dependent or addicted to benzodiazepine drugs through long-term use. Furthermore, patients with long-standing or severe anxiety are likely to respond less well to these drugs than patients with recent onset of acute anxiety. Patients with chronic anxiety are therefore likely to increase their own dose or frequency of administration, thus further favoring the potential for addiction. The benzodiazepine compounds have a long half-life.[2] Chlordiazepoxide has a half-life in the range of 7 to 28 hours. Diazepam has an even longer half-life of 20 to 50 hours. The half-life of oxazepam tends to be a bit shorter—3 to 21 hours. Because of the long half-life of these drugs it is unnecessary to administer them frequently throughout the day. It is generally preferable to advise patients using benzodiazepines to use them on an "as needed" basis, limiting their frequency of administration to once or twice daily. This will generally provide a satisfactory clinical effect and at the same time minimize the risk of drug dependency. Advising patients that they may not need to take these drugs every day will further add to the safety of their use. It is important to limit the quantity of benzodiazepines given in each individual prescription and to limit the patient's ability to refill prescriptions for these drugs. Patients should also be told to discuss their response to medication with the prescribing physician before increasing the dose or frequency of administration. Before increasing the dose of these drugs, it is important for the physician to clarify whether the symptoms experienced by patients are a result of their anxiety or an effect of the drug, since some patients occasionally experience muscle twitching or dysphoric mood states while using benzodiazepines.

Ideal patients for whom benzodiazepine antianxiety agents may be useful are individuals who have relatively acute onset of anxiety, particularly in association with life crises. For such patients the use of 5 mg of diazepam, 10 mg of chlordiazepoxide, 7.5 mg of chlorazepate, or 15 mg of oxazepam once or twice daily for 1 or 2 weeks may be beneficial. Since these drugs do not exert clearly specific pharmacological effects to counteract anxiety, they should be seen as adjuncts to psychotherapy in the treatment of anxiety rather than as "magic bullets." Patients needing to use progresively larger doses of benzodiazepines or desiring to use them over prolonged periods generally should have their medication changed early in the course of treatment in order to avoid eventual dependency. In some individuals the use of small doses of these drugs, such as 5 mg of diazepam two or three times weekly for a prolonged period of time, may be therapeutically beneficial and safe, as opposed to long-term daily administration of these medications.

Antihistamines, such as hydroxyzine, may produce drowsiness that is often considered an unwanted side effect. In some patients who are anxious, however, the use of drugs such as hydroxyzine in doses of 10 to 25 mg, one to four times daily, may produce a mild calming effect as a beneficial spin-off of the drowsiness-inducing side effect. Hydroxyzine does not produce tolerance or physical dependence and therefore is nonaddicting even when used over prolonged periods of time. Furthermore, unlike the antipsychotic agents, extrapyramidal effects have not been attributed to hydroxyzine. Therefore, in anxious patients, particularly with long-standing symptoms, a therapeutic trial of hydroxyzine may prove worthwhile, safe, and beneficial.

Patients with long-standing chronic anxiety or those individuals who do not benefit from limited use of benzodiazepines may respond satisfactorily to low doses of phenothiazine drugs. Admittedly, the use of antipsychotic drugs may be associated with the development of extrapyramidal symptoms. However, in choosing antipsychotic agents for the treatment of anxiety, those drugs with higher sedative potential and therefore lower extrapyramidal symptom–producing potential are the agents of choice. Furthermore, since anxious patients often respond well to very low doses of antipsychotic agents, the risk of unwanted parkinsonian side effects may be further minimized. Antipsychotic agents do not exert a specific pharmacological effect to counteract anxiety; however, they do exert a variety of antagonistic effects on the autonomic nervous system that play a role in the mediation of the physiological symptoms of anxiety. Additionally, the sedative side effects of the antipsychotic agents may contribute to their beneficial effect in anxiety. Since the antipsychotic agents do not produce tolerance or physical dependence there is no risk of addiction, even with long-standing use of these drugs.

The antipsychotic drugs of choice in the treatment of anxiety in the nonpsychotic patient are thioridazine and chlorpromazine. Both of these agents produce moderate sedation along with a minimal extrapyramidal effect as compared with other antipsychotic drugs. Generally, thioridazine is preferable to chlorpromazine for anxiety; however, either may be used, generally in a dosage of 10 to 25 mg, one to four times daily. Since the sedative effect of these drugs is important in their ability to alleviate anxiety, and since this effect is rather short-lived, their use in the treatment of anxiety should involve multiple doses throughout the day as opposed to the single daily dose that is most often employed in the treatment of psychosis with these agents. The dose of phenothiazines employed in the treatment of anxiety generally does not require coadministration of antiparkinsonian medications. In some patients thioridazine and chlorpromazine induce too much sedation; in such cases, trifluoperazine in a dose of 2 mg taken one to four times daily may be used to alleviate anxiety. The disadvantage of using trifluoperazine for anxiety is that it possesses a relatively low degree of sedating effect along with a greater potential for induction of parkinsonian symptoms.

Some chronically anxious patients with phobic or obsessive personality features may have pronounced alleviation of their anxiety symptoms when treated with tricyclic antidepressant drugs or such monoamine oxidase (MAO) inhibitor drugs as phenelzine. The dose and proper clinical use of these drugs for phobic anxiety states follow similar guidelines to their use in the treatment of depression, which is discussed at length later in this chapter.

The most pronounced disturbing symptoms of anxiety are often those of excessive sympathetic nervous system activity, including persistent sinus tachycardia, excessive sweating, tremors, urinary urgency, and diarrhea or abdominal cramping. Many of these physiological symptoms of anxiety respond favorably to the beta-adrenergic blocking drug, propranolol.[3] This drug is widely used in the treatment of cardiac arrhythmias, angina pectoris, and hypertension. Although use of propranolol is not approved in the United States for the treatment of anxiety, it has been extensively used experimentally in the United States and abroad and has been shown to be specifically beneficial in alleviating many of the physiological symptoms of anxiety, thereby reducing the patient's perception of this dysphoric state. A major advantage of the specific effect of propranolol for certain anxious patients is that it does not produce central nervous system depression or clouding of consciousness except as an idiosyncratic effect that is rarely seen. This drug has no addicting potential, which is, of course, an advantage for any agent that may be used over a prolonged period of time in a given patient. Propranolol is contraindicated for patients with a history of bronchial asthma, and may produce or worsen congestive heart failure for susceptible individuals. If propranolol is used for anxiety, the patients should be carefully examined by an internist, and it is preferable that they be followed simultaneously by an internist and psychiatrist because of the potential unwanted medical complications of this drug. Nevertheless, some patients who have failed to respond to a variety of medications have achieved satisfactory control of their anxiety through judicious use of propranolol. In the treatment of anxiety, propranolol is generally effective in a dosage range of 10 to 20 mg taken three to four times daily. Because of the relatively short half-life of this drug it is necessary to administer it in divided doses throughout the day in order to achieve a consistently beneficial effect. Propranolol is also of interest to the psychiatrist because it has a specific ability to reduce tremors, particularly essential tremor and the tremor induced in some patients by lithium carbonate therapy.[4] The effective dosage of propranolol for control of essential tremor and lithium-induced tremor is generally 10, 20, or 40 mg, three to four times daily.

## ANTIPSYCHOTIC DRUGS

Psychoses are among the least understood and most devastating illnesses to affect mankind. Psychotic illness causes serious disruption in the lives of individuals and has a major impact on society by incapacitating significant numbers of people. The introduction of chlorpromazine a quarter-century ago was one of the most significant advances in the understanding and treatment of psychotic illness. Since chlorpromazine first became available for clinical use, significant advances have been made in understanding the mechanisms and etiologies of psychosis. It is unlikely that a single cause will explain what appears to be a rather divergent group of related maladies. Genetic[5] and biochemical studies[6-9] have added significantly to our ability to understand and treat serious psychiatric illnesses.

The present section of this chapter will discuss drugs that are useful in the treatment of psychotic illness. For simplicity of understanding these agents are best referred to as antipsychotic drugs. These compounds have also been called neuroleptics, particularly in Europe. The term "neuroleptic" refers to the ability of these agents to produce psychomotor slowing, emotional quieting, and extrapyramidal symptoms in conjunction with their ability to alleviate specific psychotic symptoms. Antipsychotic drugs are also often called "major tranquilizers." This latter term is confusing, however, because a similar term, "minor tranquilizer", has been used to describe antianxiety drugs. The similarity in these terms suggests a similarity in their pharmacological effects. The antianxiety drugs, previously discussed in this chapter, differ from the antipsychotic drugs both in their mechanisms of action and in their therapeutic effects. An understanding of these pharmacological differences would be facilitated by avoiding the use of the terms "minor tranquilizer" and "major tranquilizer." Although antipsychotic drugs have some value in the treatment of selected patients with severe anxiety and certain agitated patients with organic brain syndromes, their primary clinical utility is in the treatment of schizophrenia, manic-depressive illness, and psychotic depression.

Antipsychotic drugs, as delineated in Table 26-1, exert a specific antagonistic action against the fundamental symptoms of schizophrenia.[9,10] These beneficial effects of antipsychotic drugs extend beyond mere sedation since they are capable of benefiting both withdrawn patients and those who are hyperactive and agitated. Furthermore, a variety of sedative drugs have been employed in psychotic patients without producing the impressive clinical improvement seen in such patients treated with neuroleptic drugs.[6,9] In addition to the beneficial effects of neuroleptic drugs in the treatment of schizophrenia, these agents also have an important role in the treatment of affective illness, both in alleviating certain symptoms of psychotic depression and in calming acutely agitated manic patients.[11] The diversity of patients who benefit from antipsychotic drugs and the failure of sedatives to bring about major improvement in seriously ill psychiatric patients suggests specific biochemical and pharmacological mechanisms of these serious psychiatric illnesses that in turn are affected by discrete pharmacological actions of the antipsychotic drugs.[9]

In addition to a wide variety of behavioral effects observed with antipsychotic drugs, numerous physiological changes are also associated with their use. There is considerable evidence to suggest a correlation between the physiological and behavioral effects of these drugs and their ability to antagonize a variety of endogenous neurochemical substances.[9] Antipsychotic drugs appear to exert their clinically beneficial effects in the treatment of psychosis as a result of their ability to block the action of dopamine, a naturally occurring chemical transmitter substance in the brain.[6] There is a general correlation between clinical potency of antipsychotic drugs and their specificity and potency as dopamine receptor blocking substances.[6,9,10,12] Among the phenothiazines the aliphatic derivatives, such as chlorpromazine, and the piperidine derivatives, such as thioridazine, exert less specific antipsychotic effects while the piperazine phenothiazines, such as trifluoperazine and fluphenazine, have a more potent and specific antipsychotic effect and likewise greater activity as antagonists of brain dopamine receptors.[6,13] Haloperidol, a butyrophenone compound, appears to be the most specific and effective antipsychotic drug in current use, particularly for the agitated schizophrenic or manic patient. Haloperidol produces strong clinical evidence of dopamine blockade that correlates with studies of dopamine and haloperidol binding to haloperidol binding sites in the brain.[12] It is conceivable that in acute phases of psychotic illness the brain receptor sites are flooded with dopamine, norepinephrine, or other neurotransmitter substances. Perhaps blockade of these receptor sites by neuroleptic drugs accounts for their effectiveness in alleviating signs and symptoms of psychosis. In addition to the dopamine blocking potential of neuroleptic drugs, these agents are also capable of blocking alpha-adrenergic receptors and cholinergic receptors.[8,9,14] The reader is referred to Chapter 27 for a more thorough discussion of the importance of alpha-adrenergic blockade and cholinergic blockade and the role that they play in the production of antipsychotic drug side effects.

Therapy with antipsychotic drugs can be divided into three phases. The initial phase of treatment is generally aimed at providing behavioral control and reducing agitation, fear, anxiety, disturbed thinking, and often hallucinations and delusions.[13] If one conceptualizes acute psychosis as a disorder involving excessive action of dopamine or related neurotransmitters, one may think of treatment in the acute phase as being aimed at producing dopaminergic receptor blockade in the brain.[6,9] Achievement of this pharmacological effect may well parallel the initial phases of clinical improvement. The term "pharmacolysis" seems applicable to describe the acute phase of drug treatment of psychosis. A rapid antipsychotic effect may best be achieved by administration of rather large doses of specific antipsychotic medications.[15,16]

The next phase of antipsychotic chemotherapy involves stabilization of the patient and the gradual reduction of dosage of medication in order to achieve the best possible control of symptoms using the lowest dose of medicine, thereby reducing the patient's vulnerability to drug side effects.

The third phase of treatment of the psychotic patient may be referred to as maintenance therapy and involves long-term continuous administration of the lowest possible dose of effective medication in order to prevent recurrence of the illness.[17]

In the schizophrenic patient these three phases of treatment are generally best accomplished by starting and continuing treatment with a single antipsychotic drug, provided that the patient is able to tolerate this medication without incapacitating side effects. If side effects do develop, they may be managed by dosage adjustment, addition of an antiparkinsonian medication in the case of extrapyramidal side effects, or in some cases changing to another antipsychotic drug.[13]

In the treatment of the acutely manic patient, treatment is usually best initiated with an antipsychotic drug in conjunction with lithium carbonate.[11] In the subsequent phases of treatment and maintenance of the manic patient, antipsychotic agents are generally given in decreasing doses until they are discontinued and the patient continues maintenance medication with lithium carbonate.

Treatment of the psychotically depressed patient usually is best initiated with antipsychotic drugs alone, followed by the addition of tricyclic or monoamine oxidase inhibitor antidepressants. Following the acute phase of treatment, the patient with psychotic depression should generally continue to receive maintenance medication consisting either of antidepressant drugs alone or in combination with antipsychotic agents or lithium carbonate.

The various antipsychotic drugs currently available for use differ significantly in their potency with respect to their ability to inhibit target symptoms of psychosis—specifically agitation, disordered thinking, hallucinations, and delusions. The available antipsychotic agents also differ significantly in the extent to which they produce a variety of side effects.[13,14] In accordance with the definition of neuroleptic drugs, all of the available agents in this class produce extrapyramidal effects. The drug-induced extrapyramidal reactions include the development of a syndrome that is identical to naturally occurring Parkinson's disease as well as the development of akathisia and dystonic reactions. The development of these extrapyamidal reactions appear to be related to the ability of antipsychotic drugs to block dopamine in the basal ganglia.[1,13] The agents that exert the most specific antipsychotic effect, such as piperazine phenothiazines and haloperidol, tend to produce more pronounced parkinsonian reactions that parallel their apparent greater dopamine-blocking potency.[9] Those neuroleptic drugs that produce more pronounced anticholinergic effects, such as thioridazine, are less likely to produce extrapyramidal reactions.[8] Elderly patients, as well as very young patients, tend to be particularly sensitive to drug-induced extrapyramidal reactions. On the other hand, those antipsychotic drugs that are more potent anticholinergic agents are more likely to produce unwanted atropine-like toxic psychoses, again particularly in the elderly patient.[9] Chlorpromazine possesses less specific antipsychotic effect and is likewise less likely to produce extrapyramidal reactions than the more potent neuroleptics. On the other hand, chlorpromazine is the most potent alpha adrenergic blocking drug among this class of therapeutic agents and is most likely to induce hypotension when the patient is at rest or with postural change. Thioridazine is essentially equal in potency to chlorpromazine both in terms of its antipsychotic effect and in terms of its ability to produce pronounced alpha-adrenergic blockade and hypotensive reactions. For all practical purposes, chlorprothixene is comparable to chlorpromazine in its spectrum of therapeutic activity, potency, and side effects. The piperazine thioxanthene derivatives, such as thiothixene, are comparable to the piperazine phenothiazines in their spectrum of therapeutic action, potency, and side effects.[1,13,14] The butyrophenone antipsychotic agent, haloperidol, appears to be the most specific antipsychotic agent currently available for clinical use.[6,13] Although haloperidol is associated with a significant incidence of extrapyramidal reactions, these unwanted effects can generally be easily dealt with in exchange for achieving rapid control of psychotic symptoms. Haloperidol has relatively little anticholinergic potency[8,9] and virtually no alpha-adrenergic blocking potential and therefore is associated with minimal risk of hypotensive reactions.[1,13,16]

The newest additions to the antipsychotic armamentarium are two compounds that are chemically unrelated to previously available antipsychotic drugs. Molindone is an indol derivative, structurally reminiscent of the endogenous neurotransmitter substance serotonin. Loxapine (Loxitane) is a dibenzoxazepine derivative, structurally somewhat similar to the more commonly known tricyclic antidepressant drugs. Thus far, both molindone and loxapine have been studied only to a limited extent. There is at this time insignificant evidence to suggest their superiority over already available and well-known, antipsychotic, chemotherapeutic agents.[18] Both molindone and loxapine have been shown in controlled studies to exert antipsychotic effects superior to placebo but insignificantly different from available effective drugs.[18] Although it was hoped that these two new compounds would provide therapeutic benefit with fewer side effects than currently available therapeutic agents, unfortunately this hope has not been realized. Both molindone and loxapine produce significant extrapyramidal effects when used in antipsychotic doses; the extent of these effects thus far appears to be intermediate between the parkinsonian-producing potency of chlorpromazine and trifluoperazine. A variety of autonomic side effects, including cholinergic and adrenergic blockade, may be produced by both molindone and loxapine. At the present time it would appear that the primary area of utility of these two new agents is in the treatment of patients who have been intolerant to other available antipsychotic drugs. Patients with prior histories of allergic or idiosyncratic reactions to antipsychotic drugs may be most likely to benefit with minimal risk when treated with drugs whose chemical structure is as unrelated as possible to the chemical structure of the compounds that produced the previous unwanted idiosyncratic reactions.

The psychiatrist who is asked to recommend treatment for an acutely psychotic patient on a medical ward should be familiar with the nature of the patient's other medical problems and should be aware of any medications that the patient may be receiving. Medical psychiatric drug interactions are discussed in detail in Chapter 27. In the medical-surgical ward setting, if the patient is severely agitated and there are no contraindications to antipsychotic chemotherapy, treatment should be instituted with the antipsychotic agent that will produce the least offensive side effects in that particular patient. Generally, the agent of choice is haloperidol in a dose of 2 to 5 mg orally or intramuscularly initially. Certainly for the elderly or very ill patient low doses should be employed, with doses of 1 to 2 mg every hour, if need be, in order to provide satisfactory behavioral control. For the patient without serious medical problems, larger doses of haloperidol may be employed after the initial dose. The patient may then be started on a regular regimen of 5 to 10 mg three to four times daily, with additional doses being given on an "as needed" basis. If the patient is particularly agitated or belligerent, larger doses of haloperidol may need to be employed, by either the oral or the intramuscular route.

When agitation or belligerence are the prime presenting symptoms a more sedating antipsychotic agent such as chlorpromazine may be beneficial. In starting treatment with chlorpromazine it is preferable to use small doses initially, again particularly for the elderly or very ill patient. The initial dose of chlorpromazine should be 25 to 50 mg orally or 25 mg intramuscularly. If the patient tolerates the drug without significant hypotension, the dose may be increased, and chlorpromazine may be administered in a dosage of 50 to 200 mg orally, three or four times daily, or 50 to 100 mg intramuscularly three or four times daily, again with additional doses given on an "as needed" basis. In the more withdrawn psychotic patient seen in the medical setting it is preferable to use antipsychotic agents with lower sedative potential, such as haloperidol, trifluoperazine, or thiothixene. Following an initial dose of 2 to 5 mg orally of trifluoperazine or thiothixene, the patient may then be stabilized on a regular dose, generally in the neighborhood of 5 mg three or four times daily, with additional doses of medication being given on an "as needed" basis. These last two agents may be particularly desirable for the withdrawn patient whom the physician prefers to sedate as little as possible. In more agitated patients, if trifluoperazine or thiothixene are chosen, it may be necessary to use chlorpromazine intermittently as well in order to achieve adequate calming and sedation. In the event that significant hypotension develops, the consultant should be prepared to lower the dose of medication or change to a different, less hypotensive drug. If extrapyramidal reactions occur, an antiparkinsonian medication such as benztropine or trihexyphenidyl in a dose of 1 to 2 mg two or three times daily may be added to the regimen. In elderly patients or those with organic brain syndrome who may be particularly sensitive to the psychotogenic effects of antiparkinsonian medication, amantadine in a dose of 100 mg twice daily may significantly reduce parkinsonian symptoms with minimal risk of worsening psychotic symptoms.[19]

The psychiatric consultant encountering an acutely manic patient on a medical-surgical ward should initiate treatment with an antipsychotic compound in order to achieve behavioral control. Although lithium carbonate is highly effective in reducing the symptoms, it tends to act rather slowly, requiring 1 to 2 weeks for a beneficial effect to be observed. Haloperidol is more rapid in its onset of action and is likely to produce significant behavioral control of the acutely manic patient within 1 to 3 days. Haloperidol is more effective in normalizing the acutely manic patient than is chlorpromazine, although the latter may achieve significant sedation with a less pronounced improvement in the manic quality of behavior.[11] In acute mania, the initial starting dose of haloperidol should be 5 mg orally or intramuscularly; however, patients with manic psychoses often require even larger doses of haloperidol or other antipsychotic agents than schizophrenic patients. It is not uncommon for acute manic patients to require 40 to 80 mg or more of haloperidol daily in the early phase of treatment.

Knowing when not to use psychotropic drugs is often as important to the consultant as an understanding of their proper use. In the general hospital setting one is apt to meet a number of patients presenting with psychotic symptoms that are in fact drug-induced or drug-related. Toxic psychoses and deliria are not uncommon adverse manifestations of nonpsychotropic drugs that are discussed in detail in Chapter 27. Almost invariably, the treatment of choice for drug-induced adverse behavioral symptoms is to discontinue administration of the offending agent if it is known or to discontinue all drug administration if the specific cause of the reaction is unclear. Generally antipsychotic medications should not be used in the treatment of toxic psychoses and deliria because they may well worsen these unwanted symptoms. Occasionally however, in order to manage the patient on the hospital ward it is necessary to administer modest doses of sedative type-drugs. Anticholinergic drug–induced psychoses likewise may be worsened by the addition of an antipsychotic agent and may best be managed by discontinuing administration of the medication; however, in some cases the administration of 1 mg of physostigmine slowly intravenously is helpful as a test to delineate and clarify the diagnosis of anticholinergic psychosis, as is discussed in Chapter 27.

Drug withdrawal states are often associated with psychotic symptoms that may not appear too dissimilar from those of naturally occurring psychoses. It is important for the consultant not to initiate treatment of such patients with antipsychotic medication. Patients withdrawing from barbiturates, sedatives, and alcohol may have a toxic delirium, they may hallucinate, and they also may have grand mal seizures or various types of atypical seizures. If one treats such a patient with chlorpromazine, one may produce two serious complications. First of all, chlorpromazine has a significant effect in lowering seizure threshold and may therefore precipitate the occurrence of seizures in a patient withdrawing from other drugs. On the other hand, chlorpromazine may produce serious hypotension in a patient being withdrawn from alcohol or sedatives. Patients being treated for drug withdrawal are best managed by the administration of barbiturate or sedative drugs as described elsewhere in this book. Antipsychotic drugs should be avoided in such patients because they do not help and may produce potentially dangerous adverse reactions. Patients who are withdrawing from barbiturates, sedatives, or alcohol may occasionally be given haloperidol for hallucinations, along with appropriate sedative medications, with relatively minimal risk of adverse reactions. Haloperidol has only limited effects in lowering seizure threshold and has very minimal potential for the induction of hypotension. Haloperidol may be a useful adjunct in the treatment of drug withdrawal, but it should never be used as the sole agent because of the potential life-threatening seriousness of some drug withdrawal syndromes, especially those associated with sedative-type drugs. More detailed discussions of these withdrawal states will be found elsewhere in this book.

## ANTIDEPRESSANT DRUGS

In the same way that antipsychotic drugs have helped us to understand chemical and pharmacological mechanisms of psychoses, pharmacological agents have also helped to extend our understanding of the mechanisms of affective illness. In the early 1950s, clinical use of iproniazid to treat tuberculosis led to the development of agitation and manic-like psychoses in a number of patients. Studies of this problem revealed iproniazid to be a potent monoamine oxidase inhibitor capable of increasing brain catecholamine concentration. Around the same time the introduction of reserpine for the treatment of hypertension was associated with the development of serious depressive illness in a number of patients, some of whom subsequently committed suicide. Studies of reserpine revealed that it was capable of depleting brain catecholamines such as norepinephrine and other biogenic amines such as serotonin. These accidental clinical discoveries helped to pave the way for an understanding of the correlation between decreased brain neurotransmitter activity and depression and also helped to clarify the parallel between increased brain neurotransmitters and manic-like psychoses.[1] Numerous more recent studies have helped to clarify the relationships between biogenic amines and mood states.[9,20,21]

Early in the history of drug treatment of depression, stimulants such as amphetamine derivatives were used clinically. These drugs are structurally similar to naturally occurring catecholamine substances. Amphetamine compounds provide stimulation and may make the patient appear better clinically; however, there is no evidence to support their ability to exert a true antidepressant effect comparable to the clinical effects observed with more widely used therapeutic agents. Drugs of the amphetamine type may induce a toxic psychosis, particularly with high dose or long-term administration, and may produce drug dependency marked by a withdrawal syndrome consisting of hypersomnolence and excessive appetite when treatment is discontinued. Occasional patients may benefit from brief courses of small doses of amphetamine-type drugs; the stimulation that these agents provide for such patients may be temporarily beneficial. Nevertheless, with the availability of a variety of effective antidepressant drugs, stimulant-type drugs should play only a minor role in the overall scheme of treatment for depressed patients.

The tricyclic antidepressant drugs, such as amitriptyline, imipramine, and doxepin, form the mainstay of the drug treatment of depression. There are a variety of tricyclic drugs that are effective in the treatment of depression. The mechanism of action of these compounds depends on their ability to block nerve reuptake of norepinephrine and thereby presumably to increase its availability at synaptic endings in the brain.[22] The tricyclic antidepressant drugs primarily differ in the extent and severity of their side effects.[13,14] In addition to inhibiting nerve reuptake of norepinephrine, all available tricyclic antidepressant drugs exert a significant anticholinergic effect. The ability of these drugs to block acetylcholine and consequently to inhibit the parasympathetic nervous system varies among the available compounds. Amitriptyline has the greatest anticholinergic effect and doxepin and desipramine the least anticholinergic effect among the tricyclic drugs. Imipramine is intermediate in its anticholinergic potency. Cholinergic blockade by tricyclic drugs is responsible for blurred vision, dry mouth, reduced sweating, constipation, urinary retention, and tachycardia. Patients with cardiac conditions or other medical problems such as prostatism that would make them particularly vulnerable to anticholinergic drugs should be treated cautiously with tricyclic antidepressants. For such patients it would generally be preferable to use doxepin or desipramine because of their lower anticholinergic potency as opposed to a drug such as amitriptyline.

Sedation is another side effect commonly associated with tricyclic antidepressants. This effect may be inconvenient or unpleasant in that it may interfere with the life functions of patients, particularly when they take such drugs during the daytime. On the other hand, the sedative side effect of tricyclic antidepressants may be beneficial in helping to induce sleep since a significant proportion of depressed patients do have sleep disturbances. Amitriptyline has the most pronounced sedative effect, while doxepin has somewhat less sedative potential and imipramine and desipramine both produce less sedation than the former two drugs. None of the tricyclic antidepressant compounds is truly stimulatory and it is misleading to consider these antidepressant agents as stimulants. In patients who have sleep disorders amitriptyline may be the drug of choice because of its greater sedative potential. Likewise, doxepin would be likely to benefit the sleep pattern. Depressed patients who tend to be excessively drowsy with or without drug therapy may do better with the less sedating antidepressant agents, such as imipramine and desipramine. It should be kept in mind that tricyclic drugs may interact with a variety of other medications, as discussed extensively in Chapter 27. The sedative effect of tricyclic antidepressants may be increased when they are used in combination with a variety of central nervous system depressant drugs. All tricyclic antidepressants interfere with the antihypertensive action of guanethidine and clonidine, as discussed in Chapter 27. The anticholinergic effects of tricyclic drugs are additive with anticholinergic effects of other therapeutic agents that medical patients may be receiving. Tricyclic antidepressant drugs also have the capacity to produce or worsen cardiac arrhythmias in susceptible individuals, as discussed in Chapter 27. Patients with known cardiac disease should be treated cautiously with tricyclic drugs, preferably using doxepin because of its lower arrhythmogenic potential. The risk of cardiac arrhythmias may also be minimized by using small doses divided throughout the day when instituting therapy and gradually increasing the dose as required for therapeutic benefit with occasional monitoring of pulse rate and electrocardiogram.

Some patients receiving tricyclic antidepressant drugs may become confused or agitated. This effect is linked either to their anticholinergic action or to the ability of these drugs to uncover a previously unrecognized psychotic disturbance. Larger doses of tricyclic drugs may produce a toxic psychosis and some patients with unrecognized, bipolar, affective illness may develop acute manic psychoses following treatment of depressive illness with tricyclic drugs. Occasional confusion and less well-defined memory defects have been associated with tricyclic antidepressants.[23]

In some patients the concomitant administration of phenothiazines, such as small doses of trifluoperazine (5 to 15 mg per day), may reduce the likelihood of agitation and confusion occurring during the course of tricyclic antidepressant drug treatment. Another potentially useful reason to combine phenothiazines and tricyclic antidepressants is the ability of the former group of drugs to inhibit the metabolism of tricyclic compounds. It is conceivable that this kind of drug interaction would favor the achievement of higher blood levels of the tricyclic antidepressants.[24] Clinical observations suggest that patients may respond more rapidly in some cases when small doses of trifluoperazine are added to tricyclic drugs. In addition, some patients who fail to respond favorably to tricyclic antidepressants in full therapeutic doses will show significant clinical benefit when small doses of phenothiazines are added to the tricyclic drug regimen. Nevertheless, these data and observations do not support the use of fixed dosage combinations of phenothiazine and tricyclic drugs. In administering one of the commonly available fixed dosage combinations of perphenazine and amitriptyline one will have to provide the patient with an excessive dosage of phenothiazine in order to provide a therapeutic dosage of amitriptyline (150 mg daily). It is therefore preferable when treating patients with phenothiazines and tricyclic drugs together to use single drug preparations and reserve the ability to adjust dosage of the two therapeutic agents independently. Another value of combining phenothiazines and tricyclic drugs in the treatment of depressed patients is that the phenothiazine may relieve anxiety early in the course of treatment, often within a few days, while it is necessary to wait 2 to 3 weeks to achieve a therapeutic response to tricyclic antidepressants.

The treatment of patients with tricyclic antidepressants is very much dependent on providing adequate doses of these drugs. In general, most studies indicate that 150 mg of tricyclic antidepressant must be administered daily in order to achieve and maintain a satisfactory antidepressant response.[13,22,25] Doxepin appears to be less potent in its antidepressant effect than other tricyclic compounds. Clinical data suggests that 200 to 300 mg of doxepin must be administered in order to produce the same response as 150 mg of amitriptyline.[13] Nevertheless, even with the use of relatively high doses, doxepin may produce less disturbing anticholinergic and arrhythmogenic effects than equivalent therapeutic doses of amitriptyline.

Tricyclic antidepressant drugs work quite effectively when administered in single daily doses, and generally they are best given at bedtime in order to minimize unwanted effects. Although 150 mg is the usual effective daily dose of these drugs, it is inadvisable to initiate treatment with this dose of medication. It is preferable to start treatment with tricyclic antidepressant drugs by administering 50 mg at bedtime for one to three nights followed by 100 mg of the drug at bedtime for an additional similar period of time with a subsequent increase by the end of the first week of treatment to a full therapeutic dose of 150 mg. Since some patients will respond to 150 mg daily of doxepin it is worth treating the patient at this dosage level for 2 weeks (unless the circumstances are urgent) before increasing the dose further. Since most patients require 2, 3, or 4 weeks to show a beneficial response to tricyclic drugs, one needs to look out for the safety and welfare of the patient while awaiting therapeutic response to medication. Patients who have failed to achieve a satisfactory drug response after 2 to 4 weeks of treatment may then benefit by having their dosage of tricyclic drug increased to 200 mg nightly for an additional week or two, and subsequently the dose may be increased even further to 250 or 300 mg per night in patients whose initial response has been unsatisfactory.

Patients who have failed to respond adequately to tricyclic antidepressants may be given a trial of small doses of phenothiazines added to the regimen as described before. Some patients who fail to respond to tricyclic antidepressants may eventually develop a favorable response to these drugs when lithium carbonate is added to the treatment regimen. Some patients who fail to respond to tricyclic antidepressants may achieve satisfactory improvement in their depression when treated with monoamine oxidase inhibitor–type antidepressants.

A variety of monoamine inhibitors have been shown to be clinically beneficial in depression. These drugs appear to exert their therapeutic effect by increasing the availability of norepinephrine at synapses in the brain by inhibiting one pathway of catecholamine metabolism.[21] Monoamine oxidase inhibitor antidepressants were introduced into clinical therapeutic use shortly before the availability of tricyclic drugs. The early experience with monoamine oxidase inhibitors preceded an understanding of their potential interaction with tyramine-rich foods and phenylethylamine compounds. Because this problem was not understood initially, patients were not warned about dietary restrictions associated with their drug treatment. As a consequence of this problem, some patients taking monoamine oxidase inhibitors developed hypertensive crises, at times severe enough to produce cerebrovascular accidents or even death. These serious misadventures in the early use of monoamine oxidase inhibitor drugs led to their being seen as dangerous. When tricyclic antidepressants became available they were generally recognized as being safer than monoamine oxidase inhibitors and largely displaced the latter drugs from common therapeutic use.

Several clinical studies have demonstrated the therapeutic efficacy of monoamine oxidase inhibitor–type antidepressants.[26,27] Clinical experience and reports in the literature also suggest that some patients who fail to respond to tricyclic antidepressants will respond favorably to monoamine oxidase inhibitors with satisfactory clearing of depressive symptoms. Hypertensive reactions in patients taking monoamine oxidase inhibitors are the result of potentiated responses to tyramine and sympathomimetic agents under the influence of catecholamine metabolism blockade. Therefore, in selected patients monoamine oxidase inhibitor–type antidepressants may be used safely if the physician adequately explains to the patient the risks of adverse reactions and the need to avoid certain foods and medications. In prescribing monoamine oxidase inhibitor antidepressants it is necessary for the physician to provide the patient with a typewritten sheet of instructions that clearly delineates the foods and medications to be avoided in conjunction with monoamine oxidase inhibitor drugs. An example of an appropriate list of instructions is presented here.

The major disadvantage of the MAO antidepressants is that people taking them need to avoid eating certain foods or taking certain other medications. Patients taking MAO antidepressants must not eat or drink the following foods:
1. Fermented cheese, specifically cheddar or other strong tasting cheeses
2. Pickled herring, sardines, and anchovies
3. Chicken livers
4. Canned or processed meats
5. Pods of broad beans
6. Canned figs
7. Yeast extract
8. Wine and beer

Patients taking MAO antidepressants should either drink decaffeinated coffee or limit their intake to 2 cups of regular coffee per day. Patients on these medications should not eat more than 2 ounces of chocolate per day. Alcoholic beverages should be avoided while taking MAO antidepressants; however, one may occasionally have a single cocktail or 2 or 3 ounces of white wine. While being treated with MAO antidepressants, one should not eat more than 2 ounces of sour cream, yogurt, cottage cheese, American cheese, or mild Swiss cheese per day. All other cheese products or food products whose manufacturing process involves fermentation should be avoided in the diet.

Patients being treated with MAO antidepressants should not, under any circumstances, use nose drops, cold remedies, cough syrups, diet pills, or any kind of stimulant drug.

The problem of hypertensive crises associated with monoamine oxidase inhibitors is discussed in further detail in Chapter 27. Phenelzine and tranylcypromine are both monoamine oxidase inhibitor–type antidepressants that produce clinically beneficial responses.[26,27] Monoamine oxidase inhibitors tend to exert their antidepressant effect generally after a lag time of about 1 week after starting treatment. Tranylcypromine appears to have some stimulant qualities and indeed bears some structural resemblance to amphetamine-like compounds and may exert an antidepressant effect within 1 to 3 days of instituting treatment. The usual starting dose of tranylcypromine is 10 mg daily, increased to 10 mg twice daily after the initial week of treatment. Many patients will respond adequately to 20 mg of tranylcypromine daily; however, in some patients the dosage may be gradually increased up to 40 mg as required to achieve a therapeutically beneficial result. Phenelzine is usually started in a dose of 15 mg daily with subsequent dosage increases at weekly intervals up to 30, 45, or occasionally 60 mg daily until an adequate therapeutic result has been attained. Monoamine oxidase inhibitor drugs may produce a mild degree of postural hypotension and indeed one such compound, pargyline, has been used successfully in the treatment of hypertension, as discussed in Chapter 27. Monoamine oxidase inhibitors are free of anticholinergic effects and may be used safely in many patients who have previously developed urinary retention or other adverse anticholinergic effects while treated with tricyclic antidepressants. Some investigators have suggested that despite what sounds like a potentially dangerous pharmacological interaction, tricyclic antidepressants may be used simultaneously with monoamine oxidase inhibitor drugs.[28] Thus far, the evidence to support significant increased benefits from combining may be tried cautiously in selected patients who are able to be carefully monitored and followed. If monoamine oxidase inhibitors and tricyclic drugs are combined simultaneously in treatment of depressed patients, the potential risks of this combination should be discussed in detail with patients, who should most probably be asked to sign a consent acknowledging that they understand these potential risks. It is particularly important to obtain such informed consent from patients because at the present time the Food and Drug Administration of the United States has not approved the combined use of these two antidepressant drugs.

## MOOD-STABILIZING DRUG: LITHIUM CARBONATE

Unlike other psychotropic drugs, which are complex organic molecules, lithium carbonate is a simple compound that may be classified chemically as a salt. Following observations of the sedative potential of five lithium compounds used for nonpsychiatric indications, Cade first demonstrated the efficacy of lithium salts in controlling agitated psychotic states in ten manic patients.[29] In the intervening years since Cade's dramatic discovery, a vast number of studies have been conducted to explore the psychotropic effects and therapeutic potential of lithium carbonate, the most commonly used lithium salt.[30] The clinical actions of lithium are quite variable under different circumstances. Indeed, it seems paradoxical that the same substance can both calm agitated patients and alleviate depression. It is for this reason that the term "mood-stabilizing drug" seems to be the most appropriate description of the actions of this compound. This descriptive term implies the ability of lithium to stabilize or normalize mood whether the starting point be a "high" (mania) or a "low" (depression). The term "mood-stabilizing drug" also implies the ability of lithium carbonate to act prophylactically in preventing recurrent episodes of both mania and depression.

The biphasic effect of lithium carbonate on mood states makes its mechanism of action difficult to understand. Indeed, the pharmacological means by which lithium exerts its beneficial effect is not well delineated. There is evidence to suggest that lithium affects the flow and balance of electrolytes across cell membranes. Some data suggest that lithium may help to correct the reportedly elevated intracellular sodium concentration associated with severe affective illness.[31] Considerable data exist to show that clinically attainable lithium concentration can exert an antagonistic action at catecholamine-mediated synapses in the brain. Lithium may also interfere with norepinephrine and dopamine release at central nervous system synapsis.[31] These latter findings seem to reasonably explain the antimanic qualities of lithium if mania is understood as a disorder involving excessive catecholamine effects in the brain. The beneficial effect of lithium in depressive illness is difficult to relate to these latter mechanisms of action, but may well involve the effect of lithium on the synthesis and release of other neurotransmitter substances such as acetylcholine.[31] Studies of the interaction of antipsychotic drugs with receptor sites in the brain have postulated that dopamine receptors, and perhaps other receptors as well, may exist in two conformational forms.[12] Perhaps changes in receptor site conformation in the brain may also help to explain the biphasic effects of lithium on mood states.

The therapeutic use of lithium as a highly beneficial treatment for acute manic psychoses is well established.[11,30,32] In such acutely agitated patients lithium is capable of gradually diminishing the agitated and manic symptoms, returning the patient to a more stable, normalized mood state. Lithium when given alone may require 1 to 2 weeks in order to provide satisfactory behavioral control in such patients. A more rapid response may be obtained by treating acutely manic patients with a combination of an antipsychotic, such as chlorpromazine, or haloperidol, along with lithium carbonate.[11,30]

Although studies are currently in progress to understand the correlation between therapeutic effects and serum concentration of a variety of psychotropic drugs, the relevance of this relationship has been recognized almost from the beginning of lithium therapy in psychiatry. Lithium serum concentrations in the range of 0.6 to 1.2 mEq per liter are generally associated with beneficial therapeutic and prophylactic results with this drug.[30] Since the range of therapeutic blood levels is derived from studies of a large and heterogeneous population, it is easily understandable that some patients may benefit from serum lithium levels somewhat below the suggested therapeutic range while other patients will require concentrations somewhat above the usually accepted limits. In acutely manic patients it is often desirable to achieve blood lithium concentrations of 1.0 to 1.5 mEq in order to facilitate more rapid improvement. It must be noted, however, that higher serum concentrations of lithium tend to be associated with an increased incidence or severity of lithium side effects. Occasionally, patients may be seen who appear to be unable to tolerate prophylactic lithium maintenance because of side effects. Sometimes the management of such patients can be facilitated by reducing the dose of lithium carbonate and consequently its blood concentration. Maintaining patients at lower lithium blood levels may require more frequent observations and laboratory tests, but it frequently allows patients to reap the benefits of lithium therapy and avoid unpleasant side effects.

In addition to the demonstrated value of lithium in the treatment of acutely manic patients, extensive studies support the prophylactic efficacy of lithium carbonate in patients with recurrent manic illness.[33] Some studies have supported a beneficial effect of lithium in the prophylaxis of recurrent depression.[30,32,34] The prophylactic value of lithium against recurrent depression seems less well established than its beneficial effects in preventing recurrent attacks of mania. It appears clinically that a significant number of patients with recurrent depressive illness may benefit from lithium prophylaxis; however, if these patients are followed over a prolonged period of years, perhaps a third of them will require specific antidepressant drug treatment at some point in their course. Even in many patients who do require such specific pharmacological treatment there appears to be some decrease in both the frequency and the severity of depressive episodes during lithium prophylaxis.

The therapeutic value of lithium as a single agent in the treatment of depression is less well established; however, some studies have supported the antidepressant effect of lithium.[30,35] The therapeutic value of lithium in depression appears primarily to exist in patients with bipolar illness rather than those with unipolar disorders. Some patients with long-standing or recurrent depressive illness that has failed to respond to adequate trials of tricyclic or monoamine oxidase antidepressants may benefit from a combination of lithium carbonate and therapeutic doses of antidepressant drugs. In patients with persistent depression apparently unresponsive to drugs, a trial of combined lithium carbonate and antidepressant therapy should be considered prior to electroconvulsive therapy if a clinical emergency does not exist. There is some evidence to suggest that the therapeutic and prophylactic value of lithium in depression may be enhanced by attaining serum lithium concentrations somewhat higher than those usually employed (0.8 to 1.2 mEq per liter).[34]

Lithium carbonate has been tried in a variety of atypical psychiatric disturbances with variable results.[30] Premenstrual tension and its attendant emotional lability and distress may be benefited by a trial of lithium carbonate if the condition is sufficiently bothersome to the patient and not improved with more conservative measures.[30] The syndrome of emotionally unstable character disorder (EUCD), generally occurring in adolescent females and marked by chronic maladaptive behavior patterns associated with rapid mood swings, may benefit significantly from lithium treatment and prophylaxis.[36]

The use of lithium therapeutically and prophylactically, whatever the indication, must follow certain guidelines in order to facilitate effective and safe treatment with this potent and valuable drug. Prior to the administration of lithium carbonate certain baseline laboratory studies should be performed. A baseline electrocardiogram is important since therapeutic doses of lithium may be associated with minor electrocardiographic changes, particularly in the ST segment and T-wave.[30] If the electrocardiographic changes occur during lithium treatment, the baseline electrocardiogram is useful to document their relationship to lithium rather than to intercurrent coronary disease. Since lithium intoxication can be associated with abnormalities of cardiac conduction and rhythm, the pretreatment electrocardiogram is of further value in the long-term management of the patient. Lithium carbonate treatment may be associated with abnormalities of the thyroid gland, as discussed in Chapter 27; for this reason treatment and follow-up of the patient on lithium are facilitated by obtaining measurements of serum thyroxine (T4) and triiodothyronine (T3). Prior to starting lithium therapy, pretreatment measurement of thyroid-stimulating hormone (TSH) may be of value in helping to clarify a thyroid abnormality in the rare event that it may occur during lithium treatment. It is of utmost importance to obtain serum creatinine or blood urea nitrogen measurements, or both, prior to starting lithium treatment. Abnormalities in these tests imply renal functional impairment that may give rise to excessive lithium concentrations in the presence of usual therapeutic doses of lithium. In patients with cardiac, respiratory, or renal disease or in those patients receiving diuretics, it is important to measure serum electrolytes prior to instituting lithium treatment.

Lithium is removed from the body almost entirely by renal excretion. The half-life of lithium in normal healthy adults is generally about 18 hours, while in elderly or infirm individuals the lithium half-life may double. Sodium and lithium are reabsorbed competitively by the proximal tubules of the kidney. Sodium is further absorbed in the distal tubules although lithium is not.[31] Salt restriction will increase lithium retention and may lead to toxic serum concentrations. Diuretic drugs that act at the distal tubules will facilitate the excretion of sodium but not that of lithium; therefore, diuretics tend to facilitate lithium retention and may lead to lithium toxicity. With the exception of salt restriction and diuretic drugs other dietary changes or medications have little effect on the therapeutic or toxic actions of lithium carbonate.

In order to make lithium treatment as safe as possible it is preferable to start with relatively low doses. In healthy individuals with normal renal function lithium carbonate may be prescribed in doses of 300 mg three or four times daily. In elderly patients or those with renal disease, lower doses should be employed; however, such individuals may be safely treated with lithium if low enough doses are selected and blood levels are adequately monitored. It is important in instituting lithium treatment to advise patients never to take the drug on an empty stomach. If lithium is taken at meal time or with small snacks, the likelihood of gastric irritation, nausea, and epigastric distress will be minimized. Lithium is absorbed rapidly from the stomach over a period of 3 to 6 hours following each dose. Because serum lithium concentrations tend to peak within a short time following lithium ingestion, it is important to measure serum lithium concentrations at a stable interval following drug administration. For practical purposes, it is generally advisable to measure serum lithium concentrations approximately 12 hours after the previous dose of lithium. Lithium levels may be measured at intervals somewhat shorter or longer than the suggested 12 hour period; however, this will affect the measured serum level of lithium. Lithium serum determinations done within the first 6 hours following lithium dosage may provide erratic results because of the ongoing process of lithium absorption. It is often helpful to note in the patient's record the time interval between the last dose of lithium and the time of blood-drawing in order to clarify laboratory results that appear inappropriate. During the initial phases of treatment with lithium in the acutely manic or depressed patient, serum determination should be done once and preferably twice weekly. Once the patient demonstrates the ability to tolerate lithium, lithium blood levels should be done at weekly intervals during the first month of treatment. Subsequently, lithium concentrations may be measured every 2 weeks during the second month of treatment. After the second month of treatment, lithium levels may be measured somewhat less frequently, at intervals of 3 to 4 weeks. Patients who have been treated with lithium for a period of several months and have maintained relatively stable serum lithium concentrations may then be safely followed with serum lithium determinations done at intervals of every 6 to 8 weeks. Although some clinicians favor infrequent serum lithium measurements during long-term management, it seems preferable to determine serum lithium levels at intervals of no less than every 2 or 3 months even over periods of years of treatment with this drug. Aside from the advantage of spotting an abnormal lithium level or perhaps an abnormal behavior pattern, the regular measurement of lithium levels is beneficial subjectively because it helps to facilitate the patient's understanding of the importance of regular medication use and follow-up to continued well-being.

Most patients in the initial phases of treatment with lithium experience relatively few side effects. Unlike other psychotropic drugs, lithium does not interact with the autonomic nervous system, nor does it produce measurable sedation except in the manic or hypomanic patient. Occasional patients experience anorexia, nausea, or epigastric distress with lithium treatment; the symptoms usually abate rapidly either spontaneously or by rearranging lithium dosages to coincide with meals. These gastrointestinal symptoms may also appear in patients as early signs of lithium toxicity, and this problem must be explored by measuring lithium blood levels if the symptoms persist. Some patients experience dryness of the mouth or a metallic taste when starting lithium treatment; often these symptoms disappear, but in some cases they persist throughout treatment and the patient learns to tolerate or ignore them. Muscle tremors are often seen at the outset of lithium treatment, but they generally disappear within the first week or two. Persistent tremors of the hands and fingers in association with lithium treatment may be benefited by reducing the dose of lithium or by changing the pattern of administration so that peak lithium levels reached following each dose are minimized as a result of giving multiple smaller doses. In some patients persistent tremor associated with lithium may disturb the day to day functioning of the patient and require treatment with propranolol, as mentioned earlier in this chapter. The association of tremor with ataxia, muscle weakness, or muscle hyperirritability may be a sign of lithium intoxication and should be investigated by measuring the serum lithium concentration. A variety of neurological symptoms, including vertigo, slurred speech, incontinence, and seizures, may be associated with lithium toxicity and should be evaluated and treated promptly by discontinuing lithium and administering adequate volumes of fluid. Additional medical aspects of lithium are discussed in detail in Chapter 27.

Unlike antipsychotic and antidepressant drugs, there are insufficient data to support the administration of lithium carbonate in a single daily dose. On the other hand, in light of the average 18-hour half-life of lithium carbonate, it is not necessary to administer this drug in multiple divided doses throughout the day after the initial phase of treatment. Lithium prophylaxis can be adequately accomplished by dividing the total daily dose of lithium into two parts, administering approximately one-half of the dose in the morning and one-half in the evening, preferably with breakfast and supper.

The daily maintenance dose of lithium carbonate varies among individual patients. The required dosage of lithium does not necessarily vary directly with body size. Some elderly individuals may be maintained adequately with satisfactory blood levels of the drug by administering 300 to 450 mg of lithium daily. On the other hand, some patients require daily maintenance doses of 1,800 mg or occasionally more. Both the therapeutic and maintenance dosages of lithium should be guided by clinical observation of the patient along with measurements of serum lithium concentration. Patients taking lithium should be encouraged to phone their physician in the event of the development of any intercurrent illness that may increase the likelihood of lithium intoxication. Patients taking lithium should also be encouraged to discontinue their medication for a day or two in the event of the development of nausea, vomiting, or diarrhea. The development of these symptoms in a previously asymptomatic individual should signal the need for obtaining lithium blood level measurements. Indeed, any change in behavior or symptoms in a patient being maintained on lithium should be investigated by measuring the serum lithium concentration and observing the patient clinically.

## SUMMARY

The following principles should be helpful in avoiding therapeutic misadventures involving medical-psychiatric drug interactions:

1. Avoid combining multiple sedative-type drugs and use the lowest possible doses of these medications in elderly or medically ill patients, particularly those with pulmonary disease. Limiting the dose and duration of treatment with antianxiety (sedative) drugs will minimize the risk of dependency and addiction.

2. Use strongly hypotensive phenothiazines such as chlorpromazine or thioridazine with caution, if at all, in elderly patients or those with cardiovascular disease. Haloperidol or piperazine phenothiazines such as trifluoperazine are preferable in such patients. Chlorpromazine and thioridazine can produce electrocardiographic changes that may be confused with the changes of coronary heart disease.

3. Remember that antipsychotic drugs, antidepressant drugs, and antiparkinsonian agents all produce anticholinergic effects. These effects are additive when these medications are taken simultaneously. Unpleasant or dangerous physiological or behavioral reactions may occur. Patients receiving tricyclic antidepressant drugs along with antipsychotic drugs rarely require antiparkinsonian medication.

4. Tricyclic antidepressants should be used with caution in cardiac patients because of the arrhythmogenic potential of these drugs. Doxepin tends to be somewhat less anticholinergicand arrhythmogenic than other tricyclic antidepressants. Doxepin may be used safely in cardiac patients when administered in small divided doses with gradual dosage adjustment being made until the desired therapeutic response is achieved.

5. Tricyclic antidepressant drugs should never be used in hypertensive patients being treated with guanethidine because they interfere with the hypotensive action of the latter drug. Reserpine should never be used to treat hypertension in a depressed patient or in an individual with a prior personal or family history of depression.

6. Monoamine oxidase inhibitor antidepressant drugs may be used safely and produce desirable clinical improvement if the patient is properly educated and provided with a printed list of foods and medications to avoid during treatment with these drugs.

7. Lithium carbonate is a beneficial and safe drug in the treatment and prophylaxis of affective disorders if used in conjunction with careful monitoring of serum lithium levels. Patients must be screened for the absence of renal disease prior to lithium treatment and should maintain adequate dietary salt intake and generally avoid diuretics during lithium administration.

8. A wide variety of drugs including atropine, synthetic anticholinergic drugs, digitalis, quinidine, lidocaine, pentazocine, indomethacin, and steroid hormones may produce toxic psychoses or delirium. Treatment of such adverse reactions must begin by discontinuing the offending drug and changing to a different therapeutic agent. Antipsychotic medication may facilitate improvement in drug-induced toxic psychoses; however, new medication should not be added to the regimen until the offending agent is discontinued.

**REFERENCES**

1. Byck, R.: Drugs and the treatment of psychiatric disorders. In Goodman, L.S., and Gilman, A.: The pharmacological basis of therapeutics, New York, 1975, The Macmillan Co.

2. Greenblatt, D. J., and Shader, R. I.: Benzodiazepines in clinical practice, New York, 1974, Raven Press.
3. Wheatley, D.: Comparative effects of propranolol and chlordiazepoxide in anxiety states, Br. J. Psychiatry **113**:1411-1412, 1969.
4. Winkler, G. F., and Young, R. R.: The control of essential tremor by propranolol, Trans. Am. Neurol. Assoc. **96**: , 1972.
5. Matthysse, S. W., and Kidd, K. K.: Estimating the genetic contribution to schizophrenia, Am. J. Psychiatry **133**:185-191, 1976.
6. Snyder, S. H.: The dopamine hypothesis of schizophrenia: focus on the dopamine receptor, Am. J. Psychiatry **133**:197-202, 1976.
7. Gillin, J. C., Kaplan, J., Stillman, R., and Wyatt, R. J.: The psychedelic model of schizophrenia: the case of N, N-Dimethyltryptamine, Am. J. Psychiatry **133**:203-208, 1976.
8. Snyder, S. H., Greenberg, D., and Yamamura, H. I.: Antischizophrenic drugs and brain cholinergic receptors, Arch. Gen. Psychiatry **31**:58-61, 1974.
9. Snyder, S. H., and others: Drugs, neurotransmitters and schizophrenia, Science **184**:1234-1253, 1974.
10. Seeman, P., and Lee, T.: Antipsychotic drugs: direct correlation between clinical potency and presynaptic actions on dopamine neurons, Science **188**:1217-1219, 1975.
11. Shopsin, B., Gershon, S., Thompson, H., and Collins, P.: Psychoactive drugs in mania: a controlled comparison of lithium carbonate, chlorpromazine, and haloperidol, Arch. Gen. Psychiatry **32**:34-42, 1975.
12. Creese, I., Burt, P. R., and Snyder, S. H.: Dopamine receptor binding: differentiation of agonist and antagonist states with $^3$H-dopamine and $^3$H-haloperidol, Life Sci. **17**:993-1001, 1975.
13. Hollister, L. E.: Clinical use of psychotherapeutic drugs, Springfield, Illinois, 1973, Charles C Thomas, Publisher.
14. Shader, R. I., and DiMascio, A.: psychotropic drug side effects, Baltimore, 1970, The William & Wilkins Co.
15. Donlon, P. T., and Tupin, J. P.: Rapid "digitalization" of decompensated schizophrenic patients with antipsychotic agents, Am. J. Psychiatry **131**:310-312, 1974.
16. Anderson, W. H., Kuehnle, J. C., and Catanzano, D. M.: Rapid treatment of acute psychosis, Am. J. Psychiatry **133**:1076-1078, 1976.
17. Davis, J. M.: Overview: maintenance therapy in psychiatry: I. Schizophrenia, Am. J. Psychiatry **132**:1237-1245, 1975.
18. Davis, J. M.: Recent developments in the drug treatment of schizophrenia, Am. J. Psychiatry **133**:208-214, 1976.
19. Fann, W. E., and Lake, C. R.: Amantadine versus trihexyphenidyl in the treatment of neuroleptic-induced parkinsonism, Am. J. Psychiatry **133**:940-943, 1976.
20. Maas, J. W.: Biogenic amines and depression: biochemical and pharmacological separation of two types of depression, Arch. Gen. Psychiatry **32**:1357-1361, 1975.
21. Schildkraut, J. J.: Catecholamine metabolism and affective disorders. In Usdin, E., and Snyder, S., editors: Frontiers of catecholamine research, New York, 1974, Pergamon Press, Inc., pp. 1165-1171.

22. Glassman, A. H., and Perel, J. M.: The clinical pharmacology of imipramine: implications for therapeutics, Arch. Gen. Psychiatry **28**:649-653, 1973.
23. Cole, J. O., and Schatzberg, A.: Memory difficulty and tricyclic antidepressants, McLean Hosp. J. **1**:102-107, 1976.
24. Gram, L. F., Overo, K. F., and Kirk, L.: Influence of neuroleptics and benzodiazepines on metabolism of tricyclic antidepressants in man, Am. J. Psychiatry **131**:863-866, 1974.
25. Raskin, A.: A guide for drug use in depressive disorders, Am. J. Psychiatry **131**:181-185, 1974.
26. Lurie, M. L., and Salzer, H. M.: Tranylcypromine (Parnate) in the ambulatory treatment of depressed patients, Am. J. Psychiatry **118**:152-155, 1961.
27. Robinson, D. S., and others: Controlled clinical trial of the MAO inhibitor, phenelzine, in the treatment of depressive-anxiety states, Arch. Gen. Psychiatry **29**:407-416, 1973
28. Spiker, D. G., and Pugh, D. D.: Combining tricyclic and monoamine oxidase inhibitor antidepressants, Arch. Gen. Psychiatry **33**:828-830, 1976.
29. Cade, J. F. J.: Lithium salts in the treatment of psychotic excitement, Med. J. Aust. **36**:349-352, 1949.
30. Gershon, S., and Shopsin, B.: Lithium: its role in psychiatric research and treatment, New York, 1973, Plenum Press.
31. Baldessarini, R. J., and Lipinski, J. F.: Lithium salts: 1970-1975, Ann. Intern. Med. **83**:527-533, 1975.
32. APA Task Force: The current status of lithium therapy, Am. J. Psychiatry **132**:997-1001, 1975.
33. Davis, J. M.: Overview: maintenance therapy in psychiatry: II. Affective disorders, Am. J. Psychiatry **133**:1-13, 1976.
34. Prien, R. F., and Caffey, E. M., Jr. :Relationship between dosage and response to lithium prophylaxis in recurrent depression, Am. J. Psychiatry **133**:567-570, 1976.
35. Noyes, R., Jr., Dempsey, G. M., Blum, A., and Cavanaugh, G. L.: Lithium treatment of depression, Compr. Psychiatry **15**:187-193, 1974.
36. Rifkin, A., and others: Lithium carbonate in emotionally unstable character disorder, Arch. Gen. Psychiatry **27**:519-523, 1972.

# 27

# Medical-psychiatric drug interactions

**JERROLD G. BERNSTEIN**

The psychiatric consultant frequently encounters a variety of pharmacologically related problems. Although such problems are not unusual in the practice of office psychiatry, they tend to be more common and more complex when the psychiatrist is called as a consultant in the general hospital. In this setting, the psychiatrist is likely to see patients with a variety of complicated medical problems that may create greater vulnerability to the medical consequences of psychotropic drugs. Furthermore, the medical or surgical patient is likely to be taking a variety of medications that may interact with pharmacological agents prescribed by the psychiatrist. In addition to these kinds of pharmacological problems, the psychiatrist acting as a consultant in the medical setting is apt to come upon psychiatric signs and symptoms that may be directly related to other medications that the patient is receiving, not to mention, of course, that certain medical conditions may include psychiatric manifestations. This chapter will focus on some of these problems and their management.

## MEDICAL COMPLICATIONS AND SIDE EFFECTS OF PSYCHOTROPIC MEDICATIONS

In addition to producing certain desired pharmacological effects, all medications produce some unwanted effects, commonly referred to as side effects. These unwanted effects may be directly related to the specific pharmacology of the drug under consideration or may not be pharmacologically specific—in which case they are considered idiosyncratic. While these latter effects usually are not predictable and tend to be relatively infrequent, they may nevertheless be very disturbing. An example of an idiosyncratic reaction to a psychotropic drug would be the development of cholestatic jaundice in a patient receiving chlorpromazine. In addition to side effects, psychotropic drugs may exert pharmacological effects that interact with a coexisting medical problem.[1-3]

In order to discuss psychotropic drug side effects, it is necessary to have a clear understanding of the classification of psychotropic drugs. For practical purposes, psychotropic drugs may be divided into four separate groups.

1. *Antianxiety drugs* (sedatives) (minor tranquilizers)
2. *Antipsychotic drugs* (neuroleptics) (major tranquilizers)
3. *Antidepressant drugs*
4. *Mood-stabilizing drugs*

This classification of psychotropic drugs is shown in greater detail along with specific representatives of each group in Table 26-1, p. 452.

**Antianxiety drugs (minor tranquilizers)**

Since anxiety is perhaps a ubiquitous aspect of human existence, a variety of drugs have been used in attempting to alleviate it. Generally, this group of psychotropic agents includes sedative-type drugs such as the barbiturates, the propanediols (for example, meprobamate), and the benzodiazepines (for example, chlordiazepoxide). Generally speaking, these drugs exert a central nervous system depressant effect and excessive sedation is the most frequently encountered unwanted effect.[4] Indeed, in certain susceptible individuals even small doses of these drugs may produce respiratory depression. Although sedative drugs such as alcohol and barbiturates are widely recognized as producing addiction, addiction to meprobamate and the benzodiazepine compounds is less widely known. It is important for the clinician to be aware of the fact that meprobamate and the benzodiazepine drugs such as chlordiazepoxide, chlorazepate, diazepam, and oxazepam may produce addiction.[5] Indeed, these drugs are capable of producing both tolerance and physical dependence, marked by the development of a withdrawal syndrome when their use is discontinued after a prolonged period of moderate to high dose drug intake. The withdrawal syndrome associated with benzodiazepines is identical to the withdrawal syndrome associated with barbiturates.[6] The parameters and treatment of sedative addiction are discussed more fully in Chapter 3.

It is important to understand that a variety of drugs may produce central nervous system depression and may interact in an additive fashion when used together in the same patient. Such drug interactions may simply be uncomfortable or unpleasant to the patient. An example of this is the excessive drowsiness in a patient receiving a hypnotic agent at bedtime and an antianxiety drug during the day. On the other hand, such additive effects may have more serious consequences, including the possible development of addiction or fatal respiratory depression when a patient takes multiple central nervous system (CNS) depressant drugs simultaneously, even though the dose of each individual drug may be rather modest.

Drugs in groups 1, 2, and 3, as well as antihistamines and a variety of other medications, may exert additive sedative effects, and therefore their combination may produce unexpected and unwanted drowsiness or sedation. Essentially, all drugs in group 1 may produce tolerance and physical dependence. Furthermore, drugs in group 1 produce cross-tolerance within the group so that small doses of several different group 1 drugs may combine to produce an addictive problem. Drugs in groups 2, 3, and 4 do not produce tolerance or physical dependence, nor do they participate with group 1 drugs in the phenomenon of cross-tolerance. Lithium carbonate (group 4) does not produce sedation or drowsiness under normal circumstances, although lithium will of course calm an excited manic patient, and CNS depression may occur when toxic blood levels of lithium are achieved.

### Antipsychotic drugs (major tranquilizers)

The antipsychotic drugs exert specific pharmacological effects that reduce or obliterate many of the symptoms of psychotic illness,[7] as discussed in Chapter 26. As shown in Table 26-1, the antipsychotic drugs may be divided into five separate chemical groups: phenothiazine, thioxanthene, butyrophenone, dihydroindolone, and dibenzoxazepine. The pharmacological characteristics of the various antipsychotic drugs can be predicted by knowing to which chemical group they belong. All antipsychotic drugs exert some anticholinergic effect.[1] This effect is based on the ability of these compounds to block the action of acetylcholine at receptor sites in the body. This may also be called parasympatholytic effect because it represents a blockade of the parasympathetic section of the autonomic nervous system. Anticholinergic effects are most commonly manifested physiologically by the development of dry mouth, blurred vision, urinary retention, constipation, and tachycardia in patients receiving these drugs. Among the antipsychotic drugs, thioridazine (Mellaril) is the most potent anticholinergic agent. Chlorpromazine (Thorazine) is also a very potent anticholinergic agent. Trifluoperazine (Stelazine), fluphenazine (Prolixin), and thiothixene (Navane) are relatively weak in their anticholinergic effects. Haloperidol (Haldol) is the least potent anticholinergic agent among the antipsychotic drugs. Those antipsychotic drugs that produce more pronounced anticholinergic effects are less likely to produce extrapyramidal (parkinsonian) symptoms.[8]

In addition to the physiological effects of cholinergic blockade, there also may be behavioral consequences of this effect. Specifically, drugs with strong anticholinergic effects may produce a toxic psychosis. Such an effect has been recognized for more than a century in certain susceptible individuals receiving atropine or in patients taking overdoses of atropine-like drugs. Paradoxically, existing psychotic symptoms in some patients may worsen when these patients are given antipsychotic drugs, particularly those with strong anticholinergic effects.

Furthermore, it is important to realize that all of the antiparkinsonian medications such as benztropine (Cogentin), biperiden (Akineton), and trihexyphenidyl (Artane) produce strong anticholinergic effects.[2] Therefore, a patient receiving antipsychotic medication along with antiparkinsonian medication can be expected to have an additive anticholinergic effect and may complain of excessive dryness of the mouth, blurred vision, urinary retention, constipation, or tachycardia. In addition to the anticholinergic effects of antipsychotic and antiparkinsonian medications, all of the tricyclic antidepressant drugs such as imipramine (Tofranil) and amitriptyline (Elavil) produce pronounced anticholinergic effects and may produce an additive effect when given along with antipsychotic medications so that patients may develop excessive symptoms of parasympathetic blockade. In fact, the anticholinergic actions of the tricyclic antidepressant drugs may be therapeutically beneficial in allowing one to avoid the administration of antiparkinsonian medications when patients are receiving tricyclic antidepressants along with antipsychotic medication.

It is often useful to perform a physostigmine test on a patient who develops psychotic symptoms while receiving anticholinergic medication.[9] In such a situation—a patient developing behavioral signs suggestive of an atropine-like (anticholinergic) psychosis—physostigmine may be administered intravenously, preferably by diluting 1 mg of physostigmine to a total volume of 10 ml with saline and slowly injecting the solution over 2 to 5 minutes. If this dosage is adequate, the patient will develop peripheral signs of parasympathetic stimulation such as increased salivation, abdominal cramping, or the desire to urinate or defecate. When these signs develop following administration of physostigmine, if the previously observed mental symptoms have been related to anticholinergic excess, the mental symptoms should clear partially or completely within a few minutes of the intravenous injection. If symptoms do not clear and the patient does not develop pronounced signs of peripheral parasympathetic stimulation, the same dose of physostigmine may be repeated in 15 to 20 minutes. If physiological signs of parasympathetic stimulation occur and there are no behavioral changes, the physostigmine test should be considered negative; that is, the behavioral effects are not related to anticholinergic toxicity. A positive physostigmine test is manifested by both development of physiological symptoms and improvement in the mental symptoms.

Elderly patients, particularly those with even minor degrees of organic brain disease, may be particularly sensitive to the behavioral manifestations of anticholinergic drugs.[1,2] Therefore, in such patients it is generally preferable, when using antipsychotic medication, to choose those agents with the weakest anticholinergic effect. Furthermore in such patients, the use of antiparkinsonian medication should be avoided if at all possible, again because of the risk of behavioral toxicity. Antiparkinsonian medications should never be used prophylactically along with antipsychotic drugs in elderly patients. If such patients develop extrapyramidal symptoms, it is preferable to administer individual doses of diphenhydramine (Benadryl), generally 25 to 50 mg orally, intramuscularly or intravenously. If extrapyramidal symptoms persist in an individual who has been shown to be particularly sensitive to the behavioral effects of antiparkinsonian medication, amantadine (Symmetrel) may be the antiparkinsonian medication of choice. Amantadine appears to have minimal anticholinergic effect and to exert its antiparkinsonian effect largely through a central dopaminergic mechanism.[10] Generally, 100 mg of amantadine once or twice daily will provide clinical benefit for drug-induced extrapyramidal reactions.

Some patients may be extremely intolerant to the physiological manifestations of cholinergic blockade by antipsychotic drugs. Often the symptoms of blurred vision, dry mouth, urinary retention, and constipation are very annoying and may be minimized by choosing an antipsychotic agent of lesser anticholinergic potency. On the other hand, in an individual who is responding well to a particular antipsychotic drug, but who complains of excessive anticholinergic symptoms, a peripherally acting cholinergic stimulant may be a useful adjunct to therapy.[11] Continued complaints of blurred vision may be minimized by the use of 1% pilocarpine eye drops two or three times daily. Ocular symptoms related to psychotropic drugs may, at times, be managed by arranging for ophthamologic consultation and the prescription of corrective lenses. Persistent dryness of the mouth may be both annoying and disadvantageous from the standpoint of dental health; indeed, some individuals believe that reduced salivary flow, which may be produced as an anticholinergic manifestation of a variety of psychotropic medications, may predispose individuals to a greater incidence of oral pathology—both dental caries and disruption of the integrity of the gums and oral mucosa. Oral dryness, as induced by psychotropic agents, may be improved by prescribing 1% pilocarpine solution and recommending that patients use approximately 1 teaspoonful of this solution to rinse the mouth several times daily. Persistent constipation and difficulty in urinating, in association with psychotropic drugs, may improve in response to the oral administration of bethanechol (Urecholine), generally in a dose of 10 to 25 mg three or four times daily.[11] Certainly, the prescription of any of these cholinergic agents should follow only after thorough evaluation of the patient to rule out any organic causes for the symptoms. Furthermore, potential complications of cholinergic stimulant drugs must be considered before they are prescribed.

Individuals with cardiac disease may be particularly sensitive to the anticholinergic action of antipsychotic drugs because this effect is manifested by vagal blockade and increased heart rate.[1] The heart rate increase generally presents as sinus tachycardia related to vagal blockade. Anticholinergic agents, however, may effect impulse conduction within the myocardium and thereby worsen an already existing atrial or ventricular arrhythmia. The arrhythmogenic potential of antipsychotic drugs in most patients is relatively minimal as compared with the greater arrhythmogenic potential of tricyclic antidepressant drugs to be discussed later in this chapter.

The beneficial effects of antipsychotic drugs are generally correlated with their ability to produce blockade of catecholamines, specifically, dopamine in the brain.[7] In addition, antipsychotic drugs also tend to produce peripheral alpha adrenergic blockade. Antipsychotic drugs vary in their dopamine blocking potency. They also vary in their ability to produce peripheral alpha adrenergic blockade.[1,7,12] The central and peripheral adrenergic blocking effects of these drugs are generally not parallel. For example, haloperidol (Haldol) is the most potent dopamine blocking agent but it produces the least amount of peripheral alpha adrenergic blockade among the antipsychotic drugs.[12]

The major clinical concern with respect to alpha-adrenergic blocking actions of the antipsychotic drugs is that this is the mechanism by which these agents produce hypotensive reactions.[1] Blockade of adrenergic receptors in peripheral vascular beds leads to vasodilation, a fall in peripheral resistance within the circulatory system and a consequent fall in blood pressure. This hypotensive effect tends to be most pronounced when the patient moves from a sitting or a reclining position to a standing position. Patients with cardiovascular disease and elderly patients, in general, are most sensitive to this hypotensive effect. In some individuals it is of relatively minor consequence and can be detected only by measurement of the blood pressure. On the other hand, many individuals have a marked hypotensive response that may be associated with fainting or falling, and, indeed, such individuals may sustain serious physical injuries. Among the antipsychotic drugs, chlorpromazine (Thorazine) has the most pronounced hypotensive effect. Thioridazine (Mellaril) is fairly close to chlorpromazine in hypotensive potency. The piperazine phenothiazines such as trifluoperazine (Stelazine) and the piperazine thioxanthene derivatives such as thiothixene (Navane) are far less potent in their alpha-adrenergic antagonism and hypotensive effect. Of the antipsychotic agents Haloperidol (Haldol) is least likely to produce hypotensive reactions even when used in very large therapeutic doses by oral or parenteral administration.

Peripheral adrenergic blockade produced by antipsychotic drugs may become more problematic in patients receiving other therapeutic agents with adrenergic blocking effects. Patients with peripheral vascular disease may be treated with a variety of vasodilator drugs including alpha adrenergic blocking agents such as phenoxybenzamine (Dibenzyline) and direct acting vasodilator agents such as isoxsuprine (Vasodilan). Coronary vasodilators such as isosorbide (Isordil) and nitroglycerin may also produce vasodilation of other vascular beds. Cerebral vasodilator drugs such as the ergot-containing agent Hydergine may also produce some generalized vasodilation. Any of these vasodilator or adrenergic blocking drugs may produce an additive effect when used along with antipsychotic drugs with hypotensive potential. This is of particular importance in that the patient may develop excessive dizziness or fainting when one of these vasodilator agents is combined with antipsychotic treatment. Furthermore, in some situations, such as the elderly confused individual who is being treated with an agent such as Hydergine and who then receives a phenothiazine, the clinical circumstances may worsen, with the development of both hypotension and possibly decreased mental function due to decreased cerebral blood flow in the presence of hypotension.

Beta-adrenergic blocking drugs such as propranolol (Inderal) have become very important therapeutic agents for a variety of indications including the cardiac arrhythmias, angina pectoris, hypertension, and anxiety. A patient receiving full therapeutic doses of propranolol will have fairly complete beta-adrenergic blockade.[13] If such a patient now is given an antipsychotic agent with potent alpha-adrenergic blocking effect, complications may arise from the combined peripheral adrenergic blockade. Such a patient may develop a hypotensive reaction of greater magnitude than if he had received either agent individually. Furthermore, because of both alpha-adrenergic and beta-adrenergic blockade, this patient will be less responsive to the usual adrenergic stimulant drugs used in the treatment of profound hypotension. Generally patients developing hypotensive reactions to therapeutic doses of antipsychotic agents are best managed by allowing them to lie flat and await eventual disappearance of the offending medication's effect, which generally occurs within an hour or two. Patients developing more profound hypotensive reactions to antipsychotic medication either alone or in combination with other hypotensive drugs may require more intensive supportive treatment, including the administration of intravenous saline or other fluid replacement. Less commonly, patients having profound hypotensive reactions to antipsychotic agents alone or in combination with other drugs or to psychotropic drugs taken in overdose attempts may require intravenous infusion of pressor agents in order to counteract the fall in blood pressure. Generally, the pressor agent of choice in such a circumstance is phenylephrine (Neo-Synephrine). This agent is generally preferred because it is a direct acting alpha-adrenergic stimulant that produces primarily a vasoconstrictor effect with relatively little inotropic or chronotropic effect. Infusion of isoproterenol (Isuprel) or dopamine would be contraindicated as treatment for antipsychotic drug–induced hypotension, since these agents produce beta-adrenergic stimulation, peripheral vasodilation, and a more intense cardiostimulatory effect than would be desired.

Some antipsychotic drugs may produce abnormalities in the electrocardiogram.[14] The primary electrocardiographic changes seen in association with antipsychotic drugs include prolongation of the QT interval, ST segment changes, and lowering, flattening, and notching of T waves. It is possible to confuse these drug-induced repolarization changes with electrocardiographic changes that may occur in the presence of coronary heart disease. There is no clear evidence, on the other hand, that antipsychotic agents produce myocardial damage. Electrocardiographic changes are most commonly associated with thioridazine (Mellaril) and with chlorpromazine (Thorazine). Electrocardiographic changes are less likely to occur with piperazine phenothiazines and have not been documented to occur with either thiothixene or haloperidol.

## Antidepressant drugs

The clinically useful antidepressant drugs are divided into two subcategories, the tricyclic drugs and the monoamine oxidase inhibitors. Both groups of antidepressants appear to exert their beneficial effect by increasing the availability of catecholamine substances such as norepinephrine at synaptic endings in the brain.[1] Greater availability or improved action of this neurotransmitter substance in the brain presumably counteracts what may be a pathophysiological substrate of certain clinical varieties of depression. The tricyclic drugs act by blocking nerve reuptake of norepinephrine, thus increasing its availability, while the monoamine oxidase inhibitors block one of the pathways for metabolic breakdown of norepinephrine, the enzyme monoamine oxidase. Tricyclic antidepressants exert an adrenergic effect in the brain as well as at other sites in the body. Tricyclic antidepressants may produce or worsen existing cardiac arrhythmias in susceptible individuals, particularly in those with underlying coronary or valvular heart disease.[15] In such individuals, therapeutic doses of tricyclic drugs may produce atrial or ventricular premature beats or may increase the frequency of such abnormal beats if they are present prior to drug therapy. The arrhythmogenic effect of these drugs appears to be related to two mechanisms, adrenergic action and anticholinergic effect.[15] Tricyclic drugs that block the reuptake of norepinephrine in brain tissue exert a similar effect in the peripheral autonomic nervous system, the myocardium, and other sites throughout the body. It would appear that the ability of tricyclic drugs to inhibit norepinephrine reuptake would give rise to increased norepinephrine in the myocardium and thereby increased myocardial irritability, as manifested clinically by atrial and ventricular arrhythmias.

Tricyclic antidepressants are potent anticholinergic agents.[1] The physiological and behavioral manifestations of cholinergic blockade have been discussed in detail previously in this chapter. Tricyclic drugs are among the most potent anticholinergic agents prescribed clinically. The anticholinergic effects of these compounds are associated with blurred vision, dry mouth, urinary retention, constipation, and tachycardia.[1] The anticholinergic effect of tricyclic drugs appears to be the major mechanism of their ability to produce sinus tachycardia. Furthermore, this anticholinergic effect appears to interact with the adrenergic effect previously described, in the production or worsening of cardiac arrhythmia. The anticholinergic potency of the tricyclic antidepressant drugs varies considerably. Doxepin (Sinequan) and desipramine (Norpramin) produce the least pronounced anticholinergic effect and are least likely to be arrhythmogenic among the tricyclic drugs. Amitriptyline (Elavil) produces the most pronounced anticholinergic effect and is also most likely to be arrhythmogenic among the tricyclic drugs. Imipramine (Tofranil) is intermediate between doxepin and amitriptyline from the standpoint of anticholinergic potency and tends to be somewhat less arrhythmogenic than amitriptyline.

Tricyclic antidepressant drugs may produce direct depression of the myocardium even in usual therapeutic doses, though this is more likely to occur in individuals with underlying heart disease.[15] Myocardial depression may be an important clinical manifestation associated with overdose of tricyclic antidepressant drugs. In some individuals, congestive heart failure may occur during treatment with tricyclic drugs; these agents have also been associated with worsening of preexisting heart failure in susceptible individuals.[15] Tricyclic antidepressant drugs may produce mild to moderate degrees of pedal edema in some patients. The mechanism of this edema is uncertain; it is considered by some to be a non-specific drug effect, while others think of it as a manifestation of mild congestive heart failure.

In most healthy individuals, the total daily dose of tricyclic antidepressant may be given as a single dose at bedtime. However, in patients with cardiac disease or in elderly individuals, this single daily dosage regimen should generally be avoided. In such patients, it is preferable to start tricyclic antidepressants using very small doses, 10 to 25 mg two or three times daily, with periodic monitoring of blood pressure, pulse, and electrocardiogram. If no untoward effects occur, the dosage of tricyclic drugs can be gradually increased to whatever dosage level is necessary to provide a beneficial therapeutic effect. Generally, one should continue to administer that medication on a long-term basis in divided doses throughout the day, since this kind of regimen would reduce the likelihood of a major adrenergic or anticholinergic response occurring following a large single dose of medication. In a patient with cardiovascular disease, generally doxepin (Sinequan) or desipramine (Norpramin) would be the preferable agent among tricyclic drugs from the standpoint of lesser likelihood of cardiac complications.

The tricyclic antidepressants may produce postural hypotension. The mechanism of this effect is uncertain.[15] It is generally believed to be related to peripheral vasodilation, with or without an associated myocardial depression. Tricyclic antidepressants do not have pronounced adrenergic blocking effects, and it is not likely that adrenergic blockade explains their ability to produce postural hypotension.

All tricyclic antidepressant drugs, though they vary somewhat in efficacy and side effects, appear to work by a similar mechanism of blocking nerve reuptake of norepinephrine. The ability of these agents to block the reuptake of norepinephrine is of importance in that it is by this mechanism that these agents antagonize the hypotensive action of guanethidine (Ismelin) and clonidine (Catapres).[15,16] Both of these antihypertensive agents are taken up in nerve endings by a process similar to that responsible for nerve uptake of norepinephrine. These drugs exert their blood pressure–lowering effects by inhibiting release of norepinephrine at nerve endings.

In a patient whose hypertension is being treated by either guanethidine or clonidine, the addition of a tricyclic antidepressant to the regimen will block further nerve uptake of the antihypertensive agent and thereby give rise to progressive elevation in blood pressure.[15,16] The physician prescribing an antihypertensive drug who is unfamiliar with this interaction or unaware that the patient is receiving a tricyclic agent may progressively increase the dose of antihypertensive agent in order to attempt to control blood pressure. If the tricyclic drug is withdrawn, the patient is now subjected to an excessive dose of antihypertensive medication in the absence of tricyclic drug effect and, therefore, the blood pressure may dramatically fall, quite possibly even to shock levels. Tricyclic antidepressants should never be used in conjunction with guanethidine or clonidine because of this potentially dangerous interaction. There is no evidence to demonstrate tricyclic antidepressant drug interference with the efficacy of other antihypertensive medications, such as methyldopa (Aldomet), hydralazine (Apresoline), or thiazide diuretics.[15]

Monoamine oxidase inhibitor drugs also play an important role in the treatment of depression. These agents appear to produce their beneficial effect by interfering with one of the enzymes important in the metabolic breakdown of norepinephrine, thereby increasing the availability of norepinephrine in the brain. The major disadvantage of monoamine oxidase inhibitor antidepressants is that they may produce serious hypertensive reactions.[17,18] These hypertensive reactions appear to develop only when patients taking these medications consume tyramine-rich foods or other medications containing phenylethylamine compounds.[18] It is, therefore, of utmost importance when prescribing monoamine oxidase inhibitor drugs, such as phenelzine (Nardil) or tranylcypromine (Parnate), to provide patients with detailed instructions regarding this potential interaction. The most effective way of providing adequate information to patients is to present them with a printed or typewritten sheet of instructions along with the prescription for the monoamine oxidase inhibitors. The printed instructions should describe, in some detail, the kinds of adverse reactions that may be experienced. It also should clearly state that patients should avoid eating or drinking the following tyramine-rich foods:

1. Fermented cheeses, specifically cheddar and other strong cheeses
2. Picked herring, sardines, and anchovies
3. Chicken livers
4. Canned or processed meats
5. Pods of broad beans
6. Canned figs
7. Yeast extract
8. Wine and beer

Patients taking monoamine oxidase inhibitors should limit their intake of coffee to 2 cups per day; if they drink large quantities of coffee, they should use decaffeinated coffee. Alcoholic beverages should generally be avoided in combination with monoamine oxidase antidepressants. However, a single cocktail or 2 to 3 ounces of white wine may occasionally be consumed. Small quantities, not exceeding two ounces per day, of sour cream, yogurt, cottage cheese, American cheese, mild Swiss cheese, or chocolate may be consumed while a patient is receiving monoamine oxidase inhibitors; however, larger quantities of these foods may provoke a hypertensive reaction.

Patients taking a monoamine oxidase inhibitor antidepressant should be told specifically to avoid the use of any nose drops, cold remedies, nasal decongestants, cough syrups, diet pills, or any other stimulant drugs. It is generally the best policy, when prescribing these potent antidepressant agents, to discuss in detail with the patient the restrictions that these therapeutic agents impose on them. Furthermore, it is important in prescribing these medications to be readily available to patients should questions arise. It is generally advisable to tell patients that if any medical problem develops during the use of monoamine oxidase inhibitor antidepressants, they should consult the prescribing physician before contacting any other physician or receiving other medical care so that the prescribing physician can inform other health-care providers of potential drug interactions involving monoamine oxidase inhibitor antidepressants. Patients should also be advised to contact the prescribing physician if they believe that they have eaten any of the prohibited foods or consumed any of the contraindicated medications. Generally, small quantities of these foods or medications will not provoke a serious reaction and the physician's role may simply be to provide the patient with reassurance. The hypertensive reactions that may occur in conjunction with monoamine oxidase inhibitors frequently are relatively mild—that is, systolic blood pressure elevations of only 30 mm or less. They are often associated with a sensation of jitteriness or the development of a headache. On the other hand, more serious hypertensive reactions may occur and some individuals may have a cerebrovascular accident in association with a severe hypertensive crisis.[1,18] More severe hypertensive reactions may occur and require treatment. Generally, mild sedation and rest combined with medical observation are the only treatment required if a patient develops an adverse reaction while receiving a monoamine oxidase inhibitor. More significant blood pressure elevations in association with monoamine oxidase inhibitor antidepressants may be treated with an alpha-adrenergic blocking drug such as phentolamine (Regitine) or chlorpromazine (Thorazine). Occasionally, the beta-adrenergic blocking agent propranolol (Inderal) may be beneficial in the treatment of a monoamine oxidase inhibitor–associated hypertensive reactions. If patients are chosen carefully, antidepressant drugs of the monoamine oxidase inhibitor type may be used safely and efficaciously. One virtue of this group of antidepressant drugs is that they do not produce the significant anticholinergic effects that are produced by the tricyclic antidepressants.

The most commonly observed adverse effect of monoamine oxidase inhibitor antidepressants is the development of mild to moderate degrees of postural hypotension.[18] Most patients taking these medications will show a 10 to 25 mm fall in systolic blood pressure during treatment. This postural hypotension may produce mild degrees of dizziness; however, more commonly, it goes unnoticed except for sphygmomanometric measurement. Indeed, the hypotensive side effect of monoamine oxidase inhibitor drugs has been used to therapeutic advantage in hypertensive patients. One monoamine oxidase inhibitor drug, pargyline (Eutonyl), has been marketed primarily as an antihypertensive agent.[19] Indeed, pargyline is quite effective in lowering blood pressure in hypertensive patients. One advantageous side effect of pargyline as an antihypertensive agent is the fact that it is also capable of elevating mood in depressed patients. Patients presenting with both hypertension and depression may be uniquely benefited by the use of pargyline because of its combined antihypertensive and antidepressant action. In such patients it is usually advisable to initiate treatment of the hypertension with a thiazide diuretic such as chlorothiazide (Diuril) in a dose of 500 mg once or twice daily. Subsequently, pargyline may be added along with the thiazide diuretic, generally starting pargyline in a dose of 10 mg daily and gradually increasing the dose in increments of 10 mg daily at weekly intervals until satisfactory blood pressure control is achieved.[19] Most patients treated with this regimen will demonstrate significant reduction in both systolic and diastolic blood pressure along with significant improvement in their depression in the absence of major drug-induced side effects. It is, of course, important in prescribing pargyline as well as all other monoamine oxidase inhibitor drugs, to provide thorough instructions to patients and to present them with a printed list of instructions including foods and medications to avoid. Pargyline, like all other monoamine oxidase inhibitors, may precipitate a hypertensive crisis when used in conjunction with tyramine-rich foods or phenylethyl amine derivatives.

Because of the adrenergic effects produced by monoamine oxidase inhibition, antidepressant drugs of this category may exert an arrhythmogenic effect, particularly in the presence of underlying coronary or valvular heart disease. In the absence, however, of tyramine-rich foods or phenylethyl amine–containing medications, monoamine oxidase inhibitors appear to be less arrhythmogenic than tricyclic antidepressants. This difference in arrhythmogenic potential may well be explained by the relative absence of anticholinergic effect among the monoamine oxidase inhibitor antidepressants. In addition to the interactions between phenylethyl amine compounds and monoamine oxidase inhibitors, it is also important to realize that monoamine oxidase inhibitors may potentiate the sedative and central nervous system depressant effects of alcohol, narcotics, and other sedative drugs.[4] Levodopa, used in the treatment of parkinsonism, if given to a patient receiving monoamine oxidase inhibitors, will produce a hypertensive reaction. The respiratory depressant and apneic effects of succinylcholine are potentiated by monoamine oxidase inhibitors. The hypoglycemic effects of insulin and oral hypoglycemic agents tend to be potentiated and prolonged by monoamine oxidase inhibitors.

Reserpine should never be given to patients receiving monoamine oxidase inhibitors since when reserpine is combined with these agents, excitement, agitation, and hypertension are likely to occur. Other hypotensive agents such as guanethidine and clonidine may produce hypertensive reactions in the presence of monoamine oxidase inhibitors. There is controversy regarding the safety of coadministration of tricyclic antidepressants and monoamine oxidase antidepressants. Some investigators believe that monoamine oxidase inhibitors and tricyclic antidepressants may be used together with increased beneficial effects and without undue risk; however, a hypertensive reaction is possible.[20] If the combination is used therapeutically, caution should prevail and the physician should be aware of their potentially dangerous interaction.

**Mood-stabilizing drug: lithium carbonate**

Lithium carbonate is a valuable addition to the pharmacological armamentarium of the psychiatrist. This drug is useful not only in controlling acute manic psychoses, but also in the prophylaxis of recurring episodes of mania.[21] Lithium may also exert a beneficial effect in conjunction with antidepressant drugs in the treatment of depression and lithium is useful alone or in combination with antidepressants in the prophylaxis of recurring bouts of depression. Although not attempting to exhaustively discuss the adverse effects of lithium, this chapter will focus on some medical aspects of this important therapeutic agent.

In some patients, lithium may produce impairment of thyroid function with the development of goiter in the presence of normal thyroid function tests.[22] Lithium carbonate may also be associated with the development of hypothyroidism with or without the presence of clinically detectable goiter. Lithium appears to interfere with the iodine-trapping mechanism of the thyroid gland as well as with the synthesis and release of thyroid hormone within the thyroid gland. Clinically significant abnormalities of thyroid function or structure are rarely encountered with the therapeutic use of lithium carbonate.[22] If at all possible it is generally advisable to obtain baseline measurements of T3 and T4 as well as thyroid-stimulating hormone (TSH) prior to instituting lithium carbonate treatment. In the event that there is reason to suspect thyroid abnormalities in association with lithium treatment, these tests may then be repeated. Clinically significant lithium interference with thyroid gland function will most often be marked by the presence of elevated serum TSH levels generally in the presence of normal T3 and T4 measurements. Lithium carbonate may, in some patients, produce decreased glucose tolerance.[22] Though there is no clear-cut evidence to support a diabetogenic effect of lithium, this possibility should be kept in mind. In a diabetic patient being maintained on lithium carbonate whose diabetic regulation becomes more difficult, it may be worth considering the question and perhaps offering the patient a trial period without lithium treatment.

Polydipsia and polyuria are frequently associated with lithium treatment. Most often these effects are transient and disappear as the patient becomes stabilized on lithium carbonate.[22] These effects may also occur in the presence of excessive serum lithium concentrations. Both polydipsia and polyuria generally disappear when lithium carbonate treatment is stopped and they may or may not reappear after reinstituting lithium therapy. More severe disturbances of fluid balance may occur in rare individuals taking lithium carbonate with the development of a diabetes insipidus–like syndrome. This syndrome is usually reversible with the discontinuance of lithium. However, in some individuals who have benefited significantly from lithium therapy, it may be desirable to continue treatment with lithium. In such cases, thiazide diuretics, such as chlorothiazide in doses of 500 to 1000 mg per day, may exert a paradoxical antidiuretic effect with the virtual disappearance of the diabetes insipidus–like syndrome.

Some patients, particularly in association with persistent excessively high serum lithium levels, may develop impaired renal function while receiving lithium carbonate. This may be associated with increased serum creatinine and an interference with renal tubular function. The reversibility of this latter syndrome is uncertain at the present time because it is so rare that clinical experience in its management is limited.[22]

It is of critical importance to measure blood urea nitrogen and/or serum creatinine prior to instituting therapy with lithium. Furthermore, any significant change in serum lithium concentration, thirst, or urinary output, in the presence of stable lithium dosage, should guide the physician in requesting further determinations of renal function. Patients being treated with lithium carbonate should be cautioned against restricting their salt intake and they should be advised to eat a normal amount of salt in their diet.[22] Since salt restriction will lead to excessive lithium retention and, therefore, excessive serum concentration of lithium, patients should be advised not to undertake any kind of special diet while taking lithium without consulting the prescribing physician. Diuretic drugs, generally, should not be used in conjunction with lithium for the same reason; they too may cause excessive renal reabsorption of lithium and therefore increased serum lithium levels. If an individual taking lithium requires concurrent treatment with thiazide or other diuretic agents, serum lithium should be monitored carefully and more frequently than would normally be done. Furthermore, patients taking diuretics along with lithium should have frequent measurements of serum potassium as well, since hypokalemia may increase the likelihood of lithium toxicity, particularly from the standpoint of cardiotoxicity of lithium. Lithium therapy may be associated with weight gains of 5 to 10 pounds, much of which appears to be secondary to fluid retention. This weight gain and fluid retention may be minimized by the cautious use of diuretics. Lithium-related fluid retention may be safely managed by the use of chlorothiazide in a dose of 500 mg every other day with periodic measurement of both serum potassium and serum lithium levels.

Lithium carbonate treatment may be associated with leukocytosis. White blood cell counts in the neighborhood of 11,000 to 16,000 per cubic millimeter are frequently observed during the course of lithium treatment.[22] The significance of this finding is not known nor can any pathological significance be attached to this finding. There is no evidence of abnormality of blood-cell morphology or of the hematopoietic system in association with lithium treatment.

Minor electrocardiographic changes may be seen in the presence of lithium treatment. These changes primarily consist of T wave flattening and inversion as well as widening of the QRS complex.[22] These electrocardiographic changes associated with lithium tend to resemble electrocardiographic changes associated with hypokalemia. The lithium-induced changes are reversible and disappear when lithium therapy is stopped. There is no association between these electrocardiographic changes and other evidence of myocardial damage. Since these electrocardiographic changes may also resemble those of coronary heart disease, and because it is possible to produce cardiac arrhythmias if toxic levels of lithium are reached, it is generally advisable to obtain a baseline electrocardiogram prior to instituting lithium therapy so that in case electrocardiographic changes develop during the course of treatment with lithium, a pretreatment electrocardiogram will be available for comparison.

## NONPSYCHIATRIC MEDICATIONS WITH BEHAVIORAL EFFECTS

In addition to the inconvenient and often unpleasant or dangerous medical and psychiatric sequelae of psychotropic medications, the psychiatric consultant in the general hospital setting is likely to encounter a variety of unwanted behavioral effects produced by nonpsychotropic medications that patients are receiving. Many reports of such reactions appear in medical literature and it is impossible to cover exhaustively each drug that has been implicated. Furthermore, it would be a disservice to report here uncertain or inadequately documented adverse reactions. This discussion will focus on a number of well-documented unwanted behavioral complications of medications in common clinical use.

## Anticholinergic agents

In addition to the pronounced anticholinergic effects of most psychotropic drugs that have been discussed previously in this chapter, a variety of medications are used specifically because of the desire to achieve cholinergic blockade. Atropine and a variety of other anticholinergic medications are used in the treatment of peptic ulcer disease because of their ability to reduce gastrointestinal tract secretions and motility. These drugs may have pronounced central nervous system effects and may produce a toxic psychosis or delirium.[2,3] Atropine and scopolamine are most notorious in this respect. It is also important to realize that the latter drug is frequently a component of a variety of over-the-counter tranquilizers and sleep remedies.[3] Furthermore, anticholinergic drugs, most notably atropine, are widely used in the treatment of patients who develop bradycardia following myocardial infarction. A good general rule to follow in minimizing behavioral toxicity of anticholinergic drugs is to advise the use of anticholinergic agents that do not cross the blood-brain barrier. Quaternary ammonium compounds are unable to enter the brain when administered to patients orally or parenterally. The drug propantheline (Pro-Banthine) is a potent anticholinergic agent that may be used in the treatment of gastrointestinal disorders without the risk of atropine-like psychosis because of its inability to enter the brain. Patients requiring anticholinergic agents for the treatment of bradycardia may also benefit from propantheline in doses of 15 to 30 mg given intramuscularly or orally. Propantheline exerts a significant anticholinergic effect that will benefit the bradycardia but avoid the toxic delirium often so characteristic of atropine.

## Cardiovascular drugs

**Digitalis.** Digitalis and its glycosides may produce a variety of unwanted psychiatric symptoms. Patients may develop headache, visual disturbance, trigeminal nerve pain, weakness, apathy, anorexia, nausea, and vomiting. Digitalis may also produce hallucinations, depression, and delirium.[23] Elderly patients or those with underlying organic or functional psychiatric illness may be particularly susceptible to these unwanted effects.

**Antiarrhythmic drugs.** Quinidine, which is an effective antiarrhythmic agent, may produce a variety of unwanted mental effects. Confusion and delirium are most prominent among the behavioral complications of quinidine.[24] This useful agent may produce considerable disorientation in some patients either in therapeutic doses or when excessive doses have been prescribed. Often, early signs of an adverse reaction to quinidine include tinnitus, headache, nausea, visual disturbance, hearing disturbance, vertigo, apprehension, and excitement.[24] However, patients have been observed to show none of these premonitory signs of quinidine toxicity and present with confusion, disorientation, and delirium. If such reactions are suspected, quinidine should be carefully withdrawn and another antiarrhythmic drug should be substituted.

Unfortunately, substituting another antiarrhythmic drug for quinidine is not always easy since other antiarrhythmic drugs also have been associated with adverse behavioral effects. Procainamide may also produce a variety of unwanted mental effects including weakness, giddiness, depression, delirium, hallucination, and toxic psychosis.[24] Lidocaine is a local anesthetic agent that has proved very valuable in the management of ventricular arrhythmias when administered intramuscularly or intravenously. Lidocaine may produce central nervous system stimulation, restlessness, and tremor. Clonic convulsions may develop in some patients. Disorientation, confusion, and delirium have also been reported to occur with lidocaine.[24]

Propranolol (Inderal), a beta-adrenergic blocking agent, is clinically very useful in the treatment of cardiac arrhythmias, angina pectoris, hypertension, and anxiety. Although behavioral toxicity with propranolol is relatively uncommon, a small number of patients have been reported to develop clinical signs of depression while receiving propranolol.[13] Confusion, disorientation, hallucination, and toxic psychosis are known to occur rarely in individuals being treated with propranolol.[24] More common, though less problematic, behavioral complications of propranolol may include lassitude, insomnia, and nightmares.

### Antihypertensive drugs

Reserpine, which is still occasionally used in the treatment of hypertension, may produce a severe depressive reaction in many patients. Patients with a prior history of affective illness may be particularly sensitive to the depressogenic effect of reserpine and related *Rauwolfia* alkaloids. However, patients with no such prior history have been known to become severely depressed and attempt suicide while receiving this drug. Reserpine, in doses as small as 0.25 mg per day, may produce nightmares and depression.[25]

Methyldopa (Aldomet), perhaps the most widely prescribed antihypertensive agent in current use, appears to act by interfering with norepinephrine synthesis and nerve transmission. Methyldopa may produce a clouding of consciousness in some individuals as well as confusion and may be responsible for a significant incidence of depression in patients using it for treatment of hypertension.[26,27]

Thiazide diuretics, which are commonly used to reduce the accumulation of edema fluid and as adjuncts in the treatment of hypertension, may produce lassitude, and clinical symptoms resembling mild depression.[4] Similar symptoms are also occasionally seen with high-ceiling diuretics such as ethacrynic acid (Edecrin) and furosemide (Lasix). These symptoms often correlate with slight to moderate reductions in serum potassium that may be linked to more significant depletions of intracellular potassium. Development of lassitude and depressive symptomatology in association with diuretic use may be managed clinically by the addition of potassium supplementation. This is often found to be beneficial even when serum potassium is reduced only to borderline levels.

### Anticonvulsants

Phenytoin (Dilantin) is the most commonly used anticonvulsant drug and also finds a place in therapeutics as an antiarrhythmic agent, particularly in the management of digitalis toxicity. Phenytoin may produce a variety of behavioral effects including hyperactivity, silliness, confusion, dullness, drowsiness, and hallucinations.[3,24] These behavioral effects of phenytoin may be seen with normal therapeutic blood levels though they tend, more often, to be associated with toxic blood levels of this drug. Phenytoin, in addition to its direct behavioral toxicity, interferes with the intestinal absorption of a vitamin, folic acid. Folic acid deficiency, occurring either with improper diet or in association with phenytoin therapy, may be marked by a variety of behavioral symptoms including irritability, sleeplessness, forgetfulness, depression, and dementia.[28] Therapeutic administration of folic acid in a dose of 1 or 2 mg daily may be beneficial in alleviating the behavioral complications of folic acid deficiency and may minimize the likelihood of the development of these behavioral symptoms in association with therapeutic use of phenytoin.

**Hypoglycemic drugs**

Treatment of diabetes with oral hypoglycemic agents such as tolbutamide (Orinase) and phenformin (DBI) as well as parenterally administered insulin may produce significant degrees of hypoglycemia. Hypoglycemia may be associated with a variety of mental symptoms including anxiety and agitation.[3,4] Should these symptoms develop during the course of diabetes management, frequent blood glucose determinations are necessary in order to clarify the possible relationship between these symptoms and the presence of abnormally low blood glucose levels.

**Antibacterial agents**

Two antibacterial agents commonly used in the treatment of urinary-tract infections are of interest to the psychiatrist from the standpoint of their potential for neurological and psychiatric complications. Nalidixic acid (NegGram) may produce headaches, drowsiness, malaise, vertigo, and visual disturbances. In susceptible individuals, seizures may occur. Infrequently, mental clouding and confusion have been associated with the use of nalidixic acid.[4] Nitrofurantoin (Furadantin) may produce headaches, vertigo, drowsiness, muscular aches, and nystagmus. A flu-like syndrome occasionally occurs with nitrofurantoin that may also produce confusion or clouding of consciousness.[4]

The antituberculous agent isoniazid (INH) may produce psychiatric and neurological symptoms including muscular twitching, dizziness, ataxia, paresthesias, optic neuritis, stupor, and toxic encephalopathy. Patients receiving INH may develop euphoria, transient impairment of memory, impaired reality testing, loss of self-control, and florid psychosis.[3,4] This drug inhibits the enzyme diamine oxidase and may produce agitation in some individuals. Some investigative studies have suggested that INH may exert a useful antidepressant effect. Because of the ability of INH to interfere with the metabolism of phenytoin, patients receiving these drugs in combination may develop excessive sedation and incoordination because of their impaired ability to metabolize the anticonvulsant, phenytoin.[4]

**Analgesic and antiinflammatory drugs**

Two analgesics of interest to the psychiatrist are propoxypene (Darvon) and pentazocine (Talwin). Propoxyphene is very widely prescribed and closely similar chemically to the narcotic agent methadone. When propoxyphene is used over a prolonged period of time in relatively high doses, it may produce dependency and a true addiction.[4] Patients abusing large doses of propoxyphene orally or intravenously may develop hallucinations and acute psychotic reactions.[4] Clouding of consciousness is a not infrequent side effect experienced by patients using propoxyphene as an analgesic.

Pentazocine is technically classed as a nonnarcotic analgesic agent. This drug was believed to be non addicting when it was initially introduced for clinical use. Extensive experience with pentazocine when used either orally or intramuscularly has demonstrated that this agent is truly addicting and patients abusing it over a prolonged period of time may develop a withdrawal syndrome similar to that seen following narcotic drug withdrawal.[3,4] Some individuals develop an acute psychotic reaction when given pentazocine even in limited doses for short periods of time.[3,4] Patients may develop hallucinations, delusions, and a full-blown acute psychotic reaction following even a single dose of pentazocine. Although the available data are rather limited, there is reason to suspect that patients with prior psychotic illness may be more susceptible to the psychotogenic effect of pentazocine.

Indomethacin (Indocin) is an antiinflammatory drug that is used therapeutically primarily in the treatment of rheumatoid arthritis and related disorders. This drug not infrequently produces headache, dizziness, vertigo, light-headedness, and mental confusion. Indomethacin may produce depression and suicide attempts have been reported among patients taking this drug.[3,4] Indomethacin is also capable of producing hallucinations and may produce a psychotic reaction in some patients. Indomethacin is an indole derivative, chemically somewhat similar to the naturally occurring neurotransmitter substance, serotonin. There is reason to suspect that patients with underlying affective illness or prior histories of psychotic illness may be more susceptible to psychiatric complications of indomethacin therapy.

**Hormones**

Adrenal corticosteroid hormones are of interest to the psychiatrist from several standpoints. Adrenal insufficiency (Addison's disease) is in part manifested by psychiatric symptoms including inability to concentrate, drowsiness, restlessness, insomnia, irritability, and apprehension.[29] Treatment of such patients with adrenal corticosteroids produces rapid clearing of these psychiatric symptoms. Hyperfunction of the adrenal blands (Cushing's syndrome) is likewise associated with a variety of psychiatric symptoms including confusion, anxiety, insomnia, delusions, and hallucinations.[29] Indeed, many patients treated with adrenal corticosteroid hormones for a variety of medical conditions, develop iatrogenic Cushing's syndrome including the constellation of medical symptoms previously mentioned.[4,29] Affective disturbances are particularly prominent in the presence of hypercortisolism. It is interesting to note that depression is most often associated with spontaneously occurring Cushing's syndrome, while euphoria, at times progressing to mania, is more often seen as the result of administration of exogeneous corticosteroids.[30] There is a significant risk of suicide with both endogenous and exogenous hypercortisolism.

Hypothyroidism often includes behavioral manifestions among its clinical symptoms. Indeed, a syndrome called myxedema madness has been associated with inadequate availability of thyroid hormone. These behavioral symptoms generally disappear following adequate thyroid hormone replacement.[29] Hyperthyroidism, either spontaneously occurring or induced by administration of excessive thyroid hormone, may be associated with a variety of psychiatric symptoms. Hyperthyroidism is most often marked by agitation and anxiety; however, patients may present with psychosis and it may be difficult to differentiate psychotic reactions associated with hyperthyroidism from manic or schizophrenic illness.[31] Thyroid hormones are also of interest to the psychiatrist from the standpoint of the fact that triiodothyronine (T3, Cytomel) in doses of 25 $\mu$g daily along with tricyclic antidepressants may be of benefit in enhancing and facilitating the antidepressant response.[32]

Sex hormones may exert a variety of behavioral effects. Testosterone tends to facilitate aggressive behavior.[29] Recent data suggest that serum testosterone levels may be diminished in association with long-term methadone maintenance of narcotic addicts as well as long-term use of heroin by addicts. Estrogens tend to produce a sense of well-being and may improve the mood in some women, especially following menopause.[2] Estrogenic hormones are able to inhibit the enzyme monoamine oxidase and this may, in part, explain their mood-elevating effect. Progesterone derivatives tend to be depressogenic in some individuals.[2] Various oral contraceptives that combine estrogen and progesterone hormones may induce depression.[33] Depressive reactions to oral contraceptives are more pronounced with those agents that contain higher concentrations of progesterone-like hormones.[3]

## REFERENCES

1. Shader, R. I., and DiMascio, A.: Psychotropic drug side effects, Baltimore, 1970, The Williams & Wilkins Co.
2. Shader, R. I.: Psychiatric complications of medical drugs, New York, 1972, Raven Press.
3. Hollister, L. E.: Psychiatric syndromes due to drugs. In Meyer, L., and Peck, H. M., editors: Drug induced diseases, vol. 4, Amsterdam, 1972. Excerpta Medica, pp. 571-584.
4. Goodman, L. S., and Gilman, A., editors: The pharmacological basis of therapeutics, New York, 1975, MacMillan, Inc.
5. Essing, C. F.: Addiction to non-barbiturate sedative and tranquilizing drugs, Clin. Pharmacol. Ther. **5:**334-343, 1964.
6. Smith, D. E., and Wesson, D. R.: A new method for treatment of barbiturate dependence, J.A.M.A. **213:**294-295, 1970.
7. Davis, J. M.: Recent developments in the drug treatment of schizophrenia, Am. J. Psychiatry **133:**208-213, 1976.
8. Snyder, S., Greenberg, D., and Yamamura, H. I.: Antischizophrenic drugs and brain cholinergic receptors, Arch. Gen. Psychiatry **31:**58-61, 1974.
9. Granacher, R. P., and Baldessarini, R. J.: Physostigmine, Arch. Gen. Psychiatry **32:**375-380, 1975.
10. DiMascio, A., Bernardo, D. L., Greenblatt, D. J., and Marder, J. E.: A controlled trial of amantadine in drug-induced extrapyramidal disorders, Arch. Gen. Psychiatry **33:**599-602, 1976.
11. Everett, H. C.: The use of bethanechol chloride with tricyclic antidepressants, Am. J. Psychiatry **132:**1202-1204, 1975.
12. Snyder, S. H.: The dopamine hypothesis of schizophrenia: focus on the dopamine receptor, Am. J. Psychiatry **133:**197-202, 1976.
13. Greenblatt, D. J., and Koch-Weser, J.: Adverse reactions to propranolol in hospitalized medical patients, Am. Heart J. **86:**478-484, 1973.
14. Ban, T. A., and St. Jean, A.: The effect of phenothiazines on the electrocardiogram, Can. Med. Assoc. J. **91:**537-540, 1964.
15. Jefferson, J. W.: A review of the cardiovascular effects and toxicity of tricyclic antidepressants, Psychosom. Med. **37:**160-179, 1975.
16. Briant, R. H., Reid, J. L., and Dolery, C. T.: Interaction between clonidine and desipramine in man, Br. Med. J. **1:**522-523, 1973.
17. Lurie, M. L. and Salzer, H. M.: Tranylcypromine (Parnate in the ambulatory treatment of depressed patients, Am. J. Psychiatry **118:**152-155, 1961.
18. Editorial: Today's Drugs: monoamine oxidase inhibitors, Br. Med. J. **1:**35-37, 1968.
19. Levy, B. F.: Treatment of hypertension with pargyline hydrochloride, Curr. Ther. Res. **8:**343-346, 1966.
20. Spiker, D. G., and Pugh, D. D.: Combining tricyclic and monoamine oxidase inhibitor antidepressants, Arch. Gen. Psychiatry **33:**828-830, 1976.
21. Davis, J. M.: Overview: maintenance therapy in psychiatry II. Affective disorders, Am. J. Psychiatry **133:**1-13, 1976.
22. Shopsin, B., and Gershon, S.: Pharmacology—toxicology of the lithium ion. In Gershon, S., and Shopsin, B., editors: Lithium: its role in psychiatric research and treatment, New York, 1973, Plenum Publishing Corp., pp. 107-146.

23. Church, G., and Marriott, H. J. L.: Digitalis delirium, Circulation **20**:549-553, 1959.
24. Moe, G. K., and Abilbskov, J. A.: Antiarrhythmic drugs. In Goodman, L. S., and Gilman, A., editors: The pharmacological basis of therapeutics, New York, 1975, MacMillan Inc., pp. 683-784.
25. Quetsch, R. M., Anchor, R. W. P., Litin, E. M., and Faucett, R. L.: Depressive reaction in hypertensive patients: a comparison of those treated with Rauwolfia and those receiving no specific antihypertensive treatment, Circulation **19**:366-375, 1959.
26. Adler, F.: Methyldopa-induced decrease in mental activity, J.A.M.A. **230**:1428-1429, 1974.
27. McKinney, W. P., Jr., and Kane, F. J., Jr.: Depression with the use of alpha-methyl-dopa, Am. J. Psychiatry **124**:80-81, 1967.
28. Howard, J. S., III: Folate deficiency in psychiatric practice, Psychosomatics **16**:112-115, 1975.
29. Williams, R. H.: Textbook of endocrinology, New York, 1974, W. B. Saunders Co.
30. Relkin, R. : Effects of endocrines on central nervous system, N.Y. State J. Med. **69**:2133-2145, 2247-2265, 1969.
31. Whybrow, P. C., Prang, A. J., Jr., and Treadway, C. R.: The mental changes accompanying thyroid gland dysfunction, Arch. Gen. Psychiatry **20**:48-63, 1969.
32. Wilson, I. C., and others: Thyroid hormone enhancement of imipramine in non-retarded depression, N. Eng. J. Med. **282**:1063-1067, 1970.
33. Malek-Ahmadi, P., and Behrmann, P. J.: Depressive syndrome induced by oral contraceptives, Dis. Nerv. Syst. **37**:406-408, 1976.

# 28

# Role of nurse clinicians in liaison psychiatry

**CAROLYN B. BILODEAU and SUZANNE O'HARA O'CONNOR**

Providing psychological support is an integral part of comprehensive nursing care. In response to an increased awareness of the emotional impact of illness on the patient, family, and staff, the nursing profession developed the role of psychiatric nurse clinician. The purpose of this chapter is to describe the evolution and scope of this role as it is currently practiced, with specific emphasis on the unique contribution the nurse clinician makes to liaison psychiatry.

## WHAT ARE NURSE CLINICIANS?

Reiter,[1,2] who coined the term "nurse-clinician," described these nurses as master practitioners who could provide care based on their perceptive understanding of the patient's psychobiological needs. With their discriminating judgment they assess nursing problems, determine priorities of care, and identify the measures necessary to achieve both immediate therapeutic objectives and long-term goals for rehabilitation. In addition, they are committed to nursing care of the highest quality and have the professional responsibility for extending their judgment and care to an ever-increasing number of patients.

Peplau[3] stated that clinical specialists should be experts in the clinical area who are able to serve as role models in the practice of nursing. They are sensitive observers and conceptualize their observations within a theoretical framework. They have mastered methods to analyze problems and possess a broad base of intellectual competencies.

Others state that nurse clinicians should be practitioners with expertise in a special area and should serve as consultants, educators, change agents, and researchers.[4-7]

□ We gratefully acknowledge the assistance of Christa Brown, B.S.N., M.S. and Jeanine Angell, B.S.N., M.S., in preparing this chapter.

The specific ways in which nurse clinicians function vary with their education and experience, the specific skills they possess, the setting in which they work, and the needs they identify. Yet, regardless of these differences, the primary purpose of nurse clinicians is to improve the quality of patient care.

## Development of nurse clinician role at Massachusetts General Hospital

The position of nurse clinician at Massachusetts General Hospital was an outgrowth of a 9-month experiment begun in 1965 by the Department of Nursing.[8] Through the cooperation of the psychiatric and medical head nurses and nursing administration, a plan was devised whereby one experienced staff nurse at a time was rotated from the psychiatric unit to a medical unit to serve as consultant. The psychiatric head nurse provided daily supervision to the nurse consultant.

Evaluation of the experiment identified the following effects:

1. As communication improved, the nursing staff on the medical unit developed increased awareness of patients' and staff's needs, greater skill in meeting these needs, and heightened job satisfaction.

2. Those who served as consultants became increasingly cognizant of the stresses and demands inherent in a medical setting and skillful in providing support and offering concrete suggestions for nursing intervention.

3. Those serving as consultants to the medical unit also recognized their need for more formal preparation for this role.

Based on these results, a full-time psychiatric nurse clinician position was created in 1966. The role of the nurse clinician involved collaborating with the head nurse and other health disciplines in identifying the emotional needs of patients and in designing an integrated patient care plan. The nurse was employed in a staff position under the direction of the medical nursing supervisor and worked with patients, families, and staff members on six medical units.

Creating and introducing a new and unfamiliar position within the Department of Nursing was not without its difficulties. Members of the health care team needed to learn how the psychiatric nurse clinician would function and what she would accomplish. Some members of the medical staff wondered how she could function without upsetting, antagonizing, or frightening patients. Some nursing staff members thought the clinician would take over the "talking" aspect of their work, would notice they were not competent in interpersonal relationships, and would become aware of their "negative" reactions to patients. Others were envious of her relative freedom and autonomy, her ability to choose her own hours within a 40-hour week, and her lack of direct patient assignment. At times, the clinician herself felt isolated and uncertain in developing this new role. She had no explicit administrative authority but had to gain authority indirectly from nursing staff through her competence, her ability to establish rapport, and her genuine concern for the problems of patients, families, and staff.

Despite these initial reactions, the position became accepted and integrated into the health care delivery system. Gradually, additional psychiatric nurse clinician positions were created throughout the hospital.

### Current status of psychiatric nurse clinicians

Psychiatric nurse clinicians are expert practitioners in psychiatric nursing, committed to upholding the highest standards of nursing. They have master's degrees and possess a comprehensive theoretical understanding of the principles of mental health consultation and of psychiatric assessment and treatment. They have a working knowledge of the institution's organizational structure, operational policies and practices, and directional goal.

However, their expertise alone does not effect change. Staff members must respect the clinicians as knowledgeable persons and want to implement their suggestions. The vehicle to the consultative process is a collaborative relationship based on trust, respect, and equality between two professionals in which both contribute to problem solving.[9]

The responsibility for initiating this relationship lies with nurse clinicians. Through their frequent presence and contacts with nursing staff, they share their genuine interest in helping identify patient and staff needs and in formulating interventions. Their visibility and availability during a patient crisis can further enhance the development of the collaborative relationship.

Knowing that, for some nurses, asking for help implies inadequacy, the psychiatric nurse clinicians remain nonjudgmental when their assistance is requested. They also acknowledge the perceptive observations staff have made, the appropriateness of their referral, and the complexity of the situation. They do not cross-examine staff members or imply blame by questions such as, "Why did you do that?"

but rather "That's interesting; can you tell me more?" Until the relationship is secure, clinicians give help on the level at which it is requested rather than confront the nurse with the purpose of the request.

The recommendations by nurse clinicians should reflect their understanding of the demands and pressures felt by the nursing staff over a 24-hour period. They must be aware of the staff's capabilities and be able to translate their psychiatric knowledge into realistic and useful suggestions that can be integrated into the patient's care.

The staff's anxiety about caring for a patient often serves as a catalyst for consulting with the clinician. However, their stereotypes of psychiatric personnel (weird, able to read your mind or "psych you out") can inhibit the collaborative relationship. Clinicians attempt to dispel these through the use of humor, a neat and appropriate appearance, avoidance of psychiatric jargon, and clarification of the scope and limitations of the role.

Some nurses may wonder whether clinicians report their observations to nursing administration. To foster trust and to support their verbal assurances that they are not a "hotline" to administration, they respect confidentiality and are in a staff rather than a line position.

While there are many facets of the psychiatric nurse clinician's role, emphasis in this chapter will be on work with patients, families, and nursing personnel. There are unique features in the experience and practice of each clinician. The following is not meant to describe exclusively the functioning of one nurse clinician but rather to present a composite picture.

## THE SETTING

There are some aspects of the hospital setting that affect patient and family responses. Massachusetts General Hospital is a major medical teaching center located in a busy, metropolitan area. It is viewed by many as a hospital for the acutely ill where one goes for the latest in diagnostic, medical, and surgical treatment. Due to the severity of illness, some patients require extensive surgery, radical treatments, and long-term hospitalization. Both patients and relatives may expect miracles and become angry and upset if they do not occur. Many patients are uprooted from their community and family supports and travel long distances for this hospitalization. The costs of telephone calls to significant others and the cost of lodging and meals for relatives who accompany the patient add to the financial burden the patient has to bear. Within the hospital setting, patient and family may be confronted with unfamiliar equipment, procedures, environment, and people. Multiple transfers to and from specialized units requiring continual adjustment often occur. Each of the stressors mentioned heightens the patients' and families' anxiety and increases their need for support.

## NURSE CLINICIANS IN THEIR WORK WITH PATIENTS

Nurse clinicians become involved with an individual patient by either a referral or by case-finding. A request may come from:

1. A nurse
   *Head nurse:* "She's really getting to the staff. She's so sicky sweet with her constant 'Thank you's' and 'Oh, you're so wonderful.' Yet we don't feel she is that pleased with her care. In fact, she seems quite displeased. Can you help us understand her better?"
   *Nurse caring for patient:* "He repeatedly takes his chest leads off and says he has not had a heart attack. I don't know how to approach him."
   *Supervisor:* "We have received several incident reports about Mr. Doe getting up at night when he is confused and then falling. Can you look into this?"

2. A physician
   *Cardiologist:* "She is frightened and depressed. She may need cardiac surgery and would benefit from your attention."
   *Psychiatrist:* "I'd be interested in your opinions and suggestions concerning management."

3. Another member of the health care team
   *Respiratory therapist:* "She hasn't been responding well to weaning. I'm beginning to question her motivation; I don't think she is trying hard enough. I wonder if her mother babies her too much."
   *Dietitian:* "He tells me he is not going to follow his diet. He says he would rather die than go without the foods he likes."

4. Families
   "My son has problems with drugs. Can you do anything about this while he is here for his operation?"

After receiving the request, the clinician discusses the referral with the charge nurse. After they mutually agree on involvement, the clinician talks with the patient's primary nurse and reviews the patient's record and care plan. In order for the intervention to be pertinent, the clinician attempts to determine the "hidden agenda" for the referral. On the basis of this, the clinician decides to either indirectly or directly become involved with the patient.

**Indirect intervention.** In working primarily with the staff the nurse clinician serves as a resource to the patient's primary nurse. The clinician may interpret the nurse's observations and commend the nurse's accomplishments in meeting the patient's psychological needs. Through discussion the clinician helps the primary nurse identify areas for future exploration and nursing intervention. The use of this indirect approach is founded on assessment of the staff nurse's experience with similar issues, perceptiveness, and, most significantly, willingness to work with the patient and clinician.

> Miss S., a 34-year-old patient well known to the staff on an orthopedic unit, was admitted with a self-induced infected elbow. Previous psychiatric consultations had diagnosed her as "malignantly masochistic" and "borderline personality." Only a few hours after admission, her demanding, manipulative behavior had begun to divide staff and disrupt their ability to be consistent and therapeutic. The staff's perceptive observations of the patient's behavior coupled with the clinician's awareness of previous unsuccessful direct psychiatric intervention led to the clinician's decision to work directly with the staff. The clinician and the psychiatrist coordinated their efforts in helping staff members formulate a consistent unified approach and deal with their feelings in response to the patient's behavior.

The psychiatrist and psychiatric nurse clinician together recommended that one physician who was well acquainted with Miss S.'s medical and psychiatric history, who could set limits consistently, and who was willing to visit Miss S. frequently, be responsible for writing all medication orders. In addition, a written note in her chart and order book indicated that no changes in the medication schedule be made unless agreed on by this physician. The psychiatrist met with the physician who accepted this responsibility to discuss the details of the plan.

With the nursing staff members, the psychiatric nurse clinician explained the rationale for the plan and enlisted their cooperation for making it successful. She recognized the difficulties in dealing with the type of behavior manifested by Miss S. and praised their efforts and willingness to accept the challenge of providing appropriate nursing intervention.

The clinician recommended that one nurse per shift be the *only* person on that shift to provide care to Miss S. and answer her call light. This nurse should meet with Miss S. early in the shift to communicate mutual expectations and establish with the patient a specific plan for that shift. This method would enhance the development of a routine and consistent approach to Miss S. and hopefully lead to increasing her feeling of security, decreasing her tendency to manipulate many staff members, and diminish her inclination to sabotage her care.

The clinician also suggested that the nurse caring for Miss S. communicate with the next shift clearly and explicitly any changes in the established routine or orders as well as in the patient's level of independence. This would enhance coordination and consistency of care between shifts. Finally, the clinician recommended that the nurse assigned to Miss S. encourage the patient to express directly any negative feelings within their relationship but avoid discussing Miss S.'s feelings toward other staff members. This direct expression of feelings and acceptance of the feelings shared might lessen Miss S.'s need to act out against herself or staff members.

**Direct intervention.** The most prevalent reason for direct intervention by the clinician is to evaluate patients' adjustments to their illness. Other indications include providing support to a patient and gaining insight into the nurses' experience in caring for a patient. The clinician encourages the patient's primary nurse to be present, when appropriate, during the interview to:

1. Help the patient feel less anxious
2. Foster the patient's relationship with the nurse and not with the clinician
3. Provide an opportunity for the nurse to learn interviewing skills and enhance the nurse's sensitivity and perceptiveness
4. Assist the patient's nurse to take responsibility for the patient's care
5. Facilitate a realistic and mutual assessment of the interview

The clinician makes nursing diagnosis* on the basis of their observations and the information they have obtained. The clinician documents their observations in the patient's chart and offers pertinent suggestions for patient management and recommendations for other-referrals, such as chaplain, social worker, or recreational therapist. The primary nurse generally incorporates these ideas into the patient's nursing care plan. In addition, the clinician will contact the patient's physician directly if the observations warrant the physician's

---

*"Nursing diagnoses, or clinical diagnoses made by professional nurses, describe actual or potential health problems which nurses, by virtue of their education or experience, are capable and licensed to treat."[10]

immediate attention—for example, if the patient appears actively suicidal.

The clinician routinely follows the patient's progress with the primary nurse. On the basis of the initial interview as well as of the ongoing information received, the clinician determines whether and how many subsequent visits to the patient are necessary. Some patients are seen only once; others require several visits. A few patients require continued support throughout their hospitalization and into the immediate discharge period. The following are examples of the clinician's direct intervention.

> Miss O., a 50-year-old obese woman with diabetes, chronic obstructive pulmonary disease, and peripheral vascular disease, was admitted for an aortic graft. Postoperatively in the intensive care unit she developed pulmonary emboli and pneumonia and, following a tracheotomy, was placed on a respirator. Several attempts to wean her from the respirator resulted in respiratory distress and arrest. She became so apprehensive, angry, and depressed that she refused all treatments and begged staff to let her die. The nursing staff asked the clinician to intervene, and she decided to see the patient.

On the basis of the information she obtained from the nursing staff and the observations she made during her initial interview with Miss O., the psychiatric nurse clinician made the nursing diagnoses of (1) anxiety due to fear of dying, (2) depression due to loss of hope for survival, and (3) anger due to a loss of control. She planned further visits with Miss O.

Her relationship with Miss O. developed gradually through perseverance, willingness to listen to the patient's fears and complaints, and commitment to alleviate some of the patient's emotional strain and isolation. Since Miss O. was initially reluctant to communicate verbally, the clinician verbalized the feelings that other patients had often expressed under similar circumstances. As trust with the clinician developed, Miss O. began to share feelings of despair, apathy, anger at her lack of control, and fear of dying by suffocation. During periods of heightened emotional stress, Miss O. spoke rapidly and inarticulately. When lip reading became too difficult for the clinician, Miss O. resorted to writing, pantomime, or pointing to a word chart to convey her message.

Miss O. was very hesitant to discuss her negative feelings toward staff. She responded to the clinician's reassurances that most patients experienced these feelings but were reluctant to express them because of dependency on staff and fear of retaliation by them. The clinician reaffirmed the confidentiality of their discussions by stating that only general issues and suggestions that could improve nursing care would be shared with staff. She encouraged Miss O. to raise any issues of concern with specific staff members.

The clinician's involvement with the patient coincided with frequent staff conferences to devise methods to improve patient care. Initially, the conferences focused on the nurses' feelings of frustration, anger, and guilt because "the patient isn't getting better." Nurses discussed their individual attempts to prevent Miss O.'s regression and realized that these had been sporadic and had not involved the patient or other staff members.

After staff acknowledged their previously unexpressed need for control over Miss O.'s care, they were able to discuss reasons for and ways of allowing the patient some flexibility and control over her own care. When Miss O. expressed resentment over lack of privacy and constant interruptions from staff, the nurses acknowledged the importance of privacy to her. One nurse met with Miss O. to formulate a schedule that included definite times for planned procedures and time to rest.

Nursing staff members appeared more aware of Miss O. as an individual after the clinician discussed pertinent aspects of the patient's prehospital life. The staff members demonstrated their interest in Miss O. by encouraging her to talk about her prior experiences in politics, her vocational achievements, and her varied hobbies. Miss O. responded favorably to the staff's admiration of her capabilities and seemed more motivated and confident in getting well.

During the stressful periods of weaning from the respirator, the staff and clinician instituted methods to ease Miss O.'s anxiety. Diversions (newspaper, radio, television, music, visits from a volunteer, backrubs) and attention from staff (frequent brief visits, arranging for Miss O. and staff members to be in view of each other, encouraging Miss O. to use her call light if she needed them, telling her when her nurse would return to her, and reassuring her that she was doing well) appeared to be major factors in increasing Miss O.'s confidence and ability to breathe without the respirator.

Through multidisciplinary team efforts, Miss O. reinvested herself in life. Before she was discharged home, she said, "If you all had not pushed so hard and been interested in me, I would have completely given up."

A 24-year-old woman, Miss B., was admitted from another hospital to the respiratory intensive care unit with multiple complications and infections following peritonitis, uncontrolled diabetes, and pancreatitis. Her nursing care was demanding and was further complicated by her extreme obesity, confusion, lethargy, and open abdominal wounds requiring isolation precautions. The staff requested that the clinician see the patient to help with her confusion. Since it was well documented that her high ammonia level was the prime cause for her confusion, the clinician found the nurses' insistence that she see the patient puzzling. However, when she entered the patient's room, she realized that the staff wanted her to experience how difficult it was to care for this patient. As the clinician participated with the nurses in giving care to this patient, she could empathize with their stress of caring for a young, dying patient with pungent and grotesque draining wounds. The clinician's suggestions and support were more credible after she had participated in their experience.

The clinician's interventions included:

1. Recommending that two nurses be coassigned daily on a rotating basis to care for Miss B.

2. Suggesting that the nurse primarily responsible for Miss B. be given permission to leave the patient in the care of the coassigned nurse for short, frequent intervals during time on duty

3. Organizing biweekly staff conferences to provide support for all disciplines (especially nursing leadership staff)

4. Encouraging staff to assist one another willingly both physically and psychologically in the care of Miss B.

5. Reassuring staff who were concerned about the trauma the patient experienced that (1) Miss B. probably was only slightly aware of what she was experiencing, (2) that as her condition deteriorated, she would become even less aware of her experiences, (3) that staff members were doing nothing to contribute to or foster her confusion that could be avoided, and (4) that staff members were providing the most humane, supportive care that could be given

In addition to working with individual patients, the psychiatric nurse clinician utilizes the group setting for both hospitalized and recently discharged patients. There have been groups for burn patients, cardiac patients,[11,12] and patients with neurological and dermatological problems.

One psychiatric nurse clinician led twice weekly group meetings of hospitalized patients convalescing from myocardial infarction. The purposes of these meetings were to provide patients the opportunity to share with nursing personnel and one another their concerns, needs, and reactions to illness and hospitalization; to anticipate what difficulties they might encounter after discharge; and to receive support from the group. Patients eagerly participated and were reluctant to have the meetings end. They unanimously agreed that these discussions broadened their understanding of relevant issues, led them to seek specific information, and prepared them for coping with posthospitalization difficulties. Staff nurses, who attended as observers, learned more about patients' concerns, coping behavior, and assimilation of teaching.

Another example of patients helping patients is the use of peer counseling. The medical team serves as a catalyst in initiating this technique by introducing a patient who has successfully coped with an illness to a recently disabled patient with the same problem. The veteran patient hopefully becomes a credible role model through sharing of feelings, experiences, and practical suggestions with the newly disabled patient.[13]

## NURSE CLINICIANS AND FAMILY MEMBERS

The nursing staff is concerned not only with the patient's emotional needs but also with the effects of the illness on the family. Nurse clinicians may meet with family members directly to:

1. Offer support during a specific crisis such as death
2. Elicit their help when a patient is resistant to nursing care
3. Evaluate their responses and facilitate their adjustment to the patient's illness and nursing intervention

The clinicians share their observations with nursing staff and help them integrate the family into the patient's care. They may also recommend a referral to other members of the health care team for ongoing support.

> Mr. B., a 26-year-old single male, had been hospitalized several days in an intensive care unit following extensive abdominal surgery for pancreatitis and its complications. His former life-style, including alcohol abuse, prompted many nurses to believe that he had contributed greatly to his current state of ill health. Some, thinking he was a drug addict being supplied by his mother, refused to allow her to visit him alone. They were annoyed by his mother's almost constant presence in the waiting room and her frequent requests to visit. They felt that her close emotional bond with her son contributed to his emotional instability. Nurses requested the clinician's assistance in helping them cope with the overwhelming demands of the mother.

The psychiatric nurse clinician met with Mrs. B. to learn more about the mother's own needs, feelings, and reactions and to gain further information about the patient. Based on her nursing diagnosis of Mrs. B.'s overwhelmiming anxiety the clinician's interventions included:

1. Convening with the staff to discuss their reactions to patient and mother and to communicate information about the patient from his mother

2. Recommending the social worker and chaplain be called to provide additional support to the mother

3. Suggesting that the mother, on her arrival, talk daily with the primary nurse to develop rapport with at least one nurse and to receive consistent information

4. Suggesting that the patient's mother be allowed to visit her son without a nurse in constant attendance

5. Meeting briefly with the patient's mother three times weekly to assess her response to nursing measures and to provide additional nursing support

Although the patient died, nursing personnel felt more comfortable caring for him and meeting Mrs. B.'s needs. She was able to accept her son's death more calmly than anyone had expected and stated that she was grateful for the tremendous amount of support she had received.

The group setting has been effectively utilized with family members also. For example, one clinician led twice weekly meetings for the relatives of patients hospitalized in a surgical intensive care unit. The purpose of these meetings was to provide a forum for sharing concerns, asking questions, and giving and receiving support. Another psychiatric nurse clinician and a social worker currently colead a group twice weekly for families and close friends of cardiac surgical patients. This group is designed to offer support and general cardiac information.

## NURSE CLINICIANS AND THE STAFF

While discussion to now has been on the role of psychiatric nurse clinicians in patient and family situations, the predominance of their time and efforts is directed toward staff. The clinicians' ultimate goal is that of working themselves out of a job. While in reality there is an ongoing need for the position, having this goal helps clinicians set priorities. They assist staff members in developing their expertise and autonomy in evaluating coping mechanisms, assessing emotional needs, and planning appropriate intervention. Clinicians step into a situation only when it cannot be handled equally well by a member of the nursing staff. They are concerned with promulgating their role as resources to nurses rather than as independent practitioners.

The group method of consultation has been an effective and time-saving vehicle in helping clinicians achieve their goals with staff members. They meet weekly at a scheduled time with nursing staff on each of their units. The meetings are nonstructured and focus on issues raised by the staff such as feelings toward a particular patient or family member, the psychological needs of a specific patient, or intrastaff conflicts. The degree of rapport and trust among themselves and with the clinicians affects the extent to which the group feels comfortable in exploring and sharing feelings and working toward a resolution of the problem raised. Ideally, the meetings offer the individual staff member insight, support, and recognition from colleagues and foster group creativity and cohesiveness.

The meetings are not to be considered as group therapy, and only issues that have relevance to the work setting are appropriate for discussion. Feelings about staff members can only be discussed if both parties are present. The clinician recognizes that the more internal conflict is present, the less energy is available for external goal activity. Energy that could be channeled into improving patient care is spent on interpersonal struggles.[14]

In addition to scheduled weekly meetings, the staff may request a meeting to deal with an immediate crisis, such as a combative patient, a demanding patient, or a patient who is dying.

On an individual basis, staff members consult the clinician not only to discuss patients but also to raise issues of personal concern or to request assistance in initiating psychiatric treatment for themselves. The clinician serves only as a referral source, not as a therapist to staff. Members of nursing administration periodically consult the psychiatric nurse clinician for ideas and recommendations concerning improvement of patient care and minimizing resistances inherent in change.

Many nurses attend the numerous workshops taught by the clinicians on the integration of psychological aspects into patient care, such as suicidology, anxiety, depression, or human sexuality. Recently, one clinician videotaped a patient interview to further enhance the nursing staff's awareness of the emotional needs of patients. Through the use of this technique, the clinician serves as a role model for nursing practitioners and makes a lasting contribution to nursing education.

## FACTORS INFLUENCING FUNCTIONING OF NURSE CLINICIANS

Psychiatric nurse clinicians receive satisfaction from seeing improved patient care and staff relationships as well as from being accepted and respected members of the health care team. Both nurses and physicians recognize the need for and utilize the clinicians' skills as they plan and implement care. Patients and families often communicate their appreciation for support the clinicians have given them.

Yet there are many frustrations clinicians can face in their work; too high or diversified expectations of themselves, difficulties in setting priorities, loneliness, lack of feedback, resistance, lack of authority, and lack of time. It is important for clinicians to identify the sources of frustration operant in their work setting and to actively seek a support system to continue and enhance job effectiveness and satisfaction.

Administrative support, demonstrated by encouragement and sanction of the role through support for the clinicians' ideas and projects, recognition of their expertise, and active defense when they are under fire, has been identified as vital to their success and satisfaction.[15,16] In addition, weekly peer group meetings reduce isolation and offer innovative ideas and support to the individual clinicians.

The psychosomatic-liaison service's weekly seminars and walk rounds have helped to enhance and update psychiatric nurse clinicians' knowledge of liaison psychiatry. Their close working relationship with members of the liaison service enables them to receive informal support and suggestions for approaching specific situations as well as to involve these members in conferences with staff when indicated.

Supervision, especially for the beginning clinician, can be a great source of support and learning. Serving as an individual or group psychotherapist independent of the clinician role can be an additional source of stimulation.

## UNIQUE CONTRIBUTION

Psychiatric nurse clinicians make a unique contribution to the field of liaison psychiatry. While psychiatrists are primarily concerned with evaluating patients to determine the presence or absence of pathology, psychiatric nurse clinicians are involved with contributing to the ongoing nursing assessment of patients' needs, concerns, responses to illness, nursing care, treatments, and methods of coping. Unlike psychiatrists they do not prescribe medication, order treatments, or make recommendations for medical management. They do provide direct support to patients if indicated or offer suggestions for nursing intervention.

Because they are nurses, other nurses can directly request their intervention with patients. Their familiarity with the demands placed on nursing personnel enables them to be realistic and relevant in their recommendations. At times, patient referrals may be more appropriate for a psychiatrist; however, patients, their families, or their physicians may resist such a consultation. Often the nurse clinician's intervention paves the way for acceptance of a psychiatrist.

In a collegial relationship with the liaison service, psychiatric nurse clinicians bring to the team their knowledge of nursing, their sensitivity to the difficulties inherent in giving quality nursing care, their long-term relationship with members of the nursing staff, and nursing's observations of the patient over a 24-hour period. During psychosomatic and walk rounds, they can contribute their observations and impressions of the patient, the family, and the staff interaction. They help team members be realistic, practical, and specific so that their suggestions can be readily implemented by nursing personnel.

Their continual presence on the nursing units contributes to the acceptance and integration of psychiatric concepts into general nursing and medical practice. Through the psychiatric nurse clinician, psychiatry becomes more accessible, acceptable, and vital in the management of patient care.

**REFERENCES**

1. Reiter, F.: Improvement of nursing practice. In Riehl, J. P., and McVay, J. W., editors: The clinical nurse specialist: interpretations, New York, 1973, Appleton-Century-Croft.
2. Reiter, F.: The nurse-clinician, Am. J. Nurs. **66:**274-280, 1966.
3. Peplau, H.: Specialization in professional nursing. In Riehl, J. P., and McVay, J. W., editors: The clinical nurse specialist: interpretations, New York, 1973, Appleton-Century-Croft.
4. Riehl, J. P., and McVay, J. W., editors: The clinical nurse specialist: interpretations, New York, 1973, Appleton-Century-Croft.
5. Huether, S. E., editor: Symposium on the clinical specialist in action, Nurs. Clin. North Am. **8:**683-764, 1973.
6. Rodgers, J. A.: The clinical specialist as a change agent, J. Psychiatr. Nurs. **12:**5-9, 1974.
7. Little, D.: The nurse specialist, Am. J. Nurs. **67:**552-556, 1967.
8. Bilodeau, C. B.: The nurse clinician, Quarterly Record of the Massachusetts General Hospital Nurses Alumnae Association, Inc. **61:**5-8, 1971.
9. Caplan, G.: The theory and practice of mental health consultation, New York, 1970, Basic Books, Inc.
10. Gordon, M.: Nursing diagnoses and the diagnostic process, Am. J. Nurs. **76:**1299, 1976.
11. Bilodeau, C. B., and Hackett, T. P.: Issues raised in a group setting by patients recovering from myocardial infarction, Am. J. Psychiatry. **128:**73-78, 1971.

12. Bilodeau, C. B.: Nursing intervention in adaptation to stress following myocardial infarction, unpublished report of Grant no. 2-69-022 from American Nurses Foundation, 1970.
13. Guggenheim, F. G., and O'Hara, S.: Peer counseling in a general hospital, Am. J. Psychiatry **133:**1197-1199, 1976.
14. Deloughery, G., and others: Consultation and community organization in community mental health nursing, Baltimore, 1971, The Williams and Wilkins Co.
15. Shaefer, J. A.: The satisfied clinician: administrative support makes the difference, J. Nurs. Admin. **3:**17-20, 1973.
16. Culnan, M.: Role strain experienced by the nurse clinician, Master's Thesis, Cleveland, Ohio, 1971, Case Western Reserve University.

# 29

# The Private Psychiatric Consultation Service

**FREDERICK G. GUGGENHEIM**

The Private Psychiatric Consultation Service (PPCS) at Massachusetts General Hospital (MGH) was developed in 1967, a decade after the founding of the Psychiatric Consultation Service at MGH.[1] It was designed to meet a set of specific patient and attending staff needs; some of these needs were parochial, but many are common to most general hospitals. This chapter analyzes the historical background leading to the formation of the PPCS, its original and subsequent developmental phases, and some practical methods the PPCS has been using to deal with the increasingly important third-party payers. Finally, the role of the Director of the PPCS, the consultation rate for a private service, and some of the differences between a private consultation service and a resident-run ward consultation service are discussed.

## BACKGROUND

In the decade after the Psychiatric Consultation Service was established, requests for consultations from medical and surgical house staff and attendings increased. Reasons for a private consultation service are enmeshed in facts and traditions surrounding delivery of care at MGH. Briefly, the Massachusetts General Hospital is a 1,100 bed, community-based university hospital. In many ways it is similar to other large American community hospitals. Eighty percent of all admissions come from the metropolitan Boston area (within the Route 128 circumferential highway). Half of its beds are occupied by semiprivate and private* medical and surgical patients. Although resident physicians do admission work-ups on private patients, attending physicians (mostly geographic part-time) are personally re-

---

*Semiprivate and private patient status, aptly described in Duff and Hollinshead's *Sickness and Society*,[2] will be referred to here as private patients.

sponsible for and generally perform ongoing nonemergency care. Medical specialty consultations on private patients are performed by geographic full-time, geographic part-time, and part-time attending staff.

Without any formalized mechanism for obtaining private psychiatric consultations, the increasing number and urgency of requests for attending staff psychiatrists to consult posed a major problem for the Department of Psychiatry. Those psychiatric attendings well known in the hospital community already had full schedules with teaching, research, administration, and private practice commitments. The intermittent nature of the need for service made it impractical for staff psychiatrists to save a few hours each week for orderly scheduling of consultation work. Many psychiatric attendings with available time were little known in the hospital and often were not comfortable with intermittent forays into the general hospital. Thus, attending surgeons and internists often had to plead (or at least search around for a considerable period of time) for well-recognized and respected psychiatric consultants to help with difficult patients.

Added to the psychiatric staff's problems of tight scheduling were other factors that also increased resistance to doing consultations.[3] For example, consultants with offices distant from the hospital had to contend with cross-town traffic and tight parking accomodations. In the hospital they faced a rapid turnover of young nursing staff and largely unknown medical staff, making it unlikely that any treatment team would ever work together again. Finally, financial reimbursement for consultations often proved to be inadequate or lacking. The Blue Cross/Blue Shield policies, developed by surgeons in the 1940s were aimed at compensating surgical procedures rather than concomitant medical care. Moreover, those patients requiring intensive and urgent psychiatric intervention were often delirious, remembering details of the psychotic episodes poorly (either because of repression or the amnestic properties associated with diazepam) by the time the psychiatrist's bill for services arrived. Compounding difficulties was the fact that some patients complained that the consultant's bill was too high, basing their grievances on the amount of time spent with the consultant (direct care). The consultant, however, argued the need to base charges on total time consulting on the case (direct and indirect patient care).

Despite these resistances, there were enough dramatically useful psychiatric consultations performed to create a demand for consults—a demand that outstripped available manpower. In a setting of some frustration, the PPCS was set up in 1967 as a way of resolving this dilemma. At first it was a part-time endeavor, handled by a staff psychiatrist primarily involved in private practice. He agreed to be available for three half-days per week. Within a 2 year period it became clear that a full-time salaried staff psychiatrist and secretary were needed to deal effectively with the psychiatric problems on the private medical and surgical services.

**Initial development of the service**

When it became a full-time service, the PPCS had three overt goals:

1. To provide emergency psychiatric staff consultation for the private services from 9:00 A.M. to 5:00 P.M., 5 days a week (in much the same way that medical and surgical services handle in-house emergencies with a staff member available on call)

2. To furnish backup and follow-through for emergency consults seen by psychiatric residents at times when attending staff consultations were not readily available, that is, outside the 5 day work week

3. To respond promptly to requests for elective psychiatric consultations

In the handling of the nonemergency cases, the Director of the PPCS was assisted by other staff psychiatrists who expressed interest and were intermittently available. As a backup for the PPCS, staff members were put on a rotating roster for 1 week each year to be available for one to three elective consult requests, should the need arise. Of course the existence of the PPCS did not interfere with requests from individual internists and surgeons to specific staff psychiatrists for consultation. The PPCS was set up to guarantee prompt care of high quality and to respond to each simple telephone call.

Initial goals were relatively easy to meet. The weekly work load often consisted of one to three elective consults plus one emergency request. Emergencies requiring within-the hour response generally numbered less than one every 2 months. Fig. 29-1 shows the number of requests for inpatient consultations each year from 1969 to 1975 growing from 148 to 339 consult requests per year.

Although the quantity of patients served was not impressive, the fact that the department was providing service on demand was helpful to the departmental image in the hospital. The establishment of the PPCS in itself helped to dispel some of the negative feelings about psychiatry such as: "The fantasy promises a lot; the reality provides

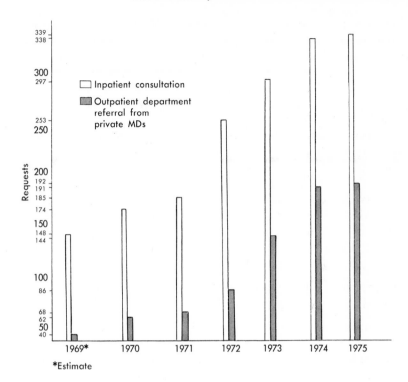

**Fig. 29-1.** Requests for service from private physicians.

little!" "Its basic tenets are unconscious, and so are its results!" Thus an initial unstated goal of the PPCS was defensive—to eradicate discontent within some echelons of the hospital staff.

Over the first 3 years of the PPCS, the medical and nursing staff gradually developed confidence that pleas for help would be met promptly and effectively. Requests for help early in the course of an illness and positive expectations helped to decrease frantic angry first calls at 5:00 P.M. on Fridays: "Come help now." Thus, the Director of the PPCS needed less often to interrupt tutorials with residents, psychotherapy sessions, or other functions for "nonemergency emergencies."

### Subsequent development

The decision in 1971 to do more thorough follow-up visits rather than to concentrate on "one-shot" consultations resulted in a considerable gain in consultation requests (Fig. 29-1). Not only was there an increase in the number of physicians served, but there was also an increment in outpatient referrals for psychotherapy (Fig. 29-1).

Gradually, during the tenure of several directors and half a decade, the PPCS began moving into a positive recognition phase. Consultees stopped complaining about poor or tardy consultations and began commenting spontaneously about the good quality of care. PPCS consultants also began to talk about how enjoyable it was to do consultations—a far cry from the angry resistance that consultants doing the 1 week rotation on the yearly roster had manifested at first. Some of the nonpsychiatric physicians then began asking the Director and others of the PPCS to present at their Grand Rounds and to participate in research projects. After several years physicians began to give the PPCS advance notice when troublesome or troubling patients were to be admitted.

### PROBLEMS IN RUNNING A PRIVATE PSYCHIATRIC CONSULTATION SERVICE

Problems and conflicts for the PPCS do not stop with the initiation of a service. Instead, suddenly the ill-defined "they" (who don't provide service, don't provide it promptly, or don't provide it for the length of the patient's crisis) become the occupants of one office with one telephone number (and two telephone lines—to increase availability for quick ingress and egress of calls).

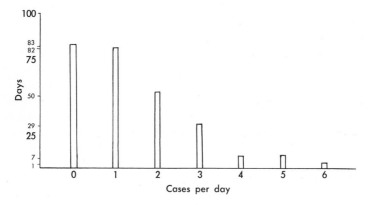

**Fig. 29-2.** Number of consultations requested per day.

## Help from colleagues

On some days it is physically impossible for one person to cover all the complicated new consultation requests, and to provide the necessary follow-up on old consultations, and to attend to the administrative, teaching, and outpatient psychotherapy commitments of the day. It is well known in consultation work that an unevenness in the number of consultation requests is the rule and not the exception: feast or famine.

Fig. 29-2 documents the distribution of 338 consultation requests over 250 working days of the PPCS during 1974. This represents approximately 1.4 consultation requests per day. As can be seen, it is rare that there are six consultation requests per day. As expected, a majority of requests are received on days when there are only one or two requests. Nonetheless, 44% of all requests are made on days in which there are three to six such requests. One quarter of these requests are explicit about same-day service because of plans for next-day surgery, disruptive ward behavior, suicidal threats, or staff anxieties.

It is on days when consultation requests are most bountiful that the PPCS has to rely not only on those physicians who enjoy doing

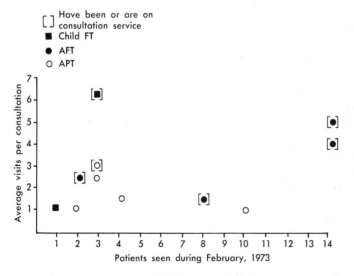

**Fig. 29-3.** Practice patterns of full-time staff versus part-time staff.

consultations (should their schedule have an available 1 or 2 hours) but also on the physicians on the weekly staff roster who have agreed in advance to be available to do consultations should the need arise. Indeed, on busy days, often to get one attending for an urgent (but not an emergency) consultation, the PPCS secretary has to place four nearly simultaneous calls to different potential consultants, such are the vagaries of office schedules and response time.

One difficulty is inherent in relying on psychiatrists not primarily involved in consultation work. Such consultants tend to perform "one-shot" consultations, relating primarily to the patient, secondarily to the consultee, and little if any to the nursing staff. Fig. 29-3 displays a survey of total consultation visits to private medical and surgical patients during a typical month in 1973. It can be seen that those actively doing consultation work made four to six visits per patient (one exception: a consultant doing diagnostic evaluations for a neurosurgeon specializing in pain), while those less currently involved in consultation work rarely saw their patients on return visits. This latter pattern of behavior can lead to disillusionment on the part of consultees and staff: "What's the point of calling a psychiatrist? Even if he's good, he still comes in anonymously, sees the patient once, and leaves. It just doesn't make any difference!"

Because of quality of care and image issues[3] it becomes important to review (randomly, systematically, sporadically, directly, or indirectly) the work of other consultants on the PPCS. One must use tact, however, as some colleagues remain sensitive to the implications of peer review when not organized through a Utilization Review Committee or a Quality Assurance Program.

### Insurance forms, billing, and other nuisances

Most physicians are not good accountants and have little patience for following the changing rules and regulations from third-party insurers such as Blue Shield and Medicaid. Not only are there negative reinforcers (incomprehensible bulletins), but also a lack of positive reinforcers (prompt financial reimbursement) because payment for services is slow in coming and erratic in amount.

There are a number of simple though constructive activities that the PPCS can engage in to assist consultants in their initial struggles with the bureaucratic maze of forms:

1. Following the performance of a consultation, the PPCS secretary can send the consultant a sample form from the correct insurance company giving guidelines for code numbers and services rendered,

types of diagnoses currently accepted, and extent of necessary explanation about the urgency of intervention and "amount of good work done by the consultant," and the like.

2. The PPCS secretary can maintain a supply of insurance companies' blank forms, filling in the material that the consultant may have neglected to collect, such as name of subscriber (if other than patient), policy number, date of birth, and address.

3. Infrequent consultants can receive suggestions on the current fee schedule from the secretary.

4. A prepared form to each consultant at the time of service will serve to remind the consultant that prompt submission of forms to the insurance carrier (at times, even before the patient has been discharged from the hospital) will enhance the likelihood of payment for services rendered. Many insurance policies still pay for only one consultation of any kind, so payment is often on a first-come, first-served basis.

The Director of the PPCS can:

1. Collate the fees that various frequently used psychiatric consultants are actually collecting on average per hour for the consultation work and share this information with colleagues.

2. Remind consultants of the necessity to update billing profiles on a year-by-year basis, keeping up with the rate of inflation. Most physicians forget that underbilling a "deserving patient of little means" ends up by lowering their Blue Shield profile and their insurance company payment. It is far more advantageous to the physician—from a financial point of view with the current system—to keep an appropriate "usual and customary" basic fee schedule and, like clinics in general hospitals, give financially insolvent patients an abatement of that portion of the bill for which they are responsible.

The Director of the PPCS' activity on statewide medical or psychiatric fee committee can also be very useful. The interests of inpatient and outpatient groups are usually well represented, but seldom are the needs of the psychiatric consultant considered. In some states, this involvement seems to have allowed consultation work billing to be appropriately based on time spent in direct and indirect care, rather than simply on time spent in a one time "consultation" procedure.

**Working with insurance companies**

Physicians are not the only ones mystified by the complexity of the fee schedules. The patient and the third-party payers, especially Blue

Shield vice presidents in charge of implementing fee schedules and payouts, are often unclear about the role of the psychiatric consultant. The best teaching device, in this regard, is a vice president's medical hospitalization with a psychiatric complication well handled by an astute consultant. Short of that unlikely event, visits to the usually receptive insurance company vice presidents can be considered as a piece of liaison work useful to the field. Another type of approach in this vein is that currently used by the Liaison Fellows' Program at MGH: weekly luncheons with Fellows and legislators, providing each side with a better understanding of the difficulties and problems of the other.

### Relating to the hospital administration

Another group mystified by the functioning of psychiatrists in general and the PPCS in particular are the hospital administrators. Here the psychiatrists' use of liaison skills can again be helpful. This is particularly important because I believe strongly that the Director of the PPCS needs to work on a salary rather than on a fee-for-service basis. This latter system usually works well in an office or clinic setting where the psychic dysfunction lies mainly within one person, one couple, or one family and direct care is billable and often adequate. However, in general hospital consultation work the disturbance usually lies not only within the patient, but also within the general system giving care.[3] As such, certain indirect services may not be billable and direct service is often not appropriately compensated. Certainly no insurance company should be expected to pay for the consultant's time if the consultant meets a head nurse's request to talk to the floor staff about management of the paranoid or confused patient "so that the next time we can detect the problem early and do a better job." As such, the psychiatrist working on a fee-for-service basis is placed in an inevitable conflict of interest: the need to use time to earn money versus the floor staff's need for information about primary prevention.

Adding to the administrator's perplexity about the functions of the PPCS is the fact that the PPCS is a money-losing unit. Although no survey is extant on the proportion of salary that the Director of a PPCS can earn from fees generated by the service if paid back to general hospital funds, it may be that only one-fourth of the Director's salary will be recovered from such billing because of other nonbillable tasks that have to be performed. Individual consultants who see an occasional patient and bill on a fee-for-service basis can count on recovering about 35% to 75% of their appropriate billable charges, either from insurance companies or from the patient (provided that contact has been seen by the patient as helpful or relief-giving).

Hospital and departmental funds are tight and getting tighter. Thus, at budget-cutting time, hospital administrators tend to question those services that are not productive, do not pay their own way, or are poorly understood. Yet the presence of an available skilled set of hands, not overburdened with administrative responsibilities, can do much to help keep the day-to-day running of certain aspects of hospital service relatively smooth. The Director of the PPCS can briefly run an inpatient service and deal with urgent psychiatric problems that occur within the general hospital. Although resident power is essential to the functioning of most university hospitals, the few gray hairs of an experienced Director of the PPCS can often calm down a disquieted or disquieting system.

## ROLE OF THE DIRECTOR

The Director of the PPCS functions in a number of roles:
1. Fireman—to put out and deal with inpatient psychiatric emergencies
2. Curbstone consultant—for indirect consultations for physicians, psychiatric nurse clinicians, and other staff
3. Psychotherapist—brief, individual, family, group
4. Resource person—for other psychiatrists doing consultations, allowing others to bail out occasionally when their vacation time approaches or when their countertransference problems get the best of them in consultation cases
5. Initiator of peer review—by informal and formal surveys (it becomes important to learn which consultants have a tendency to alienate a fair proportion of cases or consultees that they see)
6. Counselor—to other departments in dealing with emotional problems in their staff
7. Researcher
8. Inpatient and outpatient referral source—knowing who on the staff has available time; does hypnosis; is skilled at working with elderly patients, with homosexuals, with borderline patients; speaks Italian/Spanish/Greek; can give electroconvulsive therapy; does well with drug addicts, dying patients, primadonnas; and who across the United States is a good dynamic psychotherapist (in Albany), a skilled psychopharmacologist (in

West Palm Beach), or who will make house calls on a dying psychotic patient (in Pride's Crossing)

Additionally the Director of the PPCS represents the department in a variety of formal and informal functions relating to interdepartmental committee work and image.[3]

As can be seen, more than half of the working hours spent by the director of the PPCS are not spent in direct patient contact and will not result in billable time to third-party payers. Rather, time is spent serving as a spokesman for psychiatry in the general hospital, administering the placement of patients in treatment, teaching, hearing complaints, and intervening at a consultee level. It is necessary that the position of Director of the PPCS be a salaried position and not funded on a fee-for-service basis.

## CONSULTATION RATE

How many patients are or should be reached by a private psychiatric consultation service? No good answer seems to exist. First, no comprehensive report had addressed itself to a private consultation service. When no distinctions between nonprivate and private are made, there seems to be a wide variety of experiences. Expressed as a proportion of admissions, the consultation rate varies from 0.5% to 13% of all admissions. Consultation rates from American services are higher than for European ones.[4] Referral rates for specialized liaison services may be as high as 35%.[5]

Against this background, it is interesting to note that the PPCS increased its proportion of admissions serviced from 1.5% to 4% by the fourth year of full-time service. The proportion of cases serviced by the PPCS has remained stable at about 4% of all admissions since that time.

## CONCLUSION

Now in its tenth year of operation, the PPCS began by offering emergency "fireman" service to the private services. Gradually it has emerged as an important element in dealing with the complex and subtle problems of compliance and existential depression; as another hand in differential diagnosis and treating the dying; as a data-collecting base of the comparison of care; as an adjunct to the study of patients with specialized conditions (such as ileojejunal bypass,[6] limb reimplantations); and most recently, as a setting for the education of medical students in the techniques of psychiatric consultation.

## REFERENCES

1. Weisman, A. D., and Hackett, T. P.: Organization and function of a psychiatric consultation service, Int. Record Med. **173:**306-311, 1960.
2. Duff, R. S., Hollinshead, A. B.: Sickness and society, New York, 1968, Harper & Row, Publishers.
3. Guggenheim, F. G.: A market place model of consultation psychiatry in the general hospital, Am. J. Psychiatry, in press.
4. Lipowski, Z. J.: Review of consultation psychiatry and psychosomatic medicine: II. Clinical aspects, Psychosom. Med. **29:**201-224, 1967.
5. Cassem, N. H., and Hackett, T. P.: Psychiatric consultation in a coronary care unit, Ann. Intern. Med. **75:**9-14, 1971.
6. Malt, R., and Guggenheim, F. G.: Surgery for obesity, N. Engl. J. Med. **295:** 43-44, 1977.

# 30

# The Hypnosis and Psychosomatic Medicine Clinic

DAVID V. SHEEHAN and OWEN S. SURMAN

## HISTORICAL BACKGROUND AND RATIONALE

Two trends in contemporary psychiatry influenced the foundation of the Hypnosis and Psychosomatic Medicine Clinic. There is a growing demand for short-term multimodal and empirically based treatment approaches in psychiatry. This demand reflects an awareness that such therapies are often more predictably effective than lengthier and costlier treatments and that a larger and more diverse population can be treated by these methods in a one-class system of care. There is a growing realization that any form of national health insurance and accountability for cost-effective treatments will herald and end to the extended and expensive treatments of the past.

There is also a growing trend to treat psychiatric problems in general hospitals, rather than segregating them in mental health clinics and psychiatric hospitals with the attached social stigma that such isolation brings. This, along with other factors, has led to the rapid dissemination of inpatient psychiatric consultation services[1-7] for the brief evaluation and treatment of medical and surgical inpatients whose management is complicated by psychiatric problems.

However, the great majority of general hospital patients are outpatients. Consequently, an outpatient counterpart to the inpatient psychiatric consultation service and psychosomatic service at MGH was planned to serve the needs of this population. As many as 20 to 50% of patients seen in medical and surgical clinics are found to have no demonstrable organic pathology to explain their symptoms.[1] Psychosocial stresses contribute heavily to the onset and maintenance of these symptoms.[8,9] Patients with anxiety-hysteria, anxiety neurosis, hysterical conversion symptoms, psychosomatic symptoms such as cardiac neurosis, illness phobias, hypochondriasis, or isolated symptoms that are depressive in origin but that mimic medical illness are

536

prominent in this population. Such patients return repeatedly for time-consuming evaluations in spite of repeated reassurances. Medically oriented physicians referring such patients expect comprehensive evaluation, pragmatic recommendations, and treatments with rapid and predictable outcomes rather than universal recommendations of insight-oriented psychotherapy.

As Director of the Psychosomatic-Liaison Service, Dr. Thomas P. Hackett and his team had responded to an ever-growing number of these requests. Foreseeing the need for an outpatient clinic organized to provide short-term multimodal treatments, Dr. Hackett entrusted this responsibility to the current clinic director. The clinic was expected to generate enough revenue from patient care to pay all its staff salaries and expenses. After 4 months the patient load and waiting list were sufficient to engage a second psychiatrist. At the end of the first year a behaviorally oriented psychologist joined the clinic staff full time. Near the close of the second year, because of the growing demand for more service, two part-time psychiatrists and a behaviorally oriented psychologist, all with subspecialty interests, were appointed to the clinic. Since its first day of operation the clinic has

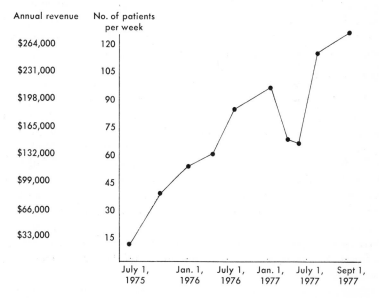

**Fig. 30-1.** Growth rate in patient population and revenue for first 26 months.

continually generated surplus income after all expenses are met (see Fig. 30-1). In spite of rapid patient turnover there is a current waiting list of over 300 patients.

## STAFFING

The unit is staffed by four psychiatrists who devote one-half to two-thirds time each to clinical care and two psychologists who provide full-time clinical care. Secretarial assistance has been central to the success and planning of the unit in maximizing time utilization, in coordinating schedules, and especially in a public relations capacity with referral sources and patients. This function is now capably provided by three half-time secretaries. A third-year psychiatric resident devotes 4 hours per week to patient care, and the clinic's involvement in residency training and the training of psychosomatic fellows will expand in the future. An undergraduate devotes 12 hours per week to research and evaluation of patient care as part of an independent studies program. Psychiatrists with sub-specialty interests and expertise may join the group when they can bring an established patient population with them through steady referrals and when enough continued demand for such sub-specialty treatments exists. The present staff members each have special interests that have already moved the clinic in this direction. Owen S. Surman, for example, has served as psychiatric consultant to the MGH Transplant and Dialysis Service. All outpatients referred in this context are seen within the psychosomatic clinic setting.

## ORGANIZATION

The Hypnosis and Psychosomatic Medicine Clinic currently provides 6,000 patient-care hours per year. It offers service for a mixture of patients: (1) those who can afford full fees (2) those who receive coverage by third parties (Blue Cross/Blue Shield, Medicaid, Medicare, and private insurance firms) and (3) those who cannot afford full fees. The proportion of each is maintained so that the clinic does not operate at a net loss. The average number of visits per patient is six, and therapy requiring more than twelve visits is unusual unless there are extenuating circumstances. One unexpected development is our finding that most patients seen in the unit were referred by former clinic patients. All patients once seen are followed by the same person until treatment is completed.

Patients are scheduled to arrive 1 hour early for the first appointment. During this time they complete standardized test batteries, for example, Hopkins SCL-90, anxiety and depression scales, and a computerized psychiatric history and mental status examination at a video terminal specially simplified and adapted for this purpose. This computer system, developed by two of the unit's psychiatrists, is the first standardized psychiatric mental status examination to use the advanced computer technology of a microprocessor. When the patient completes the last question, it provides an immediate printout of all the relevant positive and negative findings, with an interpretation of these findings and a psychiatric diagnosis. This is available to the consultant on first seeing the patient; it has resulted in a more rapid, thorough, and standardized initial evaluation. The time saved by this operation allows for earlier therapeutic intervention and more time for the therapist to focus on the patient's central problems in a humanistic way.

Considerable thought was given to the name of the unit. Since it is primarily a multimodal behaviorally oriented unit, the "Behavior Therapy Clinic" was considered. "Hypnosis Clinic" or "Psychosomatic Clinic" or "Biofeedback Clinic" are names too narrow in focus. The final name, "Hypnosis and Psychosomatic Medicine Clinic," although not without its shortcomings, serves three important purposes.

1. It alerts lay patients and referring physicians to the assortment of problems and symptoms that we treat.
2. It suggests a short-term approach to evaluation and treatment.
3. The term "hypnosis" provides a more socially acceptable entree to psychiatric treatment for those physicians and patients wanting to avoid such a stigma.

We continue to be surprised at how many patients come with innocuous requests such as hypnotherapy to stop smoking, yet rapidly reveal distressing psychosocial concerns or other symptoms with which they want assistance.

> A 27-year-old unmarried schoolteacher requested hypnotherapy to stop smoking. She proved an exceptional hypnotic subject, and her initial request was readily accomplished in a single visit. When a small weight gain ensued, that too was easily reversed.
>
> In the course of her two visits Miss H. reported symptoms of a posttraumatic neurosis. Three years earlier, while living in Europe, she had an affair with a psychotic young man who repeatedly attacked her during a bizarre accident from which she escaped with minor injury. In the months that followed she developed a dread of strangers. On returning to the States she was again a victim, first of a purse snatching and then of an attempted car theft. Her fear generalized to common objects, television shows, movies, and even verbal

expressions that might be construed as having some connection with violence. At times she experienced anxiety attacks accompanied by vivid recall of her assault. She also avoided dating.

Miss H. was intelligent, had a stable job history, came from an intact family, and had a network of close friends. In the course of three further clinic visits Miss H.'s hypnotic capacity allowed for rapid desensitization of her phobic symptoms. Positive imagery was employed for reciprocal inhibition of anxiety-laden scenes coupled with repeated suggestion that despite her previous ordeal, she had escaped unharmed and was now safe.

On routine follow-up 2 months later, Miss H. was asymptomatic. It is of special interest that she was one of our earliest patients and that her gratitude was a source of numerous clinic referrals. All of her referrals requested hypnosis for smoking.

Since this treatment comes under the guise of obtaining "hypnosis for smoking," patients feel free to discuss their visits with friends and family without the fear of being labeled a "neurotic." These factors may all contribute to the larger numbers of upper middle-class and middle-class patients seen, compared to psychiatry clinics in general hospitals. The setting for the clinic is a quiet area with a private office atmosphere with no other patient traffic or staff traffic.

Two weekly conferences for the entire staff are scheduled to discuss administrative problems, to review cases of interest, and to exchange ideas on patient care and proposals for research projects. Occasionally guests with special expertise are invited to discuss their areas of interest and to provide for our continuing education. A research conference is held to formulate, study, and develop research projects in the area of psychosomatic medicine and behavior therapy being conducted at the unit. In this manner the clinic staff collaborates on the constant refinement of methods and peer review to uphold the quality of patient care.

## ECONOMICS

A business manager is employed by the unit to advise on budgetary and other business planning. She meets with the staff and department chairman regularly to review each month's income and expenses from computer printouts. Organizationally the clinic is one of several psychiatry outpatient clinics at Massachusetts General Hospital. Financially and organizationally it is an independent module with an income and expense budget of its own. The income is generated from patient visit fees. Expenses are direct staff salaries and fringe benefits, equipment, hospital overhead, rent for space, supplies, billing costs, and expenses for medical records.

Each staff member is budgeted to deliver a specific number of patient care hours per week at a fixed hourly rate, to generate a fixed revenue. The staff member is expected to deliver this budgeted number of hours in direct patient care, compensating and making up for patient appointment cancellations by scheduling extra patients.

Over the past year there has been a reasonably steady attrition rate of 15% of patient care hours per month—through dropout, "no shows," cancellations, and patient rescheduling. This is constant from therapist to therapist and has been reduced by behavioral methods. The clinic is not paid for "no shows." The therapist is further rewarded financially for each hour's service delivered above the budgeted quota. (The clinic is behaviorally oriented!) Failure to make the budgeted quota results in proportionate salary loss. (In the history of the clinic this case has never arisen.) Each therapist is free to abate any or all of the patients' clinic fees. This is done at the therapist's expense and is reflected each month in the individual monthly patient revenue. These measures encourage individual accountability and provide a model for responsible fiscal management of the module.

The budget is set up with a flexible financial base providing a sliding salary to staff members, depending on grant money available for research. Thus, in lucrative times when research grant money is available to pursue specific projects, any of the team may reduce patient care hours and liberate time for research and writing. Conversely, in leaner periods, the staff member may immediately increase patient care hours to compensate for loss of research funds. In this way academically oriented psychiatrists may achieve some measure of financial security and stability.

## TREATMENT METHODS

The unit is a multimodal, behaviorally oriented, short-term treatment clinic. A wide range of treatments loosely categorized as behavior therapy are used, including systematic desensitization, flooding and response prevention, thoughtstopping, covert behavioral methods, cognitive restructuring, and aversive conditioning. Methohexital assisted (Brevital) desensitization or augmented respiratory relief desensitization and other such adjunctive techniques are used when appropriate.

> A typical example is that of a 32-year-old married woman referred by her physician and her psychiatrist because of a long-standing, resistant breast cancer phobia and a compulsive ritual involving breast examination. For 10 years she had undergone countless med-

ical examinations for cancer, especially of her breasts. Appropriate reassurance and her own insight into the absurdity of her persistent concern failed to provide symptom relief. In psychotherapy for 2 years, she had gained considerable insight into her symptoms and had made much personal progress without symptom relief. She was congenial, motivated, very intelligent, and insightful on examination. She described persistent episodic spontaneous panic attacks throughout the day. Sometimes they were triggered by seeing or hearing something that reminded her of her concern, such as a television commercial from the American Cancer Society or a newspaper article describing someone's death from cancer. More often they occurred suddenly, without warning. Immediately a fear of impending doom occurred and the conditioned thought, "I'll die from breast cancer," followed. As this intensified she felt compelled to examine her breasts. Finding areas of suspicious nodularity triggered alarm and a call to her physician for an appointment. Failure to follow this sequence lead to prolonged anxiety. Usually the breast checking was followed by relief. As the symptoms generalized she was fearful of even seeing her breasts and began wearing her day clothes to bed at night, much to her husband's dismay. She had a constellation of other anxiety and somatic symptoms, with elevated scores on subscales of the SCL-90 and the Zung and Taylor manifest anxiety scales. Her anxiety syndrome was treated with phenelzine sulfate, which was increased to 60 mg per day after 3 weeks, with a complete remission of her anxiety syndrome after the fourth week. However, her fear and ritual persisted. Since her habituation response was now within a more normal range, hierarchies were set up for desensitization of the illness phobia. Systematic desensitization was then done in the usual manner described by Wolpe—assisted by a 2.5% solution of methohexital sodium intravenously. After three sessions of this desensitization she could tolerate all scenes—even very anxiety-provoking ones—without anxiety (SUD score = 0). These scenes were then followed by two sessions of flooding and response prevention (not checking the breasts or going to a physician) on the same hierarchy as scenes already desensitized, again using methohexital. Over the six sessions there was a progressive decrease in the frequency and intensity of her fears and rituals, which stopped completely after the sixth session. At 1 year follow-up she remains completely symptom free with no substitution.

Biofeedback training, particularly electromyographic biofeedback, an application of operant conditioning, is employed and will probably be more widely applied in the future to train patients in self-control techniques.

Hypnosis is used extensively for diagnostic and treatment purposes for a wide range of problems from wart removal to control of stress-related asthma and also for habit control, as with smoking. It is probably most effective when a behavioral model is followed to guide technical maneuvers under "hypnosis." Patients are instructed in self-hypnosis and tapes are usually made of the induction for further home training between sessions. Sodium amobarbital (Sodium Amytal) interviews are done occasionally, principally for diagnostic purposes, and have been useful in some investigative work, such as for hysterical amnesia in witnesses or victims of violent crime.

Not infrequently various psychotropic medications are called for in treatment. Short-term therapy may be necessary to clarify some problem or conflict or to support a patient through a life crisis or loss. When long-term therapy is indicated, the patient is referred to the outpatient psychiatry clinic, where this is provided.

## PROBLEMS TREATED

Various clinical problems that respond to the techinques mentioned are treated. In the initial phase of the clinic's growth, referrals for hypnotherapy for habit control problems like smoking and obesity predominated. Over time referrals became more diversified. Although the treatment of obesity was often met with an initially gratifying response, extended follow-up revealed that this was followed by frequent exacerbation.

A breakdown of cases seen currently by the clinic is as follows:

| Type of case | Total % of cases seen |
|---|---|
| Anxiety, hysterias, phobias | 35 |
| Habit control—hypnotherapy | 25 |
| Psychiatric complications of medical illness | 15 |
| Diagnostic evaluations | 15 |
| Behavior therapy and biofeedback | 10 |

These include habit control problems such as smoking, obesity, and nail biting, particularly when these problems are immediately life-endangering to the patient—as in patients with chronic bronchitis and emphysema and following myocardial infarction. Psychosomatic symptoms like migraine, chronic pain syndromes including headache, sexual dysfunctions, and a wide array of hysterical conversion symptoms such as paralysis, blindness, aphonia, tics, and paresthesias are found with some frequency. Anxiety states, especially anxiety hysteria with hyperventilation syndrome, palpitations, and neurasthenia, and phobic and obsessive-compulsive disorders are seen in large numbers. Patients without apparent organic pathology to explain their symptoms are referred for evaluation and treatment by their physicians. Not infrequently patients in psychoanalysis or long-term psychotherapy are referred for brief "symptomatic" treatment when their symptoms resist recovery after good insight and detailed exploration of the symptoms' origin have been achieved. They are referred back to their analysts for continued therapy when those limited goals have been achieved.

The medical clinics have been a frequent source of referral for brief outpatient consultation. The following is an example.

> A 33-year-old unmarried salesman was referred to the clinic after a 2 week general hospital admission failed to relieve him of intractable vomiting.
>
> Mr. J. complained of "stomach trouble since the age of 6 months." As a child he was a "poor eater" and was restricted in play activity by abdominal distress. Upper abdominal pain, intermittent vomiting, flatulence, and eructation persisted throughout his adolescent and adult years. Despite considerable business and financial success he continued to live with his parents and depended on them for simple functions.
>
> As a college freshman, Mr. J. became acutely depressed and developed protracted vomiting after breaking off with a girlfriend. The episode responded transiently to a brief course of electroconvulsive therapy. In the years that followed the patient underwent repeated medical evaluations at several centers without positive findings. On one occasion he was said to have a lactose intolerance, on another, anorexia nervosa. An attempt at psychotherapy was unsuccessful.
>
> One year prior to his clinic visit, Mr. J. underwent laparotomy with the finding of mild chronic cholecystitis and pancreatitis. A cholecystectomy was performed along with pancreatic sphincteroplasty and selective vagotomy. Surgery was followed by acute pancreatitis. After a 3-month convalescence he noted transient improvement, but his symptoms soon reappeared.
>
> Mr. J.'s recent hospital admission was preceded by daily bouts of bilious vomiting and abdominal pain described as aching and constant. Onset of symptoms was associated with loss of a relationship with a young woman whom he had dated for 2 years.
>
> On examination the patient was a depressed, wasted, anxious man. Despite his medium height and frame he reported a weight of 125 pounds. There was evidence of severe sleep disturbance, frequent crying spells, and suicidal ideation.
>
> An interview with the patient's father revealed a family history of depression responsive to electroconvulsive therapy.
>
> Treatment consisted of a combination of hypnosis, supportive psychotherapy, and imipramine (Tofranil), 150 mg daily. Hypnosis was employed for both direct suggestion and experience of positive imagery to enhance self-esteem. The response to treatment was

gratifying. After approximately 2 weeks, Mr. J. noted that he could eat any type of food without distress. At 1 year follow-up he had increased his weight to 160 pounds. He is active at work and his mood has stabilized on a maintenance dose of antidepressant.

Individual clinic staff members have special consultation interests and work closely with medical specialists in those areas. Psychiatric symptoms that interfere with medical management, such as illness phobias, hypochondriasis, and poor compliance to medical regimens, are now seen with increasing frequency. Since the unit was conceived as the outpatient counterpart to the inpatient psychiatric consultation and psychosomatic service, patients seen on that service who require special management are followed after their discharge from inpatient status.

## SUMMARY

Our experience suggests that there is a growing demand for clinical expertise in the outpatient evaluation and treatment of stress-related symptoms and illnesses in a general hospital. The clinic described meets the needs of this patient population (and their physicians) who had not found suitable treatment opportunities in other settings. With careful business management, such a clinic can avoid the tradition of deficit budgeting that has been customary for so many psychiatric outpatient clinics. We hope others will be encouraged by our experience to establish similar units.

### REFERENCES

1. Weisman, A. D., and Hackett, T. P.: Organization and function of a psychiatric consultation service, Int. Record Med. **173**(5):306-311, 1960.
2. Lipowski, Z. J.: Reveiw of consultation psychiatry and psychosomatic medicine: II. Clinical aspects, Psychosom. Med. **29**:201-224, 1967.
3. Lipowski, Z. J.: Consultation-liaison psychiatry in a general hospital, Compr. Psychiat. **12**:461-465,1971.
4. Lipowski, Z. J.: Psychosomatic medicine in a changing society: some current trends in theory and research, Compr. Psychiat. **14**:203-215, 1973.
5. Lipowski, Z. J.: Psychiatric consultations in medical and surgical out-patient clinics, Can. Psychiatr. Assoc. J. **14**:239-245, 1969.
6. Peterson, H. W., Martin, M. J.: Organic disease presenting as a psychiatric syndrome, Postgrad. Med. **54**:78-83, 1973.
7. Lipowski, Z. J.: Consultation-liaison psychiatry: an overview, Am. J. Psychiatry **131**(6):623-630, 1974.
8. Stoeckle, J. D., and Davidson, G. E.: Bodily complaints and other symptoms of a depressive reaction, its diagnosis and significance in a medical clinic, J.A.M.A. **180**:134, 1962.
9. Stoeckle, J. D., and others: The quantity and significance of psychological distress in medical patients, J. Chron. Dis. **17**:959, 1964.

# 31

# Legal aspects of consultation

JAMES E. GROVES and JAMES M. VACCARINO

The law respects and protects the physician who acts as a good doctor but a poor lawyer far more than the one who acts as a good lawyer but a poor doctor. Consultants—whether lawyers or psychiatrists—to physician-consultees have as their first and major task that of convincing consultees that their safest haven within the law is good faith, common sense, and the highest standard of clinical care of the patient. Physicians confronted with legal problems tend suddenly to see the law and lawyers as adversarial to good patient care. They become constricted, defensive, and convoluted in their logic; they panic and become arrogant.

Such situations are not uncommon. During his first 8 days as a consultant to our Medical and Surgical Services, a psychiatric resident was asked by five different physicians some seven questions of a medicolegal nature:

1. "Is commitment to a mental hospital a possible disposition for this demented old man?"
2. "What do I do with this guy who wants to sign out against advice but won't sign the AMA form?"
3. "What is the liability of a house officer who forgets to note in the chart that the patient is leaving the Emergency Ward against advice?"
4. "What is 'brain death' anyway?"
5. "Is this woman competent to manage her own funds?"
6. "What is the Service's liability for actions by an intern who treats a patient in that patient's home?"
7. (From a female physician) "Do I have to transfer this man to a male physician's care just because he doesn't happen to like women doctors?"

Such questions portend matters of some delicacy, and consultants not only must be familiar with relevant legal concepts but also must use this knowledge to diminish consultees' anxiety and enhance their effective functioning. When consultation requests have legal overtones, psychiatric consultants have to expand their purview beyond that to which they are accustomed. Consultees are seeking help in combating anxiety and gloom arising not only from lack of knowledge of a medical specialty not their own but also because of unfamiliarity with facts entirely outside medicine—and to these facts of law they attach fearful, sinister import.

Since statutes vary from state to state and change from year to year, the following pages represent an attempt to articulate durable principles applicable to the psychiatric consultation rather than to list specific fine points of law.

## PHYSICIANS' RIGHTS AND OBLIGATIONS

1. *Negligence, malpractice,* and *liability* are terms that are often misunderstood by physician-consultees. What they mean and what they imply are simply a physician's responsibility to a patient for failure to adhere to the accepted standard of medical practice that resulted in a compensable injury. The accepted standard of care is not inflexible or unreasonable, but a deviation from it must be justified in court by the use of testimony of unbiased observers or experts.

2. *Confidentiality* between patients and physicians is usually demanded and protected by statute and custom. Exceptions occur when keeping such confidences could reasonably be expected to endanger the life of the patient or other persons. In a California case[*] this concept was affirmed when it was held: "The Court recognizes the public interest in supporting effective treatment of mental illness and in protecting the rights of patients to privacy. But this interest must be weighed against the public interest in safety from violent assault." An exception to the obligation for confidentiality may occur in the case of physicians being sued by patients when the confidences are needed by the physicians for their own defense.

3. *"Good Samaritan"* laws exist in most states. They are an attempt to ensure that no liability will ensue to practitioners who volunteer their expertise at the scene of an accident. Although it is of some comfort to physicians to have such safeguards, it is, in most cases, an untested concept and quite possibly unnecessary since there exist other common law principles that afford similar protection.

4. *Refusal to treat patients* in the hospital or out is a right that most physicians are unaware that they possess. This right obtains when no

---

[*]Tarasoff versus the Regents of the University of California, December, 1974.

agreement to treat, implied or expressed, has been consummated. For example, maintaining a walk-in clinic or emergency room can be construed as an implicit agreement to treat. If no "contract" such as this exists, then physicians cannot be legally compelled to consider a patient's case. In a situation in which a prospective patient discusses his or her history with a physician, it may be difficult to assert that no relationship has been established, particularly if the patient is under the impression that such exists. Physicians must clarify at the outset that they may or may not accept a case. Clearly this situation does not embody the emergent or even urgent medical problem. When the physican elects not to treat an individual, the physician should make every effort to provide an alternative course to avoid claims of abandonment, which is similar to negligence. The optimal care of the patient is the first consideration. Whenever a physician desires to dismiss a patient from treatment or to transfer the patient to another physician, the transferring physician must ensure a continuity of care by specific arrangement with the physician who is going to treat the individual. Also the physician should enter in the medical record the course pursued and the reasons and indications for such a transfer of care.

These notions about transfer of patients or not electing to treat are important for consultants because, often, the knowledge that a physician can cease the care of a particular patient allows enough "give" in a confrontation so that the physician's anxiety diminishes and negotiation can begin.

5. *The dying patient and the care of the hoplessly ill* are receiving such attention in the media that consultants may expect high-voltage requests for help from physicians who find themselves in situations in which the question of patients' competence to understand the nature of their acts is raised. Primarily, it should be remembered that although patients can request that no heroic efforts be employed to preserve them in the case of hopeless prognosis, this is clearly distinct from requests for active intervention to precipitate death, hence euthanasia, which is absolutely illegal. In the former case, such requests are, in their proper perspective, helpful to physicians in making their decisions with regard to future treatment modalities. Consulting psychiatrists in such circumstances should be concerned with determining whether such requests stem from depression or pain and whether or not patients are capable of understanding the nature of their acts and therefore capable of understanding the nature of their requests. Finally, the psychiatrist should do what he or she can to ensure the

comfort of the patient, such as seeing that treatment of clinical depression and alleviation of tractable pain are not overlooked in the anxiety that surrounds the dying patient (see Chapter 32).

## THE CIVIL RIGHTS OF PATIENTS

Much needed and long-awaited measures for the protection of the civil rights of mentally ill and medical patients are sometimes poorly comprehended by physicians, who may view these protections as intrusions into their domain of clinical judgment and as instruments that hamstring them in their attempts to provide optimal clinical care. The American Hospital Association has set down some guidelines for physicians and patients in their published statement, "A Patient's Bill of Rights." This is appended at the end of the chapter. Food and drug laws, new and experimental treatments and procedures, commitment and restraint laws—all recently modified—enlarge the area of anxiety for physicians who previously had to concern themselves with only consent, competency, and refusal of treatment against medical advice.

1. *New drugs, treatments, and procedures* should not be used without informed consent by patients or next of kin where indicated and proper authority from hospital and governmental agencies. Even a commonly used drug may not be administered for an uncommon or not officially recognized indication without approval by the Food and Drug Administration and hospital committees on ethics and experimentation. Examples at present are the usage of lithium carbonate for prophylaxis of recurrent depressions without mania and the use of aspirin as a anticoagulant.

2. *Commitment and physical restraint* are areas generally poorly understood by patients and physicians alike. In most states psychiatrists can restrain patients to examine them against their wills, provided the examination takes place immediately. In some states, psychiatrists are empowered to commit patients to a mental hospital for evaluation without themselves having examined those patients. This power, however, is best left unused except by the courts. Usually, if a physician restrains a patient and then decides that the patient is not committable, the physician is not liable to civil or criminal action, provided the physician had reasonable cause to restrain and acted in good faith. In a general hospital, if a medical or surgical patient is psychiatrically committable but requires medical or surgical treatment, the wisest course is to enact commitment procedures and request the mental health facility to accept the patient but allow him

or her to remain in the general hospital for care. This commitment action must later be reassessed when the clinical status of the patient changes.

One of the most common questions for psychiatric consultants concerns delirious, demented, or psychotic patients who are being treated on a medical or surgical ward. Patients with such conditions as delirium tremens, postoperative psychosis, presenile dementia, and acute or chronic psychotic illnesses with a concurrent medical illness are often frightened, confused, disoriented, and assaultive; they tend to lash out at staff, try to leave their beds or the ward, and create general havoc. Frequently the psychiatric consultant is called after patients have been restrained, not only because management recommendations are sought, but also because the staff wishes the consultant to lend sanction to the physical restraint of these patients.

The nursing care, psychotropic medications, and physical management of psychotic patients are covered in Chapter 9. The legal aspects of restraint of patients on a medical or surgical ward are the concern here. In situations in which patients are incapable of understanding the nature of their acts, are in need of hospitalization, and yet are not committable under any relevant statute, it is defensible as in the best interest of patients to protect their own personal integrity by customary and acceptable methods, including restraint. In these cases the consent of the patients' next of kin should be apparent. The justification for such, including history and formal mental status examination, should be clearly documented in the medical record, along with psychiatric differential diagnosis, treatment, and management recommendations.

While restraining patients may open a physician to charges of "battery" (the unpermitted, unprivileged touching of another person) or of "false imprisonment," not restraining may lead to charges of negligence (failure to follow accepted standards of practice). Although exposure to an action for battery is possible, if the action of restraint was reasonable under the circumstances and the medical record reflects such justifications, the chances for successful litigation against a physician are remote. Alternatively, a failure to restrain where such is indicated carries a greater risk of loss, both to patients who injure themselves (or others) and to the physician who is sued for negligence.

3. *Leaving treatment against medical advice* is the prerogative of the competent, nonconsenting patient. If patients are able to understand the nature of their acts and are unimpaired in judgment beyond those

stresses commonly imposed by the hospital situation, they can leave against advice (provided they are able to understand and judge such advice) whether or not they sign an instrument acknowledging that they are leaving against advice. The consultant frequently arrives to find a patient detained on a ward by the security police not because he or she wishes to leave against advice but because the patient refuses to sign a form acknowledging that. If patients appear competent and nonconsenting, they may be asked for their signature, but must be released even if they will not give it. Patients who are not competent and for whom it would be dangerous to leave should, of course, be restrained.

The threat to sign out against medical advice is generally more a psychological problem than a legal one (see Chapter 12). If there is time for the consultant to work with the patient, the consultant often finds that there has been some interruption of communication between physician and patient; if this can be healed, the patient will often be dissuaded from leaving. If the patient leaves, major tasks for the consultant are to mollify the staff so that the patient may return later if necessary and to reassure the patient that return is permitted. This provision of some "give" in a confrontation is sometimes effective in aborting a threat to leave against advice.

## CONSENT AND COMPETENCY—UNDERSTANDING AND JUDGMENT

Considerations of commitment and restraint lead logically into issues of consent and competency, of understanding and judgment. Patients may be competent and not give consent; they may be incompetent but try to give consent; they may be incompetent and not give consent; or they may be competent and give consent. But the crux of the matter is that there can be no consent unless there is first competency.

There is one instance, however, in which neither consent nor competency should be considered. That is the case of dire and obvious medical emergencies. If patients are brought to the hospital or encountered outside it with life-threatening medical emergencies and physicians, in the pressure of time, act with their best judgment and in good faith, they should not fear civil or criminal action. In an obvious medical emergency a physician must act without studying the legal aspects unless a next of kin to the patient is there and actively staying the physician's hand. Even in such an instance, physicians who act in good faith and with good clinical judgment are not very likely to suffer more than some inconvenience after the fact. Nonetheless, once the emergency is over, it is wise for the physician to chart immediately in the medical record or office notes what occurred and why the physician acted as he or she did.

Now to return to consent and competency, there can be no consent unless there is first competency. About the question of competency to stand trial, for example, most statutes are comparatively clear— individuals must be able to understand the charges against them and must be able to participate in their own defense. For competency in medical issues, such as diagnostic procedures, treatment, and leaving the hospital against advice, the patient's competency must be evaluated in the context of the situation at hand. That is, patients may be competent in some situations but not in others. Patients are often not capable of deciding complex and intricate medical and surgical questions without adequate explanation. On the other hand, a patient may have been deemed by a court incompetent to manage his or her own funds, to make a will, or to enact a contract (such as marriage), and yet still be quite competent to refuse an operation that might save the patient's life. Competency in this instance hinges on the patients' ability to understand the illness, treatment, and consequences—in other words, to understand such concepts as "live or die," "find out what's wrong with you," and "take the pain away." Consent depends on competence, which in turn depends on judgment and understanding sufficient to the context of the decision.

It is not the physician's task to answer questions about financial competency, testamentary capacity, competency to enact contracts, and the like. If such questions arise in the consultation, the psychiatrist's only task is to inform the consultee so that such decisions may be properly left to the courts or to the patient's legal representative. Similarly, the physician may not pronounce a patient "incompetent" in the legal sense; this pronouncement requires a formal court proceeding. A physician may not opine on issues of a patient's general legal competency unless asked to do so by the courts. Consent depends on the patient's ability to make an understanding, informed judgment on the particular question at hand. Patients who are uninformed because of communication difficulties, such as a foreign language, deafness, or aphasia, and patients who are ignorant of important aspects of their care cannot technically give consent, whether or not they are competent.

Since unconsented treatments or procedures are in most states considered battery and are more frequently considered negligence, and since consent hinges on understanding, it is at his or her own peril that a physician goes through with a procedure or treatment on a passive, confused, or fearfully mute patient who seems compliant or willing. The ancient maxim *Qui tacet consentire videtur* (silence gives assent) will not protect physicians and is not defensible. Physicians must obtain informed consent from competent patients or from their next of kin if the patients are incapable of granting it.

Most states accept the psychiatric definitions of understanding and judgment, but these should be documented in the chart or office notes

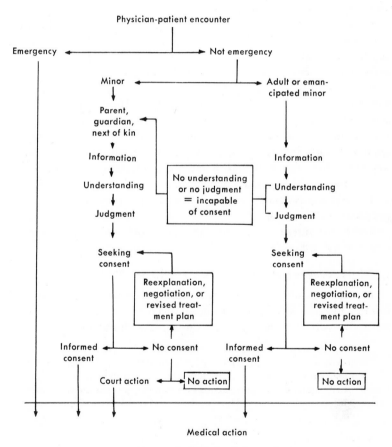

**Fig. 31-1.** Seeking and obtaining informed consent.

of the physician in the form of a mental status examination. Impairments of intellect, memory, attention, and consciousness flaw understanding; impairments in reality testing, sense of reality, impulse control, and formal logic flaw judgment. The presence or absence of any and all of these flaws should be noted in the formal, recorded mental status examination and their bearing on the context of an illness, procedure, or treatment should likewise be elaborated.

There are important exceptions to these guidelines for seeking and obtaining informed consent. The instance of the medical emergency has been mentioned. Another is the case of an emergent medical situation coupled with a psychiatric condition that would make the patient committable—such as the suicidal patient who refuses treatment as a means to a suicidal end.

The issue of obtaining informed consent is complicated in the case of minors. First of all, the age of minority varies from state to state. Second, the rights and consentability of minors vary from state to state and from medical condition to medical condition. Massachusetts, for instance, permits minors to give consent for treatment of drug addiction irrespective of parental authority. Third, the reason for denial of consent by a parent may protect the physician's actions—such as life-saving measures prohibited by the parents on religious grounds. Finally, there is the notion of the "emancipated minor," a minor who is free from parental control and dominance. Generally, informed consent by an emancipated minor, carefully documented in the record, protects the physician's action from criticism by the parent or guardian of that minor.

The decision-tree for seeking and obtaining informed consent is summarized in Fig. 31-1.

## THEORY VERSUS PRACTICE: LAW AND MEDICINE

This is a hypothetical case example on which most physicians would agree among themselves and most lawyers would agree among themselves—but one group would not agree with the other.

> Mrs. R. was a 30-year-old woman without previous psychiatric history who suffered acute onset of abdominal pain. In the emergency ward she showed signs and symptoms of an acute abdomen that was clinically diagnosed as gangrenous bowel. She rapidly became comatose as signs of shock developed and she was rushed to the operating room for exploratory laparotomy. Just before the induction of anesthesia she returned to consciousness, jumped from the operating table, and ran down the hall, saying that she refused to be operated on. The surgeon, who was scrubbing at the time, ordered the patient

to be brought back, strapped to the table, and anesthetized. Gangrenous bowel was found, resected, and the patient recovered uneventfully from the surgery.

Under the law the surgeon's actions constituted battery. The patient may well have been incompetent and certainly was not consenting, but she was not examined for competency and no consent was sought from her next of kin. Fortunately the patient was happy with the result, as was her family, but had she not been or had she died, the outcome for the surgeon could have been serious indeed. Had this surgeon been sued, his best defense would probably have been that this was a medical emergency and that he acted in good faith to save the patient's life in absence of informed consent. The plaintiff might have argued that the patient was able to run from the operating room and so was in fact not in imminent danger of death and that there was time for seeking consent. And so the arguments might have gone, back and forth, and the outcome is anyone's guess. Juries in general would probably find for the surgeon, but not always. The best rule is, if at all possible, seek informed consent from the patient or next of kin.

We would like to conclude this chapter as we began it, saying that the best friend under the law that a physician possesses is the best standard of clinical care of the patient. But from the hypothetical case it may be seen that there is sometimes—and we wish to stress, rarely— an apparent conflict between optimal clinical care of the patient and the law.

What we wish to stress is that such apparent contradictions are rare, that they occur under the pressures of time and anxiety, and that anticipation, communication, compromise, and common sense often are effective in reconciling such differences. When anticipation, communication, compromise, and common sense are lacking in an apparent contradiction between the law and good clinical care, it is the job of the consultant to try to provide them.

> Dr. B. was a brilliant, dedicated surgical intern. She called for a psychiatric consultant for Mr. J. one night because the patient had refused to allow her to examine him on the grounds that he didn't like women. She was strongly reluctant to place him in the care of a male physician on another team, but was concerned about what might occur if his clinical condition worsened. Mr. J. was a 50-year-old hemophiliac patient who had been hospitalized with a large inguinal hernia with question of incarcerated bowel. The psychiatric consultant found him to be a healthy-looking man who was frightened, demanding, and angry but not psychotic or suicidal. He was rational and had intact formal judgment. He told the consultant that he had "a

grudge" against women because "they are carriers of hemophilia but can't get it themselves. My mother gave me this disease and made me miserable when I was little, and now this dame comes along and wants to poke around in me. No dice." The consultant discovered on talking with the patient that what he feared was the rectal examination, which was used periodically to make sure that he had not begun to bleed into his bowel. The consultant then took the following steps: (1) He got a supply of rubber gloves, lubricant, and guaiac papers and taught the patient how to do his own test for occult blood. (2) He informed the patient that he considered him not insane and not incompetent, but that the hospital was not obligated to provide a male physician in such a nonemergency situation. He told the patient, in short, that he might have to choose between the female surgeon and no physician at all. (3) He told the surgeon about the fear of the rectal examination and that the patient was able to do his own monitoring for occult bleeding. He also told her that she was not obligated to transfer the patient nor liable if she did not. (4) But he did ask her to "compromise" with the patient. The surgeon and the patient agreed on an interim solution for the night: the physician could examine him if she believed he needed it but he could do his own rectal examination.

In this instance the physician and the patient backed away from a confrontation. Enough "give" was placed in the system so that they could compromise. The consultation involved the patient's consent, which he would not at first give and then later did in a somewhat qualified way. It involved his competence to make judgments on the basis of his understanding of his clinical condition. It involved the physician's liability in the case, by which she had at first felt trapped. If the patient had begun to hemorrhage or decompensate emotionally (or both) during the night, the consultation might have come to involve a decision on restraint. If a solution had not been worked out, the situation might have come to a threat to leave against medical advice, which would have necessitated another assessment of the patient's clinical status against his ability to understand and make judgments. A changing clinical course might have altered the physician's liability in the face of a possible change in the patient's competence to consent.

Whatever might have happened, it still would have come down to an informed judgment on the part of the consultant set against the backdrop of the changing fact-patterns of the case—a weighing of the clinical course against the mental status of the patient against the physician's rights and responsibilities against probable outcome and, finally, against what was humanly workable. The consultant's ability to see what was humanly workable helped to resolve the apparent conflict between law and medicine. As Alfred North Whitehead once remarked, "Reason is the horse we ride after we have decided which direction we want to go."

## CONCLUSION

The psychiatric consultant to the physician having a medicolegal problem should, in addition to the usual consultation, take the following steps:

1. Know the clinical facts of the consultation.
2. Know or find out the salient facts of law concerning the consultation.
3. Know the nature of any apparent conflict between clinical care and the law.
4. Know the hospital attorney; share information and attempt to develop a multidisciplinary team approach to patient care.
5. Try to gain some time for resolution; for example, attempt to push back deadlines for procedures, treatment, leaving the hospital against advice, and the like.
6. Know the personalities of the physician and the patient.
7. Know the next of kin to the patient, their understanding, fears, biases, personalities, and the probabilities of informed consent from them.
8. Act as go-between, diminishing anxiety and communication gaps among physician, patient, family, and try to find areas for compromise and agreement.
9. Search out covert disagreements and hidden fears in the physician and patient; try to find common-sense measures that would remedy these and search for "loopholes" and areas in which conflicts can be mended or avoided.
10. Provide detailed documentation in the patient's medical record or chart of the patient's understanding, judgment, consentability, and clinical and psychiatric status, as well as the course pursued.
11. Use such consultations to teach physicians that they have little to fear from the law and to teach patients that they have little to fear from their physicians.

# Appendix

## A PATIENT'S BILL OF RIGHTS

The American Hospital Association Board of Trustees' Committee on Health Care for the Disadvantaged, which has been a consistent advocate on behalf of consumers of health care services, developed the Statement on a Patient's Bill of Rights, which was approved by the AHA House of Delegates February 6, 1973. The statement was published in several forms, one of which was the S74 leaflet in the Association's S series. The S74 leaflet is now superseded by this reprinting of the statement.

The American Hospital Association presents a Patient's Bill of Rights with the expectation that observance of these rights will contribute to more effective patient care and greater satisfaction for the patient, his physician, and the hospital organization. Further, the Association presents these rights in the expectation that they will be supported by the hospital on behalf of its patients, as an integral part of the healing process. It is recognized that a personal relationship between the physician and the patient is essential for the provision of proper medical care. The traditional physician-patient relationship takes on a new dimension when care is rendered within an organizational structure. Legal precedent has established that the institution itself also has a responsibility to the patient. It is in recognition of these factors that these rights are affirmed.

1. The patient has the right to considerate and respectful care.

2. The patient has the right to obtain from his physician complete current information concerning his diagnosis, treatment, and prognosis in terms the patient can be reasonably expected to understand. When it is not medically advisable to give such information to the patient, the information should be made available to an appropriate

person in his behalf. He has the right to know, by name, the physician responsible for coordinating his care.

3. The patient has the right to receive from his physician information necessary to give informed consent prior to the start of any procedure and/or treatment. Except in emergencies, such information for informed consent should include but not necessarily be limited to the specific procedure and/or treatment, the medically significant risks involved, and the probable duration of incapacitation. Where medically significant alternatives for care or treatment exist, or when the patient requests information concerning medical alternatives, the patient has the right to know the name of the person responsible for the procedures and/or treatment.

4. The patient has the right to refuse treatment to the extent permitted by law and to be informed of the medical consequences of his action.

5. The patient has the right to every consideration of his privacy concerning his own medical care program. Case discussion, consultation, examination, and treatment are confidential and should be conducted discreetly. Those not directly involved in his care must have the permission of the patient to be present.

6. The patient has the right to expect that all communications and records pertaining to his care should be treated as confidential.

7. The patient has the right to expect that within its capacity a hospital must make reasonable response to the request of a patient for services. The hospital must provide evaluation, service, and/or referral as indicated by the urgency of the case. When medically permissible, a patient may be transferred to another facility only after he has received complete information and explanation concerning the needs for and alternatives to such a transfer. The institution to which the patient is to be transferred must first have accepted the patient for transfer.

8. The patient has the right to obtain information as to any relationship of his hospital to other health care and educational institutions insofar as his care is concerned. The patient has the right to obtain information as to the existence of any professional relationships among individuals, by name, who are treating him.

9. The patient has the right to be advised if the hospital proposes to engage in or perform human experimentation affecting his care or treatment. The patient has the right to refuse to participate in such research projects.

10. The patient has the right to expect reasonable continuity of care.

He has the right to know in advance what appointment times and physicians are available and where. The patient has the right to expect that the hospital will provide a mechanism whereby he is informed by his physician or a delegate of the physician of the patient's continuing health care requirements following discharge.

11. The patient has the right to examine and receive an explanation of his bill regardless of source of payment.

12. The patient has the right to know what hospital rules and regulations apply to his conduct as a patient.

No catalog of rights can guarantee for the patient the kind of treatment he has a right to expect. A hospital has many functions to perform, including the prevention and treatment of disease, the education of both health professionals and patients, and the conduct of clinical research. All these activities must be conducted with an overriding concern for the patient, and above all, the recognition of his dignity as a human being. Success in achieving this recognition assures success in the defense of the rights of the patient.

## SUGGESTED READINGS

Albert, H. D., Kornfeld, D. S.: The threat to sign out against medical advice, Ann. Intern. Med. **79:**888-891, 1973.

Beresford, H. R.: Legal issues relating to electroconvulsive therapy, Arch. Gen. Psychiatry **25:**100-102, 1971.

Butler Hospital Symposium: Human rights, the law, and psychiatry, Bull. Am. Acad. Psychiatry Law **2:**1974.

Consents to medical or surgical procedures. In Hospital law manual, attorney's volume, Health Law Center, Aspen Systems Corporation, February, 1973. (See especially Sec. 4-9, Mental incompetents, and Sec. 6, Refusal of consent.)

Curran, W. J.: Malpractice by psychiatrists in a private hospital, Am. J. Pub. Health **60:**1528-1529, 1970.

Curran, W. J.: Legal psychiatry in Massachusetts: another step forward, N. Engl. J. Med. **284:**713-714, 1971.

Curran, W. J.: Insanity defense in the District of Columbia: end of an era, N. Engl. J. Med. **287:**702-703, 1972.

Curran, W. J.: The first mechanical heart transplant: informed consent and experimentation, N. Engl. J. Med. **291:**1015-1016, 1974.

Curran, W. J.: Confidentiality and the prediction of dangerousness in psychiatry, N. Engl. J. Med. **293:**285-286, 1975.

Curran, W. J. and Shapiro, E. D.: Law, Medicine and forensic science, Boston, 1970, Little, Brown and Co.

Daedalus: Ethical aspects of experimentation with human subjects, J. Am. Acad. Arts Sci., Spring, 1969; also Proc. Am. Acad. Arts Sci. **98:**(2): 1969.

Dawidoff, D. J.: The malpractice of psychiatrists, Springfield, Ill., 1973, Charles C Thomas, Publisher.

Guttmacher, M. S.: The role of psychiatry in law, Springfield, Ill., 1968, Charles C Thomas, Publisher.

Hamilton, J.: Malpractice from the private practice and institutional psychiatric viewpoints, Md. State Med. J. **19:**69-74, 1970.

Hoch, P. H., and Zubin, J.: Psychiatry and the law, New York, 1955. Grune and Stratton, Inc.

Joost, R. H., and McGarry, A. L.: Massachusetts mental health code: promise and performance, Am. Bar Assoc. J. **60:**95-98, 1974.

Katz, J., Goldstein, J., and Dershowitz, A. M.: Psychoanalysis, psychiatry, and law, London, 1967, Collier-Macmillan Ltd.

Moore, M.: Some myths about "mental illness," Arch. Gen. Psychiatry **32:**1483-1497, 1975.

The principles of medical ethics with annotations especially applicable to psychiatry: official actions, Am. J. Psychiatry **130:**1058-1064, 1973.

Rothblatt, H. B., and Leroy, D. H.: Avoiding psychiatric malpractice, Cal. West. Law Rev. **9:**260-273, 1973.

Saxe, D. B.: Psychiatric treatment and malpractice, Med. Leg. J. (London) **37:**187-196, 1969.

Schwartz, V. E.: Civil liability for causing suicide: a synthesis of law and psychiatry, Vanderbilt Law Rev. **24:**217-255, 1971.

Slawson, F.: Psychiatric malpractice: a regional incidence study, Am. J. Psychiatry **126:**136-139, 1970.

Slawson, F.: Patient-litigant exception, Arch. Gen. Psychiatry **21:**347-352, 1969.

Stone, A.: The right to treatment, Am. J. Psychiatry **132:**1125-1135, 1975.

# 32

# Treatment decisions in
# irreversible illness

## NED H. CASSEM

Urs Peter Haemmerli, Chief of Medicine at the Triemly City Hospital in Zurich, a man of stature and impeccable credentials, was arrested at his home in Zurich on January 15, 1975, accused of murdering by starvation an unspecified number of unnamed elderly patients at his hospital. The accusation was brought by a journalist, whom he told in an interview that patients in irreversible coma were maintained on saline and water alone.[1] Providers of critical care have been under increasing fire from public and private sectors because of the technology we possess to provide advanced life support. Occasionally professionals in intensive care settings, like Dr. Haemmerli, are accused of murder. More often they are accused of prolonging dying, being sadistic, or misusing technology for inhumane ends. In short, we are damned if we use our skill and damned if we do not.[2]

Is there a time when "heroics" should stop? Because explosive hostility and accusations may be the initial response to such inquiries, the presence of a psychiatric consultant can help sort out and redirect feelings so that some responsible decision about patient care can be made. Such decisions include medical, ethical, and legal issues, as well as emotional ones, and therefore the psychiatrist is not the only consultant required by the physician who faces these treatment decisions. A discussion of some of these issues precedes specific guidelines for the psychiatric aspects of the consultation.

## BASIC ETHICAL ISSUES
### The patient's role in decision-making

In the Hippocratic oath two ethical principles dominate decision-making about treatment. The first is negatively expressed, namely, do no harm (*primum non nocere*). The second is to restore health (or maximize it). If an 85-year-old man with tight aortic stenosis, in otherwise good health, suddenly decompensates, an aortic valve replacement will ordinarily reverse his illness. As such, the aortic valve replacement is medically indicated. Ethically speaking, treatment that will reverse illness and restore health (within a certain margin of error), when available, is regarded as necessary—that is, it would be unethical to withhold it from the patient. It is never given to the patient without the patient's consent. If the 85-year-old man with suddenly decompensated aortic stenosis also had a widely spread metastatic cancer, both he and his physician might be quite reluctant to pursue aortic valve replacement. In this case, the patient would have many questions for the physician, such as likelihood of surviving surgery and possibility that the risks and suffering of the procedure might outweigh its benefits. The patient cannot demand just any treatment against medical advice—that is, the physician is not the "automated tool" of the patient. Likewise, the patient has the right to refuse any treatment, even one that would be deemed necessary (that is, capable of curing his disease).

What can the physician do if the patient refuses a curative or genuinely helpful treatment (such as aortic valve replacement)? In such cases, a psychiatric consultation may be requested. There are only four conditions under which the physician may proceed against the will of the patient. First, if the patient is in intractable pain and would like to die just to get rid of the pain, then pain relief should be administered intensively until the patient has a relatively pain-free chance to reevaluate the situation. Second, if the patient is psychotic and not in his right mind, the physician may proceed in the best interest of the patient, ordinarily with the consent of the patient's family. Third, if the patient is treatably depressed, the depression should be treated first and the situation rediscussed. If there is not time, then the physician may proceed with the help of the psychiatrist and the consent of family. Fourth, there are situations in which there is not time for a discussion, most commonly in emergency ward settings. In emergency situations where the patient is comatose or cannot respond and no one is around, the physician must act in what is assumed to be the best interest of the patient.

There are times when situations are difficult because of emotionally charged issues, but not because of ethical issues. A recent and significant article by Imbus and Zawacki[3] described the experience in a burn unit with patients whose burns were so extensive that survival was unprecedented. By application of certain criteria, the physician was able to determine when a burned patient first arrived whether or not there was precedent for survival. When there was not, the nurse and physician involved had the courage to tell this to the patient and family and present them with a choice of full fluid replacement therapy or comfort measures. Twenty-one of twenty-four such patients chose comfort measures, and they and their families were grateful to the burn unit team for helping them face the inevitable death. In these cases, the ethical principles were quite clear. There was no obligation to treat the burns. However, psychologically it was extremely difficult to become accustomed to telling patients and families the truth. There are other cases where the prognosis is not so clearly known and both psychological and ethical factors become increasingly complex.

### Committee consultation for more complicated treatment decisions

In late 1973 at Massachusetts General Hospital a subcommittee of the Critical Care Committee was formed to study the treatment of irreversibly ill patients. The initial task of the subcommittee, named the Optimum Care Committee, was to compile data. Eventually the committee became official and now functions on a regular basis in the hospital.[4]

The number on the committee was deliberately kept at a minimum and consists of a psychiatrist as chairman, an oncologist, a general surgeon, the nursing supervisor of all the intensive care units, the hospital lawyer, and a patient, a woman who had undergone a shoulder disarticulation for a rare and highly malignant bone tumor. The psychiatrist (the author) is a Jesuit priest with formal training in ethics, the nursing supervisor is a religious sister, and the patient is a physical therapist at another hospital. Of the members, three are women, three men; five members are white, one is black. Representation of varying disciplines was important in the selection of this committee, but more important in selection of the physician members were two things: that they be widely respected by the members of their own specialty and that they be known for their ability to get along with practically everybody. Whenever committees are involved, primary physicians are likely to feel criticized. Individuals who are least threatening in this way are therefore most valuable because a wide basis for trust has already been established.

This committee is available to serve *in an advisory capacity* to physicians in situations where difficulties arise in deciding the appropriateness of continuing intensive care therapy for critically ill patients.[4] Although the intensive care unit (ICU) director may suggest a review by the committee, the ultimate request must come from the responsible physician. The committee's role is advisory and the responsible physician may accept or reject its recommendations.

After the committee had been in operation for approximately 2 years, the data were reviewed and several observations made about decision-making in critical care. Ethical and psychological aspects that may be helpful for the psychiatric consultant are emphasized.

## ETHICAL ASPECTS OF DECISION-MAKING

Ethically speaking, treatment that will reverse illness and restore health is regarded as necessary. All treatments that are not medically indicated are not necessary. (They may be *justifiable*, but they are not necessary.) It is with this in mind that Paul Ramsey has made the distinction between *imperative* and *elective* treatments.[5] In another place[6] he has argued that the terms "ordinary" and "extraordinary" be dropped entirely and replaced by the newer terminology. It goes without saying that treatments that do not restore health and that inflict additional suffering on the patient are often medically contraindicated. Since necessary treatments that reverse illness, like the aortic valve replacement in the 85-year-old suddenly decompensated man—are imperative, it is unethical to withhold them. Consequently, difficult decisions focus on elective treatments—those that cannot reverse the illness but may still be indicated.

## JUDGING REVERSIBILITY

Whether, in fact, the illness can be reversed or *how far* it can be reversed is the most basic and most difficult of all the questions. This is a purely medical question best answered by physicians. Will an individual recover from coma? What are the chances that an aneurysmectomy will restore cardiac function and viability in a person? These are not ethical but clinical questions based on facts and experience. Persons with the most advanced and best clinical judgment are best qualified to answer them. In our experience we quickly learned that the first and most urgent question raised by patients, families, and medical staff focuses on the severity of the illness. Is it reversible? What and how much will the treatments accomplish? Some of the ethical literature assumes that this question has already been answered. In fact, the problem is actually worsened by discussion of "hopelessly" or "irreversibly" ill patients, because the label assumes the outcome is already known. In most cases in intensive care units, the confidence with which the label "irreversible" can be applied depends entirely on the clinical judgment of the primary physician along with the best consultations he or she is able to acquire. Nor is any committee equipped to give this expertise unless it is explicitly designated as a prognosis committee (such as a committee of neurological specialists). Whenever necessary, a specialist has already been consulted and has expressed opinions. So a considerable question remains, and it is often difficult, for this reason, to distinguish imperative from elective treatments. Many times the role of the committee is to support the primary physician and consultant while everyone honestly awaits the best clinical judgment about reversibility. Once the physician makes a clinical judgment that the illness can no longer be reversed by any treatments available, then all treatments become elective.

## ELECTIVE TREATMENTS

For all elective treatments, the relative risks and benefits to the patient must be weighed by both physician and patient. Since in critically ill patients the line separating positive from negative treatment effects can be quite thin, decisions about appropriate treatment can be exceedingly difficult. Faced with a difficult elective decision (for example, a gastrectomy to stop gastrointestinal hemorrhage of a patient wih metastatic cancer), the committee's role is not to search for principles, but to clarify as much as possible with the treating physician, the patient, and the family all the benefits and hazards likely to result from the treatment. If the best judgment indicates that the hazards outweigh the benefits (for example, the chances of surviving gastrectomy are only fair and the downward trajectory of the metastatic cancer is so steep that the postoperative period appears likely only to increase the angle of decline), then the treatment is judged unnecessary or even contraindicated. Since these are always prudential judgments, certainty can only be maximized by maximizing knowledge of the consequences. This is done by medical consultation about treatment efficacy, review of the entire course of the illness, and thorough assessment of the patient's objective and subjective reserves to respond to the treatment. In every case, the primary physician's role is greatly facilitated both medically and ethically by having a conscious and communicative patient. In almost all the cases our committee is called to see, the patient is semicomatose · or worse.

## THE DILEMMA OF STOPPING TREATMENT

Choosing to start an elective treatment can be difficult, but it is much easier than stopping a treatment already begun. Deciding to start or stop the use of the respirator is a most difficult and frequent problem. Ethically, stopping the respirator is no different from choosing not to start it. The difference is psychologically great, but no different in principle. This can be best illustrated by comparing cessation of the respirator with that of the intraaortic balloon pump (IABP). A patient with a massive anterior myocardial infarction may require the IABP for support of a damaged ventricle. There is a limited amount of time on the IABP during which the injured ventricle may recover sufficient function for idependent contraction. Because of the danger of infection and hemorrhage, use of the IABP is ordinarily limited to about 1 week (even though patients have been maintained on them for 3 weeks or more). Even for patients who cannot be helped by cardiac surgery, the decision to stop the use of the IABP is very straightforward. Once it has become clear in 3 to 5 days that the balloon has been unsuccessful in bringing about restoration of independent ventricular function, plans for its removal are made and the patient and family informed. This usually means that the patient will die, and maximum support of both patient and family is imperative.

The same logic applies to the use of the respirator, which appears to be the most controversial of all treatments to stop. Fletcher[7] has argued for a legal identity between omission and cessation, the latter applying to removal of instruments like respirators. He argues that cessation should not be classified as an act, but as an omission because the principles are the same. Ethically, the use of the respirator is no different from the use of the intraaortic balloon pump.

My own present reasoning is based on reversibility of the illness. What justifies the initial use of the respirator for any patient is the belief or at least hope that the condition of the patient is reversible. This basis for treatment (the medical indication) justifies the use of the respirator. If, in fact, at the onset of coma it were known that the victim's damage was beyond repair, then the respirator's use would not be medically indicated. It would be an unnecessary treatment and might even be contraindicated. Its use is justified by the belief that the basic disease process of the patient is reversible. If, after a sufficient period, it becomes clear that the patient on the respirator has an illness that is not reversible, then the use of the respirator becomes unnecessary. (It may be justified, but it is not necessary.) At this point there are critics who say that the respirator may not be withdrawn because its withdrawal will result in the death of the patient. They argue that the use of the respirator is mandatory because it is an obstacle between the patient and death. However, what justified the use of the respirator in the beginning continues to justify its use throughout treatment: namely, the reversibility of the patient's illness. When the best-informed medical judgment is that the patient's condition is no longer reversible, the respirator becomes an unnecessary treatment. To say that its continuation is required because it is preventing death is an effort to change the premises on which it was justified in the first place. As such, this argument is invalid, a sort of moral double-cross. If the use of the respirator was justified by the potential reversibility of the patient's illness on admission, its use ceases to be justified when the medical judgment finds the illness irreversible.

## OTHER FACTORS COMPLICATING TREATMENT DECISIONS

Socioeconomic aspects of decision-making continue to haunt patients, families, and medical staff. While it is true that many families will worry about the costs of intensive care, the time is steadily approaching when the interests of the individual will be opposed to those of society. Cullen and others[8] studied the outcome of 226 critically ill patients of whom 164 did not survive. Of $617,710 spent for blood and blood fractions in this group of patients, $515,000, or 83%, went to the 164 nonsurvivors and 17% to the survivors. Of seventeen patients in the intensive care unit following elective cancer surgery, only one survived. Of seventy-seven patients who developed acute renal failure, 89% died. The authors conjectured that if each terminally ill patient of the 2 million who die each year "benefited" from hospitalization for his or her terminal illness at an average cost of $14,000, the total cost, including physician fees, would amount to $28 billion. One could also argue that a nation that spends $40 billion annually on alcohol, $20 billion on cigarettes, and more than both combined on pets could afford these "benefits" if they were indicated. Socioeconomic pressures were nonexistent in our own hospital at the scene of individual treatment decisions. For this we were grateful. Needless to say, however, considerable pressure outside hospitals is being exerted to control hospital budgets and reduce spending. Therefore, the time may not be far off when an individual's treatment costs will be challenged as unwarranted on the sole basis of the amount spent.

## PSYCHOLOGICAL FACTORS COMPLICATING TREATMENT DECISIONS

The psychiatric consultant's task (aside from the consultation on competence to refuse treatment, p. 563) may be no more than to help provide an atmosphere where communication is possible, enabling some clarity to emerge. In fact, the obstacles to this almost entirely result from the emotions of the participants, not from their cognitive incompetence. In the early months of the existence of the Optimum Care Committee, conflict over treatment decisions was by far the most common precipitant for consultation. Wherever these conflicts existed, psychological factors played the key role. Seldom was the objective medical status of the patient the main issue. These psychological difficulties can be classified under five headings.

1. *Physician-nurse conflict caused by consultants.* It came to our attention in a few disputed cases that even where primary physicians had made their treatment wishes known and had given the reasons for their decisions quite clearly, they were bitterly criticized by the nursing staff. It came to light that either the consultants (in the case of private physicians) or the interns (in the case of the Chief Resident) undermined the confidence of the nurses in the primary physicians' judgment by making bedside comments like "What a waste of time," or "This man's electroencephalogram is no more active than a grapefruit's." The nurses, who were in effect performing 24-hour resuscitation on the sicker patients, were demoralized by these remarks, concluded that their own efforts were meaningless, and questioned the value of therapeutic procedures. They also doubted that the primary physicians regarded treatment as worthwhile.

2. *Interdisciplinary conflict.* One disputed case brought to light a feeling of conflict between surgeons and anesthesiologists in an intensive care unit. When a surgeon's patient, whose planned gastrostomy generated considerable protest from the ICU physicians, was taken to the operating room for the procedure, he arrived with a systolic blood pressure of 40 mm Hg and arterial pH of 7.09. The surgeons were furious and saw the inadequate ventilation of the patient in transit as the intensive care unit's way of thwarting their own plans to treat the patient, thereby bringing about his death. Subsequent discussion revealed that feelings of mutual mistrust were deeper than the conflict over the care of this patient. His care became the occasion for expressing the preexisting animosity. The two groups were willing to meet jointly so that the conflicts could be minimized.

3. *Distortion of facts.* When a dispute arose over the further intensive care treatment given to an elderly physician, the committee, as is customary, questioned several persons about the man's condition. The nurses angrily protested that treatment was extreme and unwarranted. The first four nurses who were questioned said that the patient

who was being treated had metastatic cancer. However, the operative note in the chart revealed that all margins of the resected portion of the stomach were free of tumor and metastasis was not suspected. In another case a specialty physician leaving the bedside of a critically ill woman about whom treatment was in dispute was asked his opinion. "Oh, it's terrible. She's comatose." At the time this patient was not comatose but curarized. Once disagreement began, it seemed quite simple for factual distortions such as these to multiply, always in the direction of supporting the treatment decision wanted by the individual who was twisting the facts.

4. *Patients who don't die "on time."* A woman with end-stage cardiac disease, dependent on the IABP, could no longer use this device and it was removed. Death was expected, but she lingered for several days. On the tenth day there was an outburst among the nursing staff coupled with severe criticisms of the inhumane medical treatment of the woman. When asked what they considered inhumane, they said levarterenal (Levophed) should not be continued. Because they knew, on reflection, that stopping the pressor was followed by pulmonary edema (a terrible way to die), further explanation was sought for their feelings. It turned out that the patient had a rather difficult and contentious personality and remained alert and contentious after the IABP was stopped. The psychological set on the part of both the nursing staff and the patient's family geared them for a short rather than a long vigil. When the time began to drag on, both family and staff became quite irritable and blamed "overtreatment" for the problem.

5. *Impatience in harried house staff.* It also appeared in the later phases of the committee function that there was some impatience on the part of some medical house staff with the deliberation phase of decision-making deemed essential by the committee. Not liking the uncertainty involved in making a medical judgment about reversibility of illness and insecure at the thought of meetings with the patient and family, some house officers showed a tendency to make hasty decisions not to treat. The most common objection was lack of time for such meetings. Such insecurity is to be expected and the consultant can be very helpful by joining such meetings so both consultant and family can support the house officer's honest communication about the patient's prognosis.

**INTERVENTION**

The major source of all the psychological conflicts comes from the uncertainties of the illness. It simply is rare to be able to speak of a case as being "100% hopeless." Psychological stress can be minimized by the following efforts:

1. Decrease uncertainty as much as possible by disseminating all available information (on diagnosis, progress, and prognosis) among physicians, staff, and family.
2. Make every effort to decrease conflict between groups—nurses, physicians, different specialists, family.
3. Specifically emphasize increasing tolerance of uncertainties, especially since the patient's condition can change.

Patient-centered conferences where treatment considerations are honestly aired seemed to have provided the best means for doing this.

## A PROTOCOL FOR DIFFICULT DECISIONS

Whether or not a committee is necessary in aiding decision-making for very difficult cases, there are certain guidelines that we have come to follow after the experience of the past 4 years. The following recommendations have been formulated as a result of that experience.

1. When the patient is admitted to an intensive care setting, the patient and family should be told of the ethical aspects of the physician's concern that the patient gets the best care. This is usually done by reassuring the patient and family that whatever can be done to reverse the illness will be aggressively pursued. At the same time, however, the family is assured that we are aware that intensive care settings are criticized for treating people too aggressively when there is no benefit to be gained from treatment. We say that we are concerned to avoid this also and that we even have a committee available if people are worried about this. The aim is to help, not harm.

2. Honesty about prognosis at all times is an absolute requirement. Because it is so important to issue no false promises to a family, simple, daily, honest communication about the patient's progress or lack thereof should be given to the family. Even though the question is frequently asked about discussing prognosis with the patient, this is a distortion of the therapeutic relationship. The patient is far less interested in a theoretical prognosis than in what a specific treatment can or cannot do. This is the ordinary basis for discussion with the physician. When treatments appear to have diminishing benefits, this should be shared with the patient. Again, it is a question of reassuring the patient that anything that can reasonably be done to help will be secured, while equal vigilance will be maintained to do nothing harmful. In many of these instances the inevitability of death will

emerge from discussion of the treatments and their diminishing returns. This is the appropriate way for discussion about death to emerge. If the physician *begins* by discussing prognosis with the patient, it is often seen by the patient as the physician's way of looking for a chance to escape. Thus, a physician does not go in and say, "I think we've done everything we can for you." In this instance a physician is actually saying he or she is about to depart. However, the physician may have to say something like the following: "I'm very worried about our ability to stop bleeding if it starts again. In your condition you can't tolerate another abdominal exploration, and gastrectomy is out of the question. We have an indwelling catheter in one of the arteries to your stomach and the Pitressin drip stopped the bleeding last time. Right now the cimetidine is holding you. But the Pitressin has already compromised your circulation severely and we are very reluctant to use it again. Therefore, we hope that you don't have another hemorrhage. If you do, we'll keep you comfortable, but may not be able to stop it." This sort of conversation can be very threatening to the physician, who needs maximum support from everyone to facilitate it.

3. When a question arises about stopping a treatment that has become unwarranted, it is usually time for a meeting. If the physician can have a discussion with the patient, this may not be necessary. When the patient is comatose, it is imperative. It is much better to have this meeting before the fact than when the crisis arises. For example, a semicomatose woman in severe respiratory failure had gangrenous feet. The reversibility of her lung disease was a question that hung in the balance. In order to avoid above-the-knee amputations, her feet would soon have to be amputated below the knee before infection spread. On the other hand, if she were not going to survive, the family wanted no amputations done. At this point the primary physician, family, representatives from the nursing staff, the infectious-disease consultant, and the committee chairman all met to discuss what was happening. The general message conveyed in such a meeting is that the hospital team has nothing to hide. The questions are all legitimate and very difficult ones, and their resolution in decision must be a mutual process with full understanding on all sides. In this particular meeting the primary physician, a respiratory physician, was pushed to give his clinical judgment of the reversibility of the patient's lung disease. His experience was extensive in this area and buttressed by some recent research. He had discovered that for patients like her, survival was without precedent when the age of the

patient was above 40 and if fibrotic changes had occurred in the lung. It was agreed that a lung biopsy would be done to determine her survival possibilities and that the amputation decision would depend on the findings. The biopsy showed fibrosis and all agreed no amputation should be done. She died of respiratory failure, and the family was grateful for the openness and support of the ICU team.

4. Periodic, even daily, meetings with all or some of these members may be necessary. It is important that communication be maintained at a maximum between the primary physician and the entire staff so that everyone is not only informed, but can share information with the family about each new phase of the patient's condition and the plans for treatment.

5. Once the physicians and nurses have had a meeting with the family, the entire staff needs to be alerted to importance of supporting the family in the presence of such serious illness. Specific discussion in rounds about the status of family members and what can be done to help them is essential.

6. The chart should reflect all of the preceding points. That is, all consultants should write their honest opinions about prognosis. Evidence of prolonged serious discussion about suitable treatments and all the reasoning involved should appear in the chart. The chart should also include daily statements about individual family members, so that the staff will not lose sight of comprehensive care. This also alerts other staff members to what is happening to the family as well as to the patient.

## AFTER A DECISION TO STOP: AGGRESSIVE PURSUIT OF COMFORT AND SUPPORT

In the words of Abelson, "Death of a loved one was bad enough when it was in the hands of God. Now it is often a much more distressing experience."[9] Even though this discussion has focused on decision-making, it would be incomplete were the reader left with the impression that the work is over when the decision to maintain or limit life-supporting measures is reached. When a decision to limit or stop certain treatment measures has been made, overall treatment must be intensified, if anything, so that the patient and family are enabled to meet the patient's death as peacefully and comfortably as possible.

One final practical reminder is in order. After the primary physician has decided that certain treatments are not appropriate (for example, further surgery, resuscitation after ventricular fibrillation), then *all* orders on the patient must be reviewed. Some need to be curtailed (for example, pressors are maintained but not escalated if blood pressure starts to fall) or omitted (painful debridement of wounds or dressing changes), so that all treatments are aimed at making the patient as comfortable as possible. Specific family needs are included, such as: Do family members want to be present at the moment of death? Should pain and other medication be held so the family can speak to the patient for a last time? Would they like beverages or food at the bedside so they can maintain a vigil?

While it has been accurately said that modern critical care technology provides many miracles, Groves[10] observed that it is an even greater miracle to have medical staff members who, when ordinary technologies have failed to reverse an illness, are still willing to stand by the patient as life ends. The responsibility for making decisions to continue or omit treatment measures is awesome enough. After they have been made, the delicate and sensitive issues of human suffering and loss demand even more compassion and courage to continue care under those circumstances. Even when we decide that our advanced technologies are no longer indicated, we can still agree that certain extreme measures are indicated—extreme responsibility, extraordinary sensitivity, heroic compassion.

Finally, a common objection to proceeding in the best interest of the patient is the fear of legal reprisals against those who make such decisions. In commenting on those physicians who rush to court in order to protect themselves in advance from the hazards of legal action, Justice Jacob Markowitz had this to say: "Men and women such as Semmelweis, Jenner, Curie, Sanger, Salk, Walter Reed, Lister, Pasteur and Wasserman would not be deterred by the mere fear of possible legal consequences of their acts. Many of them risked martyrdom to perpetuate the principles and ideals of the Hippocratic oath."[11] If the best interests of the patient were clear and the prognosis always evident, these decisions might be easy to make. The best any physician can do is, on the one hand, consult any and all experts at hand who can advise about the illness and its treatment, and, on the other, convey to the patient and family the risks and benefits of embarking on possible treatment courses. The consultant's objective is not to make recommendations that can protect the physician from litigation, but to support him or her fully in determining what course of treatment best serves the good of the individual patient. As with any other treatment decision based on best available judgment, the profession and hospital should be willing to defend this in court.

**REFERENCES**

1. The Haemmerli affair: is passive euthanasia murder? Science **190**:1271-1275, 1975.
2. Cassem, N. H.: Controversies surrounding the hopelessly ill patient, Linacre Q. **42**:89-98, 1975.
3. Imbus, S. H., and Zawacki, B. E.: Autonomy for burned patients when survival is unprecedented, N. Engl. J. Med. **297**:308-311, 1977.
4. Critical Care Committee of the Massachusetts General Hospital: Optimum care for hopelessly ill patients, N. Engl. J. Med. **295**:362-364, 1976.
5. Ramsey, P.: Prolonged dying: not medically indicated, Hastings Center Rep. **6**:14-17, 1976.
6. Ramsey P.: "Euthanasia" and dying well enough, Linacre Q. **44**:37-46, 1977.
7. Fletcher, G. P.: Prolonging life, Wash. Law Rev. **42**:999-1016, 1967.
8. Cullen, D. J., and others: Survival, hospitalization charges and follow-up results in critically ill patients, N. Engl. J. Med. **294**:982-987, 1976.
9. Abelson, P.: Anxiety about genetic engineering, Science **173**:285, 1971.
10. Groves, J.: Personal communication, 1974.
11. Markowitz, J.: Petition of Nemser, 51 Misc. 2d 616, 273 N.Y.S. 2d 624, Superior Court, 1966.

# Index